Language Disorders in Children

An Evidence-Based Approach to Assessment and Treatment

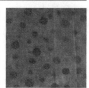

M. N. Hegde
California State University, Fresno

Christine A. Maul
California State University, Fresno

PEARSON

Boston • New York • San Francisco
Mexico City • Montreal • Toronto • London • Madrid • Munich • Paris
Hong Kong • Singapore • Tokyo • Cape Town • Sydney

Executive Editor and Publisher: *Stephen D. Dragin*
Editorial Assistant: *Meaghan Minnick*
Marketing Manager: *Kris Ellis-Levy*
Editorial Production Service: *Omegatype Typography, Inc.*
Composition Buyer: *Linda Cox*
Manufacturing Buyer: *Andrew Turso*
Electronic Composition: *Omegatype Typography, Inc.*
Interior Design: *Carol Somberg*
Cover Administrator: *Linda Knowles*

For related titles and support materials, visit our online catalog at www.ablongman.com.

Between the time website information is gathered and then published, it is not unusual for some sites to have closed. Also, the transcription of URLs can result in unintended typographical errors. The publisher would appreciate notification where these errors occur so that they may be corrected in subsequent editions.

Library of Congress Cataloging-in-Publication Data

Hegde, M. N. (Mahabalagiri N.)
   Language disorders in children : an evidence-based approach to assessment and treatment
/ M. N. Hegde, Christine A. Maul.
     p.   cm.
  Includes bibliographical references and index.
   ISBN 0-205-43542-4 (alk. paper)
   1. Language disorders in children. 2. Evidence-based medicine. I. Maul, Christine A. II. Title.

RJ496.L35H443 2006
618.92'855—dc22

                    2005048862

Printed in the United States of America

10   9   8   7   6   5   4   3   2   1   10   09   08   07   06   05

For

Adam

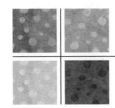

Contents

chapter	Evidence-Based Treatment Techniques	173

6

chapter	Establishing Basic Language Skills	209

7

chapter

8

Expanding Language Skills   238

chapter

9

Maintaining Language Skills: A Family Partnership   274

chapter

10

Supporting Academic Performance: Language and Literacy   300

chapter
11

Children in a Multicultural Society: Implications for Assessment and Treatment   330

PART III
Language Disorders in Specific Populations of Children

chapter
12

Children with Developmental Disability   359

chapter
13

Children with Autism and Other Pervasive Developmental Disorders   387

chapter

14

chapter

15

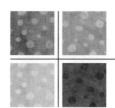

Preface

Language disorders create serious social, educational, and personal problems for children. Their academic success depends largely on their language skills. If the problems are allowed to persist into adolescence and early adulthood, higher educational potential is severely curtailed. Consequently, adults who have limited language skills experience lower occupational opportunities and realize only a limited economic benefit. Therefore, language disorders pose a serious threat to overall quality of life.

Assessment and treatment of language disorders in children is a major responsibility of speech-language pathologists. Whether they work in public schools, private clinics, or pediatric hospitals, clinicians are likely to work with a significant number of children who have failed to learn language in their typical home environment. The clinicians realize the importance of remediating language disorders in children to minimize or eliminate the negative educational, social, and occupational consequences of limited language skills. We wrote this book with a view to assist both the professional and student clinicians in gaining expertise in the assessment and treatment of language disorders in children.

By design, our book is mainly practical, although it also offers sufficient explanatory and theoretical concepts to understand the clinical conditions. We know that clinicians at all levels need evidence-based methods to treat communication disorders in children and adults. Above all, we know that clinicians need a set of practical methods that have been shown to be effective in experimental evaluations. Furthermore, we know that clinicians need a set of guidelines to select treatment procedures and classify them according to a hierarchy of evidence. Finally, we know that clinicians need a comprehensive source of information on a wide variety of children who have language disorders or language disorders in addition to other impairments.

Our aim was to write a book that fulfills the multiple needs of language clinicians and students in both undergraduate and graduate courses on language disorders. We have organized the book into three parts. In three chapters, Part I offers an overview of language, a description of language disorders in children, and a discussion of children with specific language impairment. Part II, the bulk of the book, is devoted to assessment and treatment of language disorders. One comprehensive chapter promotes child-specific assessment procedures, and the six following chapters are concerned with treatment. First, we offer an evidence-based treatment framework in Chapter 5. In subsequent chapters, we fill in this framework with specific, experimentally supported treatment techniques (Chapter 6) that may be used in establishing basic language skills (Chapter 7), expanding those basic skills into more complex language skills (Chapter 8), and promoting generalized production and maintenance of skills in natural environments (Chapter 9). In view of the importance of integrating language treatment with literacy skill-enrichment in the schools, we have written a separate chapter (Chapter 10) on supporting academic performance. Part II ends with a discussion of assessment and treatment of language disorders in children with diverse cultural backgrounds (Chapter 11).

Part III of the book describes language disorders in varied groups of children. We have described assessment and treatment modifications needed to serve children with developmental disabilities or mental retardation (Chapter 12), children with autism and other pervasive developmental disorders (Chapter 13), children with neurological impairment or hearing loss (Chapter 14), and children who need augmentative and alternative communication treatment (Chapter 15).

Throughout the book, the emphasis is on detailed information on treatment. We trust that the clinicians and instructors who use this book will find the assessment and treatment emphasis and the description of experimentally evaluated methods consistent with current professional expectations.

Acknowledgments

This text is the result of collaboration between the two of us with the help of many others. It would not have been completed without the patience and support we received from our families. The following reviewers gave us excellent, thoughtful, and constructive criticism to which we did our best to respond: Donna J. Crowley, Florida State University; Kerri R. Phillips, Louisiana Tech University; and Roberta L. Wacker-Mundy, State University of New York at Plattsburgh. The support we received throughout this venture from Allyn and Bacon's Executive Editor, Steve Dragin, and his staff has been outstanding. One of our students, Jelyn Gaskell, provided us with interesting information on augmentative communication. Another student, Amanda Fitts, worked diligently to put together the reference list and glossary; her help has been invaluable in finishing the book on target. Families of children enrolled in various programs at our clinics were gracious in allowing us to include photographs of their beautiful children in our text. Our colleagues at California State University, Fresno, in the Communicative Disorders and Deaf Studies Department supported and cheered us on throughout this year-long project. Finally, the book has been richly illustrated with Dan Hemesath's beautiful photos and Gwen Conville's striking figures.

To all of you, a very warm thank you!

chapter

1

Language and Verbal Behavior

outline

- Rational versus Empirical
  Approaches

- Language versus Verbal Behavior

- Linguistic Analysis of Language

- Linguistic Explanations of Language
  and Language Learning

- Analysis of Verbal Behavior

- Language and Communication

- Verbal and Nonverbal
  Communication

- Chapter Summary

- Study Guide

This book is about children who have impaired communication skills because of their language disorder. The limited language repertoire in these children makes them relatively ineffective in social situations. Their language disorder typically has minimal or unintended effects on others. Similarly, these children realize only partial benefits or effects from the language others produce. Their academic learning is negatively affected. When these children grow up, their persistent language difficulties affect their occupational performance, income, and quality of life. In most societies, good verbal (language) skills offer advantages that poor skills deny. Therefore, limited language skills are a serious social problem. That this problem can be treated to a significant extent is the main theme of this book.

To understand language disorders we need to understand the nature and properties of language itself. Understanding language, however, has varied meanings to people of different perspectives, which are as varied as the disciplines that study it. Language has been a subject matter of many disciplines, including philosophy, linguistics, psychology, neurology, and lately, speech-language pathology. It has long been idealized and debated by poets and philosophers. And language has been the fabric of social communication, in particular, and social life in general. Apparently, oral language is an elaborate, sophisticated, versatile, and creative skill that sets human beings apart from the rest of the animal world.

In virtually all societies, children learn language with little or no effort on the part of the parents. Although social isolation, limited exposure to language, and exposure to language of poor quality may hinder normal acquisition of language, most children learn language without strenuous, systematic, and formal parental teaching. Everyday, language that parents and others in the environment exhibit, coupled with typical social interactions that take place, seems to be sufficient for most children to learn language (Hart & Risley, 1995).

Some children, however, do not learn listening and speaking skills as effortlessly as the majority. In many cases, a failure to learn language skills is associated with additional clinical conditions or disabilities. For instance, a child with developmental disability, cerebral palsy, or hearing impairment has difficulty learning language in the typical environment. Other children may fail to acquire language in the absence of any associated clinical condition. Such children seem to be developing normally in all respects, except for speech and language. Without direct intervention, some children with a mild language disorder may eventually achieve language skills that approximate those of their typically developing peers. Others, however, will continue to exhibit significant deficiencies in language skills with negative social and educational consequences. These children need intervention as early as possible to maximize their potential to become good communicators.

Speech-language pathologists (SLPs) are the professionals who offer that intervention to children with language disorders. To best serve families and children with language disorders, SLPs must have a good understanding of varied perspectives on language and its disorders, and techniques of assessment and intervention. The objective of this book is to offer such perspectives and describe techniques of assessment and treatment for students and professionals. In this chapter, we will summarize various views on the nature of language, the varied aspects of language, and the divergent approaches to studying it. The remaining chapters in the book will address language disorders, their assessment, and treatment.

Both in scientific and popular literature the term *language* is widely used. Almost all speakers seem to understand what it means. The scientific definitions of language, though, are as varied as its investigators. There are those who question the usefulness or validity of the term *language* as used in its study. The major differences in definitions and perspectives are related to two broad approaches to the study of language. We will begin with those two approaches.

Rational versus Empirical Approaches

Rationalism, a branch of philosophy, is the belief that reason is the source of knowledge. Rationalists accept statements as valid if they are rational and consistent with the rules of logic and reasoning. They discount the importance of other means of generating knowledge. For example, they would not insist that what is rational should also stand the test of sensory experience. The most influential school of thought in linguistics—the prominent academic discipline studying language—has been rationalist. The soon-to-be described transformational generative grammar of linguist Noam Chomsky is essentially a rationalist theory.

> What branch of philosophy states that reason is the source of knowledge?

Linguistics is the study of language. Although nothing prevents linguists from going beyond rationalism, they typically stay within its confinements. Rationalist approaches to language (and other aspects of human experience) tend to be heavily theoretical. Rationally consistent theories of linguistics, for instance, enjoy widespread recognition and acceptance. In linguistics, the rational approach results in structural analysis of language. In a structural analysis, the form of language is of great interest. Words, phrases, and sentences are forms of language. Different sentence forms are different structures of language. In analyzing sentence forms, the structural and rational linguist is not typically interested in who says what, when, and why. The social conditions under which someone said something is less important than the rules that generate structures of language. Therefore, the emphasis in linguistics has been on the rules of grammar that help generate varied sentence forms. Different rules may be formulated for speech–sound combinations and meaningful sentences, but rules are the main object of rational analysis.

> Linguistics emphasizes language forms and rules of grammar.

Empiricism, another branch of philosophy, is the belief that sensory experience is the source of knowledge. Empiricism is the basis of natural sciences. Empiricists will not accept a proposition as valid because it is rational, consistent, and coherent; they demand that rational propositions be put to empirical test before they are accepted or rejected. An empirical test is a condition that scientists arrange to experience the truth value of statements. Arrangement of such a condition is called a scientific experiment. In essence, rational propositions are plausible scientific hypotheses, but they should be shown to be true in sensory experience. Empirically true statements are logical and rational, but not all logical and rational statements may be true.

> What is an empirical test scientists arrange to experience the truth value of statements?

An example of the difference between rational and empirical approaches to evaluating the truth value of statements may help clarify the difference being discussed. In an effort to understand how children acquire language, one might hypothesize—as indeed did Chomsky—that children are born with an innate language-acquisition device that helps them construct the rules of the language they hear in their environment. Chomsky advanced this view because in his opinion nobody explicitly teaches complex grammar (which, in his view, is the essence of language), and children learn language very fast. Presumably, learning of behaviors is slow, whereas innately determined blossoming is very fast. This is a perfectly logical and rational hypothesis. But is it true? Do children have a language-acquisition device in their head (or somewhere else)? To show that this is true, one would have to conduct empirical research involving children in whom the existence of a language-acquisition device is demonstrated. Various logical assumptions or reasons that led to the hypothesis cannot be pointed out as proof of the hypothesized device. Rationalists, though, typically point out as proof the reasons they first thought of as suggestive of the hypothesis: that nobody teaches grammar to children and that they acquire language very fast. Structural linguists have generally made little or no effort to study language-learning children in their families and social context.

> A story that has been told in different sources illustrates the difference between the rationalist and the empiricist. Centuries ago, faced with the question of whether horses have teeth in their mouths, rationalists began to argue on the basis of opinions of authorities, reasoning, and established beliefs. After listening to the arguments for hours, an empiricist asked, "Why not find some horses and look into their mouths?"

An empirical scientist, facing the same question of how children acquire language, may have some plausible ideas, but will select children and families and study their interactions to understand the language-acquisition process. Empirical scientists need to see and hear children (sensory experience) before making assumptions about their language. Rationalists are satisfied with logic and reasoning. Empirical scientists may support the hypotheses of a rationalist, but they will insist on observations. Empiricists have to see and hear and feel to believe. A scientific experiment is a way to "see" if hypothesized relationships are indeed true.

Language versus Verbal Behavior

In the study of language, structural linguists have been the rationalists who advanced complex theories about the nature of language and how children learn language. Linguists generally believe that language is a mental system or structure, mostly innately given (i.e., the child is born with it). Speech-language pathologists have generally accepted the linguistic view of language. The influence of rationalist theories in the analysis of language (including phonological analysis) is marked. Students and professionals generally know more about the linguistic analysis than about the behavioral analysis of language. Often, the representation of the behavioral view of language in sources SLPs consult is both incomplete and biased. Nonetheless, the clinical intervention with children who have language disorders is mostly behavioral, as there is no linguistic treatment of language disorders. This schism between the understanding of language and clinical intervention for language disorders has created a conceptual inconsistency in speech-language pathology.

Behavioral scientists, on the other hand, have argued that rational theories do not represent children who learn to speak and listen at home and beyond. Behavioral scientists suggest that social interaction itself is more powerful than innate mechanisms in teaching and learning language. They even suggest that language as a mental system of rules is the result of a formal linguistic analysis and does not represent speaking and listening skills of children and adults. Therefore, they prefer the term *verbal behavior* to *language*. Verbal behavior is both observable and modifiable, whereas a mental structure, being unobservable, is only presumable.

> What term do behavioral scientists prefer in place of *language*?

In the subsequent sections, we will offer descriptions of both the linguistic and behavioral views of language. Our descriptions will be brief, because generally, students will have taken academic courses on language and its development before they study language disorders in children.

Linguistic Analysis of Language

Linguistic definitions of language vary. Different definitions emphasize somewhat different aspects of this complex phenomenon. Most linguists define **language** as an arbitrary system of codes and symbols used to express ideas. Inherent to many linguistic definitions are the assumptions that (1) language is a set of symbols or codes that represent ideas, events, and experiences; (2) the system is arbitrary; and that (3) language is rule-governed.

> Etymologically, the origin of *language* is tongue, for the word is derived from *lingua*, Latin for *tongue*.

That words stand for ideas, objects, and experiences is an old assumption about language. Because the elements of a language represent something else, they are said to be codes or symbols. For instance, the word *cat* stands for, or represents, a certain domestic four-legged creature. That the sound sequence *c-a-t* should stand for that particular animal is said to be arbitrarily agreed on by a community of people because there is no inherent reason why some other word could not do the same. Obviously, the symbols for the same objects, organisms, or experiences are different in different languages, underscoring the nature of arbitrariness of symbols used in language.

Language is not a haphazard collection of symbols; it is an organized system that is governed by certain rules. For example, there are rules for combining sounds into words and words into sentences. In different languages, the same or similar sounds may be combined in different ways to represent the same object or experience. Similarly, languages differ in the way the words are combined into phrases or sentences. In English, for example, it is correct to place an adjective before the noun it modifies (e.g., *the green house*). In Spanish, however, the adjective follows the modified noun (*la casa verde*). Linguists believe that it is the innate rules of language that make language use creative. Speakers can generate an infinite variety of sentence structures from the rules of their language.

Many linguists also suggest that language is a mental system in that all speakers have a mental structure of their language. According to the influential transformational grammar of Chomsky (1957, 1965), this mental structure is mostly innate and consists of a knowledge of the universal features of grammar. Because of this innate mental structure, children know the rules of their language beforehand and construct the rules of their specific language from what they hear around them. It is that innate knowledge that helps adults speak their language with expected regularity. It is also believed that children acquire their language with amazing speed because they already know the universal rules of grammar.

The linguistic analysis of language is structural in the sense that the various parts of language are described as the topographic (formal) elements that make up its totality.

According to linguists, language is not only a mental system, but it also is a mental structure. Generally, language is described as a structure that holds it contents—meaning. Language is described in terms of its structural components and modalities. While the components include the phonologic, semantic, syntactic, morphologic, and pragmatic features of language, the modalities include production and comprehension.

What the linguists typically describe under each of the structures of language is a set of rules that presumably govern the production of various aspects of language. Therefore, the language structures are indeed rule structures. For instance, one set of rule structure governs the sequence, combination, and production of speech sounds. Another set of rule structure governs meaning, and yet another rule structure governs grammar, and so forth.

Phonologic Component and Speech

The larger language system has a speech component. It is through the production of speech sounds that an oral language is realized. Narrowly defined, **speech** is the production of sounds of a language. More broadly defined, speech is the actual production of oral language; it is a specialized kind of movement made to communicate through oral language. Speech is a building block of the larger unit called language.

The sounds of a language are thought to be organized into a system. **Phonology** is the study of that sound system—of speech sounds, speech production, and the rules for combining sounds to form meaningful words and sentences. The **phonologic component** of a language includes the production of speech sounds and the organization of sounds according to the rules of the sound system of a language.

The root of the word *phonology* is *phone*. A **phone** is any sound a vocal tract is capable of making. When a phone is a part of a language and helps convey meaning, it is called a **phoneme.** A tongue click, for example, is a phone but not a phoneme in the English language. However, it *is* a phoneme in some African languages in which it conveys meaning (Lyovin, 1997). Similarly, the sound represented orthographically by *th* and phonetically by /θ/ is a phoneme in the English language, but does not exist as a phoneme in Russian.

> A nasal snort is a phone but, in the English language, *not* a phoneme.

A phoneme is traditionally defined as the smallest unit of sound that conveys meaning within a language. The words *hit* and *bit*, for example, convey different meanings because a single phoneme distinguishes the two words. There are rules that govern how phonemes can be combined to form words. In English, sound combinations such as /ptw/ never occur, and the phoneme /ŋ/ never occurs in initial word position.

A phoneme is actually a family of similar sounds. The production of a phoneme varies depending on the phonetic context in which it is used within a word or sentence during connected speech. The /l/ phoneme, for example, is pronounced differently in words such as *like* (the "light" /l/), *call* (the "dark" /l/), and *bottle* (the "syllabic" /l/), and all these varying productions are the **allophones** of the phoneme /l/. Similarly, in the word *rat*, the /r/ phoneme is produced with the lips in a flat, neutral position, but in the word *root*, the /r/ is produced with rounded lips, due to the rounded nature of the /u/ phoneme which follows it. These allophonic variations do not change the meaning of the word. Listeners typically do not distinguish allophonic variations of phonemes; people

> What are slight differences in the production of a particular phoneme that do not affect meaning?

respond to speech mostly on the basis of such other variables as context and meaning of the words.

Individual speakers have their own slight variations on the pronunciations of the phonemes they speak. If those variations are slight, listeners do not take much notice. The speech of an individual speaker who badly distorts a phoneme, omits a phoneme, or substitutes one phoneme for another, may be unintelligible to the listeners. If a child commits errors on only one or just a few phonemes, it is likely that an articulation disorder will be diagnosed, which is a type of disorder that is not related to language. A child who exhibits an articulation disorder may have normal language skills. In other words, a child may have a speech disorder and normal language. There are many children, however, who have both a speech and a language disorder, exhibiting poor articulation and atypical development of language.

Some children make many errors in speech production, and, as a consequence, the phonemic contrasts collapse, and meaning is negatively affected. In these cases, if the errors made are consistent with recognizable patterns, a phonological disorder is likely to be diagnosed. Unlike isolated speech–sound errors, phonological disorders are thought to be related to language. The speech–sound error patterns these children produce are called **phonological processes,** which have been defined in various ways, most usefully as common patterns children display when acquiring the sound system of their language. These patterns, or phonological processes, are a normal part of the acquisition of speech sounds, unless they persist beyond certain age levels (3–5 years, depending on the particular process). For example, many children younger than the age of 3 delete the final consonant of a word, resulting in such productions as [bu] for *book* or [da] for *dog.* This problem is called the phonological process of final consonant deletion. Another common phonological process, called cluster reduction (also called cluster deletion or cluster simplification) is illustrated by such productions as [bɛd] for *bread* and [tov] for *stove* (refer to Table 3.1 in Chapter 3 for a description of common phonological processes). If a child's production of phonological processes persists beyond the age of 3, intervention to improve intelligibility of speech may be warranted.

> Diagnosing a phonological disorder is dependent in part on the child's correct production of phonemes in other contexts. For example, if a child has good articulation of consonants in initial and medial positions, but deletes them in final word position, it is assumed to be a phonological disorder, rather than a motor-based articulation disorder.

The phonological component and speech production are addressed in detail in courses on phonological and articulation disorders. Therefore, this text elaborates on the remaining four components of language (semantic, syntactic, morphologic, and pragmatic).

Semantic Component

Semantics is the study of the meaning of words and word combinations of a language. The **semantic component** of a language is the element of meaning in language. In linguistics, even the meaning of utterances is a matter of structure. The semantic component is a structural unit of language.

The number of words (**lexicon** or **vocabulary**) a child produces and understands is a common but basic measure of a child's knowledge of meaning. However, semantics as a study of meaning in language includes more than a simple count of the number of different words a child produces and understands. Word meanings vary depending on the context and

What is the element (or component) of meaning in a language?

usage. They may be complex, multiple, abstract, or metaphoric. Children master the more direct, concrete, and simple meanings of words before they master the indirect, abstract, and complex meanings. Children with language disorders typically have difficulty mastering the complex and the abstract meaning of words, phrases, and sentences.

Although an exhaustive description of the semantic component of language is outside the scope of this chapter, we will briefly take note of a few common types of meanings semanticists (linguists who specialize in semantics) describe. According to linguists, words refer to (stand for) objects, events, persons, and so forth. **Referential meaning,** therefore, is a simple, concrete meaning of a word that points to (refers to) an object, person, or event. In addition to other kinds of meanings, dictionaries give referential meaning. The referential meaning of the word *mother,* for example, is "a woman who conceives, gives birth to, and raises a child" (American Heritage College Dictionary, 1997).

The **connotative meaning** is the emotional meaning the words suggest. Few people can hear and say the word *mother* (especially when it refers to their own mothers) without experiencing an emotional reaction. Depending on the past experience with the mother, the word may provoke a warm and pleasant feeling or a sad and unpleasant one.

Words that express relation between objects and events are said to convey **relational meaning.** For example, prepositions (*in, on, under,* etc.) suggest relation between objects (e.g., "The ball is on the desk" versus "The ball is under the desk"). Other relational terms refer to kinship (*mother, son*), dimension (*big/little, high/low*), or time (*before/after, now/then*).

Inferential meaning is that which is not explicitly stated but deduced (presumed) from what is said. For example, if someone said that, "Mary went to a restaurant and ordered chicken chow mein and fried rice," it may be inferred that she went to a Chinese restaurant, even though that has not been directly said.

Figurative meaning is the meaning phrases convey that the words used in that phrase do not convey. When words are used figuratively, they convey a meaning other than the one the words themselves convey. **Idioms** are a common type of figurative language. An idiom such as, "It's raining cats and dogs," only means that it is raining hard, not that cats and dogs are falling from the sky, as the words in the sentence literally state. Irony, metaphor, and similes are other forms of figurative language. Statements of **irony** mean the opposite of what the words themselves suggest. Most often, irony is understood by the context of speech, intonation, and facial expressions of the speaker. A statement such as, "Oh, that's so nice!" might not be recognized as ironic unless one understands that the driver who uttered it had another car cut in dangerously close. A **metaphor** makes a comparison between two or more objects, which are unlike each other (e.g., "The moon was a ghostly galleon . . . "). **Similes** do the same thing, but include either the word *as* or *like* (e.g., "My love is like a red, red rose"). Children typically learn to understand and produce figurative language around 7–9 years of age, although competence in their understanding and production improves throughout the adolescent and early adult years (Nippold, 1996, 1998). Children with receptive or expressive language disorders often have difficulty producing and understanding figurative language.

To summarize these various types of meanings, consider the word *house.* Its referential meaning is "a structure used as a residence." Its connotative meaning might convey feelings of contentment and security. In a sentence such as, "The house where Mr. Jones lives is located in Beverly Hills," the word *where* expresses relational meaning (the location of the house). Because Beverly Hills is a commonly known wealthy neighborhood, one might infer that Mr. Jones is wealthy. The woman who says, "My house is your house," is figuratively offering her generous hospitality, not literally granting co-ownership of her real estate.

The examples in the previous paragraph show that the same word, phrase, or sentence may convey **multiple meanings.** The word *bat,* for example, can refer to a nocturnal flying mammal or a long cylindrical club used to hit a ball in the game of baseball. When used as a verb, it can mean hitting that ball (e.g., "*bat* it into left field") or to flutter (e.g., "to flirt successfully, learn to *bat* your eyelashes"). Such words, which are identical in pronunciation but have different meanings, are referred to as **homonyms** or homophones. Sometimes homonyms are spelled the same (e.g., "I *saw* the show"; "He cut the wood with a *saw*"), and sometimes they are not (e.g., "We went to the movies last *night*"; "He was a *knight* in shining armor"). Produced in isolation and without a context, such words are ambiguous; their meanings remain obscure.

> Give more examples of homonyms or homophones.

Words not only have multiple meanings, but they are also related to each other in multiple ways. The different ways in which words are related to each other are subsumed under **lexical relationships.** Different words that convey the same meaning are called **synonyms** (e.g., *big/large/enormous*; *destroy/obliterate/annihilate*; *pretty/beautiful/lovely*). Pairs of words that convey directly opposite meanings are called **antonyms** (e.g., *love/hate, in/out, up/down, near/far*).

> What is the lexical relationship of the words contained in the following pairs: *rock/stone; neat/messy?*

Some researchers of child language acquisition have classified meanings that children seem to acquire into **semantic relations,** which are contrasting units of meaning that are expressed in different forms of words, phrases, and sentences. For example, children who correctly name objects are said to have acquired the semantic relation of nomination; those who produce a phrase such as *my kitty* are said to have mastered the semantic relation of possession. See Table 1.1 for semantic relations reflected in the two-word utterances children typically produce by the age of 2.

Linguists and cognitive specialists believe that mastering semantic concepts requires the ability to categorize. That is why many tests designed to measure a child's developing language include at least one or two items that assess whether a child will give a category name for a group of pictures (e.g., saying "furniture" when shown pictures of a sofa, a table, a chair, and a bed). A child who cannot categorize individual items has difficulty with abstract concepts. This may indicate the presence of a language disorder as well.

Syntactic Component

A collection of rules about word combinations and sentence structures within a language is called **syntax.** The part of language that refers to syntactic rules is called the **syntactic component.** In Chomsky's theory of transformational grammar, universal syntactic rules that apply to all languages are innately given (Chomsky, 1957, 1965). Children are presumed to know the rules of universal grammar from birth. Because of this innate knowledge of syntactic structures, both adults and children know the acceptable sentence structures in their language.

table 1.1

Semantic Relations and Children's Two-Word Utterances

Semantic Relation	Expressed as a Linguistic Structure	Example of Two-Word Utterance	Possible Intended Meaning*
Nomination	Demonstrative + Noun	That baby!	That is a baby.
Nonexistence	Negative + Noun	No kitty	There is no kitty here
Agent-object	Noun + Noun	Doggie food	The dog is eating his food.
Agent-action	Noun + Verb	Daddy sleep	Daddy is sleeping.
Action-object	Verb + Noun	Kick ball	Let's kick the ball!
Action-indirect object	Verb + Noun	Drink baby	Give baby a drink.
Action-locative	Verb + Noun *or* Verb + Locative	Go home. Jump here!	Let's go home. Jump right here!
Possessor-possession	Noun + Noun	Mommy hat	That is Mommy's hat.
Entity-locative	Noun + Noun *or* Noun + Locative	Horsie barn Granma here!	The horse is in the barn. Grandma is here!
Entity-attribution	Noun + Adjective *or* Adjective + Noun	Dolly pretty Pretty dolly	The dolly is pretty.
Recurrence	Adjective (*more* or *another*) + Noun	More milk!	I want more milk!
Rejection	Negative + Noun	No milk!	I don't want milk!
Conjunction	Noun + Noun	Shoes socks!	I need my shoes and socks.

*Discerned by context

Source: Compiled from Bloom (1970), Bloom and Lahey (1978), Brown (1973), and Schlesinger (1971).

At a descriptive level, the syntactic component is analyzed in terms of rules of grammar and sentence construction. A complete sentence, for example, must consist of at least two parts, a noun and a verb (or, more precisely, a subject and a predicate). The length of an utterance is irrelevant when determining whether or not a sentence is grammatically correct. "I am" is a complete sentence, while "The man who had been standing by the building in the pouring rain under an umbrella" is an incomplete sentence, or sentence fragment, because it consists of a subject, but no predicate; the noun is followed by one long adjectival phrase further describing the noun. Adding a verb to the predicate to make an assertion about the subject will make it complete: "The man who had been standing by the building in the pouring rain under an umbrella *sighed.*"

The term *syntax* is sometimes equated with the word *grammar*, because both suggest rules of sentence formation. Grammar, however, encompasses a broader concept than syntax. Besides syntactic rules, grammar also sets forth semantic restrictions. The sentence, "The patient complained of infrequent but intense headaches" satisfies the syntactic and semantic rules of grammar. However, the sentence, "The patient complained of infrequent but constant headaches" breaks no syntactic rule of grammar but is not consistent with semantic rules. This grammatically correct sentence describes a situation that is impossible; one cannot have "infrequent but constant" headaches. Besides the syntactic and semantic rules of a language, grammar also includes the morphologic component of language, which will be described later.

The rules of syntax, as a part of grammar, determine in what order words can appear in a sentence. Each language has its own set of syntactical rules. In English, for example, a basic word order is subject-verb-object (e.g., "Dan bought a computer"). Constructions such as "Dan a computer bought" or "Bought Dan a computer" are not syntactically correct in English, but the Japanese language has a basic word order of subject-object-verb (as in "Dan a computer bought"), and the Irish language has a verb-object-subject construction (as in "Bought Dan a computer") (Owens, 2004).

Language is creative because its elements can be arranged and rearranged in many different ways that still conform to syntactic rules. Once a language-learner has mastered a particular construction, an infinite number of phrases or sentences can be generated. For example, in English, adjectives precede the nouns they modify, and the noun is often preceded by an article, a syntactic rule that can be annotated as article-adjective-noun. Learning this syntactic rule means that the language-user can generate countless phrases such as *the big house, the soft pillow, a beautiful rose, an ugly building,* and so forth, without having to learn each phrase one-by-one.

Morphologic Component

Morphology is the study of word structures, and, as previously noted, is a part of grammar. The **morphologic components** are the smallest elements of grammar, called **morphemes.**

Morphemes are the smallest units of meaning within a language. Most morphemes are words, but some morphemes are even smaller than words. Linguists recognize two kinds of morphemes: free and bound. A **free morpheme** conveys meaning standing alone and cannot be broken down into smaller parts. The word *walk* is a free morpheme. It can convey some meaning by itself and it cannot be broken down into smaller parts and still retain meaning. In essence, any word with no affixes is a free morpheme, also referred to as a *root* or *base* word. **Bound morphemes** are those suffixes and prefixes which are attached to a root word. Bound morphemes cannot stand alone, as they convey no meaning until they are combined with a root word. There are two types of bound morphemes: (1) derivational bound morphemes, and (2) inflectional bound morphemes.

> An affix is a small element of language added to words. When the element is added to the beginning of the word, it is called a prefix; added to the end of a word, it is called a suffix. The word *undo* contains the prefix *un-*. The word *walking* contains the suffix *-ing.*

Derivational bound morphemes. Elements of language that help create entirely new words from root words are called **derivational bound morphemes.** Examples of derivational bound morphemes include suffixes such as *-ment* in *engagement* and *-ish* as in *foolish.* Prefixes serving as derivational bound morphemes include *un-* as in *uneven* and *dis-* as in *discomfort.* A root word can have more than one derivational morpheme attached to it, consisting of suffixes, prefixes, or both, resulting in words such as *unbelievable, miscommunication,* or *disrespectful.*

> How many morphemes are there in the following words: *disestablishment, uncoordinated, undoubtedly?*

Inflectional bound morphemes. Elements of language that are attached to a root word to add to the meaning of the root word, but not to create a new word, are called **inflectional bound morphemes.** Examples of inflectional bound morphemes include the

box 1.1   **Examples of Some Bound Morphemes in the English Language**

INFLECTIONAL MORPHEMES		DERIVATIONAL MORPHEMES	
Morpheme	Example	Morpheme	Example
present progressive -*ing*	sleep*ing*	comparative -*er*	dri*er*
past tense -*ed*	wait*ed*	superlative -*est*	warm*est*
plural -*s*	cup*s*	adverbial -*ly*	quick*ly*
possessive -*'s*	father*'s* son	agentive -*er*	farm*er*
present tense -*s*	walk*s*		

present progressive -*ing*, the past tense -*ed*, and the possessive and plural -*s*. The word *jump*, for example, is a free morpheme, or root word. When the bound morpheme -*ing* is added to it, the meaning is altered, and the word *jumping* is recognized to mean action that is presently taking place (see Box 1.1 for more bound morphemes).

Children's production of free and bound morphemes is an indication of their successful language acquisition. Therefore, an assessment of a child's language development includes an analysis of how many free and bound morphemes the child produces. This analysis results in a quantitative measure called a mean length of utterance by morphemes, which will be described in Chapter 4 on the assessment of language.

Just as there are slight variations of phonemes, called allophones, so are there slight variations of morphemes, called **allomorphs.** For example, the bound morpheme regular plural has several allomorphic variations, although they may all be spelled with the phoneme /s/. Consider the following regular plural words: *cups*, *bags*, and *oranges*. In the first word, the final -*s* suffix is pronounced as [s] where as in the second word, it is pronounced as [z]. In the third word, the plural inflection is pronounced as [ɛz]. Similarly, the regular past tense -*ed*, as in the word *waited*, also has several allomorphic variations, including [t] as in *walked*, [d] as in *cried*, and [tɛd] as in *painted*.

Pragmatic Component

The phonologic, semantic, and syntactic structures of language are a means for social communication. This aspect of social production of language is called the pragmatic component. **Pragmatics** is the study of language production in social contexts. Therefore, pragmatics places greater emphasis on the functional, as opposed to the structural, aspects of language. *Functional* in this context refers to social production of language. Even so, the linguistic analysis treats the functions of language in structural terms as the different functions are often described as pragmatic structures. We prefer to describe the pragmatic aspects of language as pragmatic skills, or even more directly, as conversational skills.

Most pragmatic skills are observed when speakers engage in social discourse (conversation). These skills may be either verbal or nonverbal. Presumably, besides learning the phonologic, semantic, and syntactic aspects of language, a child should master the conversational skills in which the other aspects of language are realized.

Verbal pragmatic skills. Various communication skills needed to initiate and sustain conversation are called **verbal pragmatic skills.** The connected and contingent flow of language during social interaction between two or more individuals is defined as **discourse,** or conversation (Roseberry-McKibbin & Hegde, 2005). The quality of discourse is dependent on the skill of conversational partners in producing utterances that are logically related to each other. Linguists also believe that speakers and listeners should know and adhere to the pragmatic rules of language for successful social interaction. Verbal pragmatic language skills include:

> What is connected, contingent flow of language during social interaction between two or more individuals?

- Initiating conversation
- Taking turns in a conversational exchange
- Maintaining a topic during conversation
- Shifting to different topics during conversation
- Requesting conversational repair
- Responding to conversational repair requests
- Producing language that is appropriate to context and situation
- Narrating experiences and events

Initiating conversation, typically described as topic initiation, involves social rituals of greeting, "small talk," and the graceful entry into a satisfying discourse that begins with the introduction of a specific topic for discourse among conversational partners. To continue discourse, the conversational partners should exhibit good turn-taking skills so that each person plays the role of a speaker and listener. Each partner in conversation takes turns to maintain discourse. Speakers maintain a topic until they have nothing more to say on it or some other topic attracts attention, at which point the conversation partners shift to a new topic of discourse. Topic shifts should be gradual, the result of cohesive utterances leading up to the introduction of a new topic.

Often during conversational discourse, a conversational partner might be misunderstood, at which point one or more speakers ask questions, request more information, or seek clarifications in various ways. Such devices listeners use (e.g., "I'm sorry, I didn't quite follow you—where did you take your vacation?") when they do not understand a speaker are called **conversational repair strategies.** When listeners make requests for clarification, speakers then respond appropriately so they are better understood. Such responses to conversational repair requests also are pragmatic language skills. Efficient speakers continuously gauge the listener responses and offer clarifications sometimes even before a request is made.

> Conversational repair is a particularly valuable skill for students who may not understand the teacher's instructions the first time they are given. A child who can gracefully ask for clarification will function better in the classroom.

A person with good pragmatic language skills will modify language expressions according to the context and social situation. Speech-language pathologists (SLPs), for example, will use nontechnical language when speaking to clients or parents but will switch to technical jargon when speaking to other SLPs. Similarly, many adolescents with good pragmatic language skills may switch from the heavily slang-laden, informal language they might use with their peers to more standard, conventional language when conversing with adults, particularly parents or teachers.

Narrative skills are another part of verbal pragmatic language. Being complex language skills, narrative skills are important in social communication. Individuals may narrate personal experiences, stories, or events in a logically consistent and sequential manner. In this skill, utterances build on each other and lead to a satisfying conclusion. In recent years, there has been an emphasis on assessing this pragmatic language skill in school children to identify possible language disorders.

Three types of narrative discourse skills may be assessed in children of elementary school age (Hughes, McGillivray, & Schmidek, 1997). **Personal narratives** require children to relate personal experiences, such as telling about what happened at their last birthday party or where their family went on vacation. **Script narratives** require children to describe a routine series of events. A properly sequenced and sufficiently detailed response to such questions as, "Tell me how to make a peanut butter and jelly sandwich" or "How do I get to downtown from here" are script narratives. **Scripts** are written or verbal descriptions of routine events. **Fictional narratives** require children to tell a story, such as a well-known fairy tale or the plot of a popular movie or television show. Children might also be asked to retell a story that has just been told to them or, most difficult of all, to create their own stories.

> A boy is asked to tell about his trip to the zoo—what type of narrative has he been asked to produce?

Nonverbal pragmatic language skills. Various physical, emotional, and gestural aspects of communication that supplement, expand, or even contradict what is said in words are called **nonverbal pragmatic language skills.** Nonverbal pragmatic skills are popularly called body language, and include:

- Maintenance of eye contact
- Physical distance maintained during communication (proxemics)
- Gestures
- Facial expressions

Nonverbal pragmatic skills are often as important as verbal skills in maintaining smooth social interactions. During discourse, the conversational partners in many societies are expected to maintain eye contact with each other. In each community, a certain physical distance may be considered appropriate during verbal exchanges. Some societies tolerate more closeness than others.

> What is the more technical term for the popular phrase *body language?*

In all communities, gestures are a significant part of verbal communication. Gestures typically supplement what is said in words, but in some special cases, they may replace words. In people with serious verbal impairments, for example, gestures may be the only means of basic communication. Facial expressions, similar to gestures, add additional meaning, reinforce what is said, or suggest something other than what is said in words. For example, when someone says, "Very good! Very good!" with a sarcastic smile, the listener knows that what is meant is the opposite of what is said.

Pragmatic language skills, both verbal and nonverbal, are heavily influenced by culture and social norms. We will describe the interrelation between communication and culture in Chapter 11.

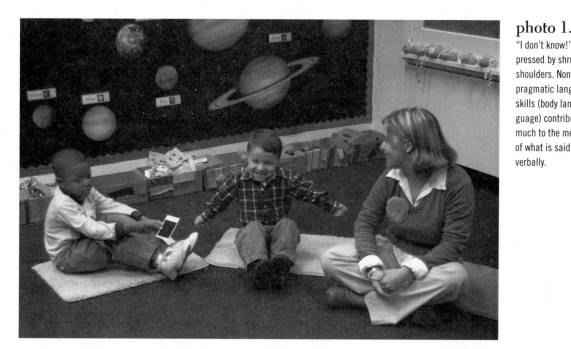

photo 1.1
"I don't know!" is expressed by shrugging shoulders. Nonverbal pragmatic language skills (body language) contribute much to the meaning of what is said verbally.

Comprehension and Production

In the linguistic analysis, comprehension and production are the two major modalities of language. Comprehension of language is also called **receptive language,** and production of language is also called **expressive language.**

The terms *comprehension* and *receptive language* are inferred when listeners pay attention and understand what is expressed either verbally or nonverbally (e.g., through sign language). Some adults understand some aspects of a foreign language, but cannot speak it. Unless it is produced out of a rote memory of phrases and sentences, those who can speak (produce) a language can usually understand it. Children who are learning a language may show great variations in comprehension and expression. Generally, young children comprehend more than they can express. On occasion, though, they may say words or phrases whose meaning they do not understand (McLaughlin, 1998).

Although comprehension and receptive language are described as passive mental states in linguistics, speech-language pathologists measure it only by actions that the listeners perform. It is only through correct verbal or nonverbal responses a client gives to commands or during conversation that a clinician can judge the client's comprehension of language. For example, to assess comprehension of single words, the clinician may ask a child to point to the correct picture placed among several pictures.

Language production is speaking or communicating nonverbally (e.g., as in sign language). Appropriate language production involves all aspects of language described so far—the phonological, semantic, grammatic, and pragmatic aspects. These aspects should be integrated into cohesive expressions to which listeners can react. Children with a language disorder may have deficiencies in producing one or more aspects of the language—typically multiple aspects.

Linguistic Explanations of Language ◼ ▨ and Language Learning

◼ ▨   Although there is no agreement among experts, explanations of language and how children acquire language abound. Various linguistic explanations of language and its learning are especially well known. The most commonly advanced explanations come from such rational linguists as Chomsky (1957, 1965, 1982, 1999) and his followers. Subsequent explanations, consistent for the most part with Chomsky's ideas, have been proposed by such rationalists as Pinker (1994).

According to Chomsky, a universal grammar is the essence of language. **Universal grammar** is a set of rules that applies to all human languages and can help generate new sentences with varied word combinations. For Chomsky, language is creative precisely because of a finite set of rules that allow for the generation of an infinite and varied set of sentences. Speakers of all languages have an innate knowledge of the universal grammar. This innate knowledge is called language competence, to be distinguished from language performance. While performance may be imperfect because of fatigue and momentary distraction, the innate competence (knowledge of universal grammar) is perfect. The classic versions of Chomsky's theories did not consider language use or performance. Even though Chomsky (1982, 1999) has revised his theories several times, the essence of his earlier ideas remains the same.

> ▨ What branch of philosophy are the theories of Chomsky (1957) and Pinker (1994) consistent with?

Language competence and language performance are related to two of Chomsky's other concepts: the **surface structure (S-structure)** and the **deep structure (D-structure)** of language. The S-structure refers to the actual order of words in a sentence. Surface structures can be seen (words as arranged on a piece of paper) or heard (as spoken by an individual). The D-structure refers to the underlying meaning the sentence conveys. Deep structures are not seen or heard; they are abstract and are understood only through a formal syntactic analysis. Surface structures are derived from the deep structures.

The meaning contained in the same D-structure may be transformed into different kinds of surface structures (different sentences with varied word order). For instance, an action an individual performs may be expressed in an active or a passive form as in "The mother brought the child to the clinic" versus "The child was brought to the clinic by the mother." Both the forms express the same meaning (the same D-structure), but the word arrangements (the S-structures) are different. Similarly, it is possible to have one S-structure with more than one D-structure. In such cases, the sentence is ambiguous because it has different meanings. For instance, the surface structure "Flying kites can be dangerous" may mean that the act of flying kites is dangerous or kites that fly can pose dangers.

Surface structures and deep structures are related to each other through Chomsky's concept of **grammatical transformation,** an operation that relates the deep and surface structures and yields different forms of sentences. Words are rearranged by deleting, substituting, or adding words to create different surface structures. Each sentence form (e.g., active, passive, question, negation) requires a particular grammatic transformation. The following illustrates how a specific surface structure can be transformed to convey different deep structures:

> Mary ate the pizza.
> Who ate the pizza? (a question-transformation)
> Did Mary eat the pizza? (a question-transformation)
> The pizza was eaten by Mary. (a passive transformation)
> The pizza was not eaten by Mary. (a negative-transformation)

Language creativity, Chomsky believed, is largely attributable to this process of grammatic transformation. Through knowledge of the rules of grammar and the use of transformations, language-users can generate countless varieties of sentences. Therefore, Chomsky's theory is also known as the **transformational generative theory of grammar.**

Chomsky does not believe that evolution contributed much to language. He considers language a creation of the human mind, an emergence at the human level. He does not believe that elements of language (i.e., basic communication) found at the animal level played a significant role in the emergence of human languages. Chomsky also does not believe that social interactions play a major role in learning and sustaining language. He assigns little or no role to learning in the acquisition of language.

How do children learn their language? According to Chomsky, it is this innate (present at birth) knowledge of the universal grammar, not specific learning or teaching, that makes it possible for children to learn language as rapidly as they do. Because children have knowledge of rules that apply to all languages, all they have to do is to figure out the particular rules that apply to their own language. Chomsky proposed that the innate knowledge children have of the universal grammar is contained in a hypothetical entity he called the **Language Acquisition Device (LAD).** The LAD receives data about the grammar of the particular language the children are exposed to. By analyzing this language input, children construct the grammar of their own language. In essence, language acquisition is the acquisition of syntactic rules, not such other aspects of language as meaning, social communication, and so forth. This acquisition is not a matter of learning, but a matter of refining or elaborating what is already known.

> Ever wonder what a Language Acquisition Device looks like? No one knows, because no one has ever seen one!

A view consistent with Chomsky's in most respects that has received much popular attention is that of Pinker (1994), who attributes language to a language instinct that only humans have. The language instinct hypothesis differs from Chomsky's theory of transformational generative grammar in one important respect: while Chomsky disregards the importance of evolutionary forces in the origin of language, Pinker believes that language indeed is due to biological forces in the form of an instinct.

Rationalists Chomsky, Pinker, and others cite several arguments to support their innately or instinctively determined view of language. Among others, they argue that (1) language is too complex to be learned by young children who cannot so easily master other skills; (2) parents do not explicitly teach language (especially the all-important grammar) to their children; (3) children acquire language too rapidly for it to be learned; (4) the universal aspects of grammar defy learning; and (5) children in different societies and cultures acquire language in roughly the same manner.

Many empirical scientists are skeptical of the argument that language is innately given or instinctively determined. The argument is typically made as a series of assertions; these assertions do not offer independent evidence. For instance, that language is too complex to be learned, children acquire it too rapidly, and that young children could not possibly learn it are all assertions before the fact. Empiricists question these assertions on the basis of both the lack of evidence to sustain them and the presence of evidence that contradicts them. For instance, there is no factual evidence that only simple things are learned and complex things have to be innate or instinctive. In fact most instinctive human behaviors are simpler, not more complex—contrast, for example, the instinctive eye blink reflex with the task of building rockets, writing a poem, or designing a beautiful building.

That language is acquired too rapidly to be learned is a questionable assertion. The rate at which something may be learned cannot be prejudged; we just have to find out. What is *rapid* acquisition and what is *slow* acquisition? These are matters of judgments, not facts. Therefore, the judgment that the rate at which children acquire language is rapid and the conclusion that it is not learned are both assertions without independent evidence.

Most of the cited observations of rationalists do not necessarily support the nativist or instinctive view of language. For instance, the universal features of language are no evidence of an innate mechanism or an instinct. Many social habits or rituals have universal features (e.g., ceremonies of birth, wedding, death), but it would be far-fetched to claim an innate mechanism or an instinct for them. Similarly, the observation that children in vastly different societies acquire a variety of languages in roughly the same sequence does not compel a claim of nativism or a language instinct. Similarities in environmental stimuli and social interactions could explain similar learning sequences across societies.

Analysis of Verbal Behavior

The behavioral psychologist B. F. Skinner (1957, 1986) provided an alternative to the linguistic description and explanation of language. Decidedly nonlinguistic in his approach, Skinner rejected the concept that language is a mental, cognitive, or any kind of rule system because such a concept was simply inferred from the behavior of individuals with no possibility of independent verification. Because language is traditionally conceived as a mental system or an entity that is inferred and beyond experimental manipulations, Skinner proposed the term **verbal behavior** to describe speaking, listening, reading, and writing.

Skinner defined verbal behavior as "behavior reinforced through the mediation of other persons" (1957, p. 2). He considered verbal behavior a form of social behavior, because all social behaviors are reinforced by persons in a community. A nonverbal behavior such as moving away from situations that cause physical harm need not be reinforced by other persons, but verbal behaviors are normally produced and reinforced only in a social milieu, receiving reinforcement from others. A verbal response like "Can I have some juice please?"

The "revolutionary" pragmatic view of language was nothing new—Skinner's ideas predated it by at least 15 years.

or "What time is it?" are reinforced and maintained only by the actions of other persons. Consequently, Skinner's view of verbal behavior is more consistent with the pragmatic view of language that emphasizes social interactions against universal grammars of the rationalists. In fact, Skinner's 1957 view of verbal behavior as a functional unit that includes the speaker and listener antedates the pragmatic view of language that was hailed as revolutionary in the 1970s and 1980s.

Skinner thought that the traditional linguistic analysis of language is too structurally oriented to offer a meaningful analysis of talking and listening that people exhibit in social contexts. He stated that such linguistic structures as phonemes, morphemes, words, phrases, sentences, and various grammatic features do not reflect the reasons why people talk. Being a natural (empirical) scientist, Skinner's interest was in analyzing the causes and effects in human communication. In essence, Skinner was asking: What kinds of causes lead to what kinds of verbal behavior? Skinner found that when the goal is to understand why people say what under specified conditions, terms like *words, sentences,* and *grammar* did not help.

In behavioral analysis, there are three kinds of causes that impel people to behave verbally. Internal states of the speaker are one set of causes that produce a class of verbal behaviors. For instance, thirst, hunger, pain, physical discomfort, sexual drive, and other physiological states of motivation may cause various kinds of verbal behaviors. External stimuli in the social and physical environment form a second set of causes of a different class of verbal behaviors. Much of everyday talk is produced in response to the social and physical world surrounding the speaker. Prior verbal behaviors of the speaker are the third set of causes that generate verbal behaviors. What a speaker just said may cause more to be said, in the manner of what is popularly called a train of thought. There also is much of this kind of verbal behavior in everyday social interactions. When an attempt is made to relate verbal behaviors to these causes, the linguistic structural terms are inadequate. This is because there are no specific and independent What are three causes of verbal behavior? causes for the production of phonemes, morphemes, words, phrases, sentences, semantic units, and pragmatic structures. In other words, a cause that forces a word from a speaker may be no different from a cause that leads to a sentence. Therefore, different linguistic structures do not necessarily have different causes. In essence, linguistic structures are not based on a cause–effect relationship. Yet, a scientific analysis of language requires a causal analysis. Therefore, Skinner proposed functional units of verbal behavior for scientific analysis.

Instead of grouping verbal behaviors on the basis of their structures (e.g., words, phrases, sentences), Skinner grouped them on the basis of their independent causes. Such groupings are functional units. In the behavioral analysis, a **functional unit** includes a category of verbal behavior and a cause that precedes it. It may be noted that the term *functional* in this case does not mean use, as it often means in other contexts, especially in pragmatics. The term *functional* means causal, and a functional unit is a cause–effect relationship. As noted before, the cause is a state within the speaker, events and objects in the environment, or the speaker's own prior verbal responses. The effect is a verbal production. When someone says something, it is expected to affect listeners who react in some way to what was just said, otherwise there is

> Because it is defined in terms of observable, measurable functional units, *verbal behavior* can be subjected to experimental research much more easily than *language,* defined as an internal, mental event that cannot be directly observed.

little or no communication. Such listener reactions are typically described as *consequences* of a verbal response. Skinner asserted that a scientific understanding of verbal behaviors requires us to specify (1) the cause or causes of verbal behaviors, (2) the behaviors themselves, and (3) the consequence the behaviors receive in terms of listener reactions.

Therefore, Skinner grouped all verbal responses that have the same or similar causes and receive the same kinds of consequences as a functional unit, which may be a word, a phrase, a sentence, or an extended utterance. With this kind of an analysis, Skinner described the following functional units of verbal behavior: mands, tacts, echoics, intraverbals, autoclitics, and textuals.

Mands

Skinner coined the term **mand** to include the kinds of verbal behaviors that are demands, commands, requests, and so forth. Mands are verbal responses that have motivational states as causes and often specify their own reinforcers. Motivational states that cause mands include thirst, hunger, discomfort, pain, and sexual drive. Therefore, most mands are driven by internal physiological states of the speaker. That a mand specifies its own reinforcer makes it easier for the listener to react to the speaker in ways that would reinforce the speaker's verbal response.

Many everyday verbal behaviors are mands. They demand immediate attention and action from the listeners because they specifically ask for reinforcement. For instance, a speaker who requests, "Would you please turn on the fan?" is suggesting that she or he is feeling too warm (a physiological-motivational state) and that the fan will help alleviate the state of discomfort. The person to whom the request is directed knows precisely what to do and what will reinforce the request: turning the fan on. This is what is meant by the statement that a mand specifies its own reinforcer. As we will see later, other classes (functional units) of verbal responses do not do that.

What is a functional unit of verbal behavior that specifies its own reinforcer?

A motivational state will not automatically cause a mand—environmental stimuli are also needed. For instance, the speaker would not ask anyone to turn a fan on if there is no fan in the room. Also, if there is no one else in the room, the person who feels it too warm will walk over to the fan and switch it on (no verbal behavior). A mand is emitted (produced) when a certain physiological state is coupled with a certain environmental condition. Therefore, to scientifically understand a mand, one needs to know or infer the physiological (motivational) state of the speaker, the coupling environmental stimuli, and the reinforcer the response specifies in the form of the actions it demands (mands) of the listener. In most everyday interactions, however, the listeners who reinforce mands do so simply on the basis of the mand alone. When someone asks for a glass of water, the person who provides it assumes thirst and does not question the speaker about his or her motivation. On the other hand, there are situations when a mand's reason (cause) is demanded. For instance, when a child asks for a cookie soon after dinner, the parent may ask, "Why? You just ate," to which the child might reply, "You know she snatched my last piece of pizza!" See Table 1.2 to better understand the nature of mands, their causes, and consequences (reinforcers). Note that:

- A mand can be a word, a phrase, or a complete sentence; therefore, structure is not as important as the class to which a verbal response belongs.
- Each mand is driven by a state of motivation and emitted under an appropriate stimulus condition.

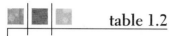

table 1.2

What Are Mands? What Causes Them? How Are They Reinforced?

Mands	Motivational State	Environmental Stimuli	Reinforcer
"Water!"	Thirst	Inside a home, sight of water, a waiter in a restaurant	A glass of water
"Salad, please."	Hunger	A person asking	A bowl of salad
"I want you to leave, right now."	An aversive state	A person who is aversive	Departure of the aversive person
"Please pass that sweater to me."	Feeling cold, an aversive state	The sweater	Handing the sweater
"Fire!"	Fear	Something burning	Flight
"Yummy!"	Deprivation, not satiated yet	"Do you want more ice cream?" "Yes, please!"	More ice cream

- Each mand specifies the reinforcer (the expected action from the listener).
- Only what is specified (or something similar) will reinforce a mand.
- All reinforcers are primary (food, drink, termination of an aversive event or state).

Mands are typically reinforced by **primary** or **unconditioned reinforcers,** which are biological in nature and do not depend on past experience. For instance, food, drink, moving away from dangerous or aversive stimuli are of survival value; hence, their effects are biologically determined. Consequently, they are immediately reinforcing without a need for past learning.

Children probably begin to mand early. A child's crying response when hungry may be a reflexive mand; it is not a learned (operant) response yet. Later on when the child says, "Cookie!" it is a mand in the form of a single word. Young children often mand with single words: "Up!" "Down!" "More!" "That!" "Milk!" and so forth, demand reinforcing actions from the caregivers. Subsequently, when parents teach more polite forms of request, the child learns to produce elaborate, subtle, and even indirect mands ("I think I'm hungry, Mom").

Teaching mands to children with language disorders is an important task. Children who cannot mand do not have verbal means to fulfill their needs. There is evidence that some children who lack mands exhibit such undesirable behaviors as fussing, hitting, snatching things from others, and exhibiting a variety of undesirable behaviors. There is also evidence that teaching them mands will reduce those behaviors.

Tacts

Another functional unit of verbal responses is called *tacts*. A **tact** is a group of verbal responses whose cause is a state of affairs in the environment and which are reinforced socially. Tacts are often descriptions and comments on environmental events and objects. Unlike mands,

What is a functional unit of behavior which is reinforced socially and whose cause is an environmental condition?

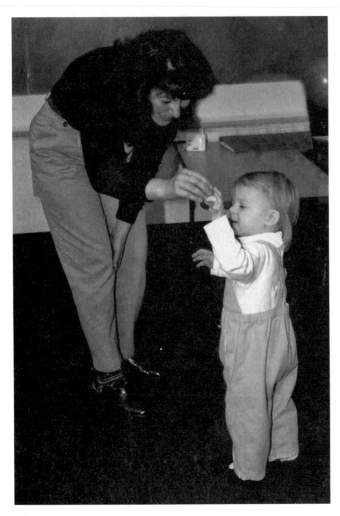

photo 1.2

Mands specify their own reinforcers—a child asks for a cookie and is reinforced by receiving the cookie.

tacts are not caused by states of deprivation or motivation and they do not specify their own reinforcers. Also unlike mands, tacts are reinforced by social (secondary) reinforcers, not primary. A listener smiling, nodding, paying attention, agreeing, and following up with similar statements may reinforce a speaker's tacts. A simple observation, such as, "My, what a beautiful day!" may be reinforced by the listener who smiles, nods, and says, "Yes, isn't it?"

Discriminative environmental stimuli or events and an audience (one or more listeners) are usually sufficient to evoke tacts. **Discriminative stimuli** are stimuli in the presence of which a response has been reinforced in the past and, therefore, the response is more likely in its presence. In the previous example of a simple tact, the speaker probably would not say anything if the person encountered has not responded to the speaker's speech in the past.

To be reinforced, tacts should bear some conventional correspondence with the stimuli and events being tacted. For instance, a tact such as "What a beautiful sunset!" produced in the morning would not be reinforced. In this case, there is no correspondence between the stimuli (sunrise) and the tact. Young children who are still learning their verbal repertoire may be treated with leniency, however. An 18-month-old child who calls a truck a "car" might still be reinforced. But as the child's tacts increase, parents may require progressively better correspondence between the discriminative stimuli and the tacts that evoke them. Thus, children learn to give more differentiated tacts.

Sometimes it may not be clear to the caregivers whether a child has produced a mand or a tact. For instance, a 2-year-old may say "car" while playing with an older child. The youngster's response may be either a mand (e.g., "Give me the car") or a tact (e.g., "I see a car" or "That's a car"). The nature of the response becomes clear when the older child asks, "Do you want it?" and the child nods or tries to reach for it. This suggests that the child's single-word production was a mand. See Table 1.3 to better understand the nature of tacts.

Unlike previously discussed semantic relations or structures, Skinner described children's early utterances in terms of functional units of verbal behavior.

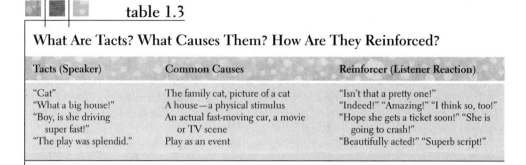

table 1.3

What Are Tacts? What Causes Them? How Are They Reinforced?

Tacts (Speaker)	Common Causes	Reinforcer (Listener Reaction)
"Cat"	The family cat, picture of a cat	"Isn't that a pretty one!"
"What a big house!"	A house—a physical stimulus	"Indeed!" "Amazing!" "I think so, too!"
"Boy, is she driving super fast!"	An actual fast-moving car, a movie or TV scene	"Hope she gets a ticket soon!" "She is going to crash!"
"The play was splendid."	Play as an event	"Beautifully acted!" "Superb script!"

Note that:

- Events and objects evoke tacts.
- To determine whether a response is a tact or not, one will have to observe the beginning and the end of an interaction. An obvious external stimulus or event is the first sign that it is a tact. But the external stimulus cannot be printed material or someone else's model. If the stimulus is printed material, the response is a textual; if it is a model, the response is an echoic.
- If the speaker, after hearing an approving comment, does not demand any further action from the listener, then it is likely a tact. To be considered a tact, the particular episode of interaction should end with a reinforcing comment from the listener.
- If the speaker demands additional action, then it was not a tact, more likely a mand. For instance, a child who says "Cookie" may not end the interaction when the mother says, "Yes! A big one!" The child may demand it in other ways (such as trying to reach for it).

It is said that compared to mands, tacts are objective, disinterested verbal responses (Winokur, 1976). Those who mand are asking others to do something for them; those who tact are sharing their experience with others.

Echoics

The term *echoic* comes from *echo*. An **echoic** is a verbal response that re-creates its own causal stimulus. More often than not, the causal stimulus is another speaker's verbal response. Therefore, echoics are verbal responses under the control of other persons' verbal responses. The reinforcement for echoic responses is usually contingent on a good match between the stimulus and the acoustic properties of the echoic itself. In other words, echoics are reinforced when they sound like their own stimuli.

> What functional unit of verbal behavior is more commonly known as an imitated response?

An echoic is more commonly described as an imitated response. An imitation is a replication of its own stimulus. For instance, when the mother says "Kitty," and the child then repeats it, the stimulus (the mother's production) and the echoic response (the child's production) have the same form; the stimulus and the response match. A stimulus that is imitated (replicated) is called a **model**. In essence, then, speakers' imitations of modeled stimuli are echoics.

Echoics may be partial and covert. **Partial echoics** are repetitions of only a portion of what is heard. Sometimes people echo only the last part of an utterance they have just heard. Such partial echoics may have the effect of requesting clarification, reinforcing the speaker's statement by suggesting agreement, or when a response is not imminent. See Box 1.2 for examples of types of echoic behavior.

Echoics are distinct from mands and tacts in that only the echoics duplicate their own stimuli. Mands and tacts take a different form from their causal variables. When a speaker exclaims "This *is* a supersized hamburger!" the verbal response and its cause (the gigantic hamburger) are totally different. When a child mands "Juice!" the verbal response and the juice are as different as they could be. But when a child echoes a clinician's modeled "Say, juice," the clinician's stimulus and the child's imitated response ("juice") are acoustically the same. Clinically, when a child learns to echo, and the clinician fades the modeled stimulus, the previous echoics may fall into other functional units. That is, a child who has learned to echo "I want juice!" may eventually produce it as a mand under conditions of deprivation or may tact "Juice!" to name it.

Linguists have generally claimed that behaviorists explain language acquisition on the basis of imitation. Presumably, behaviorists have claimed that children imitate adult speech and language productions and thus acquire language. This is certainly not the case. Larger and more complex verbal behaviors that children acquire are not echoed often enough to be the basis of their learning. Instead, echoics may help children get started in their learning of verbal behaviors (language). Young children may echo speech sounds, syllables, and simple words and get reinforced for them. A mother who reinforces her baby for echoing her "da-da" or "ma-ma" may get the child started on learning certain syllables. Later the baby will echo better approximations of *Daddy* and *Mommy*. There is observational evidence that babies do echo babbled speech sounds, syllables, and eventually words. There also is experimental evidence that when a baby's echoing of mother's productions is reinforced, the babbling will increase in frequency (McLaughlin, 1998; Winokur, 1976; see also Chapter 4).

---

box 1.2   **Examples of Echoic Responses**

Verbal stimulus:	You need to get ready for your appointment.	Verbal stimulus:	What do you think of the situation in the Middle East?
Echoic response:	Appointment? What appointment? *(requests clarification)*	Echoic response:	The situation in the Middle East . . . *(a quick response is not imminent)*
Verbal stimulus:	His wife is very pretty.		
Echoic response:	Very pretty! *(indicates agreement)*		

In everyday verbal communication, echoics play a smaller role than such other verbal behaviors as mands and tacts. What we call spontaneous speech is decidedly not echoic, and much of everyday speech is spontaneous (in control of more natural stimuli than modeled verbal stimuli). Nonetheless, echoics play a significant role in teaching verbal behavior to children with language disorders. These children often cannot spontaneously produce words under normal conditions of stimulation. They cannot mand when they are deprived of something (in need of something) or cannot tact when confronted with physical and social stimuli. Simply asking them to produce the word is often ineffective. Therefore, clinicians model the correct response for the child to echo. Echoics are then reinforced. Normally, there should be near-perfect matching between the stimulus and the echoic to reinforce the echoic. In the clinic, as well as in homes during the early acquisition of basic words (tacts or mands), some discrepancy between the modeled stimulus and the attempted imitation may be tolerated. For instance, when the clinician gives the model "truck," for a child to imitate, the echoic may sound more like "tuck," but the child may still be reinforced. In gradual steps, the clinician may require progressively better matching between the modeled stimulus and the echoic. Parents may also similarly be tolerant of imperfect echoics in the beginning stages of learning.

A form of echoics, echolalia, is seen in children who are autistic and verbal. These children often immediately repeat what they hear. Autistic children also repeat what they have heard in the past; this delayed repetition is not echoic in the behavioral analysis as the stimulus is not immediate. We will describe children with autism and their language problems and treatment in Chapter 13.

> We will describe children with autism and their language problems and treatment in Chapter 13.

Intraverbals

Much of what people say during the course of a day may not be in response to physical stimuli and events surrounding them. Often, a speaker needs an external stimulus only to trigger an initial verbal response. Once started, the speaker can go on for a while because speech produced is stimulus for more speech. In other words, one's own speech triggers more speech in a chain-like fashion. Speech caused by speakers' own prior speech is known as the **intraverbal.**

Intraverbals explain how people go on talking in the absence of a parade of physical stimuli. For a lecturer, the sight of an attentive audience is the entire physical stimulus needed to get started and then go on to speak for hours. Much of that speech is intraverbal because what the speaker just said serves as stimuli to say more, which in turn serves as stimuli for what will be said next. In this chain-like fashion, continuous and fluent speech is produced because of the power of the intraverbal control.

> What is a functional unit of verbal behavior caused by the speaker's own prior speech?

More obvious and simple examples of intraverbals include reciting the alphabet, counting, or giving telephone numbers or addresses. Certain terms that go together (learned more like a single unit) also illustrate simple intraverbals. For instance, when a speaker begins by saying "A table and a . . ." it is likely to be completed by saying "chair." In this case the production "chair" is the intraverbal, and the prior words the speaker said are the stimuli. Proverbs and idioms are also intraverbal functional units. Intraverbal control of speech is evident when a speaker begins by saying, "A stitch in time . . ." (prior speech that serves as stimuli for the final part) and finishes by saying, "saves nine" (the intraverbal).

At a more complex level, history is learned and talked about as a series of intraverbals. To name the first few presidents of the United States in their chronological order, it is helpful if the speaker can get started with the first, George Washington; if not, it may be difficult to establish the correct chain of names. The name Washington may prompt John Adams, which may prompt Thomas Jefferson, and so forth. This shows that the first name serves as a stimulus for the second, the second a stimulus for the third, and so on. When abruptly asked, "Who was the seventeenth President?" the person who responds may have to establish his or her own intraverbal control to answer it correctly. The speaker may go like this: "Well, let me see. I know Abraham Lincoln was the sixteenth President . . . and after Lincoln, oh yes, it was Andrew Johnson!" In this case, Johnson's name (intraverbal) was prompted by Lincoln's (speaker's own prior verbal response). When suddenly asked, "Which letter comes before S?" a child may overtly or covertly start reciting the alphabet to get a running start that takes the child to the correct spot. Such running starts are good examples of intraverbal control. As these examples make it clear, intraverbal responses are like verbal chains. Speakers' own verbal stimuli and responses are chained. Some chains are shorter while others are much longer.

Much of academic and technical learning is also a function of intraverbal control. A student in speech-language pathology who has been educated about it and who starts by saying, "The definition of a discriminative stimulus is . . ." can correctly say the rest of the definition because what was just said can trigger the rest of the response; it is the rest of the response that is intraverbal. But when asked to define a discriminative stimulus, someone who has not been educated in it will simply not say much, or if forced to say something, will be dysfluent (will repeat, interject, and pause).

Fluency, both in speech and oral reading, is likely a function of intraverbal control (Hegde, 1982). As in the previous example, one who talks about anything fluently will have established good intraverbal control. Lack of intraverbal control is likely to result in hesitant, interjected, pause-filled, and repetitive speech and oral reading.

Autoclitics

A common linguistic criticism of the behavioral analysis of language is that it cannot explain grammar. This criticism is unfounded because Skinner's (1957) analysis includes a nontraditional and sophisticated analysis of grammar, including syntactic and morphological aspects.

Unlike Chomsky and other linguists, Skinner did not consider grammar to be central to verbal behavior (language). Nor did Skinner consider grammar to be the cause of verbal behavior. It may be recalled that an innate grammar is the cause of language and its acquisition in the linguistic analysis. Grammar is an effect, not a cause in the behavioral analysis (Winokur, 1976). It is like other kinds of verbal behaviors—nothing special. In the behavioral analysis, grammar is secondary to the primary verbal behaviors of the kind described so far (e.g., mands, tacts, intraverbals, echoics). Speakers need to think of word order, sentence structure, morphologic inflections, and so forth only when they

What are secondary verbal behaviors that describe or comment on certain aspects of primary verbal behaviors?

have something to say. In essence, grammar depends on other aspects of verbal behavior. Therefore, Skinner coined the term *autoclitics* to "suggest [verbal] behavior which is based on or depends on other verbal behavior" (Skinner, 1957, p. 315). **Autoclitics** may be defined as secondary verbal behaviors that describe or comment on certain aspects of primary verbal behaviors. In essence, autoclitics give additional information to the listener on what the speaker says.

There are different kinds of autoclitics. Some autoclitics work like the grammatical elements of the linguistic analysis. For instance, the morphological features of English are a variety of autoclitics. These autoclitics specify aspects of the environment that caused the speaker's primary verbal behavior. For example, when the plural inflection *-s* is included in a sentence such as, "These are two cups," the quantitative aspect of the event that caused the statement is specified. The plural *-s*, being an autoclitic, informs the listener that the primary verbal behavior, which tacts (describes) the physical stimuli *cups*, are caused by more than one cup. In essence, autoclitics of this kind specify properties of stimuli that caused primary verbal behaviors. Similarly, other autoclitics specify the temporal aspects of stimuli that cause the primary verbal behaviors. For instance, when a speaker says, "The boy is running," the autoclitics *is* and *-ing* (the *verbal auxiliary* in the linguistic analysis) inform the listener that the action is contemporaneous to the primary verbal behavior. When a speaker changes it to "The boy was running," the autoclitics *was* and *-ing* inform the listener that the action that caused the primary verbal behavior (the boy's running) has a different temporal relationship (past) to the current verbal behavior. In all of these examples, the article *the* specifies the particular stimulus (perhaps in an array of stimuli) that caused the primary verbal behavior. Note that there would be no use for any of the autoclitics unless the primary verbal behavior (tacting or describing some physical stimuli) was already imminent.

Some other autoclitics clearly specify to the listener as to *why* the speaker is saying something at all. For instance, when a speaker makes a statement such as, "I see in the newspaper that it is going to rain tomorrow," one part of the statement (*I see in the newspaper*) is an autoclitic explaining why the speaker is saying that "it is going to rain tomorrow" (Skinner, 1957). Note again that there would be no need for the autoclitic *I see in the newspaper* unless the primary verbal behavior *it is going to rain tomorrow* was imminent.

Still other autoclitics inform the listener about the strength of what is being said (again, the primary verbal behavior). A speaker may say, "I strongly believe that the statement is false" or, "I am inclined to think that the statement is false." In such cases, the strength of the primary verbal behaviors (tacting a false statement or a questionable statement) are suggested by the autoclitics that precede them. The autoclitic *I strongly believe that* suggests a higher strength of the response than *I am inclined to think that*. These examples show that Skinner's autoclitics go beyond the traditional elements of grammar.

Textuals

Verbal behavior as Skinner (1957) defined it includes reading and writing. Space will not permit a more detailed description of these important aspects of verbal behavior. It may be noted briefly that **textuals** are a class of verbal behaviors that are controlled by printed stimuli or

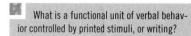
What is a functional unit of verbal behavior controlled by printed stimuli, or writing?

writing. As verbal behavior, textuals may be overt (oral reading) or covert (silent reading). Textual responses (oral or silent reading) are tightly controlled by the printed stimulus in that the reader has no choice but to name the stimulus, as each printed word has its own proper name.

Meaning in the Behavioral Analysis

As we saw earlier, semanticists consider meaning a property of language. The structure of language is supposed to hold meaning, its content. In the behavioral analysis, meaning is neither the content of language nor its property. Spoken words or sentences do not hold meaning as buckets hold water. Consistent with the emphasis on a causal analysis that characterizes the behavioral view, **meaning** may be defined as a relation between a controlling variable (cause) and a verbal production. In essence, meaning is a relation between antecedents and the responses. Listeners who do not have access to the cause of a verbal episode fail to understand its meaning. Failing to understand the meaning of an utterance means that the listeners cannot react promptly, effectively, or fully to the speaker.

If meaning were to be a property of language and if words were to hold meaning, the meaning of all words, phrases, and sentences spoken should be immediately clear to the listener who knows the dictionary meaning of those words. Knowing the dictionary definition of words, however, is not sufficient to understand everyday conversations. For example, a child playing with some toys may say "truck," and the parents who heard it may not understand the child's production, even though they fully know the meaning of the word *truck*. To understand the child's production, the parents look for what caused it: Is the child playing with a truck? Did the child see a commercial on the television for a toy truck? Did the child see the picture of a truck in a storybook? Did the child simply imitate a word heard on the radio? The child's production would be meaningful to the parents only when they understand its antecedent (cause, stimulus).

Not only the words, but phrases or sentences also illustrate that meaning lies in a controlling relation, not in linguistic structures. A listener may be puzzled when asked, "I did not see you yesterday!" although every word that was spoken was understood. The meaning would be clear only when the listener finds out that there was a meeting in which the listener was expected but did not show up, because the listener did not know about it. The cause of the speaker's statement was the meeting and the listener's expected but failed attendance. The listener needed access to this cause to understand the statement.

Skinner's analysis of verbal behavior is relevant to speech-language pathology because it (1) is empirical as is any clinical discipline; (2) reconceptualizes a mental system as observable skills that clinicians measure and treat; (3) avoids speculative theorizing that is not helpful to clinicians; and (4) is consistent with the methods of treatment used in remediating language disorders in children. Skinner's analysis considered language a form of social behavior long before pragmatists saw it that way. Much of the experimentally supported treatment procedures in speech-language pathology are behavioral.

We will close this chapter with a brief review of a few additional concepts that may be understood both from the standpoint of linguistics and behavioral science. These concepts are frequently used in speech-language pathology to describe certain distinctions in both normal and disordered communication.

Language and Communication

Language, as we have seen so far, may be thought of either as a mental system of rules or as a form of social behavior. **Communication,** a frequently used term in both linguistics and speech-language pathology, is traditionally defined as exchange of information between two or more persons in verbal, gestural, written, and other forms. Those who believe that language is a mental system of rules recognize that communication is a social act. From a behavioral standpoint, communication is speaking, writing, gesturing, signing, and so forth that affect other people. While the linguistic view of communication implies that something (information) is passed back and forth among people, the behavioral view stresses the actions of, and interactions among, speakers and listeners.

> Which view stresses actions of, and interactions among, speakers and listeners?

In a sense, communication is a more comprehensive view of social interaction than the term *language* suggests. As a social act, communication integrates all aspects of language, including written and spoken forms, verbal and nonverbal (gestural) forms, and various social conventions of interactions among people.

Verbal and Nonverbal Communication

Communication can be verbal or nonverbal because language itself may be verbal or nonverbal. **Verbal communication** is vocal language production and involves orally produced speech to affect listeners. **Nonverbal communication** is production of such nonvocal behaviors as signs, gestures, and nonvocal symbols to affect other people. Similarly, verbal language is spoken language whereas nonverbal language is production of signs, gestures, and nonvocal symbols.

American Sign Language (ASL) is an example of a nonverbal language in which the speaker manually gestures to communicate. ASL has all the features of an oral language, except that it is not oral. Like oral languages, ASL is creative, dynamic, and powerful. It has its own structural rules. ASL clearly shows that oral language is not the only means of effective communication.

Other nonverbal communication systems include *Blissymbolics, carrier symbols,* and *Mayer-Johnson* icons. All these are nonverbal systems of language that can be used as an alternative for people who, for various reasons, cannot produce oral language at all or to augment the communication of people whose oral language skills are limited. Therefore, these systems are referred to as augmentative or alternative communication (AAC). Providing a system of AAC for children who have significant difficulty with oral language is an important aspect of language treatment and will be described in Chapter 15.

Chapter Summary

To understand language disorders, it is necessary to study the nature and properties of language itself. Both rationalistic and empirical investigators have studied language and its properties.

Linguists, many of whom are rationalists, have mostly been concerned with the structure of language as a mental system. They have described language in terms of such components as phonological (related to sound systems), semantic (related to meaning), syntactic (related to word arrangements), and pragmatic (related to use of usage). Linguists recognize two modalities of language: receptive and expressive. A school of linguistic thought, influenced by Chomsky, believes that language is possible mostly because of an innate mental capacity.

Behavioral scientists, most of whom are empiricists, have described language in terms of verbal behavior and functional units. Skinner, an early behavioral scientist to study verbal behavior, described such functional (cause–effect) units as mands (commands, demands, requests), tacts (descriptive statements), echoics (imitative behaviors), textuals (reading), intraverbals (speech generated by speech itself), and autoclitics (grammatical elements). In explaining language, behavioral scientists place heavier emphasis on learning variables than on innateness.

Communication may be verbal or nonverbal. Verbal communication involves spoken language, and nonverbal communication includes gestures and such formalized systems as the American Sign Language.

Study Guide

1. Compare and contrast the philosophical approaches of rationalism and empiricism. How do they verify the truth value of their statements? What effects have these two approaches had on the study of language?

2. How are the linguistic structures described by linguists different from functional units described by Skinner? Point out the usefulness of each of these two approaches to an analysis and treatment of language disorders in children.

3. What arguments do rationalists such as Chomsky and Pinker cite to support the idea that language is innately or instinctively learned by children? Critically analyze these arguments.

4. How did Chomsky distinguish between surface and deep structures? What was his reason for distinguishing the two structures of language? What process relates the two structures in Chomsky's theory?

5. With suitable illustrations, defend the statement that "mands specify their own reinforcers."

6. Explore and justify the statement that "meaning of words is not a static, single, and invariable entity." Give examples that help justify the statement.

chapter 2

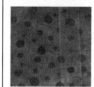

An Overview of Language
Disorders in Children

At its inception in the 1920s, the profession that we know today as communicative sciences and disorders (speech-language pathology) was concerned mainly with stuttering and articulation disorders. *Speech pathology* and *speech correctionists, therapists,* and later, *pathologists* were the well-established names. There was no particular emphasis on *language* disorders either in the name of the profession, the national professional organization, the name of the specialists, or in their scope of practice. The study and treatment of child language disorders were not a significant part of the profession until the 1960s. It was only in 1978 that, to reflect an expanded scope of practice, the American Speech and Hearing Association renamed itself the American Speech-Language-Hearing Association.

Several factors compelled speech clinicians to move into the realm of child language disorders. One factor was an escalating pressure on speech-language pathologists working in public schools to evaluate and treat children with all forms of communicative disorders. This forced them to take a closer look at language skills of children. The clinicians could no longer ignore language disorders in children, as language disorders were second only to articulation disorders in their prevalence.

Another factor was advances in the study of language and language acquisition in children. Speech pathologists of the 1960s came under the heavy influence of linguistic research on language, especially that of the generative linguists, notably Chomsky (1957, 1965). Subsequent shifts in the study of language within the pragmatic framework which emphasized the social nature of language further enriched the practical and clinical aspect of verbal communication (Halliday, 1973, 1975). Both cross-sectional and longitudinal studies of language acquisition in children (Bates, Bretherton, & Snyder, 1988; Bloom, 1970; Brown, 1973; Hulit & Howard, 2002; McLaughlin, 1998) provided a foundation for assessing child language disorders and attracted the attention of specialists in communicative disorders.

Yet another factor that influenced the profession's entry into child language disorders was a series of behavioral intervention studies—published in the 1960s and 1970s—that showed that, contrary to the nativists' claim, children with language disorders may be taught specific language skills. Some of the early studies demonstrated that such behavioral techniques as modeling, prompting, shaping, and positive reinforcement are effective in teaching semantic, morphologic, and syntactic skills to children with limited language skills (Guess, 1969; Guess et al., 1968; Hart & Risley, 1975; Lovaas, 1966; Risley & Wolf, 1967; Sailor et al., 1968; Schiefelbusch, 1973, 1978; Schiefelbusch & Lloyd, 1974). In subsequent years, treatment efficacy research, especially involving the behavioral methods of intervention, continued to provide an evidential basis of treating children with language disorders (see Goldstein, 2002; Hegde, 1998b; Warren & Rogers-Warren, 1985, for reviews of studies). As the linguistic-theoretical, developmental-empirical, and behavioral-clinical knowledge base on child language and disorders expanded, speech pathologists were the leading professionals to seize the opportunity to expand their scope of practice into child language disorders (Bloom & Lahey, 1978). Thus evolved a language pathology.

The scientific study of child language and the clinical assessment and treatment of child language disorders are now well established. Speech-language pathologists are recognized specialists in child language disorders. Nonetheless, there is no single definition of language disorders; this situation, however, is not unique to language disorders. Most disorders of communication have varied definitions. In spite of varied definitions, most clinicians can diagnose language disorders. We will first consider a few definitions and then offer a pragmatic and clinically oriented description of language disorders in children.

What Are Language Disorders in Children?

There are several reasons why there are multiple definitions of language disorders. First, language is a complex and varied phenomenon. Consequently, language disorders also are a complex and varied phenomenon. Differing orientation to this complex phenomenon can result in different definitions. Second, although linguistics is the primary discipline concerned with language, several other disciplines, including philosophy, psychology, and behavioral science also are concerned with language. Consequently, language has been conceptualized differently across these disciplines (Bloom, 1970; Bloom & Lahey, 1978; Bloomfield, 1933; Brown, 1973; Catania, 1972; Chomsky, 1957, 1965, 1980; Halliday, 1973, 1975; Hook, 1969; Julia, 1983; Lenneberg, 1967; McNeill, 1970; Salzinger & Salzinger, 1967; Skinner, 1957; Winokur, 1976). Different conceptualizations of language have led to different views of its disorders. Third, children who fail to learn skills through normal social interactions are a heterogeneous group. Some children who have language disorders also have such associated conditions as autism, developmental disability, neurological impairment, or hearing loss (see Chapters 12, 13, & 14). Many other children who have language disorders do not appear to have any other serious problems; limited language skills are their only significant problem, even though this characterization is coming under increasing scrutiny (Leonard, 1998; see Chapter 3 for details and contrasting views). Fourth, these diverse children experience varied problems in the acquisition, comprehension, and production of the different aspects of language. These and other reasons make it difficult to offer a concise definition that captures the essence as well as the variety of language disorders.

Concise definitions of language disorders are available. However, before they can be applied in diagnosing language disorders in children, such concise definitions need significant translations. Nonetheless, concise definitions are valuable in conceptualizing a clinical problem. Clinicians should understand that definitions of technical terms tend to be concise as well as abstract and, therefore, they need to be elaborated to turn them into practical tools for diagnosis and treatment.

Collective Definitions of Language Disorders

Some definitions of language disorders are collective in that committees of certain professional organizations have offered them. Definitions from the American Speech-Language-Hearing Association (ASHA) and the American Psychiatric Association (APA), are examples.

The ASHA Ad Hoc Committee on Service Delivery in the Schools (1993) states that:

> A language disorder is impaired comprehension and/or use of spoken, written, and/or other symbol systems. The disorder may involve (1) the form of language (phonology, morphology, syntax), (2) the content of language (semantics), and/or (3) the function of language in communication (pragmatics) in any combination. (p. IV-108)

ASHA's definition of language disorders is heavily influenced by Bloom and Lahey's (Bloom, 1970; Bloom & Lahey, 1978) conceptual model of the structural linguistic analysis of language. ASHA's definition implies that language has a structure or form called phonology, morphology, and syntax. The contents of this structure is meaning (semantics), and the use of language (pragmatics)[1] is distinguished from both the form and content. Although an interaction among these aspects is implied, a questionable division of form, content, and use of language is its weakness.

ASHA states that a language disorder exists when there is impaired comprehension and use of spoken language, written or symbol systems, or both. This broad-based definition implies that reading and writing skills along with expression and comprehension of other symbol systems are parts of language skills and that speech-language pathologists (SLPs) may be involved in their assessment and treatment. The definition of language disorders within such a broad scope makes sense as SLPs are now seen as specialists who have something unique to contribute to enriching preschool and school-age children's literacy (reading and writing) skills and in teaching nonverbal modes of communication. Therefore, the role of SLPs in remediating literacy problems and in teaching nonverbal systems of communication will be the topics of later chapters.

> Why is it incorrect to say that children have disorders of pragmatics?

The main limitation of ASHA's definition of language disorders is that it is based on a view of language that is too structural to be empirically meaningful. The idea that language has a structure that holds meaning in it—like a vessel that holds water—is not consistent with a clinically relevant empirical view of language as a set of skills produced under specific social conditions. Although the Bloom and Lahey's (1978) term, language *use*, implies production in social conditions, the overall form-content-use view divides language into artificial structural compartments.

The American Psychiatric Association's *Diagnostic and Statistical Manual of Mental Disorders*, 4th ed. (DSM-IV-TR; 2000), offers criteria for diagnosing various mental and behavioral disorders. Professionals in many disciplines use this manual as a standard reference. Several diagnostic categories defined and described in the DSM-IV-TR are relevant to diagnosing language disorders in children. Two diagnoses, expressive language disorder and mixed receptive–expressive language disorder, are found in children who exhibit only a language disorder and no other disorder or deficit. Expressive language disorder, according to the DSM-IV-TR, may be evident in both verbal and nonverbal forms of communication. It is characterized by limited language skills including a small range of words, slow acquisition of words and other aspects of language, limited sentence structures and variety, and limited and simple grammatical forms. Phonological disorders may be associated with language disorders in children. In addition, expressive language disorder may cause reading and writing problems in school-age children. Children with expressive language disorder may also have mild problems in language comprehension. If language comprehension problems are serious, then the child has a mixed receptive–expressive

> A problem in producing language is called an expressive disorder, whereas a problem in understanding spoken or written language is called a receptive disorder.

---

[1]The terms *phonology, morphology,* and *semantics* respectively refer to the study of sound systems, word structures, and meaning. Similarly, *pragmatics* is the study of social use of language. The terms do not refer to structures, forms, elements, components, or use of language.

box 2.1 **A Summary of Some DSM-IV Criteria for Diagnosis of Language Disorders (American Psychiatric Association, 2000)**

Characteristics of Expressive Language Disorder

- Standardized tests scores for expressive language development are significantly below scores for tests of nonverbal intelligence and receptive language skills.
- Symptoms may include a restricted vocabulary, production of errors in verb tense, problems with word recall, and difficulty producing complex sentences.
- The language difficulties negatively affect academic or occupational performance or social communication.
- The language difficulties are greater than the language problems typically associated with any other diagnosis (e.g., developmental disability, sensory impairment) that may also be present.

Characteristics of Mixed Receptive–Expressive Language Disorder

- Standardized test scores for measures of *both* expressive and receptive language are significantly below scores for tests of nonverbal intelligence.
- Symptoms include those listed for Expressive Language Disorder *and* demonstrated difficulty in comprehending spoken language, at the word or sentence level, or in regard to specific categories of words, such as prepositions.

language disorder. In addition to the expressive problems, these children have difficulty understanding spoken language. Note that according to the DSM-IV-TR, there is no purely receptive language disorder; a child's language disorder may be predominantly expressive or both expressive and receptive (see Box 2.1).

The DSM-IV-TR definition of language disorders depends on a child's performance on standardized tests of language development and those of nonverbal intelligence. The child's scores on standardized language tests must be substantially lower than his or her scores on standardized tests of nonverbal intelligence to diagnose a language disorder. To diagnose an expressive language disorder, the child's scores on expressive tests should be substantially lower than the same child's scores on receptive tests. To diagnose a mixed expressive–receptive language disorder, the child should obtain lower scores on both kinds of standardized tests.

DSM-IV-TR recognizes that language disorders may be associated with numerous clinical conditions that have, as a component, accompanying language difficulties, often severe. DSM-IV-TR criteria, therefore, will be referred to in future chapters that describe such conditions as developmental disability, pervasive developmental disorders, and attention-deficit disorders.

The main problem with the DSM-IV-TR definition of language disorders is that it relies heavily on standardized test performance. Besides test of language development, the definition requires the administration of nonverbal intelligence or other cognitive tests to children with language disorders. The practice of administering standardized tests to diagnose language (and speech) disorders is common in speech-language pathology. Nonetheless, it is fraught with too many empirical problems to be satisfactory as the sole or even the most important criterion.

> Does the DSM-IV-TR recognize a purely receptive language disorder?

Although this is not the place to critically evaluate standardized tests of language development, a few major problems can be summarized as a matter of caution in using them (Laing & Kamhi, 2003). Standardized tests of language development inadequately sample children on a national basis. They are mostly based on local samples, but clinicians inappropriately use them nationally. Even if they are standardized on national samples, the profile of test scores may be irrelevant to individual clients of different ethnocultural backgrounds. But an even more troublesome aspect of standardized tests—something rarely mentioned—is that they sample the skills inadequately. A language test may give a child one opportunity, or at best two to three opportunities, to produce a skill. Judgments based on such inadequate sampling of skills may be invalid. For instance, a child who did not produce the plural *s* on two words presented (e.g., *hats* and *books*) may still produce the plural morpheme at home in different word contexts. Standardized tests rarely sample complex verbal behavior (language skills) in naturalistic social interactions. Finally, the age-based norms that language-development tests produce are based on average performance of large groups that may bear little or no relevance to individual children clinicians evaluate and treat.

Yet another problem with the DSM-IV-TR definition of language disorders is that it requires a comparison of mental age (as determined by nonverbal tests of intelligence) with the child's language skills. The requirement that a child's language performance must be substantially lower than measured nonverbal intelligence to diagnose a language disorder in children is problematic. What if both language skills and nonverbal intelligence scores are low and roughly equal? One would then not diagnose a language disorder and offer no treatment. As Dale and Cole (1991) point out, such a stance would be inappropriate because matched language and nonverbal skills do not mean there is no problem. Furthermore, SLPs may not have the training to administer tests of nonverbal intelligence and interpret the scores. The concept of mental age as a criterion to evaluate language performance is questionable. For the SLP, a direct method of evaluating language skills without reference to other variables they cannot directly measure will be most useful.

A Behavioral Definition of Language Disorders

All definitions of language disorders refer back to typical or normal skills that are impaired. In linguistic approaches, normal skills are acceptable production of language structures. To define language disorders, the linguistic approaches specify impairment in production of those structures. Similarly, a behavioral view allows a definition of language disorders that would emphasize the impairment in what it considers the typical skill (verbal behavior). As we noted in Chapter 1, language skills are social behaviors that have an effect on the immediate listener or listeners, and in some cases, on the more remote larger segments of one or more social communities (as in the case of printed or broadcast verbal behavior). Therefore, we define **language disorders** as a lack of acceptable or effective social repertoire to affect the behaviors of other persons in social, educational, and occupational milieu, or to be affected by the verbal behaviors of other persons. However, some children's difficulty may be more pronounced in verbally affecting others, whereas other children's difficulty may be limited effects they experience from verbal exchanges. In more familiar terms, this means that a child may have a predominantly expressive language disorder (producing limited effects on others) or a predominantly receptive disorder (not experiencing the full range of intended effects of communication). Still other children may have both the kinds of problems (receptive as well as expressive disorder).

The definition hinges on the concept that language is a social skill that, when exhibited, has an effect on the listener. Similarly, persons with adequate language skills are affected by language produced around them. For instance, a child's production, "Can I have a glass of milk, Mommy?" has a typical effect on the mother; she hands a glass of milk to the child. If the message is unclear because the critical words are missing, then it may not have the expected effect on the mother. Similarly, when the mother asks, "What did you learn in school today?" the child needs to have a certain verbal skill to be affected as expected; in this case, a correct response demonstrates an expected effect of the mother's question. In children with language disorders, verbal repertoire is either lacking or ineffective. When it is lacking, the person cannot produce effects through verbal means and cannot experience effects others try to produce by the same means. When the repertoire is inadequate, the person will produce partial, ambiguous, or wrong effects on others and will experience similarly unacceptable effects from others. The basic idea is that verbal behavior (language as produced in speaking, reading, writing, or manual language systems such as American Sign Language) refers to social actions that produce effects on others and a readiness to be affected by other people's social actions. The expressive language of a person affects the actions of others and receptive language prepares the person to be affected by language others express. Therefore, the definition includes the traditional expressive and receptive language disorders, but states them in terms of what children do verbally to change people around them and how the children are changed by the verbal actions of others. The definition makes an explicit reference to verbal repertoire in academic milieu. Therefore, the behavioral definition of language disorders includes impaired reading and writing skills. In fact, as we noted in Chapter 1, verbal repertoire includes thinking as well. Therefore, impaired language skills, especially abstract language skills, may restrict a child's thinking to concrete experiences.

> It is true that any disorder of communication may limit the effects of communication on others. In this case, the reduced effectiveness is due to limited language skills (as against impaired speech or voice).

The behavioral and the linguistic definitions of language disorders will have to be ultimately translated to specific, observable, and teachable skills that are intact versus those that are lacking or deficient. Nonetheless, the differences are notable. The linguistic definition is structural and rational. It is based on theoretical compartments of language (form, content, use). The linguistic definitions are based on the view that language is a mental system. The behavioral definition of language disorders is empirical and functional. It emphasizes the actions of children as speakers and listeners. The behavioral definition is based on the view that mental systems are inferred from actions and that it is more effective to study the actions. A definition that directs the clinicians' attention to what the child does is immensely more practical than those that redirect their attention to presumed mental processes that need clinical translations.

Definitions and Diagnostic Guidelines

A limitation of all definitions of language disorders, including those stated so far, is that they are too abstract to be useful in formulating diagnostic guidelines or criteria. Within

> The term **empirical** means the statements are based on objective, observable, and measurable events or experiences.

its own theoretical framework, each definition may be valid in that it captures the essence of language disorders. Nonetheless, definitions do not automatically generate clinically useful diagnostic criteria. The need for such criteria will invariably lead to broader descriptions of observable skills and some forced compromises because of professional practice constraints.

In the United States, a majority of children's language disorders are diagnosed in public schools. Because of the legal restrictions and mandates that affect special education in the United States, language disorders (as well as other communication disorders) are diagnosed on the basis of guidelines the local school districts or state departments of education propose. Such guidelines may not strictly adhere to a scientific definition of a disorder. Many practical and funding exigencies affect the guidelines. Therefore, such terms as *deficiency, inadequacy, ineffectiveness, the degree of deviance from the normal, severity, significant impairment,* and so forth need to be operationally defined to assist in clinical decision making. The most basic question the public school clinicians face is this: To what extent should the problem be exhibited before services are mandated for a given child? The more severe the disorder is required to be before the services are mandated, the more economical the program would be for the state—this factor alone may shape many public school guidelines. This factor also requires the use of standardized tests in clinical practice in schools.

It is generally believed that standardized tests help diagnose a language (or speech) disorder in children. A closer examination shows that this is not the case, at least not in practice. Assuming the results are valid, a standardized test may show that the child's language skills are *different* from other children of the same age; the extent of this difference may be stated in terms of standard deviation from the mean performance. Compared to children of typical repertoire, children may be shown to be more or less different—giving rise to the concept of severity of a disorder. In practice, this determination alone does not suggest a language disorder that requires services; identifying a deviation that does not require services serves little social purpose. Therefore, state and local school district guidelines offer help. Depending on the adopted guidelines, for example, clinicians may qualify or disqualify a child for treatment. From a parent's standpoint, it is important to know whether their child has a disorder or not, but it is even more important to know whether the child qualifies for services or not. School clinicians may qualify a child for services only if that child's skill deviated by more than one or two standard deviations from the mean performance as shown in the test manual. Standardized tests, therefore, are used mostly to determine whether the services will be offered or not. Children who are barely above an adopted service criterion may still have a disorder and yet be denied services. From a definitional or clinical standpoint, denial of service does not mean an absence of a disorder. Therefore, the decision to offer no services to certain children who may have a disorder is a matter of institutional policy, not of science or clinical judgment.

A troublesome assumption inherent to the view that a certain degree of deviation from the norm is required to offer services is that those who deviate less will overcome their deficiencies without professional help. There is no strong empirical support to sustain this assumption; in fact, the available evidence suggests that without intervention, language disorders and their negative effects on academic performance tend to persist in children (Beitchman et al., 1996; Beitchman, Wilson, Brownlie, Walters, & Lancee, 1996; Johnson et al., 1999; Rescorla, 2002). Children who lack skills to a lesser extent may still need treat-

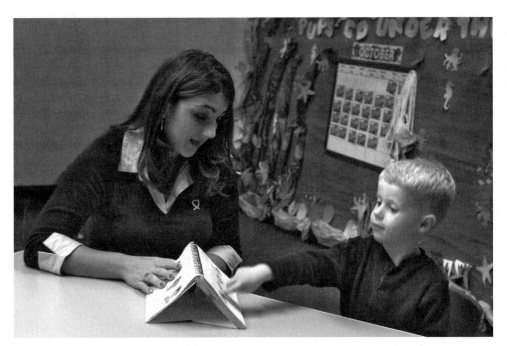

photo 2.1
Administration of standardized testing will determine whether or not the child will receive speech and language services in the public schools, but will not necessarily result in the accurate diagnosis of a language disorder.

ment. They may need less intensive and short-term treatments than those whose skill deficiencies are more serious. Children who sustain a communication handicap only for a year or two may still benefit from treatment that more quickly remediates the deficiency and thus better prepares them for academic success and social enjoyment.

Organizations, including public school districts, have sought to meet the challenge of providing services with limited funding. Of necessity, they have had to develop criteria that are based more on practical exigencies than on scientific evidence of a disorder. In some schools, many children with language disorders may fail to receive needed services because of the too high criteria adopted to qualify them for services, a situation that is in violation of the Individuals with Disabilities Education Act (IDEA) Amendments of 1997, reauthorized and revised as the Individuals with Disabilities Education Improvement Act of 2004. In recognition of this problem, the National Joint Committee for the Communication Needs of Persons with Severe Disabilities (2003) has provided a listing of arbitrary criteria that should not be used to determine eligibility for speech-language services, because they are ethically unacceptable and legally questionable. Box 2.2 lists those criteria, called a priori criteria, because they are arbitrarily applied before or without assessment.

How to deliver mandated services with limited funding is a nationwide dilemma that school administrators face. Facing their obligation to make use of their resources the best way they can, they have to rely on criteria that fit their resources—not necessarily those that fit the needs of children. It is a problem to which no immediate solution is expected. However, school SLPs are bound by a Code of Ethics that requires them to "hold paramount the welfare of persons they serve professionally" (ASHA, 2003a, p. 13). The first ethical and professional responsibility clinicians have, then, is not to the organizations they

box 2.2   **Science versus Administrative Policy—The Dilemma of the School SLP**

In an effort to provide mandated services within severe funding constraints, school districts often adapt a priori criteria to determine eligibility for speech-language services. Criteria are a priori if they are arbitrarily applied either before assessment or in the absence of assessment and are not supported by scientific evidence. Speech-language pathologists, however, are bound by ethical and legal concerns to diagnose and treat language disorders based on their independent assessment of each client's communicative skills and needs. The National Joint Committee for the Communication Needs of Persons with Severe Disabilities (2003) has set forth a list of a priori criteria that should *not* be used in determining eligibility for speech-language services. The list reflects a response to many common practices employed by school districts strapped for adequate funding for mandated services.

A Priori Criteria That Should NOT Be Used to Determine Eligibility for Speech-Language Services

- *Discrepancies between cognitive and communication functioning.* SLPs assessing children for language disorders should not require a demonstrated gap between verbal ability and nonverbal intelligence.
- *Chronological age.* Children should not be arbitrarily dismissed from services when the child achieves a particular age or grade level (e.g., many children with language disorders are summarily dismissed from services when they transition from elementary to secondary grade levels).
- *Diagnosis.* Children should not be excluded from eligibility solely because they have a particular diagnosis (e.g., children with a profound level of

developmental disability may be regarded as "uneducable" and arbitrarily excluded from speech-language services on the basis of the diagnosis alone).
- *Absence of cognitive or other skills purported to be prerequisites.* SLPs should not exclude children with language disorders because they do not have "prerequisite skills" thought to be necessary for them to benefit from therapy (e.g., some school SLPs may not qualify children with language disorders because they "cannot attend to task," without considering the possibility of teaching the children to pay attention).
- *Failure to benefit from previous communication services and supports.* Children should not be excluded from service because past therapy has appeared to be of no benefit; this does not necessarily mean they cannot benefit from a new approach or from a longer period of intervention.
- *Restrictive interpretations of educational, vocational, and/or medical necessity.* SLPs should not allow restrictive policies written by organizations they work for to override their own, independent, professional judgment.
- *Lack of appropriately trained personnel.* SLPs should not refuse to qualify children solely because caseloads are high and quality personnel hard to locate.
- *Lack of adequate funds or other resources.* SLPs should not refuse to qualify children solely because adequate funding for services is not available and resources are scarce.

A tall order, but one the SLP is ethically and legally obligated to meet.

work for, but to the children they serve. Because SLPs are valued and respected professional people, they can be effective advocates for diagnosis and delivery of services to all children who need them. In their efforts to offer needed services to all children, clinicians may consider developing strong advocacy positions based on the ASHA Code of Ethics and the recommendations of the National Joint Committee for the Communication Needs of Persons with Severe Disabilities. Working closely with parental advocacy groups within the school district also might help secure needed resources to serve children with language disorders.

A Description of Language Disorders

All definitions of language disorders—whether they are linguistic, behavioral, or some other—are likely to generate some debate among clinicians. A description of skills that may be impaired in children with language disorders is likely to be less controversial and more practical than definitions. Such descriptions are both essential and eminently useful in assessing children with language disorders. A description of language disorders may be more useful to clinicians of divergent views because the descriptions themselves are theoretically neutral and free from varied (hence, controversial) diagnostic criteria. Describing the language disorders in children they serve, clinicians may then diagnose and treat those disorders according to the guidelines accepted in their professional setting.

The heterogeneous group of children who have language disorders exhibit a set of commonly occurring deficiencies:

- *Limited amount of language.* Children with language problems almost always show a deficiency in the quantity of language learned, comprehended, and produced. These children have a sparse verbal repertoire. Limited early vocalizations, limited vocabulary, and slow learning of new words are often the first signs of a problem with learning language that is adequate to meet social and academic demands. Their descriptions of events and personal experiences will be poor, inadequate, or sparse. Children with language disorders are especially likely to have difficulty learning and producing language that refers to abstract events. Their expressions may be more often limited to the present and the concrete.

- *Deficient grammar.* Children with language disorders typically have difficulty in learning, comprehending, and producing language with adequate grammatic elements. With limited syntax, their sentences may be shorter, simpler, and often devoid of variety. The language these children produce is likely to omit various grammatic morphemes (e.g., the plural s, the possessive s, the present progressive *ing*, articles, pronouns, prepositions, and so forth). The syntactic or morphologic deficiencies may be gross or subtle, depending on the severity of the disorder.

- *Inadequate or inappropriate social communication.* Often described as pragmatic language problems, children with language disorders may produce their limited skills inadequately or inappropriately. Their social communication may not be appropriate to the time, place, person, and topic of conversation. These children may not initiate conversation, may fail to maintain the topic once initiated, may interrupt the speaker, or avoid eye contact during social interactions. The children may fail to request objects and help, may not ask questions when they do not understand

Clinician: Hi Tom, how are you today?
Tom: [no response]
Clinician: What do you see in this picture? [showing a picture of many animals]
Tom: Kitty.
Clinician: What else?
Tom: [shrugs his shoulders]
Clinician: Tell me about this one.
Tom: Doggy sleeping.
Clinician: Sleeping on what?
Tom: Bed.
Note lack of elaboration and limited amount of language Tom produced.

Clinician: Matt, what are these?
Matt: Two cup.
Clinician: What do you see here?
Matt: Boy running.
Clinician: Whose bag is this? This lady's or that man's?
Matt: Lady.
Clinician: Where is the crayon?
Matt: Box.
Clinician: Say the crayon is in the box
Tom: In box.
Note the missing grammatic morphemes and short utterances.

Clinician: Good Morning, John!
John: Hi.
Clinician: I was going to tell you that today we are going to . . .
John: Miss Jenny, you know what?
Clinician: Yes, tell me.
John: See, new shoes.
Clinician: When did you buy them?
John: Yesterday.
Clinician: Who took you to the store?
John: I want to play with the Legos today.
Note the failure to greet the clinician, interruptions, and failure to maintain the topic of conversation the clinician introduced.

spoken language, may fail to obey simple commands because of lack of understanding, and may not understand how to say things differently if they are not understood.

- *Deficient nonverbal communication skills.* Children with language disorders may exhibit limited nonverbal communication skills. Their production of gestures and other nonverbal means of communication may be deficient. Gestures that facilitate understanding of messages may not supplement their oral communication attempts. The children may fail to understand gestures and signs others use during communication. Their learning of nonverbal skills may be delayed or impaired.
- *Deficient literacy skills.* In addition to oral and gestural communication deficits, children with language impairment may experience reading and writing difficulties. Abstract use of language may be impaired as well. The children may not understand idioms, proverbs, and common sayings or may interpret them literally instead of figuratively.

1. Mother: Joe, you look tired. Why don't you hit the sack?
Joe: I don't want to hit it!

2. Mother: It is raining cats and dogs.
Joe: [looking puzzled] No, it is just raining, Mom!

Note Joe's literal interpretation of idiomatic expressions.

This brief description of the basic problems of children with language disorders is not specific to any etiology. The description is a summary of certain common difficulties children with language disorders may have. Depending on associated clinical conditions, children with language disorders also may have sensory deficiencies (e.g., hearing loss), behavioral problems (attention deficit), and idiosyncratic language features (e.g., children with autism). Language of children with such special clinical conditions are described in later chapters included in Part III of this book.

Language Disorders by Any Other Name

We prefer to use the term *language disorder* to describe a social communication deficit present in children, but there are other names for it. Although a majority of experts use that term, clinicians will come across a variety of other terms. Some are of historical significance and others may be used as synonyms for language disorders in the current literature. For instance, children's limited language skills may be referred to as childhood or congenital aphasia, dysphasia, language deviance, language impairment, language delay, or language disorder. To complicate the matter, professionals disagree not only over the definitions of these terms, but also over their appropriateness or validity.

Childhood or Congenital Aphasia or Dysphasia

Some early researchers on language disorders believed that children who have trouble learning verbal skills may be neurologically impaired (Benton, 1964; Eisenson, 1972). Researchers and clinicians saw similarities between children's language disorders and aphasia, a language disorder in adults which results from specific, localized lesion of the brain, the same sort of lesion caused by a cerebral vascular accident (stroke). Therefore, in the past, the term *childhood aphasia* was used to describe language disorders in children. There is

Why are the terms *childhood aphasia* or *dysphasia* inappropriate?

no evidence, however, that supports the view that language disorders in all children are due to neurological problems, although when such problems do exist, language disorders tend to accompany them. Many children who have language disorders do not exhibit neurological or behavioral symptoms of focal brain injury. Although subtle neurological impairments cannot be ruled out and future neurological research may prove to be more productive, there is currently no justification to use the term *childhood aphasia* to describe the language learning problems of most children.

The term *dysphasia* also carries with it the implication that children with language disorders have neurological deficits. **Dysphasia** is a language disorder with a neurological basis. This term is currently not used for the same reason that childhood aphasia is not. In addition, the term *dysphasia* was used long before the SLP's scope of practice included the assessment and treatment of **dysphagia,** defined as swallowing disorders. The two terms, *dysphagia* and *dysphasia*, though having very different meanings, are so similar as to cause confusion if they were both used. This is another reason to abandon the term *dysphasia*.

> Is dysphagia a language disorder?

Language Deviance

Some experts in the past had wondered whether in acquiring language, some children follow a deviant pattern or follow the normal patterns but progress more slowly. Those who thought that language disorders are a result of some children following unusual or abnormal patterns were more likely to use the term *language deviance*. The term implies that a child with language difficulties is not just slow to acquire language, but exhibits a pattern of language not found in children who typically learn their language.

> Do children with language disorders with no other problems exhibit a deviant pattern of language acquisition?

This is certainly true of some diagnostic categories. Children with autism, for example, may show patterns of language that are not found in other children, including those who are learning language normally or those who exhibit language disorders without any other complicating conditions. Nonetheless, the evidence is now overwhelming that many children who have language disorders follow the normal pattern of development, but the acquisition is slower and may plateau at a lower level than normal. Therefore, the term *language deviance* does not describe the language problems of most children with language disorders, and, therefore, is not currently used.

Language Impairment

A disorder may or may not have a consequence that affects normal functioning in a person. An impairment is "any disorder in structure or function resulting from anatomic, physiologic, or psychologic abnormalities that interfere with normal activities" (Anderson et al., 2002). Certainly, deficiencies in language skills interfere with normal social, academic, and occupational activities. As noted previously, it is through verbal behaviors that children and adults influence the behaviors of people in their immediate as well as remote environment. Children and adults with deficient verbal skills cannot affect others as fully, clearly, or forcefully as those with good verbal skills. A child who cannot make requests or cannot read is a case in point. The child has a social and academic impairment.

The use of the term *language impairment* is widespread and generally acceptable, although some may object to its use because of its negative connotations. It is difficult to strip negative connotations from any diagnostic term (a diagnosis of genius may be an exception!) as they do suggest some problem or limitation. In this book, we will use the terms *language disorder* and *language impairment* interchangeably. It may be noted, however, that the term *language impairment* is routinely used to describe language disorder not associated with any other clinical conditions. See Chapter 3 for a description of this condition, called specific language impairment.

> Do *language disorders* and *language impairment* mean the same?

Language Delay

A delay is an eventual, if deferred, arrival at a destination, not an absence of something or someone. Many early researchers and clinicians thought that a child who is slow to learn language will soon catch up with other children of comparable age. Therefore, the term *language delay* seemed to describe children who are "slow to talk." At their sluggish pace, slow talkers were expected to acquire at least average language skills as they advanced through school.

Whether language problems of children simply suggest a "delay" has treatment implications. Perhaps slower learning up to a point is acceptable to society, thus eliminating the need for language treatment in some children. Therefore, unlike other terminological distinctions, this delay versus disorder dichotomy has prompted much empirical research.

Although many children who exhibit mild and early language delay eventually acquire normal language skills, research has shown that some residual deficits may be evident in later childhood. Beitchman et al. (1996) found that children identified at age 5 as having low overall language skills continued to perform poorly on linguistic, cognitive, and academic measures when retested at the age of 12 years, 5 months. In a further study, Beitchman et al. (1996) found that children who had low overall language skills at age 5 were more likely to develop behavioral difficulties, including aggressive and hyperactive symptoms by age 12 years, 5 months.

Stothard et al. (1998) conducted a longitudinal follow-up of 71 adolescents who had language delay at the age of 4 years. At the age of 5, these children had been divided into two groups—those whose language delays had resolved by then and those whose language delay still persisted. The authors found that children with resolved early language problems did not differ at the ages of 15–17 years when compared to an age-matched normal-language control group on measures of vocabulary and language comprehension, but did significantly less well on tests for literacy skills. Furthermore, the children who still had language difficulties at age 5 continued to have significant deficits in all aspects of spoken and written language, and they continued to fall further behind their peer group in vocabulary growth.

Another longitudinal study by Johnson et al. (1999) also found that a group of students identified at age 5 as speech or language impaired, or both, continued to exhibit communication difficulties when compared to control groups at ages 12 and 19. Stability in language performance over time was demonstrated, with better long-term outcomes for those who had been diagnosed with speech (articulation) disorders compared to those who had been diagnosed with language disorders. Also, children who had been diagnosed with specific language impairment performed better as a group than did children whose language disorders were associated with sensory, structural, neurological, or cognitive deficits.

Rescorla (2002) examined 34 children described as "late talkers" as toddlers, comparing them at the age of 6–9 years to a matched group of 25 typically developing children. Although the late talkers performed in the average range on most language tasks by age 5, they had significantly lower scores through age 9 and were slightly less skilled in reading.

The research on residual deficits raises some important issues. First, an assessment of persistent language deficiencies in older children (e.g., adolescents) is difficult. Measures of vocabulary, language samples, and standardized tests of morphologic and syntactic skills may grossly underestimate complex and abstract language skills that are necessary to perform well in high school and beyond. Therefore, it is likely that residual deficits in older children are greater than reported so far. Second, it is possible that more effective and intensive treatment than currently offered early in life will eliminate most if not all residual effects that seem to linger in some children. Third, children with severe language disorders who are also diagnosed to have complicating clinician conditions (e.g., developmental disability, neurological impairment, and autism spectrum disorders) may continue to exhibit language deficiencies in spite of experiencing significant improvement with intensive and effective treatment. In any case, the assumption that language disorders will resolve themselves in such a brief duration as to cause no negative social and academic consequences for a child is untenable. Early intervention and parent training are essential in the case of all children with language disorders.

> What is the best policy when a 4-year-old child is diagnosed with a language disorder: (1) assume the child will catch up with other children eventually or (2) offer treatment and parent education?

Because of its inherent implication, use of the term *language delay* is avoided in favor of *language disorders*. The term is particularly inappropriate when a child's language disorder is associated with such other clinical conditions as developmental disability, autism, or neurological deficits. Families struggling to cope with such diagnoses are ill-served by the use of terms that may foster false hope and prevent them from seeking much needed professional help.

Prevalence and Incidence of Language Disorders

The number of individuals who are diagnosed with a particular disorder at a given time is its **prevalence.** The **incidence,** on the other hand, is the rate at which a disorder appears in the normal population over a period of time, typically one year. Prevalence is a current state of a disease; incidence is a rate of future occurrences of that disease.

The number of children who are communicating normally but who develop a language disorder during the course of an observational period is the incidence of that disorder (American Speech-Language-Hearing Association, 1991; Portney & Watkins, 2000; Rothman & Greenland, 1998). In this case, newborns would have to be followed for a few years to note the number of children who would be diagnosed with language disorders. Observing normal or healthy children (or adults) for an extended period of time to note the number of individuals who show a disease or a disorder is called the **longitudinal method** of research. The method is expensive and time consuming. Therefore, few such studies have been conducted.

Those who measure prevalence always start with those who already have the clinical condition of interest. In establishing prevalence, one asks a simple question: how many individuals currently have a disorder or disease? For instance, one might ask, how many children in school district X have a language disorder? To answer this and similar questions, the researchers sample clinical records across schools and other facilities (Leonard, 1998; Portney & Watkins, 2000; Rothman & Greenland, 1998). The researchers count the number of children with a language disorder. In essence, a simple head count of children in the country, state, or a region who are diagnosed with a language disorder—if that is feasible—will give prevalence data. As such, researchers use the **cross-sectional** method of one-time observation of a section of society to establish the prevalence of a disorder.

For most childhood language disorders, measures of prevalence are more relevant than measures of incidence. Most children who are diagnosed with a language disorder have it from the beginnings of social communication. Unlike in adults who have aphasia, language disorders in children are not typically preceded by a period of competent language skills. Exceptions exist, however.

How are the terms *prevalence* and *incidence* different?

Children who sustain brain injury at various stages of childhood or acquire a significant hearing loss may have a preceding and varying period of normal language skills. But in the majority of children (including those with autism, congenital hearing loss, and certain genetic syndromes), language disorders are evident from the earliest period of social communication. Therefore, prevalence is the measure to seek.

Although the method of head count is simple, counting children with language disorders in a school district, a state, or a country is progressively more complicated. The most common and practical method of counting children with language disorders is to gather statistics from various organizations (e.g., school districts), agencies (state and local child services), and clinical facilities (private clinics, hospital outpatient speech and hearing clinics).

Several factors compromise the reliability and validity of statistics gathered to establish prevalence data. First, the number of children with language disorders varies across ages. Some younger children who have had successful intervention for their mild language disorder may be free from it when they get older. Second, some children who have language disorders may be counted as those with learning disorders, emotional disturbance, autism, developmental disability, cerebral palsy, and hearing loss, without recognizing their inevitable language disorder. Third, different agencies that report statistics on children with language disorders use varied criteria for diagnosis and service delivery. Generally, children with mild language disorders are more likely to be missed than those with severe language disorders. Fourth, language disorders vary across socioeconomic groups. A skewed sampling of upper socioeconomic levels may underestimate the prevalence of the disorder in poorer sections of a society. For these reasons, it is difficult to state the number of children who have language disorders in any given year.

A few available studies report that 12 to 13 percent of children exhibit language disorders. For instance, Beitchman et al. (1986) found that among a sample of 1,655 five-year-old children in the Ottawa-Carleton region of Canada, 12.6 percent had a language disorder. The authors also found that 4.56 percent of those who had language disorders also had speech disorders. In a U.S. sample of 1,502 kindergarten children, Tomblin, Records, and Zhang (1996) found language disorders in 13.58 percent.

Reported prevalence rates of language disorders in children who have no other complicating clinical conditions are relatively consistent. A language disorder in a child who is otherwise normal is called specific language impairment (SLI), described in detail in Chapter 3. Several studies suggest a prevalence rate of 7 to 8 percent of SLI in kindergarten. For example, Tomblin et al. (1997) reported a 7.4 percent prevalence rate of SLI based on a screening sample of 7,218 monolingual English-speaking kindergarten children. The authors also reported a prevalence rate of 8 percent for boys and 6 percent for girls, somewhat higher than expected for girls. Ruben (2000) also reported an SLI prevalence of 7.5 percent for kindergarten children. Furthermore, a study by the National Institutes of Health indicated a prevalence rate of 7.6 percent among 5-year-old children (Ervin, 2001).

The overall prevalence of language disorders in children is much higher than either 7 to 8 percent reported for SLI or 12 to 13 percent reported for unselected children. None of these figures include children who have language disorders associated with diminished hearing (deaf or hard of hearing), developmental disability, autism, cerebral palsy, traumatic brain injury, and so forth. Prevalence figures for those conditions will be discussed in subsequent chapters.

Varieties of Language Disorders

Children who exhibit language disorders are a varied group. Consequently, the total clinical picture varies across children. This variation is due not only to individual differences, but also to associated clinical conditions. These variations may be classified into two broad categories: specific language impairment and language disorders associated with other clinical conditions.

Specific language impairment, as noted earlier, is not associated with another clinical diagnosis. In some children, a language impairment is their main or primary problem, although they may have additional subtle difficulties in certain sensory or intellectual functions (Leonard, 1998; also, see Chapter 3 for details).

The second category of language disorders is broad and includes diverse impairments in addition to language problems. Therefore, this category may be called language disorders with associated clinical conditions. Children who have language disorders of this second category have another primary or secondary diagnosis. In essence, children in this category are diagnosed with two clinical conditions: a language disorder and another sensory, behavioral, neurological, or intellectual impairment. For instance, an oral language disorder in some children is associated with reduced hearing acuity. In other children, a language disorder may be associated with autism, neurological impairment, or developmental disability. It should be noted however, that the dual diagnosis in these children is mostly a matter of practical and professional concerns. Speech-language pathologists tend to assess and treat language disorders in children who have a dual diagnosis while recognizing that the children have other problems. The SLPs also recognize that the language disorders are a part of the larger clinical picture which includes problems that other professionals assess and treat. Language disorders associated with another primary diagnosis are described in the third part of this book.

Historically, language disorders have been classified either etiologically or descriptively. What we have called language disorders with associated clinical conditions is traditionally described as a classification based on etiology. An **etiological classification** of disorders or diseases is based on their causes. As such, language disorders can be classified according to the presumed or demonstrated causes of the disorder. Etiologic classification is based on the medical model in which, ideally, the most effective treatment is possible when the cause or causes of a disorder are known. When known, causes, not the symptoms, are treated. For example, when a patient complains of stomach pain, the cause may be an ulcer; pain is the symptom. The effective and lasting treatment is directed against the ulcer, although the pain may be temporarily managed. When the causes of a disease are unknown, the treatment is symptomatic, not a cure; only the symptoms, not the underlying disease, are treated. Simply reducing the fever with aspirin while the disease goes untreated in a patient is an example of symptomatic treatment.

> **Etiology** is the study of causes of disorders and diseases.

As applied to language disorders, the etiologic classification implies that in some children, developmental disability, autism, deafness, and neurological deficits *cause* their oral language impairment. The argument is that if the children did not have autism, developmental disability, and so forth, they would not have had a language disorder. Therefore, developmental disability or autism is the cause of language disorders. Unfortunately, this argument, though apparently valid, has some serious limitations.

Scientifically, causes and effects are separate; they should not be simultaneous or coexisting from the beginning. In the case of several children with language disorder, the etiological classification fails to fulfill this basic tenet: demonstrated causes and their effects (language disorders), both separated in time. Consider these questions: Is developmental disability or autism the cause of the language disorder in a child? Maybe, but more likely not. How does the clinician know that a child has developmental disability or autism? The clinician knows partly because the child's language is limited or shows special characteristics. Language disorders are a part of these clinical conditions; the condition is diagnosed partly because of the child's limited or unusual language behaviors. A certain pattern of language disorder, for example, distinguishes children with autism from other children with language disorders. If language disorders are a part of the clinical condition (autism or developmental disability), then that condition cannot be the cause of the disorders.

> Is autism the cause of language disorders or a coexisting condition?

In other cases, the etiologic classification makes limited, but better sense. For example, hearing loss and language disorders may be technically separated. Hearing loss in children may become apparent before their language disorder does. Hearing loss may be measured independent of language skills. Similarly, traumatic brain injury (TBI) may be measured independent of language skills. In some cases, evidence of normal language skills may have been established before the brain injury, and the impairment of language skills may be measured after the injury. In such cases, the etiologic model may have limited sense.

It should be noted, though, that in each case where a particular clinical condition is thought to be the cause of the language disorder, that cause is never experimentally demonstrated. The presumed cause (e.g., developmental disability) and the language disorder are correlated conditions. Both are likely to have other, more important causes. These causes may include an abnormal gene, a genetic predisposition, and certain unfavorable environmental events (e.g., limited stimulation or social interaction with the child).

A **descriptive classification** of language disorders avoids explicit assumptions of causation. Those who advocate a descriptive classification believe that it is difficult to specify causes of language disorders, and, therefore, the main clinical task is to describe the language characteristics of children who have problems. A comprehensive description of semantic, grammatical, and pragmatic deficiencies of children with language disorders is considered clinically sufficient to assess and treat them.

A descriptive classification should not imply that it is unimportant to investigate or understand causes of language disorders. It is important to understand why some children have language disorders. If the causes are unknown, we still can treat language disorders. If causes are known, the effects may be prevented, however. What is critical in this debate is that it is not useful to presume causes or assign causes to correlated (coexisting) conditions whose causes remain uninvestigated.

The etiological and descriptive classifications are not mutually exclusive. If they are treated as such, neither category is useful to an understanding of language disorders in children. We need a good understanding of the causes as well as effects. Until valid causes are revealed, the clinicians and researchers will have to refrain from undue speculation.

While it may not be helpful to think of developmental disability, autism, or TBI as the causes of language disorders in a given child, it is helpful to know that the child has one of these associated clinical conditions. Such knowledge is essential for both assessment and treatment planning. Each clinical condition poses some special challenges for the clinician in assessment and treatment. A clinician who has only a superficial knowledge of autism, developmental disability, and other clinical conditions will be unprepared for a comprehensive assessment and treatment of the child.

Although the basic treatment technique will remain the same or substantially similar, the clinician will approach the treatment of a child's language disorder differently if the child is also autistic, developmentally disabled, brain injured, or hard of hearing or deaf. For example, in planning and implementing treatment, the clinician should be prepared to handle the attention deficits of children with TBI, unusual and challenging behavior problems of children with autism, limited intellectual potential of those with developmental disability, amplification needs of children with hearing loss, and so forth. Besides teaching language skills, the clinician should expect to reduce some undesirable behaviors, establish cooperative behaviors, increase attending behaviors, use amplifying instrumentation, and so forth, depending on the clinical condition of the child. No similar special concerns may exist for children who have specific language impairment.

For the reasons stated so far, an associated condition-oriented description of language disorders, adopted in this text, is necessary for clinicians to analyze the overall pattern of language and related deficits that affect treatment planning and management. This orientation acknowledges the limitations of the etiological approach based on current knowledge, recognizes the importance of finding causes of language disorders, and emphasizes the assessment and treatment relevance of the clinical conditions that may coexist with language disorders.

Risk Factors for Language Disorders

Even if specific causes remain uncertain, many factors are known to be associated with language disorders. We have noted in the previous sections that language disorders are a part of such clinical conditions as developmental disability and hearing loss. Many other factors also are associated with language disorders later in the life of children. Relevant factors that are present in persons from before the time of a clinical diagnosis are known as **risk factors.** Although there is no assurance that they caused the disorder, there definitely is an association between the presence of certain factors and later manifestation of specific disorders. In essence, such factors are correlated with the disorder and the disorder can be predicted in children who earlier exhibit those factors. In general, several prenatal, perinatal, neonatal, or environmental factors are associated with language disorders and may be thought of as contributing factors, if not the causes.

Prenatal Risk Factors

Prenatal conditions involve factors that may affect the developing fetus prior to birth, including conditions that may result in premature birth. Various maternal factors can affect the prenatal development of the human fetus. Any variable that affects the normal development of the fetus may have an adverse effect on language acquisition.

Maternal use of common teratogenic (toxic) substances such as alcohol, nicotine, illicit drugs, and caffeine can seriously interfere with the development of an embryo. Maternal drug use can produce drug-addicted babies who exhibit symptoms associated with withdrawal shortly after birth. These symptoms can include tremors, irritability, high-pitched crying, seizures, and poor feeding (American Academy of Pediatrics Committee on Drugs, 1998). Maternal infections, such as kidney or bladder infections, often result in serious fetal anomalies. The fetus can also be seriously affected by the mother's contraction of viral diseases. TORCH is an abbreviation for a group of viruses—*t*oxoplasmosis, *o*ther infections, *r*ubella virus, *c*ytomegalovirus, and *h*erpes simplex viruses—all of which are particularly harmful to the developing fetus. Any one agent or more contracted by the mother can result in the infection of the fetus or newborn, resulting in TORCH syndrome. Effects can include abortion or stillbirth, retardation of intrauterine growth, or premature delivery. If the infected infant survives, the baby is likely to have deafness, developmental disability, heart defects, visual impairment, and other anomalies such as microcephaly and retarded overall growth. There is no effective medical treatment to alleviate these effects (Anderson et al., 2002).

> Toxoplasmosis is a disease caused by protozoan parasite *toxoplasma gondii.* Rubella is also known as German measles. Cytomegalovirus is a group of herpes virus (human herpes virus 5). *Herpes simplex* viruses cause various kinds of skin diseases.

Good prenatal care is critical to the developing human fetus. Unfortunately, in the United States, 17 percent of pregnant mothers do not receive first trimester care, and 3.9 percent receive very late or no care. This may be one reason why the United States ranks number 24 among selected countries in infant mortality with a rate of 7.0 deaths per 1,000 live births (March of Dimes, 2004). Infants born to mothers who do not receive prenatal care during the first trimester have mortality rates that are significantly higher than those born to mothers who get prenatal care (Rosetti, 2001). Lack of prenatal care increases the risk of infant mortality or premature birth, or both, and is a significant risk factor in the development of language disorders in infants who survive.

Premature birth with low birth weight. Technological advances and medical research have made it possible to save many more infants born prematurely than were saved in the past. Infants who are born prematurely are at risk for the development of language disorders; the more premature the birth, the higher the likelihood that some type of disability, often with an accompanying language disorder, will exist. Children born at 22 weeks gestation have a 10 percent survival rate, and of those who survive, 65 percent will have some sort of serious handicap; at 24 weeks gestation, 50 percent will survive and of those, 33 percent will have a serious handicap; at 26 weeks gestation, 90 percent will survive and 20 percent will have a serious handicap (Rosetti, 2002). Known causes of prematurity include:

- Infection of the amniotic fluid or membrane
- Maternal drug or alcohol abuse
- Fetal distress
- Maternal age (under 16 or over 36)
- Maternal kidney infection
- Multiple gestation
- Placental bleeding
- Excessive or insufficient amniotic fluid
- Premature rupture of the membrane
- Maternal preeclampsia; symptoms include hypertension (high blood pressure), proteinuria (abnormally large quantities of protein in the urine), and edema (swelling)
- Uterine abnormalities or "incompetent" cervix

Premature birth often results in low birth weight (LBW). Infants weighing less than 1,500 grams, or approximately $3^1/_3$ pounds, are considered to be high risk for developmental disabilities, including language disorders. Often, LBW infants must experience an extended stay in a neonatal intensive care unit, which, like any extended hospital stay, may interfere with the child's development (see Box 2.3 for a description of the NICU as risk factor for developmental disability).

Perinatal Risk Factors

Perinatal conditions are factors that may affect the infant *during* birth. The term *perinatal* pertains to the time and process of giving birth or being born. Several factors relating to labor and delivery may result in a disability:

- Abnormally long labor (22–24 hours is the average for a firstborn infant)
- Precipitated or uncontrolled delivery
- Abnormal presentation of the infant (e.g., a breech birth in which the feet, knees, or buttocks are presented first)
- Delivery by cesarean section
- Fetal distress, resulting in an abnormal heart rate
- Placental abnormalities
- Any perinatal condition that causes brain injury

Neonatal Risk Factors

Neonatal risk factors are those that affect an infant's development. The neonatal period stretches from birth to 28 days following birth. This period is of critical importance to the newborn infant. It is a particularly risky time for infants: 65 percent of deaths that occur during the first year of life happen in this 4-week period (Anderson et al., 2002).

| box 2.3 | | The Neonatal Intensive Care Unit as a Risk Factor for Developmental Disability: How SLPs Can Help |

Neonatal intensive care units (NICUs) are staffed with highly trained medical personnel whose first concern is the survival of the infant. However, the environment of the NICU may contribute to a poor developmental outcome for the infant. Researchers have expressed concerns regarding sensory overstimulation of infants who are subjected to bright fluorescent lighting, high-decibel sound levels, and brusque handling by medical personnel administering the frequent invasive medical procedures necessary for infant survival (Blackburn, 1998; Bremer, Byers, & Kiehl, 2003; Slevin et al., 2000). It is thought that such overstimulation, along with isolation from the mother and other family members, may be harmful to language, cognitive, and motor development in the infant.

No direct cause–effect relationship between noise, bright light, impersonal handling, and future developmental delay has been scientifically established. However, medical personnel and administrators have suggested "developmental care" in addition to necessary medical care.

SLPs can provide instruction to medical staff in using "child-directed speech," formerly called "motherese," when interacting with NICU infants, and by advocating for a gentler, more family-friendly NICU. Robison (2003) offered the following additional suggestions for NICU staff:

- Provide a calm, relaxing environment with lighting and sound muted to the extent possible
- Avoid unnecessary alarms and silence necessary alarms as soon as possible
- Be mindful of unnecessarily loud conversation and other sounds produced by NICU staff
- Shield the infant's eyes carefully if using an over-the-bed bright light for hands-on care
- Provide as much space and comfort as possible for family caregiving and interaction with the infant
- Encourage families to personalize their infant's bed space; ask families what can be done to make the environment more "homelike"

Risk factors associated with the neonatal period include (Rosetti, 2002):

- Low or unusually high birth weight
- Hyperbilirubinemia: an excess of bilirubin (yellow bile pigment) in the blood of the newborn, marked by a yellow tinge to skin pigmentation commonly called jaundice. Mild cases require no treatment, just monitoring. In severe cases, the excess bilirubin becomes toxic, a condition called kernicterus, and brain damage may occur.
- Poor feeding
- Any kind of infection
- A collection of three or more minor anomalies: even in the absence of an identifiable congenital syndrome, a collection of three or more anatomical anomalies (e.g., webbed fingers, toes, or both; any orofacial clefts; excessively large, protruding ears, etc.) constitutes a risk factor for future developmental disability

Infants who have experienced any of these prenatal, perinatal, or neonatal risk factors must be monitored closely. Periodic assessment of these infants is necessary to determine whether or not a language disorder exists, so that intervention for the disorder may be given as early as possible.

Medical and Genetic Factors

Various medical conditions that may or may not be inherited are associated with language disorders. Congenital syphilis, for instance, will negatively affect all aspects of child development, including language learning. Various kinds of skull and brain anomalies are associated with language disorders. Children who are born with an unusually small head (microcephaly) or enlarged head due to fluid accumulation in the brain (hydrocephaly) may have difficulty learning language. Persistent and severe seizure disorders also may negatively affect language learning (see Chapter 14 for details).

Serious and chronic illness that requires prolonged hospitalization of the child may also retard language learning. Any injury to the speech mechanism including the laryngeal structures may have the same effect. Hearing loss, of course, is a well-established sensory deficiency that results in oral language impairment (see Chapter 14 for details).

Many genetic syndromes that cause developmental abnormalities also are associated with language disorders (Leonard, 1988; McCauley, 2001). A **syndrome** is a constellation of signs and symptoms that are due to morbid genetic and anatomic–physiologic processes. Syndromes may be inherited or may be congenital in the sense that the symptoms are seen at birth but not necessarily inherited. There is a long list of syndromes known to be associated with language disorders. Any syndrome that causes developmental disability results in language disorders. Down syndrome, for example, is due to a genetic abnormality that results in limited cognitive as well as language skills. Many other genetic syndromes that cause such sensory deficiencies as hearing loss also are associated with language disorders. In fact, hundreds of syndromes may affect physical growth, intellect, hearing, and speech and language (Shprintzen, 2000). See Box 2.4 for a list of some common genetic syndromes that are associated with language (and speech) disorders.

Genetic factors also seem to play a role even when the language disorder is not associated with a genetic syndrome. For instance, studies have shown that language disorders are more common in certain families than in other families, suggesting a potential

---

box 2.4   **Selected Syndromes Associated with Language Disorders**

Down syndrome: Also known as trisomy 21 because of an abnormality of chromosome 21. Developmental disability of varying degrees, otitis media, hearing loss, and speech and language problems are characteristic features.

Cornelia de Lange syndrome: A congenital syndrome characterized by microcephaly, developmental disability, and severe speech and language impairments.

Cri du chat syndrome: Caused by an abnormality of chromosome 5, cri du chat is recognized by the baby's cry that resembles that of a cat's. Developmental disability and language disorders are common.

Fetal alcohol syndrome: A congenital syndrome caused by maternal alcoholism during pregnancy, resulting in microcephaly, developmental disability, physical growth problems, and speech and language disorders.

Fragile X syndrome: This is an X-linked syndrome, caused by a fragile site on the long arm of the X chromosome, resulting in speech and language problems.

Moebius syndrome. A genetic syndrome with congenital bilateral facial palsy, mild developmental disability in some cases, reduced tongue strength, potential language disorders.

Pierre-Robin syndrome. A somewhat rare genetic syndrome with autosomal recessive inheritance in most cases, associated with cleft palate, hearing loss, and speech-language problems.

Prader-Willi syndrome: A genetic syndrome characterized by physical growth problems and speech and language disorders.

Turner syndrome: This syndrome affects only females because it is caused by a single X (sex) chromosome instead of the normal two. Some children with this syndrome may have language learning problems although intellectual deficits are uncommon.

influence of general genetic factors (Choudhury & Benasich, 2003; Tallal et al., 2001; Tomblin, 1989). The influence of genetic factors has been studied extensively in the context of specific language disorders, and the studies are reviewed in Chapter 3.

Environmental Factors

It is evident that language learning requires a favorable family and social environment (Hart & Risley, 1995; McLaughlin, 1998; Moerk, 1983, 1992, 2000). Much of the research on the verbal environment and language learning has been done with children who are acquiring language normally contrasted with those who have failed to learn language in spite of normal or near-normal intellectual and sensory functions. Certain social and family variables are known to influence language learning. For instance, children from lower socioeconomic status, children of parents with little or no education, and children of certain minority groups that experience a high rate of poverty tend to have below-normal language skills (Bruck & Tucker, 1974; Kaiser & Delaney, 1996; Kaiser et al., 2000; Kaiser, Cai, Hancock, & Foster, 2002; Tough, 1982; Whitehurst & Fischel, 2000). Consequently, language disorders are somewhat more prevalent in children from lower socioeconomic status than from upper socioeconomic status. In some cases, however, the reported higher incidence of below-normal language skills in children belonging to such minority groups as African Americans may be due to assessment biases. These children are at a disadvantage when standardized tests that are inappropriate for these children are used to assess their language skills (Laing & Kamhi, 2003; Qi et al., 2003).

Family environment is an important factor in promoting good language skills in children. For instance, families that provide a literacy-rich home environment for their children tend to promote better language skills in their children than families that do not provide literacy materials at home. Parents who spend a significant amount of time reading and writing at home tend to have children with better language skills than those who do not engage in such literacy activities. Parents who read stories to their children and who display advanced language for their children, also promote advanced language skills. As a review of research (presented in Chapter 3) shows, evidence for the influence of environmental factors that promote or retard language and literacy skills in children is substantial (Whitehurst & Fischel, 2000). Nonetheless, whether a poor environment is a cause of language disorders is still an open question.

Interaction among Factors

Although no particular factor may explain language disorders in all children, a combination of several factors may. It is evident that children who have language disorders are a heterogeneous group. Some have obvious genetic or congenital syndromes. Others are relatively healthy individuals. Some have mild to severe sensory problems; others do not. Some have an obviously impoverished home environment. Others have a normal home environment (with siblings who have normal language skills) and yet fail to learn language. Therefore, it is difficult to make generalized statements that apply to all children with language disorders.

A child's physical health, intellectual (cognitive) level, physical (neurophysiological) growth, sensory capabilities, presence or absence of genetic or congenital syndromes, parents' education and occupation, verbally enriched or impoverished home environment, all combine to produce relatively favorable or unfavorable consequences for a child who is learning a language. Although it is still important to determine the specific contribution each of those (and perhaps other unknown) variables make, it appears that language learning and a failure to learn language at the normal rate are both a result of an interaction among a complex set of variables.

In individual cases, one or the other variable, or a combination of a small set of variables may exert an overriding influence on language learning. For instance, compared to other potential variables, a genetic syndrome that creates profound developmental disability, hearing loss, and neuromuscular problems will have an overriding influence on a child's oral language learning. When genetic and neuromuscular variables are relatively normal, a severely verbally impoverished home environment may be the most critical factor. In most cases, a combination of variables—perhaps a different combination in individual cases— may be responsible for normal or impaired language acquisition.

Effects of Language Disorders

While there may be disagreement over the causes of language disorders, most would agree with the seriousness of the effects of language disorders on children, their families, and on society in general. Childhood language disorders have far-reaching consequences. Language problems affect a child's social behavior and educational achievement; many children with early language disorders are later diagnosed with learning disabilities in schools. Limited language skills in some children may lead to aggressive, uncooperative, and otherwise unsocial behaviors. Several studies have shown that such undesirable behaviors are reduced when children are taught appropriate language skills to request, to cooperate in activities, to play socially, and so forth (Parrish & Roberts, 1993).

Language disorders that persist into adulthood can cause serious occupational difficulties. During the last half of the twentieth century, the manner in which people make their living went through a fundamental shift from occupations based on manual labor to technical and professional occupations that emphasize the use of communication skills. People who have limited communication skills, then, are likely to have restricted occupational choices. Furthermore, limited language skills in adults cost the nation. Based on 1999 dollars, it has been estimated that unemployment and underemployment of adults due to their communication disorders result in a $122.6 billion annual loss to the U.S. economy (Ruben, 2000).

Because of such serious consequences, assessment and treatment of language disorders are an important part of the duties of the speech-language pathologist. SLPs are in a unique position to have a positive effect on the quality of the lives of children who have language disorders and their families.

The largest group of children with language disorders are those with specific language impairment (SLI). SLPs working with children will typically have numerous children with SLI on their caseloads. Children with SLI apparently have no additional impairments other than difficulties with language. They may therefore be assessed and treated for their language disorders with little need to modify assessment and treatment procedures to accommodate additional diagnoses. Before discussing basic assessment and treatment procedures, then, it will be useful to have a more comprehensive understanding of the characteristics of children with SLI. The following chapter will discuss this population of children, leading to chapters in Part II which will delineate basic assessment and treatment procedures—procedures which, without modification, are relevant to intervention for children with SLI.

Chapter Summary

The American Speech-Language-Hearing Association (ASHA) defines a language disorder as impairment in comprehension and/or use of spoken, written, and/or other symbol systems. The American Psychiatric Association (APA) defines language disorders in terms of a discrepancy between language skills and nonverbal intelligence. Behaviorally, a language disorder is a lack of acceptable or effective social repertoire to affect the behaviors of other persons in social, educational, and occupational milieu (*expressive* language) and to be affected by the verbal behaviors of other persons (*receptive* language). School districts and state departments of education in the United States often define language disorders using criteria that may be related to eligibility for services.

Although children with language disorders are a heterogeneous group, they commonly exhibit: (1) a limited amount of language; (2) deficient grammar; (3) inadequate or inappropriate social communication; (4) deficient nonverbal communication skills; and (5) deficient literacy skills.

A prevalence rate of 7 to 8 percent for specific language impairment in kindergarten-age children is often reported. The overall prevalence rate for language disorders is much higher, as language disorders are often associated with other conditions, such as hearing loss, developmental disability, autism, cerebral palsy, traumatic brain injury, and so forth. There are two broad categories of language disorders: (1) specific language impairment which is not associated with other clinical diagnosis and (2) language disorders associated with other clinical conditions (e.g., hearing loss or autism). Language disorders may be classified either descriptively or etiologically.

Many prenatal, perinatal, neonatal, or environmental risk factors may signal later language disorders in children. Medical and genetic factors associated with language disorders include congenital syphilis, skull and brain anomalies, chronic illness that requires prolonged hospitalization of a child, hearing loss, and many genetic syndromes that affect physical growth, intellectual functions, hearing, and speech and language. Environmental risk factors include certain social and family variables that are known to influence language learning. Low socioeconomic status, for example, may be a risk factor for language disorders. Each child's difficulty with language is probably the result of an interaction among a complex set of variables, limiting the validity of any generalized statements.

Language problems affect social behavior, educational achievement, and ultimately occupational success. Assessment and treatment of language disorders, therefore, are important duties of SLPs.

Study Guide

1. Critically evaluate the conceptual bases of the definition of language disorders offered by the American Speech-Language-Hearing Association (ASHA) and the

American Psychiatric Association (APA). What would be the main problem if a speech-language pathologist were to use the APA definition in diagnosing language disorders in children?

2. Contrast the ASHA definition with that of the behavioral definition offered in the text. Point out the limitations and strengths of each of these two definitions. Which one would you prefer and why?

3. Suppose you are employed as a speech-language pathologist in a public school that has unusually restrictive diagnostic criteria for offering services to children with language disorders. How would you present an argument to the school administration that more scientifically based criteria need to be considered so that more children who need the services are indeed offered those services? What kind of scientific argument would you make?

4. You are asked to offer a workshop to parents of school-age children on the risk factors associated with language disorders. Prepare an outline for such a presentation. What factors would you emphasize and why? Give justifications based on your own geographic area where certain risk factors may be more predominant than other factors.

5. Compare and contrast the etiological and descriptive classifications of language disorders. What is problematic about the assumption that language disorders are caused by accompanying clinical conditions? Critically examine the statement that the two classifications are not mutually exclusive.

chapter

3

Children with Specific
Language Impairment

outline

Before we begin a discussion of assessment and treatment of language disorders in children, we present a description of language disorders that are found in many children. As noted in the previous chapter, a form of child language disorder speech-language pathologists commonly treat is known as specific language impairment (SLI). An understanding of SLI will facilitate our discussion of language assessment and treatment procedures that apply to a wide variety of children.

A language problem in a child who is apparently normal in most if not all aspects is commonly called **specific language impairment.** Children who exhibit SLI do not have other significant clinical condition or conditions that would readily explain it. The term implies that the impairment is specific to language, which means that the child has only *one* impairment, which is restricted to language skills. In all except their language skills, these children are roughly comparable to normally developing children. It may be noted that this is the standard view of SLI; our characterization of children with SLI will initially follow this standard view and subsequently take into consideration some divergent views that suggest potential and perhaps subtle cognitive and motoric difficulties in these children.

In many other children, language disorders are associated with some other obvious and serious clinical condition. As we will see in later chapters, language disorders may be associated with developmental disability, autism, cerebral palsy, traumatic brain injury, hearing loss, and so forth. Such children, then, are diagnosed with both a language disorder and another, concomitant, clinical condition. Assessment and treatment procedures to be described in the next chapters are applicable, with suitable modifications, to children with concomitant clinical conditions. Therefore, these children will be addresses in the final section of the book.

We noted in Chapter 2 that in the past, the terms *congenital aphasia* or *childhood aphasia* were used to describe language disorders. Those terms typically referred to what we now call SLI. Presumed brain injury or dysfunction was an early explanation for this type of a language disorder, but such pathology was never convincingly demonstrated.

A Description of SLI

SLI is diagnosed only after age 4, as many children who show signs of slow language learning in early years are "late bloomers" who catch up with normally developing children (Rescorla, 1989). The late bloomers' language problem may be described as slow early language development (SELD). Some estimates suggest that up to 15 percent of children may be late bloomers who fail to acquire 50 single words and two-word productions by 2 years of age. In nearly half of them, language learning may be accelerated to approximate the normal. In the other half, language problems tend to persist. Consequently, SLI is present in about 7 to 8 percent of preschool and school-age children. In the absence of sustained and effective instruction, SLI will persist in these children (Leonard, 1991), although the prognosis for children with SLI who receive treatment is better than for those who have language disorders associated with such concomitant clinical conditions as autism or hearing loss (Johnson et al., 1999).

It is difficult to determine which toddlers are "late-bloomers" and which may have a persistent language problem. Early intervention is warranted if a child is slow to develop language. "Wait and see" is a risky policy for possible language disorders.

How do the scores children with SLI receive on verbal tests of intelligence compare to the scores they receive on nonverbal tests of intelligence?

Most children who are students in regular classrooms who receive treatment for language disorders are likely to have SLI. Academically, the children with SLI may perform somewhat below average, especially if their language deficiencies are not remediated. Generally, though, children with SLI have normal or near-normal intelligence. Therefore, their scores on verbal tests of intelligence are lower than their scores on nonverbal tests of intelligence.

Children with SLI learn language skills at a slower rate, but their pattern of acquisition is not grossly abnormal or deviant. Therefore, compared to children without language disorders, children with SLI exhibit lower language skills at each age or grade level. Also, children with SLI may exhibit a pattern of language development that is asynchronous; some of their language skills may be more advanced than other skills. Pragmatic language skills, for example, are often less impaired than are syntactic and morphologic skills. In general, children with SLI exhibit various combinations of phonologic, semantic, morphologic, syntactic, and pragmatic problems.

Early Communication Deficits

Infants who later develop SLI may also show deficiencies in early communicative behaviors, although, as noted earlier, SLI is typically not diagnosed until age 4. It is useful to understand the early communication deficits of children, even if some of them will not be later diagnosed with SLI. Therefore, we shall describe these deficits with the cautionary note that they may precede SLI in only some children. In any case, infants and toddlers in whom SLI is later diagnosed do exhibit early communication deficits. In essence, early communication deficits are the first warning signs of SLI.

Long before children produce their words between 12 and 18 months of age, the appearance of early communication skills signal the emergence of competent language skill. It is typical to describe an infant's early communication skills as the *prelinguistic* stage of development. However, prelinguistic behaviors are also communicative, even if they do not have a linguistic structure, emphasizing the view that linguistic structure is not the critical element in classifying a behavior as communicative.

Most early communicative behaviors of infants are shaped out of reflexive behaviors. As described in Chapter 7, infants' early reflexive behaviors that help lay a foundation for later communicative behaviors include cooing, babbling, and looking at the mother's face, turning the head toward a source of sound, especially the mother's voice, and so forth. Some researchers describe such reflexive responses that serve as a basis for later communicative behaviors as *preintentional*, and the later communicative behaviors as *intentional*. Preintentional and intentional behaviors are also known, respectively, as perlocutionary and illocutionary. Often, preintentional (perlocutionary) and intentional (illocutionary) behaviors are described as characteristics of stages in language acquisition (Bates, 1976; Hulit & Howard, 2002; McLaughlin, 1998). Although a baby who reflexively coos or babbles is not communicating anything (hence *preintentional* in linguistic terms), the parents or other caregivers react as though the baby is communicating. Thereby the parents lay the foundation for the infant's future communicative behavior. For example, physicians will explain to parents that a child's first "smile" is actually a reflexive reaction to a gassy stomach. Parents, however, react favorably to that smile-like grimace, and the infant eventually learns to curl the corners of the lips into a social smile to produce a desired result. Or, a mother might interpret a child's vegetative babbling sounds as communicative and respond to them by saying, "Oh! Do you need a hug?" followed by cuddling the child. In due course, the child's reflexive babbling will be shaped into communicative behaviors: the child is likely to make certain sounds when in need of something. In the linguistic analysis, the infant's intention to communicate is said to have emerged. What can be clearly observed, however, is that the infant's early reflexive responses are now no longer so; they are produced because they have an effect on the caregivers who react in certain ways to reinforce the child. Such parental reactions positively reinforce the child's vocalizations, which, as a result, increase in frequency. These vocalizations are the foundations for the first words that the child will produce between 12 and 18 months of age.

> It's no accident that an infant's first "word" is often an approximation of *mommy* or *daddy*. Parents enthusiastically reinforce typical CV babbling sounds (e.g., /mama/ or /dada/), and the infant responds with increased, progressively more refined, productions.

Prior to the emergence of the first true word, perhaps as early as 12 months, an infant's communicative repertoire may include such nonverbal behaviors as gestures, facial expressions, and object manipulation. Holding arms up to indicate a desire to be picked up, opening and closing hands in the direction of a desired object, and handing a cup to a caregiver to obtain a drink are all examples of early nonverbal communicative behaviors. Appropriate responses to verbal behavior of caregivers (receptive language) also dramatically increase during this time. Children between the ages of 12–18 months typically can follow one-step, simple directions given verbally and without gestural cues.

Infants and toddlers who show deficiencies in early communicative behaviors are at risk for developing SLI in later years. If an infant does not engage in mutual eye gaze, does not display typical vocalizations, produces only a few consonant sounds in babbling, does not imitate, or does not respond to caregivers' efforts to establish turn-taking skills or joint reference, then the parents and professionals (e.g., pediatricians) should consider the possibility of a language disorder. Hamaguchi (2001) described the following patterns of deficiencies in early communication skills which may indicate a child is at risk for developing a later language disorder, including SLI:

Birth to 12 Months

- Avoids eye contact
- Rarely babbles; is unusually quiet
- Does not consistently respond to whispered speech
- Shows little interest in imitating gestures, such as "bye-bye"
- Cries often, without changing pitch or intensity
- Shows little emotion

12 to 18 Months

- Avoids eye contact
- Does not say "Mama" or "Dada"
- Does not point to common body parts when asked
- Cannot follow verbally given simple one-step directions (e.g., "Go get your shoes!"), unless accompanied by a gesture

Other possible signs of a language disability from birth to 18 months include:

- Lack of a social smile
- Lack of developmentally appropriate play activities
- Reduced use of gestures, or, conversely, an over-reliance on using gestures rather than oral language
- Impaired learning of speech sounds (phonological difficulties)

These early communication deficits that an infant or toddler may exhibit may be associated with another clinical condition (e.g., autism or developmental disability). Therefore, they are not to be taken as an indication of only SLI. However, as noted before, children who later come to be diagnosed as having SLI may also exhibit these early communication deficiencies.

Language and Speech Characteristics of Children with SLI

Children with SLI are a heterogeneous group, exhibiting different combinations of deficiencies in various aspects of language comprehension and production. In addition, many children diagnosed with SLI have concomitant problems with speech production, commonly diagnosed as phonological disorders. The varieties of symptoms that may be present add to the challenge of diagnosing and treating children with SLI. The following sections describe commonly observed speech and language behaviors of children with SLI.

True or False?
Children with SLI are a homogenous group.

Phonological Disorders

By the time they are diagnosed with SLI, children are likely to exhibit phonological disorders as well. Patterned errors of articulation are typically described as phonological disorders. By and large, phonological patterns involve simplified productions of phonemes in syllables and words that most children learning to speak their language normally exhibit. As their speech and language skills improve, these phonological processes disappear. Compared to a younger child's speech, an older child's speech productions more closely resemble adult productions.

See Chapter 1 for more information on the phonological aspects of language.

Children with a phonological disorder produce unintelligible speech characterized by predictable patterns of errors that persist beyond the time when they normally disappear in other children. For example, many toddlers learning to speak might delete the weak syllable in multisyllabic words, so that *elephant* becomes "ephant" and *spaghetti* becomes "ghetti"—a phonological process known as weak syllable deletion. These are productions that are probably readily recognizable to adults who regularly work with toddlers, and, until the toddler reaches the age of 3, are not problematic. If such productions persist, however, particularly beyond the age of 5, the child might be diagnosed with a phonological disorder, a difficulty in acquiring the correct production of the sounds of a language. See Table 3.1 for examples of several phonological processes that are evident in children's speech.

Leonard (1998) has stated that phonological processes evident in children with SLI are similar to those of typically developing children with some notable differences. Prevocalic

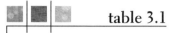

table 3.1

Phonological Processes Common in Children's Speech

Phonological Process	Definition	Examples
Unstressed syllable deletion	Omission of one or more syllables from a polysyllabic word	[ɛfənt] for *el*ephant [medo] for *to*mato
Final consonant deletion	Omission of a final singleton consonant in a word	[da] for do*g* [bɛ] for be*d*
Cluster reduction	Deletion or substitution of some or all members of a cluster	[gin] for g*r*een [tap] for *s*top [æg] for *fl*ag [dʌm] for d*r*um
Stopping	Substitution of stops for fricatives and affricates	[top] for *s*oap [tu] for *z*oo [dʌm] for *th*umb [dab] for *j*ob
Velar Fronting	Substitution of anterior-produced sounds, typically alveolar stops, for velars	[tʌp] for *c*up [do] for *g*o [bæt] for ba*g*
Backing	Substitution of a posterior-produced sound for an anterior-produced sound	[baɪk] for bi*t*e [kap] for *t*op
Liquid Gliding	Substitution of a glide for a liquid	[wæbɪt] for *r*abbit [jif] for *l*eaf

voicing and deletion of word-initial weak syllables may occur with greater frequency among children with SLI (e.g., /dap/ for /tap/ and /mændə/ for /əmændə/). Also, children with SLI might produce unusual errors (e.g., stopping of liquids as in t/r or substituting liquids for glides as in l/w) not associated with common phonological processes (Leonard & Leonard, 1985).

What two phonological processes may be produced by children with SLI more frequently than typically developing children?

Studies have shown that a majority of children referred to speech-language pathologists for the assessment of a possible phonological disorder also present with difficulties in the semantic, syntactic, and morphologic components of language (Paul & Shriberg, 1982; Ruscello, St. Louis, & Mason, 1991; Shriberg & Kwiatkowski, 1994). Rescorla and Lee (2001) reported that 40 percent of children who are diagnosed with SLI have speech problems. In some cases, a speech production problem may be contributing to the language impairment. A child who cannot articulate /t/, /d/, /s/, or /z/ will have difficulty producing missing morphological markers indicating past tense, third-person singular present tense, possession, and plurals. In other cases, it may be that the speech disorder is discovered to be the primary diagnosis, with errors in language production caused by misarticulations.

Therefore, children who are referred to professionals for assessment of a phonological disorder should also be fully assessed for a language disorder. Similarly, in a complete assessment of a child with SLI, the clinician should be alert to phonological disorders that may be present.

Semantic Problems in Children with SLI

A child's difficulty learning words and their meanings is often the first sign of a specific language disorder. Children with SLI may be slow to acquire their first few words, a milestone typically achieved between 12 to 18 months of age. These children, then, may not display the explosive increase in the acquisition of new words typical of children between the ages of 18 and 24 months. Some studies suggest that at age 2, normally developing children have a vocabulary of 200 or more words, whereas those who may be later diagnosed with SLI have a severely restricted vocabulary of about 20 words (Paul, 1966; Rescorla, Roberts, & Dahlsgaard, 1997).

Children with SLI may also persist in overextending and underextending word meanings beyond the age of 3 years (Nelson, 1993). **Overextension** is an inappropriately generalized production of a word. A child who calls all adult males *daddy* overextends or inappropriately generalizes that word production. Conversely, **underextension** is production of words in overly restricted contexts—showing lack of appropriate generalization. A child may produce the word *dog* to refer only to the family pet, but not in reference to any other dog—showing an overly restricted production of the word.

> Three-year-old Timmy could name his family's 4-door sedan as a "car," but he also referred to every other vehicle—busses, trucks, motorcycles—as a car. This is an example of what type of difficulty with generalization?

Most toddlers learn first to label concrete objects so that nouns dominate their vocabulary. Typically, children learn verbs next, and then around the age of 2 years, they begin to produce the first two-word combinations which consist of nouns + verbs. Children with SLI acquire these early appearing word combinations, but often at a later time and at a slower pace than normal. Also, children with SLI may not learn as quickly as typically developing children do that two-word combinations convey a variety of meanings beyond the noun + verb constructions (e.g., "Kitty run"), such as possession ("My kitty"), disappearance ("Kitty gone"), or rejection ("No, kitty!").

Other language problems—often described as semantic in nature—become apparent as the children with SLI enter school. Lahey and Edwards (1999) found that when compared to typically developing children, school-aged children (aged 4.3–9.7) with SLI make more errors in naming pictures of common objects. Typically, as their language skills expand, children learn words with abstract meanings. Children with SLI, on the other hand, may have difficulty with understanding abstract concepts. Therefore, such children are likely to experience academic difficulties in preschool and kindergarten. Children with SLI may not understand or produce words expressing such concepts as size, shape, color, quantity, and quality as readily as do typically developing children. Their language may typically be limited to concrete events and objects.

> Typically developing toddlers with an MLU of 2.0 do not have mastery of morphological and syntactical features. Adults have to discern the meaning of children's utterances by paralinguistic behaviors (e.g., vocal intonation, gestures, facial expressions) and contextual cues.

As the child with SLI grows, a decreased vocabulary may interfere with academic performance and socialization. As academic demands for a more extensive and abstract vocabulary increase, children with SLI may appear to have word-finding problems. However, the children may simply not know the words. Not knowing specific words, they resort to the use of such vague words as *thing, stuff, this,* or *that.* Lack of specific word knowledge may also impair speech fluency, resulting in an increase in such dysfluencies as pauses (hesitations), interjections, and repetitions. Due to their difficulties in abstract language, children with SLI in the upper elementary school grades may not understand or produce metaphors, similes, idioms, and proverbs.

> How do the receptive language skills of children with SLI compare to their expressive language skills?

In children with SLI, there is often a discrepancy between their language production and comprehension skills. Their receptive language skills are superior to their expressive skills. People may notice that children with SLI can understand many words they do not produce in speech.

Syntactic and Morphologic Problems in Children with SLI

A striking diagnostic feature of children with SLI is their deficiencies in grammar, including syntactic and morphologic deficiencies (Conti-Ramsden & Jones, 1997; Dale & Cole, 1991; Frome Loeb & Leonard, 1991; Leonard, McGregor, & Allen, 1992; Oetting & Morohov, 1997; Oetting & Rice, 1993; Paul & Alforde, 1993; Rescorla & Lee, 2001; Rice & Oetting, 1993). Generally, children with SLI speak in shorter, less complex, and less varied sentences. Their productions tend to omit various grammatic morphemes, although the sequence of learning them is the same as in normally developing children. Children with SLI take more time to learn the grammatic morphemes or may continue to omit them.

The limited syntactic skills of children with SLI result in less varied and generally limited repertoire of communication. Children with SLI are less likely to use restrictive embedded clauses (e.g., "The man *with the big suitcase* ran to catch the plane") and to manipulate, or transform, sentence structures to produce a variety of sentence types. These children may have difficulty moving from passive to active voice or changing a statement into a question. **Function words,** which include such grammatic morphemes as articles, prepositions, and conjunctions may be omitted, resulting in **telegraphic speech,** a type of condensed speech in which only essential words are used.

Morphologic problems are especially marked in children with SLI, who are either slow in learning the following morphologic features or may never learn to use some of them without intervention:

- *Regular plural morpheme and its allomorphic variations* (e.g., /s/, /z/, and /ez/ variations). Although children with SLI are slower than the normally developing children in learning plural inflections, they still master them more easily than they do main verbs, auxiliary, copula, and tense inflections.

> Some of the examples given of erred productions are examples of utterances that are consistent with the use of the African American English (AAE). Dialectical differences are *not* disorders, and children who produce AAE should not be considered to have a language disorder. A more detailed discussion of this issue will be presented in Chapter 11.

- *Possessive morpheme.* Allomorphic variations of the possessive morpheme (e.g., *Cat's tail* and *Mom's bag*), though generally delayed, may be less difficult than different classes of verbs for children with SLI to learn.
- *Present progressive -ing.* Production of verb + *ing* is generally delayed in acquisition. This one aspect of verb inflection may be less difficult to learn than some of the other morphologic skills, especially other aspects of verb inflections.
- *Third person singular* (e.g., "He play ball" for "He plays ball"). This morpheme is especially difficult for children with SLI to learn.
- *Various forms of auxiliary.* These are also especially difficult for children with SLI to learn. For example, auxiliary *is* (e.g., "He playing ball" for "He *is* playing ball"), auxiliary *are* (e.g., "They running" for "They *are* running") and their past-tense forms (*was* and *were*) may need systematic treatment before the children learn to produce them correctly.
- *Various forms of copula.* Especially difficult for children with SLI to learn are the copula *is* (e.g., "Daddy big" instead of "Daddy *is* big"), *are* (e.g., "They nice" for "They

are nice"), and their past-tense forms (*was* and *were*). These also may need systematic treatment.

- *Tense inflections.* Another especially difficult morphologic feature for children with SLI to master. Tense inflections, including the regular past tense -*ed* (as in *painted*), /t/ (as in *walked*), and /d/ (as in *begged*) may require systematic treatment.
- *Irregular plural forms.* Children with SLI may overgeneralize regular plural inflection to irregular words (e.g., *foots* for *feet*)
- *Irregular past tense verb forms.* Children with SLI may overgeneralize regular past tense inflection to irregular verbs (e.g., *goed* for *went*).
- *Distinction between the singular and plural forms of words.* Children with SLI may be confused about this distinction.
- *Distinction between the singular and plural forms of auxiliary and copula* is (e.g., *is/are*; *was/were*). Once again, the children may be confused about this distinction.
- *Subject case markings* (e.g., "Him go fast!" "Her pretty!"). Another difficult grammatic production for children with SLI to master.

Explanations for Morphologic Deficiencies in Children with SLI

Various explanations have been offered as to why children with SLI tend to have significant morphologic deficiencies. These explanations have included: (1) explanations involving perception, (2) explanations involving syntactic complexity, and (3) explanations involving semantic redundancy.

Explanations involving perception state that children with SLI do not produce morphologic features because they simply do not perceive them as well as they perceive the rest of the word or sentence. In connected speech, morphologic features are produced with less stress and lower intensity, and, therefore, not as emphasized as the rest of the word, and may simply be missed by children with SLI (Leonard, McGregor, & Allen, 1992).

Explanations emphasizing syntactic complexity identify the close relationship between syntax and morphology as the root of the problem. It is thought that children who struggle to acquire more complex syntactic structures will also have difficulty acquiring the bound morphemes that contribute to syntactic complexity, and the difficulty with morphologic features is secondary to difficulty with syntax (Watkins & Rice, 1991). There has been some speculation that children with SLI may get "stuck" in a developmental stage in which tense is treated as optional, called the extended optional infinitive explanation of the underlying cause of SLI (Redmond & Rice, 2001; Rice et al., 2000).

Explanations involving semantic redundancy state that children with SLI omit certain morphologic features because they are not critical to the meaning of an utterance. For example, semantic redundancy can be seen in phrases and sentences in the English language that convey pluralism. The phrase *two girls* contains redundant information in that the word *two* obviously implies more than one and should render the use of the plural -*s* unnecessary, as it is in many foreign languages. People who are primary speakers of many Asian languages, in which the use of a quantitative marker such as a number indicates pluralism, find it difficult to learn English usage of plural -*s*. Perhaps some children growing up in English-speaking environments also have no use for what may be perceived as redundant information and, as a result, omit a grammatically but not semantically necessary morpheme.

These are all plausible explanations for the difficulty children with SLI exhibit in the areas of syntax and morphology. None have been experimentally demonstrated to be true, however, and other unrecognized factors might also be involved.

Although no definitive diagnostic criterion of specific language impairment has been formulated, morphologic deficiencies have been described as the most "promising clinical marker" of SLI (Leonard, Miller, & Gerber, 1999). In search of that definitive "clinical marker," production of such morphologic features as past-tense marking, development of irregular past-tense and plural forms, production of auxiliary and copula *is*, and so forth has been compared across children with and without SLI. Although the studies have often succeeded in establishing such differences, none have established criteria that positively identify children who are at risk for developing specific language impairment. Children with SLI present unique diagnostic profiles with varying strengths and weaknesses. Morphologic features are often impaired in children with SLI, but no one common morphologic error can be said to exist in all or even most children with SLI.

Pragmatic Problems in Children with SLI

It is often stated that children with SLI have better pragmatic language skills than syntactic or morphologic skills. If sustained in additional research, this characteristic of children with SLI would contrast with the pragmatic language skills of children with autism (Caparulo & Cohen, 1983). Evidence on the pragmatic skills of children with SLI, however, is not consistent. In his review of studies on pragmatic language skills of children with SLI, Leonard (1998) found contradictory evidence for almost every pragmatic language skill that has been researched.

Some studies have indicated that there is little difference between the pragmatic language skills of children with SLI and other control groups. Various studies have shown that children with SLI initiate conversations, use appropriate turn-taking skills, respond to requests for clarification, and make requests for clarification (Craig & Evans, 1989; Fey & Leonard, 1984; Fey, Leonard, & Wilcox, 1981; Fujiki & Brinton, 1991; Gallagher & Darnton, 1978; Griffin, 1979; Van Kleeck & Frankel, 1981).

Several other studies have established significant differences between the pragmatic language skills of children with SLI and those of typically developing peers. Paul (1991) found that toddlers with SLI exhibited fewer interactions involving **joint attention** with their caregivers (e.g., the child and the adult looking at the same object and talking about it or manipulating it; see Photo 3.1). There has been some evidence that children with SLI are more likely to initiate conversation with adults than they are with peers, whereas typically developing children are more likely to initiate conversation with peers (Rice, Sell, & Hadley, 1991). Children with SLI have been found to talk more with language-matched peers or with other children with SLI than they talk to age-matched typical peers (Fey, Leonard, & Wilcox, 1981). Other studies have indicated that, in general, children with SLI are reluctant to initiate conversation, may initiate conversation at inappropriate times, or may interrupt or shout to gain attention before initiating conversation (Fey, 1986; Lucas, 1980; Paul, 1991).

Children with SLI might have more difficulty with social interactions in the context of group communication as opposed to one-on-one, or dyadic, communicative interactions. When groups of peers hold social discourse, children with SLI may not "break into" the

photo 3.1

Joint attention is established either when the child directs the adult's gaze to an item of mutual interest, or when the child responds to the adult's direction to attend to an object.

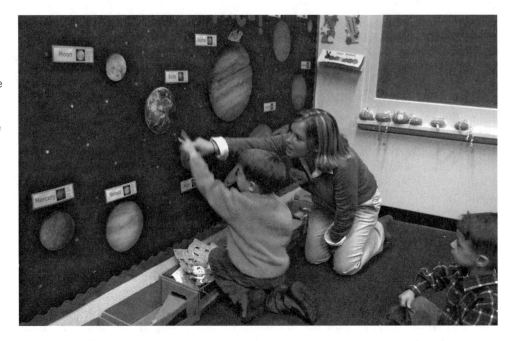

conversation (Craig, 1993; Craig & Washington, 1993). Brinton et al. (1997) reported that, when participating in conversational groups of three peers, children with SLI "talked significantly less, were addressed significantly less, and collaborated less than either of the partners within their triads" (p. 1011).

Contradictory evidence on the pragmatic language skills of children with SLI may be due to certain methodological differences between studies. Pragmatic language skills are not a unitary response class. They are a collection of different kinds of responses. Some pragmatic skills (e.g., eye contact or topic initiation) may be more basic and more easily learned than others (e.g., topic maintenance or interjecting meaningful comments at appropriate times in group interactions). Studies that have failed to show deficiencies may not have measured the more complex skills, the same skills in more complex interactions, or their measurement procedures may have been less sensitive. Even turn taking, for example, may be measured in relatively simpler one-on-one conversation or in relatively complex group interactions. Such differences could yield different results. It is reasonable to expect pragmatic language skill deficiencies in children who have other language deficiencies. Nonetheless, because of contradictory research evidence, difficulties in the pragmatic language deficiencies cannot be presumed in children with SLI. In each case, the clinician should carefully assess those skills. Progressively more complex interactions, arranged throughout language treatment sessions, may be helpful in making a final judgment on the presence or absence of pragmatic deficits in a child. In evaluating each child, the clinician should consider the following potential pragmatic deficiencies in children with SLI:

- *Fewer comments on events and persons.* Language may be generally sparse, limited in both quantity and variety.

- *Difficulty in describing events, pictures, and other stimuli.* Once again, limited or poor descriptions and repetition of a few basic descriptive terms may be the dominant characteristic of language.
- *Interactions that are limited to answering questions asked.* Children with SLI may respond to questions, but may not offer additional information and ask questions.
- *Limited use of gestures.* Various nonverbal means of communication that accompany verbal expressions may be absent or limited.
- *Passivity in conversational interactions.* Especially in group interactions, children with SLI may be passive. They may not make attempts to interject, offer quick comments, raise questions, or narrate their own experiences.
- *Inappropriate turn taking.* Children with SLI may inappropriately interrupt speakers and fail to respond when it is their turn to speak in conversation.
- *Difficulty in initiating conversation.* Children with SLI may be either slow or deficient in initiating conversation on new topics.
- *Difficulty in sustaining topics of conversation.* Children with SLI may switch topics abruptly as they may not have enough information or language skills to sustain extended conversation on topics on which typically someone else will have initiated conversation.
- *Production of irrelevant comments.* Although seen less frequently than in children with autism or developmental disability, children with SLI may on occasion make irrelevant or inappropriate comments during conversation.
- *Deficient conversational repair strategies.* Children with SLI may fail to ask for clarification when they do not understand others. These children may also fail to respond differently when others request clarification of their own messages.
- *Deficient narrative skills.* Limited vocabulary, syntax, and morphologic features can be expected to affect the narrative skills of children with SLI. Their narration of stories or personal experiences may be brief, lacking in details, and limited to a few concrete aspects of their experience or stimuli to which they respond. Chronological sequence and logical progression may be poor. Information typically inferred from stories may be missing.
- *Poor social and peer interactions.* Social and peer interactions of children with SLI may be limited to a few contacts. They may be more willing to talk to adults than to their peers.

The initial treatment targets for a child with SLI are most likely to be words and morphologic and syntactic skills. Therefore, a clinician who keeps a keen eye on these problems during language treatment may discover pragmatic problems that may become later language targets.

Causes, Correlations, and Explanations

What causes specific language impairment? How should this disorder be explained? An explanation of a disorder is a precise statement of the causes of a disorder or at the least, the conditions under which the disorder is likely to arise. Attempts at explaining SLI have led to both empirical investigations and theoretical speculations. Neither the available empirical data nor theories based on them satisfactorily explain the disorder.

That it is difficult to explain a complex disorder such as SLI whose causes remain largely uncovered is understandable. However, clinicians need to be wary of premature explanations based on incomplete or questionable evidence. In the case of human diseases and disorders, it is not possible to establish the original cause or causes through the experimental approach, which, if practical, is the best possible strategy for doing it. Such experimental research is possible to find causes of diseases in animals, but, obviously, not in the case of language disorders. Researchers cannot manipulate variables under controlled conditions to induce language disorders in human beings. Therefore, all explanations of the original or instigating causes of human communication disorders will be based on correlational data, which are weak in supporting causality. Any basic course on statistics will have proclaimed that *correlation does not mean causation*. Specific language impairment may be correlated with a certain factor but both the disorder and the factor may be caused by something else that has not been observed.

Correlation between two factors does not specify which one is the cause and which one is the effect; either one could be the cause. Furthermore, what for some seems like strong evidence based on correlation may leave the causation just as ambiguous as before. For instance, if SLI has a family history, does it mean genetic influence or family environmental influence? Many automatically assume that it is the genetic influence, but nothing in that observation rules out the influence of environmental factors. Therefore, there are only controversial causes of language disorders in children.

Certain potentially genetic, neuroanatomic, and environmental factors are correlated with SLI in children. While the presence of a single correlated factor may not always mean that the child will have SLI, the presence of multiple factors may increase the chances that the child will have SLI.

Potential Genetic Factors

Although SLI, by definition, is not associated with any other diagnosed condition, evidence suggests that genetic factors may play a role in the development of SLI in children. Genetic studies including family studies, pedigree studies, and twin studies have been made to investigate potential genetic factors that may be related to SLI in children (McCauley, 2001). Most genetic studies on SLI have been **population genetic studies** that infer the influence of genetic factors in causing clinical conditions based on differential prevalence of disorders in blood relatives contrasted with their prevalence in unrelated individuals. **Molecular genetics** isolate specific genes for specific clinical conditions. The results of molecular genetic studies are more definitive than those of population genetic studies. Until molecular genetic studies find specific genes responsible for SLI, the results of population genetic studies remain ambiguous because they cannot separate the influence of environmental variables. See Box 3.1 for a definition of selected genetic terms.

> What are three types of population genetic studies?

Family studies. Researchers conducting family studies start with a proband (the first person they see with a disorder; in this case, a child with SLI) to find out how many in that child's family have the same disorder. If the disorder is more common in the proband's family than in the general population, the researchers conclude that the disorder is familial. In such cases, the conclusion that the disorder is familial—if meant to suggest that it tends

box 3.1 | A Primer of Selected Genetic Terms

Allele: The different forms of a gene situated on a specific chromosomal locus.

Cell: The structural unit of living organisms; contains cytoplasm and a nucleus; the latter contains chromosomes on which genes are located.

Chromosomes: Structures in the cell nucleus that contain genes, the functional units of heredity.

Concordance rates: The extent to which both the members of twin pairs (identical or fraternal) have the same clinical condition. Higher concordance rates are typically thought to suggest a genetic basis for the clinical condition studied.

DNA: Deoxyribonucleic acid; the primary genetic material of living organisms.

Discordance rates: The extent to which only one member of twin pairs exhibits a clinical condition.

Dominant gene: A gene that produces an effect even when its allele is different.

Epidemiology: Study of incidence of disorders or diseases in the general or specific populations.

Family aggregation: Concentrated prevalence of diseases and disorders among blood relatives. Does not necessarily mean inherited.

Gene: A functional unit of heredity, found on a specific locus on chromosomes.

Genome: Gene + chromosome; complete set of the genetic material of a species (e.g., *human genome*).

Genotype: The genetic abnormality that causes the phenotype (expression) of a disease or disorder.

Linkage: The presence of two genetic loci on the same chromosome.

Locus: A gene's specific position on a chromosome.

Molecular genetics: Study of the DNA sequence through blood or salivary samples of individuals to isolate a specific gene that may be responsible for phenotypic abnormalities.

Mutation: A permanent change in the gene chemistry; may give a sudden rise to a new species; a cause of genetic abnormality.

Pedigree: A diagram showing the members of a family that are affected by, or are free from, a clinical condition.

Phenotype: The symptom complex of a disease or disorder as observed and measured. Phenotype is the genetic expression of a clinical condition.

Population genetics: Study of incidence or prevalence of diseases and disorders in the selected families, identical twins, fraternal twins, and unrelated individuals to identify potential genetic and environmental influences in the causation of diseases and disorders.

Recessive gene: A gene that cannot express itself because of a dominant gene's action.

Sex chromosomes: XX (female) and XY (male) chromosomes that determine the sex of an individual.

---

to run in families—is valid. If it is meant that the disorder is genetic, the conclusion is questionable, although this questionable conclusion is more the norm than the exception among population genetic researchers. Family members are typically exposed to similar environments, and characteristics of SLI may be due to something occurring in that environment rather than genetic composition. Familial incidence or prevalence does not distinguish environmental versus genetic similarities within families. Familial characteristics are not necessarily genetically inherited.

> In a family study, what is the term applied to the first person with a disorder the researchers see?

Family studies have consistently shown that the prevalence of SLI is higher in certain families than in other families (Spitz et al., 1997; Tallal, Ross, & Curtiss, 1989; Tomblin, 1989). This means that if one child (a proband) is diagnosed with SLI, there are likely to be other children with SLI among the diagnosed child's blood relatives. A weakness of most of these studies is their reliance on questionnaires completed by family members as the primary source of information on others in the family who may have SLI. The reliability of the family members' judgment about language disorders among relatives is questionable.

Other investigators have made direct assessment of family members to determine whether or not SLI is present (Choudhury & Benasich, 2003; Plante, Shenkman, & Clark, 1996; Tallal et. al, 2001; Tomblin & Buckwalter, 1994; Tomblin, Freese, & Records, 1992). In these studies, the professionals diagnosed SLI among family members; hence the diagnosis is more reliable than those supplied by untrained family members. These studies have also shown the prevalence of SLI to be higher among family members of children with SLI than among family members of unaffected children. While the prevalence of SLI in the general population is estimated at around 7 percent, the familial prevalence is estimated at 20 percent to 40 percent of members of affected families. The Choudhury and Benasich (2003) study followed 42 infants (37 families) with at least one family member already diagnosed as having SLI (affected families) and 94 infants (75 families) with no history of any kind of language impairment (unaffected families). The infants were recruited before they were 6 months of age and were administered language tests at age 3. In half the affected families, only one child had SLI. This means that in half the cases there is no other family history of SLI; the affected child is the only child with SLI. In the other half of the families with at least one child with SLI, at least two other members also were affected. Together, the authors reported an affectance rate of 32 percent. Therefore, results of several studies suggest that in about half the number of cases, the influence of genetic factors may be inferred, whereas in roughly the same number of cases, such an influence cannot be inferred.

Pedigree studies. Pedigree studies are similar to family studies, but the investigation extends back several generations of a proband. Researchers examine as many members of a proband's family as they possibly can, looking for patterns of characteristics that may be inherited. To date, the data available from pedigree studies of SLI come from a single family which has been followed by several investigators (Crago & Gopnik, 1994; Gopnik & Crago, 1991; Vargha-Kadem et al., 1995). Four generations of what has been called the KE family have been studied. Approximately half of the 30 family members have been described as having a severe form of speech and language disorder, sometimes giving the impression that the disorder is SLI.

Although the speech and language disorder found in the KE family may have a genetic basis, further investigation of the affected family members has raised questions about

> Individuals who are diagnosed with apraxia or developmental disability do not have a *specific* language impairment (SLI).

the validity of the diagnosis of SLI. The affected KE family members were found to have several accompanying deficits, most notably a profound articulation disorder that persists into adulthood. These family members exhibited severe difficulties in imitating sequenced orofacial movements (e.g., "close your lips, open your mouth wide, and stick out your tongue"). These difficulties were thought to be symptomatic of a praxic deficit, or apraxia, a difficulty in planning and executing movement. It was also found that six of the affected family members had IQ scores below 85, an intellectual deficit that precluded the diagnosis of a specific language impairment (Vargha-Khadem et al., 1995).

In a subsequent study of the KE family, Watkins, Dronkers, and Vargha-Kadem (2002) described a profile or phenotype of affected family members and existence of a core deficit. Using a variety of linguistic and nonlinguistic tasks, the authors compared the performance of three groups of subjects: (1) affected KE family members, (2) unaffected KE family members, and (3) a group of adult patients with aphasia associated with cerebral vascular accidents (strokes). The results were that deficits in speech and language profiles of the affected KE family members were similar to those of the adult patients with aphasia. Affected family members had severe orofacial apraxia and speech impairments, not typical of children with SLI. The results further revealed that affected and unaffected KE family members could be distinguished from each other on the basis of one test alone—a test of repetition of simple and complex nonwords (e.g., *rubid, hampent*). Those with language problems could not imitate nonwords as well as those with normal language skills. This finding was consistent with past research indicating that difficulties with nonword repetition may be clinically useful in diagnosing SLI (Bishop, North, & Donlon, 1996; Gathercole et al., 1994), although other multiple language deficiencies do just fine in diagnosing SLI. In any case, the suggestions that the affected members of the KE family have SLI and that that their disorder suggests a genetic basis for SLI seem inappropriate.

Twin studies. Twins, especially identical twins, have been a special target of population genetic studies. Both identical and fraternal twins may be studied to determine the concordance rate, which is the rate at which a clinical condition, found in one member of a pair, is also found in the other member of the same pair. Identical twins share the same genes whereas fraternal twins share the genes to the same extent as ordinary siblings. A higher concordance rate in identical twin pairs than in fraternal twin pairs is suggestive of a genetic basis for the clinical condition. There have been a few studies in which results have indicated a higher concordance rate for language impairment among identical twin pairs compared to fraternal twin pairs (Bishop, North, & Donlan, 1995; Tomblin & Buckwalter, 1998; Viding et al., 2004).

> In twin studies, what suggests a genetic basis for a disorder?

Until one or more genes and mechanisms of their inheritance are identified through molecular genetic research, concordance and discordance twin rates for SLI are open to opposing interpretations. Twins, especially identical twins, share more similar environments and parental reactions than ordinary siblings. A study has demonstrated that when language and cognitive skills are measured, environmental similarity for monozygotic as well as dizygotic twins is more than twice as large as it is for non-twin siblings (Koeppen-Schomerus, Spinath, & Plomin, 2003). Therefore, monozygotic twins who share genes also share a more similar environment than ordinary siblings, a fact usually overlooked in twin research. Unless twins who are reared apart are studied, environmental influences are not ruled out.

Molecular genetic studies. The genetic studies reviewed so far have all used the methods of population genetics, which analyze differential prevalence rates in different strata of society. In contrast, molecular genetic studies that seek to identify an abnormal gene or gene sequence in children with SLI are limited. A few investigations have suggested that a specific gene, FOXP2 (forkhead box P2) on human chromosome 7q31 may be involved in a specific locus of the brain (Enard et al., 2002; Fisher et al., 1998; Lai et al., 2001). However, this gene locus has been identified in the previously described KE family members with language disorders. As noted earlier, their language disorders do not resemble the pattern of deficiencies found in children with SLI. It is more likely that FOXP2 is involved in severe cases of verbal apraxia than SLI. For this and other reasons, several investigators have questioned the claim that FOXP2 is involved in SLI (Meaburn et al., 2002; Newbury et al., and the International Molecular Genetic Study of Autism Consortium, 2002; Newbury & Monaco, 2002). After a thorough analysis of children with SLI and a chromosomal analysis of FOXP2, Newbury and associates concluded that the gene was unlikely to be involved in SLI. Meaburn et al. (2002) made a genetic analysis of FOXP2 in 270 children with language disorders. Although the study was not restricted to children with SLI, their results showed no sign of FOXP2 mutation in any of the 270 children with language disorders. In essence, no particular gene that causes SLI has been isolated, although genetic abnormalities in the regions adjacent to FOXP2 may be observed (O'Brien et al., 2003). See Box 3.2 for more regarding FOXP2, the "talking gene."

Two molecular genetic studies reported in 2002 have suggested other potential genes linked to SLI (Bartlett et al., 2002; the SLI consortium, 2002). Both the studies selected participants who had SLI and obtained blood or buccal-swab samples (a sample of saliva) to make DNA analysis. The first study, reported by the SLI Consortium (2002) identified one genetic susceptibility loci on chromosome 16 and another on chromosome 19. The second study, reported by Bartlett et al. (2002), identified a susceptibility locus on chromosome 13. It should be noted that neither study replicated the results of the other. Even though molecular genetic studies sequence the genes, the different and complex statistical analyses used in identifying gene loci may result in divergent findings across studies. Until gene loci are replicated in multiple studies with different statistical analyses, the conclusions of molecular genetic studies remain tentative.

---

box 3.2   The Story of Talking Genes

Between 1998 and 2001 a group of scientists (Fisher et al, 1998; Lai et al., 2001) reported several molecular genetic studies in which the authors described a gene they called SPCH1 (speech gene). Located on the long arm of chromosome 7q, the gene was found to be mutated in 27 members of a family in Britain (the KE family) who have been a subject of much research because of their severe speech and language impairment. Later the SPCH1 was renamed FOXP2 because of the presence of a forkhead box (winged-helix) domain within the gene. Media picked up the story of SPCH1 and hailed it as the discovery of a "talking gene." Soon, the FOXP2 came to be cited as the genetic basis of SLI and autism as well. The gene was also thought to be responsible for normal language acquisition. These claims have always been questionable because the members of the KE family did not meet the criteria for SLI as they also have severe articulation problems along with oral apraxia; some members even have IQs in the below-average range. Molecular genetic studies of persons with autism did not find mutated FOXP2 in them.

Even if the FOXP2 abnormalities cause severe speech and language problems, it does not follow that the gene is responsible for normal language acquisition.

In subsequent years, genetic studies of children with SLI have suggested that gene abnormalities on chromosomes 2p, 13q, 16q, and 19q may be involved. These studies showed no linkage to chromosome 7q and the FOXP2, again contradicting its importance for SLI. Because abnormalities on 2p, 13q, 16q, and 19q have not been replicated, one cannot be sure that they are related to SLI in children. Clinicians need to watch for further research on these and other gene loci.

Reports of genetic investigation of SLI often do not make a clear distinction between SLI and other forms of speech and language impairment. Conclusions that may apply only to other clinical groups are often overgeneralized to children with SLI—a very troubling trend among some genetic researchers. Currently, the precise genetic basis of SLI or normal language acquisition is unclear.

The available molecular genetic evidence explains neither SLI nor normal language acquisition. Single gene abnormalities, such as the FOXP2 mutation, may explain simple phenotypic disorders of the kind found in the KE family. Note that the severity of a disorder does not necessarily make it genetically complex; many single genes are known to cause severe and rare disorders. To the contrary, SLI is a more common and a more complex disorder. Multiple genes that may interact with each other and with environmental factors cause common and complex disorders (Meaburn et al., 2002; Newbury & Monaco, 2002). Each of the many genes may produce only a small effect, and the effects may vary across genes, thus making the identification of defective genes more difficult than those that are mutated. As Meaburn et al. (2002) and Newbury and Monaco (2002) noted, the influence of multiple gene-environmental interactions produce disorders that vary quantitatively. That the language skills of children with SLI quantitatively differ from those of normally developing children is a reasonable characterization. That characterization also is consistent with the view of multiple gene-environmental interaction hypothesis of SLI causation.

Potential Neuroanatomic Factors

Some studies suggest that language-relevant areas of the brain in children with SLI may be structurally different from the corresponding areas of the brain in children with normal language skills. Generally, the perisylvian areas of the brain in the dominant hemisphere (structures surrounding the Sylvian fissure), and more particularly Broca's and Wernicke's areas, are involved in language production, formulation, and comprehension. The perisylvian language areas are illustrated in Figure 3.1. Studies that investigate differences in brain

figure 3.1   The Perisylvian Language Areas of the Brain

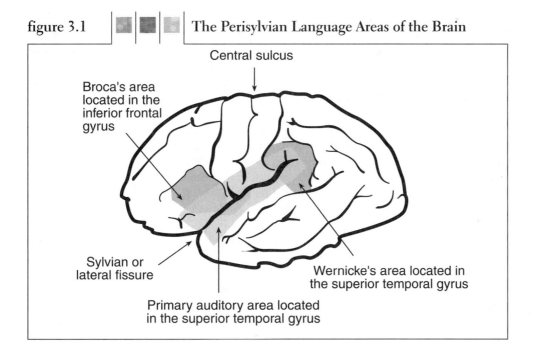

structures, known as brain morphologic studies, have mostly been done with adults with various kinds of disorders, including language disorders (Gauger, Lombardino, & Leonard, 1997; Leonard, 1998). A majority of studies conducted analyzed brain structures of adults and children with reading problems. The results, while bearing some relevance to SLI, cannot be considered direct evidence of a neurological basis for SLI. A few brain morphologic studies have involved children with SLI, however.

The left hemisphere is dominant for language in 95 percent of right-handed and up to 70 percent of the left-handed individuals. Consequently, in most people, the left perisylvian structures are slightly larger than the corresponding structures in the right hemisphere. A few studies have suggested that this is not true for children and adults with language disorders. A few studies have reported that the size of the left perisylvian region, instead of being slightly larger, may be the same as in the right hemisphere, or may even be slightly smaller in children with SLI (Gauger, Lombardino, & Leonard, 1997; Plante, et al., 1991). In addition, some children with SLI may have an extra sulcus in Broca's area, a structure not found in children and adults without SLI (Gauger, Lombardino, & Leonard, 1997). Such anomalous brain structures are described as atypical asymmetry or atypical configurations of the left and right hemispheres. Hugdahl et al. (2004) found decreased brain activation in the temporal and frontal lobes of five family members with SLI compared to a control group of six who listened to various language stimuli, including series of vowel sounds, pseudo words, and real words. The researchers concluded that these findings suggested a "functional counterpart to the structural anomalies previously reported in families with SLI" (Hugdahl et al., 2004, p. 169).

Are language disorders in children invariably associated with atypical configurations of the left and right perisylvian structures? Conversely, do typical (normal) configurations of the relevant hemispheric structures assure normal language? The answer to both the questions seems to be *no* (Plante, 1991). Some children who have atypical configurations may not have SLI. Some children who have normal language skills may have atypical configurations (larger right than the left perisylvian regions). In fact, the classic Geschwind and Levitsky (1968) study demonstrated that in nearly a quarter of normally functioning individuals, the left structures may not be larger than the right.

The meaning of brain morphologic deviations is not entirely clear, because the association of such deviations and language disorders is not consistent and is open to alternative interpretations. A typical explanation is that the atypical brain structures cause language delay. However, this is too strong a claim and too simplistic a theory. Evidence does not unequivocally support such a strong claim. Neurobiological research shows that strong environmental stimulations can promote neural growth in the brain. The possibility that a poor environmental stimulation for language skills may limit the development of connecting fibers in the brain, thus resulting in smaller perisylvian regions in the left hemisphere, has been recognized (Gauger, Lombardino, & Leonard, 1997). Therefore, atypical brain configurations may be the cause or the consequence of poor language skills. Similarly, reduced activation in certain regions of the brains of children with SLI may be a result of their poor language skills, not a cause of it.

Regardless of precise interpretations of genetic and brain morphologic findings in children with SLI, it is likely that a genetic basis may contribute to the impairment in some children. Equally likely is that without an explicit genetic basis, children can develop SLI, although future research may uncover a hitherto unknown genetic basis. Based on the available evidence, the presence of a genetic predisposition to develop SLI is a plausible hypothesis. This genetic predisposition, when combined with certain unfavorable environmental conditions, may lead to SLI.

Potential Environmental Factors

Even when a clinical condition is known to have a specific genetic abnormality, the influence of environmental factors that may combine with genetic factors to produce the condition cannot be ruled out. Indeed, the hypothesis that life events, including parent–child verbal interactions, affect the quality and quantity of language children learn and produce is beyond doubt (Hart & Risley, 1995, 1999; Moerk, 1983, 1992, 2000). However, to what extent such events play a role in the overall causation of SLI (or any other type of language disorders in children) is unclear. If clearly established, environmental factors afford a chance to treat language disorders more effectively than equally clearly demonstrated genetic factors. Several lines of research have been pursued to find out if children who develop SLI are exposed to language that is in some measure poor, inadequate, or inhibitive. Obviously, if language addressed to some children is indeed deficient, modifying it would be the primary target in treating and preventing SLI in children.

Investigation of verbal interactions. To evaluate whether verbal interactions between a child with SLI and a conversational partner are deficient in some way, researchers have arranged verbal interactions between children with SLI and their parents, siblings, peers, or unrelated adults. In many studies, verbal interactions between children with normal language skills and their parents provided a basis for comparison. In some studies, children with and without SLI were matched for chronological age; in other studies, the children were matched for language age.

Several verbal interactional variables have been of special interest to researchers. While the comparison children are those with normal language skills, the target children were those with SLI. Using both the groups of children and a variety of conversational partners (parents, unrelated adults, siblings, and peers) investigators have analyzed, among several other variables:

- The complexity of language addressed to children, measured in terms of mean length of utterance (MLU) or overall grammatic simplicity and variety
- Communication style used by partners (e.g., more or less directive)
- Frequency with which the partners initiate interaction
- Children's responsiveness to a partner's attempt to initiate communication
- Frequency with which children initiate communication
- Partner response to child initiations
- The frequency with which both the children and partners ask or answer questions
- Frequency of repeated speech addressed to children
- Eye gaze or eye contact during conversation
- Prosodic characteristics of speech addressed to children
- Partners' use of recast of sentences in which the adult changes a child production into a different form as illustrated later

The results of several studies are somewhat contradictory. The reasons for this contradiction include varied methods of investigation. More importantly, the contradictions may stem from the sheer number of somewhat poorly defined and subjectively measured variables. In one study, 70 measures were examined (Cross, 1981). Despite the contradictions, results of many studies suggest that conversational partners of children with SLI do not speak in such deficient ways as to possibly cause the language disorder (Leonard, 1998).

A few consistent findings have emerged, however. When compared to groups of mothers whose children have normal language skills, mothers of children with SLI:

- Interacted with their children less, shouted or threatened their children more, and were less likely to reason with their children (Wulbert et al., 1975)
- Were more directive and more likely to interrupt their children's play with demands (Siegel, Cunningham, & van der Spuy, 1979)
- Asked their children fewer questions (Cunningham et al., 1985)
- Used shorter, less complex utterances when speaking to their children (Bondurant, Romeo, & Kretschmer, 1983)
- Showed less prosodic variation when speaking to their children
- Used fewer recasts of their children's utterances. In recast, a child's telegraphic utterance (e.g., "want ball") is recast in a grammatic but different form (e.g., "Where is the ball?") (Conti-Ramsden, 1990; Nelson et al., 1995)

It is questionable whether the noted differences in the language addressed to children with SLI, compared to that addressed to normally developing children, are causes of the disorder. Most of the differences may be due to the disorder itself. For instance, the mothers who tended to shout at their children explained their action based on the child's unresponsiveness (Wulbert et al., 1975). More directive interactional style may have been necessary to regulate verbally deficient responsiveness. The parents' use of shorter and simpler sentences may have been reinforced because the child could respond only to such sentences. In essence, many changes seen in the speech of persons who interact with children who have limited language skills may be a way of adjusting to child's level of verbal competence. In other words, changes may be consequences, not causes, of the child's SLI.

> Caution is needed in claiming a cause–effect relation among two variables that have been shown to coexist. Even if a cause–effect relation exists, it is difficult to determine which is the effect and which is the cause.

Investigations of socioeconomic status.   There is some evidence that low socioeconomic status (SES) may offer limited opportunities to learn language skills. Low SES is correlated with poor language and literacy skills in children, as described in Chapter 10.

Low socioeconomic status of children tends to be associated with low education of parents. A portion of those who have low SES *and* limited education also may be lower in general intellectual skills. These factors may interact with the need for both the parents to work outside the home to provide for basic necessities. The parents in low SES may not talk as much to the children, and their talk may be vastly truncated and limited to meeting basic needs. The children may not be exposed to advanced spoken language. Reading and writing at home may be limited as well, and consequently, the child's language learning may suffer. Although this line of argument seems reasonable, hard empirical evidence linking SLI to low SES is lacking.

A longitudinal family study, although not involving children with SLI, has produced descriptive evidence on the relation between SES and language learning in general. Conducted by Hart and Risley (1995), the study involved systematic observation of 42 children in families divided into three SES groups: welfare, working-class, and professional. Over a period of 30 months, the researchers visited the homes once a month. "Fading into the furniture" (Hart & Risley, 1995, p. 35), the researchers observed each child's verbal interactions with his or her family. Using an elaborate coding system, the researchers recorded each communicative interaction within the household that involved the child. The resulting data revealed a direct relation between the size of the children's vocabularies at age 3 and the socioeconomic status (SES) of their homes: the lower the SES, the smaller the size of the vocabulary, and, conversely, the higher the SES, the larger the size of the vocabulary. On the average, by the age of 3, children in professional households produced 1,100 words, children in working-class households produced 700 words, and children of welfare households produced only 500 words. Further analysis of the data revealed two major differences across the three SES groups: (1) the amount parents talked to their children in general, and (2) the number of encouraging versus discouraging statements adults directed toward their children.

> What were two major differences across the three SES groups investigated by Hart & Risley (1995)?

First, the adults in the professional households simply talked *more* than did parents in other households. A linear extrapolation of the data revealed that, in a 5,200-hour year, the children in the professional families would hear 11 million spoken words, the children in the working-class families would hear 6 million words, and the children in the welfare families would hear 3 million words. Also, the utterances of the professional parents were "not only greater in amount but also richer in certain quality features" (Hart & Risley, 1995, p. 124). The professional parents used a greater variety of grammatic structures and parts of speech in their utterances, including nouns, modifiers, past-tense verbs, auxiliary-fronted yes/no questions, declarative sentences, and affirmative statements.

Second, the parents in the three SES levels differed in the number of affirmative, encouraging statements as compared to the number of prohibitive or discouraging statements directed to the children. On average, the children in the professional households received 32 affirmative and 5 prohibitive statements an hour, for a ratio of approximately 6 encouraging statements to 1 discouraging statement. Working-class children received an average of 12 affirmative and 7 prohibitive statements per hour, for a ratio of approximately 2 encouraging statements to 1 discouraging statement. Welfare children received an average of 5 affirmative and 11 prohibitive statements per hour, for a ratio of approximately 1 encouraging to 2 discouraging statements. Extrapolating the data to the first 4 years of life indicated that children growing up in professional households would have received 560,000 more instances of encouraging than discouraging feedback, children growing up in working-class households would have received 100,000 more instances of encouraging than discouraging feedback, and children growing up in welfare households would have received 125,000 more instances of discouraging than encouraging feedback.

The Hart and Risley (1995) study is monumental in that it involved a longitudinal study of a large number of children and their families. The study, however, was designed to understand everyday interactions of typical parents and their children within the selected socioeconomic groups; it was not designed to analyze potential factors related to language disabilities of any kind. While the study has important implications for parents who wish to accelerate language in their children and clinicians who plan to design home enrichment programs, it makes no claims about potential factors that could lead to language disabilities. The authors have repeatedly stated in their work that, despite the differences in the quality and quantity of talking in the home, all children were competent talkers by age 3 (Hart & Risley, 1995, 1999). Although all children's language skills were within normal variations, an important observation was that the children talked mostly like their parents.

Based on Hart and Risley's (1995) initial study and further analysis (Hart & Risley, 1999), some admittedly speculative statements can be made. Their robust observation is that parents talk to their children with vastly different quantity and quality of their speech. Nonetheless, all 42 children learned to talk normally. The authors emphasized that no special method of talking or instruction is needed for normal language acquisition. Compared to the working-class and professional parents, parents who were receiving welfare displayed language that was least in quantity and variety. Nonetheless, their children also learned normally competent language. What the study did not identify, however, is the critical core verbal interaction that is needed for normal language acquisition, as this was not the authors' purpose. What if the verbal interaction falls below that critical core necessary to learn language? What if that critical core level is higher for some children who may have a genetic susceptibility to developing SLI? In other words, what if some children need more or different interactions than needed to normally learn language? Is the need for special interactions limited to children with genetic susceptibilities? Or, is the need also based on some other environmental factors? Research designed to answer these questions can be expected to find potential environmental factors related to SLI and other forms of language disorders in children.

Is SLI Truly Specific to Language?

We have noted earlier that SLI is now a generally accepted diagnostic category in the United States and elsewhere. By definition, the diagnosis is made when no other deficits are associated with it or apparently seem to explain it. Nonetheless, the diagnosis has not stopped investigators from asking troubling questions about it, as it should not have. In spite of general acceptance, investigators have wondered whether or not SLI is a valid diagnostic category. Many researchers have questioned the basic premise that children with SLI are free from other deficits. Some researchers suggest that children with SLI almost always have related problems that preclude a diagnosis of a disorder that is specific to language. Although not at all conclusively, researchers have suggested that children with SLI may have difficulties with many types of tasks that are presumably based on cognitive skills and sensory functions.

Possible Cognitive Deficits in Children with SLI

Several cognitive skills of children with SLI have been investigated. These variables include complex reasoning tasks, presumed information processing skills, interpreting rapidly sequenced auditory or visual stimuli, haptic (touch) perception, attentional deficits, tendency toward hyperactivity, and symbolic play activities. On most variables studied, the results are inconsistent and interpretation of positive findings is controversial.

Difficulties with complex reasoning tasks. In studies designed to test reasoning skills using visual–spatial skills, children with SLI performed more poorly than did children in normal comparison groups. Tasks tested have included asking the children to predict where the water level would be in a container tilted at various angles, to select objects that match forms as seen from different orientations, and to tell whether shapes presented at different rotations were the same or different (Camarata, Newhoff, & Rugg, 1981; Johnston & Ellis Weismer, 1983). In all cases, children with SLI either did not answer correctly as often as control group children, or they answered correctly but at significantly slower response rates.

Deficits in information processing skills. Some investigators have suggested that perhaps children with SLI process various information more slowly than those with normal language skills. This slowness may be limited to linguistic tasks or may extend to both linguistic and nonlinguistic tasks. Kail (1994), for instance, proposed the generalized slowing hypothesis, which stated that the underlying cause of SLI is a slower rate of response when various kinds of linguistic, visual, and spatial information is presented with a view to evoke responses. Miller et al. (2001) suggested that a task such as picture naming "involves (minimally) the recognition of the picture, the retrieval of the name of the picture, the formulation of this name, and the actual production of the name" (p. 417). For each one of those processes, children with SLI are presumed to be proportionally slower than those with normal language skills. In addition, children with SLI are presumed to be slower in processing nonverbal information as well.

> What is the hypothesis that SLI is caused by a slower rate of response when linguistic, visual, and spatial information is presented called?

Most studies on information processing measure the response time (RT) of children with and without SLI. In some studies, RT of children with nonspecific language impairment has been included for comparison with the other two groups of children. A wide variety of verbal (linguistic) and nonverbal tasks have been presented to measure the children's RT. To measure verbal RT, children have been asked to name pictures, determine whether or not a picture matches a sentence heard, remember and describe a sequence of pictures just shown, make judgments about the syntactic correctness of sentences, identify rhyming words, judge whether two words begin with the same or different sound, and so forth. To measure nonverbal RT, children have been asked to match pictures, remember and recite a sequence of digits just presented orally, tap keys as rapidly as possible for a short duration, strike a key in response to a stimulus, strike a key if a target stimulus (e.g., a geometric shape) is present among an array of stimuli, strike one key if a rotated nonsense figure is the same as the target and another key if the two stimuli are mirror images, strike a key in response to an auditory tone, move pegs, thread beads, and so forth (Kail, 1994; Miller et al., 2001; Montgomery & Leonard, 1998; Windsor & Hwang, 1999; Windsor et al., 2001).

The results of RT studies have shown that generally, children with SLI are slower than those without SLI. The slowness has been documented in both verbal and nonverbal RT. Furthermore, children with nonspecific language disorders also have been shown to be slower compared to children with normal language skills. The degree of slowness found in children with SLI varies across studies. The variability may partly be due to differences in measuring RT and in the different methods of statistical analysis of raw data. Some studies and methods of analyses suggest that the RT of children with SLI is about 30 percent slower than the RT of children without language impairment, while other studies and different methods of analyses show about 10 percent slowness. It has even been shown that a newer statistical model called hierarchical linear modeling analysis of published data may not reveal any significant generalized slowness in children with language impairment

(Windsor et al., 2001). In essence, there is just too much variability in RT across children and studies to strongly support a generalized slowing.

In contrast to generalized slowing in information processing, some researchers have hypothesized specific forms of slowed or defective information processing. One such popular hypothesis is the temporal processing deficit proposed by Tallal et al. (Tallal, 1999; Tallal, Stark, & Mellits, 1985). The hypothesis states that children with SLI have difficulty perceiving stimuli that are presented rapidly and executing tasks that require rapidity. The children, according to the hypothesis, cannot process stimuli that are presented at relatively fast rates, hence the temporal processing deficit. Based on a complex statistical analysis called stepwise discriminant function analysis, Tallal et al. (1985) claimed that variables that measure temporal processing can correctly classify 98 percent of children with and without SLI. They described six temporal processing variables: (1) rapid production of multisyllabic words, (2) tactile discrimination (identification of two touches on two fingers), (3) discrimination of computer-synthesized syllables /ba/ versus /da/, (4) discrimination of tone versus light stimuli, (5) sequencing the letters *e* and *k*, and (6) locating touch stimuli presented to either cheeks or hands. In each case, stimuli that were presented more rapidly were difficult to perceive or produce, whereas those that were presented more slowly did not cause difficulty for children with SLI. Presumably, two variables involved tactile discrimination, two involved speech, and one involved auditory and visual stimuli. Several other studies have demonstrated that children with SLI have difficulty processing rapidly sequenced auditory or visual stimuli (see Tallal, 1999, and Leonard, 1998, for reviews of studies).

Temporal processing difficulties only mean that the children have difficulty responding accurately and promptly. Why they have such a difficulty is not evident from the data. The data that show such difficulty do not automatically mean that the difficulty is due to an auditory processing deficit. The six performance variables that Tallal (1985) describes may involve skills other than auditory processing. As pointed out by Segalowitz (2000), it is difficult to separate the effects of such other variables as "attention, working memory, distractibility, stimulus familiarity, general processing speed, and so on from specific measures" (p. 342). Interestingly, three of the six variables that Tallal et al. studied involve speech. It is not surprising that those variables distinguish children with and without SLI. Based on statistical stimulation experiments, Zhang and Tomblin (1998) also have questioned the validity of the temporal processing theory of SLI.

> Speech-language pathologists should diagnose and treat receptive language disorders. Audiologists diagnose auditory processing disorders. These are rare, and are usually the result of traumatic brain injury or stroke.

The hypothesis of temporal processing deficit has led to a commercial treatment program for children with SLI. This is a well-publicized, popularized computer program called Fast ForWord, which consists of a series of video-game-like exercises designed to slow down auditory input and then increase the rate of presentation in small increments until the child perceives auditory input presented at a normal rate (Scientific Learning Corporation, 1998). Children who have participated in this program, available only under the supervision of those who have gone through training provided by the authors, have reportedly made remarkable gains in their scores on language comprehension tests. Such claims were made on the basis of two pilot studies in which small groups of children (7 in one study and 22 in the other) were given Fast ForWord training daily for 1 month, 3 hours a day during weekdays, and 1–2 hours of "homework" during the weekends (Merzenich et al., 1996; Tallal et al., 1996). In the first study (Merzenich et al., 1996), an uncontrolled pretest–posttest design, using a variety of measures of receptive language, was used. Posttest measures showed average gains in receptive language and language comprehension equivalent to 2 years, with each child either approaching or exceeding normal limits for his or her age. Children in the second, larger study (Tallal et al., 1996) were divided into two groups, with one group receiving the computerized game training without acoustically modified speech and the other receiving the training with acoustically modified speech. Greater gains were reported for the group receiving training with acoustically or temporally modified speech (Merzenich et al., 1996; Tallal et al., 1996).

News of such significant gains made in receptive language was greeted with great enthusiasm by parents and educators, and Fast ForWord became a highly sought-after treatment for children with so-called "auditory processing disorders." However, no control groups were included in either of the pilot studies, and the research of Tallal and her colleagues has not been replicated by others. Furthermore, case studies and a limited amount of experimental research with control groups have shown gains that are far less impressive than those reported in the pilot studies (Friel-Patti, Desarres, & Thibodeau, 2001; Loeb, Stoke, & Fey, 2001; Rouse & Krueger, 2004; Troia & Whitney, 2003). There is also some evidence that there is nothing unique about the effects of the Fast ForWord program; what little effect may occur is the same effect that can be realized using other software programs (Gillam et al., 2001). Furthermore, the intensity of treatment may partly be responsible for some of the effects reported. Even if the treatment is offered only for one month, 3 hours of daily practice and 1–2 hours of weekend practice are much more intensive than any traditional (and effective) treatment offered twice weekly for about 30 minutes each. Therefore, claims of remarkable progress in receptive language skills resulting from Fast ForWord training should be interpreted with caution (Gillam, 1999; Gillam, Loeb, & Friel-Patti, 2001).

> Refer to the hierarchy of scientific evidence recommended in Chapter 4. At what level would you place evidence supporting the efficacy of the Fast ForWord program?

No clinically significant improvement has been demonstrated in expressive language skills as a result of Fast ForWord training, although some researchers have reported limited positive change in oral language immediately following treatment (Rouse & Krueger, in press; Troia & Whitney, 2003). Results of one longitudinal study also reported gains in oral language after treatment, but the gains were not maintained over a period of two years (Hook, Macaruso, & Jones, 2003).

Deficits in memory skills. Based on the assumption that memory skills are part of cognitive skills and share common properties with information processing, investigators have wondered whether children with SLI have memory deficits that negatively affect language learning. Hypothesized memory deficits may be generalized to all tasks that require learning and remembering or may be limited to verbal learning. Most investigators have investigated memory as it relates to verbal learning and remembering (Montgomery, 2002; van der Lely, 1993). Various kinds of short-term verbal memory skills examined include word recall, sentence comprehension, number recall, and recall of rote mathematical facts (Fazio, 1996; Gillam, Cowan, & Marler, 1998; Hoffman & Gillam, 2004; Montgomery, 2002; Weismer, Evans, & Hesketh, 1999). Typically, investigators have compared the performance of children with SLI (clinical group) with that of normally language-learning children (control group). The results of verbal memory investigations have been somewhat inconsistent. Short-term memory deficits are more likely to emerge in the clinical group when the clinical and the control groups are age-matched than when they are language skill-matched. Results have shown that children with SLI do not have impaired memory for single words; they are more likely to have difficulty recalling sentences in which meaning is dependent on word order.

Another task that has received much attention is nonword repetition, a task in which children are required to repeat nonsense words (e.g., /naib/, /tervak/). There is some evidence that typically developing young children's performance on nonword repetition tasks improves as they grow older, suggesting that such tasks may be valuable assessment tools for the early identification of SLI (Roy & Chiat, 2004). Several studies have shown that children with SLI have difficulty with this task (Bishop, North, & Donlan, 1996; Dollaghan & Campbell, 1998; Edwards & Lahey, 1998; Ellis Weismer et al., 2000; Gathercole & Baddeley, 1990). However, even this generally accepted finding is not without contrary evidence. Some children may repeat nonwords somewhat poorly but not to any great extent when they are matched with language-age children (van der Lely & Howard, 1993).

The meaning of verbal short-term memory deficits found in children with SLI is not entirely clear. Some investigators believe that memory deficits may be a cause of SLI (Gathercole & Baddeley, 1990; Montgomery, 2002). Because of their deficient short-term verbal memory skills, some children fail to learn language normally because they do not remember the earlier part of a sentence by the time they hear the later parts of it. Thus, the language input is not complete or processed inadequately, causing their language problem (Montgomery, 2002). Unfortunately, such explanations simply rephrase the problem to be explained: children have language problems because they forget parts of language spoken to them. Such forgetting, if present, is a part of their language problem, not an explanation of that problem. Moreover, short-term verbal memory problems are *inferred* from language problems. Inferences derived from a problem—especially when the inferred entity is measured only as a component of the problem—can hardly constitute an explanation.

Problems in haptic (touch) perception. On a haptic recognition task, Kamhi (1981) compared the performance of children with language disorders to that of normally language-learning children. The children were made to "blindly" feel geometric shapes and then were asked to point to a drawing of a corresponding shape. Results of the study indicated that language-impaired children performed significantly poorer than typically developing children matched for mental age. These results were replicated in a further study (Kamhi et al., 1984). Because success on the task was presumed by the researchers to be dependent upon "the child's ability to generate and interpret a symbolic representation of an unseen object," the poor performance of language-impaired children was interpreted to be an indication of their poor "symbolic representational ability" (p. 172). This "symbolic representational deficit" was described as being at least in part responsible for the children's language difficulties (p. 175). Again, even if deficits in haptic perception were replicated across studies done in different settings, such a finding would at most indicate that such deficits were *part* of the difficulties children with SLI experience, not a *cause* of SLI.

> The treatment implications of haptic perception deficits are unclear. Should clinicians treat haptic perception deficits? Probably not. Nothing will effectively replace direct language training for children with SLI. The same comment could be made about other presumed underlying "causes" or deficits discussed in this section.

Attentional deficits and hyperactivity. Whether children with SLI have problems in sustaining attention to various stimuli and whether the children are also prone to hyperactivity have been investigated. Researchers conducting descriptive studies have concluded that language disorders and psychiatric disorders, most commonly attention deficit hyperactivity disorder (ADHD), often coexist (Cohen et al., 1998; Love & Thompson, 1988; Oram et al., 1999; Tirosh & Cohen, 1998; Vallance, Im, & Cohen, 1999). These studies, however, were not exclusively concerned with SLI or ADHD. Some investigators included children with speech and fluency disorders as well as those with other psychiatric disorders. Furthermore, rates of comorbidity (coexistence of two or more disorders) were established through assessing groups of children who had either been diagnosed with ADHD, some other psychiatric disorder, or who had been referred for consideration of such a diagnosis. The resulting comorbidity rates were for speech disorders, language disorders in general (not necessarily SLI), or both with ADHD or some other psychiatric disorder. Therefore, currently, the precise nature of the relationship between SLI and ADHD remains unclear.

The DSM-IV-R (APA, 2000) diagnostic criteria for ADHD include descriptions of several behaviors that are also diagnostic of pragmatic and receptive language problems (see Table 3.2). Therefore, it is understandable that children with ADHD will often present with language problems as well. Because there is a possibility children with ADHD may also have undiagnosed difficulties with language, it has been suggested that a child receiving the diagnosis of ADHD should be routinely assessed for language impairment (Camarata & Gibson, 1999; Cohen et al., 1998; Tirosh & Cohen, 1998).

Symbolic play activity. By 18 months of age, children begin to engage in **symbolic play.** In symbolic play, a child uses one object during play to represent another. A child who pretends that a shoe is a telephone and uses it to chat to imaginary friends or tucks a doll into a shoe box that serves as a bed demonstrates symbolic play. Much has been made of this

 table 3.2

Overlap in Diagnostic Criteria for ADHD and Disorders in Pragmatic Language Skills and Receptive Language

The diagnostic criteria for attention deficit hyperactivity disorder (ADHD) as set forth in the DSM-IV-TR overlap with diagnostic criteria for the diagnosis of pragmatic and receptive language disorders (LD). The following is a summary of those overlapping criteria.

DSM-IV-R Criterion for ADHD That Overlap with Symptoms of Pragmatic or Receptive LD or Both	Symptomatic of Pragmatic LD	Symptomatic of Receptive LD
Has difficulty sustaining attention in tasks or play activities	Yes	Yes
Does not seem to listen when spoken to directly	Yes	Yes
Easily distracted by extraneous stimuli		Yes
Leaves seat in classroom or in other situations in which remaining seated is expected	Yes	
Talks excessively	Yes	
Blurts out answers before questions have been completed	Yes	
Has difficulty awaiting turn	Yes	
Interrupts or intrudes on others (e.g., butts into conversations or games)	Yes	

stage of child development. It is thought to be critically important to development because language is said to represent objects, events, and experiences (Piaget, 1962; Vygotsky, 1967). A child who has difficulty learning language may then be expected to have difficulty in representing nonlinguistic concepts or experiences, as revealed in impaired symbolic play.

Several studies have made a comparative analysis of symbolic play activities of children with and without language disorders. Unfortunately, it is not clear from all the reports that investigators carefully selected children who had SLI and no other form of language or speech disorder. Casby's (1997) comprehensive review of studies on symbolic play of children with SLI and those of normally developing children shows that the results are inconsistent. While some studies show that children with SLI engage in fewer instances of symbolic play than control groups of typically developing children, other studies have not revealed significant differences. Furthermore, differences found between children with and without SLI in symbolic play have been small. Documented differences may also be due partly to the communication deficits of children with SLI. Limited language skills that negatively affect social interaction may also affect all kinds of interactive play. Verbal instructions were a part of all studies in which children were asked to engage in specific kinds of play, and some children with SLI have comprehension deficits that might affect their understanding of verbal instructions. Therefore, as Casby (1997) concluded, symbolic play deficits may not be significant enough to explain SLI. Even if symbolic play deficits are significant, their treatment implications are limited.

> Two-year-old Tommy rummages in a kitchen cupboard and finds a pot which he places on his head and gleefully shows his mother his "hat." This is an example of what type of play?

Theoretical implications of underlying deficits.   A large body of theoretical literature suggests that the causes of SLI lie in the underlying cognitive and sensory deficits. For instance, some theories claim that children's short-term memory problems, difficulties in processing rapidly presented auditory stimuli, generalized slowness in processing any kind of information, a particular difficulty in processing linguistic stimuli, potential attention deficit-hyperactivity, difficulty with symbolic activities, and so forth may be the cause or causes of SLI. Of these, difficulty in processing nonverbal auditory and linguistic information as the reason for the language disorder has received much attention in the literature (for a review of studies, see Leonard, 1998; Miller et al., 2001; Tallal et al., 1985; Windsor et al., 2001).

The hypotheses that information processing difficulties cause language learning problems in children have been advanced to explain difficulties in learning specific aspects of language (e.g., morphologic or syntactic features) or language in general. One variation of the hypothesis, previously mentioned in the context of morphologic problems, states that children with SLI cannot efficiently process language elements that are brief or rapidly presented. It may be recalled that children are more likely to have problems learning such brief or unstressed grammatic morphemes as the third person singular *-s*, possessive *-s*, past tense *-ed* inflection, and articles, than such morphemes as *-ing* which are longer in duration. Because the children cannot process speech stimuli that are brief, unstressed, or rapidly presented, they have difficulty learning morphologic elements of language. Other variations of the hypothesis—specifically the generalized slowing hypothesis described earlier—suggest that an overall slowness in processing information may account for all aspects of language learning problems.

The hypothesis that the children have some inherent problem processing either particular aspects of language (e.g., morphemes of brief or unstressed durations) or language input in general presents a serious logical problem. The information processing difficulty is inferred from the observed language difficulties that need to be explained. An explanation that is inferred from the phenomenon to be explained is based on circular reasoning: it repeatedly ends up where it starts. How do we know that children with SLI have information processing problems? Because they have language learning problems. Why do they have language learning problems? Because they have language processing problems. In essence, investigators assume that children with SLI have processing problems only because of morphologic, syntactic, or general language problems. Therefore, inferred processing problems do not explain the observed language problems.

> Circular explanations may sound impressive, but they are typically invalid. One problem, inferred from another, explains no problem.

Whether cognitive and information processing deficits, if they are consistently found in children with SLI, shed any light on their language difficulty is still an open question. As scientific explanations of language disorders, they mostly fall short because, in most cases, the relation between the processing difficulty on the one hand and language comprehension and production on the other are speculative. Furthermore, such explanations do not consider the possibility that all the associated problems discovered (e.g., verbal memory, attention deficit, information processing problems) may be a part of the problem being explained (language limitations). In other words, some children may have both a language disability and not readily apparent limitations in other intellectual tasks (such as responding efficiently to rapidly presented stimuli). Just because it was historically assumed that children with SLI do not have any other problems, and just because other more or less subtle problems were later found in them, does not mean that problems found later explain those that were described earlier.

Clinical implications of underlying deficits. As the research reviewed in the previous sections suggests, children with SLI may have various cognitive and sensory deficits. Short-term memory for verbal material, speed with which the children react to various kinds of stimuli, and discrimination between similar stimuli may all be deficient to some extent in at least some children with SLI.

Nonetheless, the clinical treatment implications of such deficits cannot be taken for granted. Such underlying, coexisting, or related deficits need not be the target of treatment. If a child receives treatment for increasing symbolic play skills, strengthening visual–spatial skills, improving memory skills, or speeding up presumed auditory processing skills, there is no guarantee that such treatment will, in fact, automatically improve the child's expressive language skills. No treatment research evidence shows that underlying deficit training (1) results in expressive language skills, (2) is necessary before one can train expressive language skills, or (3) makes direct language training more efficient than when the deficit training does not precede verbal expression training. All three kinds of evidence need to be produced before one can spend valuable language intervention time treating presumed underlying processes.

Prognosis for Children with SLI

Whether children with SLI improve on their own or whether they need treatment to achieve normal language skills is the question of prognosis. The prognostic question is somewhat complicated because it is often difficult to discern whether infants and toddlers have a specific language disorder or are "late bloomers" who are slow to talk.

A prognosis for any disorder varies depending on several variables, including prompt and effective treatment and associated clinical conditions. Generally speaking, if a problem disappeared or attenuated markedly by some age, it is less likely to persist with the same force later. For instance, some evidence suggests that 39 percent of children who have SLI at age 3 may still have SLI at age 7, but 41 percent of those who still had it at age 5 will continue to have it at age 7 (Silva, 1987; Silva, Williams, & McGee, 1987). A longitudinal study by Johnson et al. (1999) has reported that children with SLI have a better prognosis than those with language *and* other problems (e.g., developmental disability, autism, or hearing loss). Also, children whose SLI is associated with attentional deficit, hyperactivity, or both have a worse prognosis than those whose problems are restricted to language problems. Generally, children with only speech impairment may have a better prognosis than those with any kind of language impairment. Other studies have shown that children with only receptive or expressive language disorders have a better prognosis than those with both receptive *and* expressive difficulties (Silva, 1987). Furthermore, children with SLI make more rapid progress in learning new words than in learning grammatic features (Rescorla, Roberts, & Dahlsgaard, 1997).

Specific rates of recovery and persistence of language difficulties vary across studies and are not entirely trustworthy. Reportedly, language difficulties may persist in 20 percent to more than 60 percent of children with SLI (Beitchman et al., 1994; Bishop & Edmondson, 1987; Stark & Tallal, 1988). A 4-year follow-up study showed that 60 percent of 196 kindergarten children who were diagnosed with SLI during their kindergarten year still had persistent language problems when they were reevaluated 4 years later (Tomblin et al., 2003). While some investigators have made efforts to isolate the recovery and persistence rates in children who only have SLI, others have included children with all kinds of language disorders as well as speech disorders in their estimates. Most troubling is that many investigators who have made longitudinal studies of children to evaluate prognosis have failed to describe the presence, extent, and efficacy of language treatment. Investigators who initially diagnose language impairment in kindergarten children have visited them over a period of 4 to 7 years to establish that their language impairment is stable. Does it mean then that the children never received any treatment in their grade school years? Does it also mean that any treatment the children may have received was ineffective? Therefore, it is not clear whether improvement is due to treatment or natural course of events in the absence of professional help. A greater percentage of children who have received early and more effective treatment may recover than those whose treatment was delayed, ineffective, or both. If the children with SLI learn to produce new words faster than new grammatic morphemes, could it be that clinicians who treat those children concentrate on easier word teaching than more difficult grammatic skill teaching? We do not know. Similarly, could it be that persistence of SLI through the grade school years only reveals a failure of language treatment offered to school-age children? Answers to these questions have important social and clinical significance.

> What type of study follows participants over a considerable duration of time?

Understanding SLI: An Integrative Discussion

The classic definition of SLI is that it is not associated with one or more obvious clinical conditions that could cause (explain) the disorder. Research in recent decades has shown that the classic view is true only in a gross sense, but not in any subtle or specific sense. Children with SLI may indeed have such other problems as impaired verbal memory, slow reaction time to various kinds of verbal and nonverbal stimuli, differential difficulty with certain aspects of language, and so forth. In essence, children with SLI may have more or less subtle impairment in certain intellectual (cognitive) skills and reaction time. While research has documented such difficulties in children with SLI, there is nothing compelling in the literature that forces one to subscribe to the view that such deficits cause their language problems.

Most explanations hypothesize specific causation while ignoring other potential causes. Even though some of the suggested causes may be invalid, it is unlikely that SLI has a single cause. Most researchers agree that it is a complex disorder that may have multiple genetic influences that interact with environmental factors. The symptom complex of SLI suggests that children with SLI have obvious difficulties in language comprehension and production, and not so obvious associated difficulties in skills that are verbal as well as nonverbal. If the associated difficulties are part of the symptom complex of SLI and not its cause, then only the genetic and environmental factors remain as potential causes.

It is possible that in the near future, molecular genetics (not population genetics that analyzes differential prevalence rates) will identify a more specific genetic basis for SLI. Even if a specific gene is identified, environmental factors may create variability in the expression of the disorder. If SLI, as some geneticists suggest, is due to the influence of multiple genes, each exerting only a small influence, then the influence of environmental variables will be significant.

The negative influence of multiple genes, none obviously defective, may create a particularly strong predisposition to develop SLI under certain environmental conditions. The high familial incidence of SLI not only suggests potential genetic influence, but possibly also a poor verbal learning environment for children whose parents or siblings have limited language skills. Genetic predisposition to limited language skills and the resulting poor language learning environment may, in some cases, combine with low socioeconomic and educational status of the family to create significant additional hurdles to language learning. Children with a genetic predisposition to limited language skills may need additional, specialized, and consistent environmental action—something sorely missing in families that are already limited in language skills, education, and means to provide additional stimulation and reinforcement for language learning in children.

A multiple gene–multiple environment interaction view just described is consistent with a hypothesis that Leonard (1991) and Dale and Cole (1991) have supported in the past. Their hypothesis stated that children with SLI are at the lower end of the normal range in language skills and reflect individual differences. Limited language skills of children with SLI are not due to any defect, disease, or damage, but to normal variation found in all kinds of skills, including language skills. Such low-normal verbal skills are problematic because of the importance of verbal skills in education and occupation. Therefore, while low-normal musical or athletic skills need not attract clinical attention, similarly low language skills would. In most cases, low-normal skills are a byproduct of multiple genetic and environmental influences.

No treatment evidence suggests that children with SLI need special kinds of assessment or treatment procedures. In spite of the popularity of indirectly treating language deficits by targeting underlying processing problems (especially auditory processing problems), direct treatment of language skills are known to be effective and efficient (Dale &

Cole, 1991; Hegde, 1998b; Leonard, 1991). Therefore, the next six chapters will describe assessment and treatment procedures shown to be efficacious through experimental research that are suitable for directly addressing the deficits children with SLI exhibit. Subsequent chapters will then describe other populations of children for whom some modifications of these procedures will be necessary.

Chapter Summary

Approximately 7 to 8 percent of preschool and school-age children have a form of language disorder that is not associated with any other kind of disability. Because the disability seems to be limited to language, it is called specific language impairment (SLI). Children with SLI have asynchronous language development that is slower, but within the typical pattern of language acquisition. Such early communication deficits as lack of babbling or eye contact are often the first warning signs of SLI.

Children with SLI may have slightly superior comprehension skills than production skills. Often the first sign of SLI is difficulty in learning words and their varied meanings. Deficiencies in grammar, including syntactic and morphologic deficiencies, are particularly marked in children with SLI. Morphologic problems of children with SLI have been explained on the basis of deficient perception, syntactic complexity, and semantic redundancy. Evidence on the pragmatic language skills of children with SLI has been inconsistent and often contradictory, but clinicians should be alert to possible pragmatic difficulties.

Genetic factors may play a role in development of SLI in children, as suggested by population genetic studies of families, pedigrees, and twins. Although molecular genetic studies have not isolated a defective gene that causes SLI, research continues. The importance of some neuroanatomic factors, especially that of differences in language-related brain structures, has been emphasized by some researchers. It is likely that such environmental factors as low socioeconomic status (SES) and limited language stimulation combine with genetic factors to produce SLI.

Some researchers have questioned the diagnosis of SLI, suggesting that children with SLI have difficulties with complex reasoning tasks, deficits in information processing skills, deficits in memory skills, problems in haptic perception, attentional deficits and hyperactivity, and difficulties with symbolic play activity.

Theoretical explanations of SLI include the hypothesis that it is due to the underlying deficits in perceptual and cognitive domains or that it is due to normal variation in language skills. Most investigators think that SLI is caused by multiple genetic and environmental influences.

Study Guide

1. The classroom teacher of Tommy, a 9-year-old child, has referred him to you for language assessment and treatment. The teacher stated that the child does not seem to have any significant sensory or intellectual deficiencies and yet does not seem to have language skills typical of 9-year-olds. Create a language assessment outline for Tommy. In this outline, specify the skills and behaviors you would

target. Why would you specifically target those behaviors? Highlight behaviors that are most critical for your diagnosis and suggest behaviors that are of secondary importance as well.

2. Describe the early communicative skills and discuss their importance in diagnosing later language disorders in children. What kinds of continuity do you see between the early communication skills and later (normal) language skills? Point out the importance of *shaping* in your answer.

3. What are phonological disorders? Discuss how phonological disorders interact with language disorders in children. Justify the statement, with suitable examples, that some morphological deficiencies of children with language disorders may indeed be due their phonological difficulties.

4. State precisely the three explanations for morphologic deficiencies seen in children with SLI: perceptual deficiency, syntactic complexity, and semantic redundancy. What kinds of evidence are cited to support these explanations? How would you evaluate the evidence and the explanations?

5. Summarize research findings on pragmatic language skills in children with SLI. Point out contradictory findings. Based on the available evidence, what conclusions do you draw about the pragmatic language skills in children with SLI? Before coming to your own conclusions, search the aggregate databases in your library (e.g., MEDLINE, PsycInfo, ERIC) to find recently published articles on pragmatic language skills in children with SLI. Discuss findings of various studies designed to investigate pragmatic language skills in children with SLI.

6. Distinguish between what is meant by *familial* and what is meant by *genetic*. Why is this distinction important in drawing conclusions from studies investigating genetic factors in SLI?

7. What did the investigations of the KE family teach us about the genetic basis of language disorders in general and SLI in particular? Did these studies support a genetic basis of SLI? Why or why not?

8. Describe interactional (environmental) variables that contribute to SLI. Include the findings of the Hart and Risley studies and findings of differences between mothers of children with SLI and those of children without SLI. What do the results of studies indicate?

chapter

4

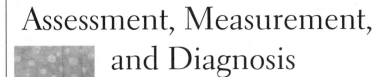

Assessment, Measurement, and Diagnosis

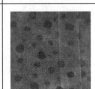

outline

W ho needs treatment for what? Before treatment can be offered, the clinician needs to establish certain facts, creating a profile of the child's pattern of communication. The clinician needs to answer such questions as the following to design a treatment plan for the child:

- Why is professional help being sought?
- What do the family members see as the problem with the child's communication skills?
- What are the concerns of a referring professional, such as a teacher or medical personnel?
- Do the referring professionals share the concerns of the family?
- What social and academic demands are made on the child?
- How well does the child meet those demands?
- What has been the child's general health and overall development?
- Are there any associated clinical conditions that should be considered in treatment planning?
- What is the child's family like?
- What are the family communication patterns?
- What are the strengths and weaknesses of the family?
- What is the family's ethnocultural background?
- What are the child's strengths and weaknesses?
- What language skills does the child have, and what language skills need to be taught?

Unless these and other questions are answered, a treatment plan designed for the child may be inadequate, ineffective, or both.

The overall clinical activities designed to understand the child and the family before a treatment program is established for that child are variously known as assessment, measurement, and diagnosis. These clinical activities help establish a profile—a detailed description—of the child, the family, and the child's social and academic environment. The profile will help design a treatment program to meet the specific needs of the child and the child's family—a treatment program that will establish language skills that are useful and relevant within the child's various environments. Such a treatment program can be designed only if the information gathered about the child and the family is accurate and reliable. Competent clinicians are highly skilled in administering pretreatment tasks to assess and measure a child's language skills, which will lead to accurate diagnosis and effective intervention.

We will begin this chapter with a discussion of the three major pretreatment tasks of assessment, measurement, and diagnosis. We will then describe in more detail procedures to assess and measure language skills, as well as ways to interpret the data collected. This interpretation will help to create a profile for the child and the family and then to make a diagnosis of the clinical problem. In the last section, procedures for diagnostic report writing will be set forth and suggestions given for presenting diagnostic information to family members.

Assessment, Measurement, and Diagnosis

The terms *assessment* and *appraisal* are often used interchangeably. We will treat them as synonyms, and we will generally use the term *assessment*. Typically, the term *diagnosis* is distinguished from *assessment* (or *appraisal*). Assessment is the activity that leads to a clinical decision called diagnosis. There is a need for emphasizing measurement within the assessment process. Reliable and valid measures obtained during assessment justify a clinical diagnosis. Therefore, assessment, measurement, and diagnosis may be distinguished as three main aspects of pretreatment tasks the clinician will have to complete.

> What are three aspects of pretreatment tasks the clinician must complete?

Assessment

Assessment of children's language disorders consists of clinical activities that precede treatment and result in an accurate, thorough description of: (1) the child's existing and nonexisting communicative behaviors, (2) the communication demands of a child's environment, (3) associated factors that may affect language skills, (4) the communication patterns of a child's family, and (5) the strengths and limitations of the child and the family.

Assessment may also be conducted during treatment to monitor progress, before dismissal to document the skill level achieved, and during follow-up appointments to evaluate maintenance of clinically established skills (Hegde, 1996a). A carefully done assessment of a child's language skills prior to treatment will lead to an accurate diagnosis and an effective treatment plan.

Although accurate assessment is a critical clinical activity, clinicians should not become "stuck" in the assessment process. Treatment should not be delayed due to inefficient assessment procedures that are extended over too many sessions. On the other hand, the assessment process should be thorough, consisting of repeated measures of language behaviors taken in various settings under a variety of stimulus conditions.

Measurement

While performing the clinical activities necessary to assess a child's language skills, clinicians gather quantitative data through measuring the communicative behaviors they observe. **Measurement** "quantifies observed objects, events, and their mathematical properties" (Hegde, 2003a, p. 185). To measure a communicative behavior, the behavior must be described in a manner that lends itself to measurement. An **operational definition** describes a behavior in observable and measurable terms. For example, vaguely defined "language compe-

> How does an operational definition define target behaviors?

tence" is neither observable nor measurable; operationally defined "production of the regular plural morpheme in conversational speech" is both observable and measurable. Measuring "auditory processing" is not possible; measuring "the number of times a child correctly responds to two-step verbal directions" is. Describing communicative behaviors in ways that are observable and measurable is important in both assessment and intervention.

Measurement is an integral part of clinical assessment. A clinician's diagnostic judgment should be based on the quantitative data generated by repeated measurement of specific language behaviors in different response modes, under varied stimulus conditions (Hegde, 1996b). Repeated measurement is necessary to establish reliability of measures. Diagnostic decisions should never be made, for example, on the basis of analysis of one language sample. Brief language samples should be collected during the first few treatment sessions to ensure reliability of measures.

Assessment Models

There are different models of assessment and clinical measurement. Although not mutually exclusive, these approaches differ in emphasizing varied means of assessment of clinically relevant skills in children with language disorders (Brice, 2002; Eisenberg, Fresko, & Lundgren, 2001; Laing & Kamhi, 2003; Plante, 1996; McCauley, 1996; McFadden, 1996; Washington & Craig, 2004). Clinicians may measure a child's language skills through (1) norm-referenced standardized tests, (2) criterion-referenced assessment tools, and (3) child-specific measurement procedures. We will take a brief look at these models of assessment and emphasize the child-specific approach, which offers certain advantages in addition to combining the strengths of the other two.

Measurement through Norm-Referenced Standardized Tests

A norm-referenced standardized test is a structured assessment tool that has been finalized on the basis of performance of a sample of children drawn from a defined population. The **norm** is the performance of the sample of children drawn from the population. The performance of an individual on the standardized test is compared to the norm to make diagnostic decisions about the individual's skill level. The clinician diagnoses a language disorder if the assessed child's scores are significantly lower than those of the children in the standardization sample.

A thorough assessment of a child's language skills can be made through procedures with little or no emphasis on standardized tests. In many clinical settings, however, clinicians are required to provide standardized test scores for children to qualify for speech-language services. Many school districts, for example, require standardized test scores for children who receive special education services, including speech-language services. Therefore, SLPs must have a thorough knowledge of how to select and administer tests, and how to interpret the resulting data. SLPs should also, however, understand the limitations of standardized tests and how to minimize the negative consequences of those limitations.

Validity and reliability are the two most important issues to consider in evaluating and selecting standardized tests. For most standardized tests, one can establish different kinds of validity and reliability.

Historically, **validity** has been defined as the degree to which an instrument measures what it purports to measure (Anastasi, 1982). In this classic sense, validity is an aspect or property of a standardized test. An alternative view of validity is that it is the extent to which interpretations of test scores are meaningful and acceptable. In this sense, validity is not a property of a test but the manner in which the results are interpreted and used to make clinical decisions (Hutchinson, 1996). As such, a test may be valid for one purpose but not for another.

The common types of validity include:

- Content validity
- Construct validity
- Concurrent validity
- Predictive validity

Content validity. Expert judgment that the contents of a test are relevant, necessary, and sufficient to measure what the test is supposed to measure is **content validity**. For example, language experts may examine the items of a morphologic test and conclude that the items do indeed measure the production of English morphemes in sufficient numbers. As another example, a test purporting to measure expressive vocabulary should contain pictured items for children to name. As the examples make clear, content validity is established through expert judgment and does not involve statistical techniques as some other forms of validity do.

> Many nationally given tests prospective students take claim to have *predictive validity.* The Scholastic Aptitude Test (SAT) is believed to predict how well a student will do in college; the Graduate Record Exam (GRE) predicts how well a student will do in a graduate program of study.

Construct validity. An expert judgment that given test scores are consistent with a theoretical expectation regarding the skill being measured is called **construct validity.** For example, theoretically, language skills measured across age groups should show a progressive increase. Two-year-olds should score higher on a language test than 4-year-olds. If an examination of scores of younger and older children do not show progressive increase with increasing age, then the test is inconsistent with theoretical expectations and, hence, invalid. Construct validity also is a matter of expert judgment.

Concurrent validity. A positive correlation between a new test and a well-established old test of the same skill is called **concurrent validity.** For example, authors may claim that the scores of their new test of receptive vocabulary are positively correlated with the scores of the well-established Peabody Picture Vocabulary Test (PPVT-III; Dunn & Dunn, 1997). Too high a correlation between the new test and the older test suggests that there is not much difference between them; a critical clinician might then question the need for the new test. Note that this is a statistically established form of validity (the method of correlation).

> If the same administrator gives the same child the same test twice, and scores are reasonably the same, what two types of reliability are assumed to have been established?

Predictive validity. Relatively accurate predictions of future performance on a related task from the scores of a test is called **predictive validity.** Many tests for child language skills claim to have predictive validity for how well children may do in language-related scholastic tasks in the future—in learning to read or write, for example. An acceptable positive correlation between the test score and the predicted performance score (sometimes called the criterion score) when it becomes available assures predictive validity. Note that predictive validity also is established statistically.

Reliability is the degree to which repeated measures of the same event are consistent. Scores obtained from a standardized test should be relatively stable across repeated administrations of the same test. Therefore, reliability also is described as stability of repeated measures. If the measures or scores fluctuate from one measurement to the next, then the method of measurement is unreliable. The common types of reliability include:

- Interjudge reliability
- Intrajudge reliability
- Alternate form reliability
- Test–retest reliability
- Split-half reliability

Interjudge reliability. Consistency of scores when two or more observers (clinicians) administer the same test or measurement procedure is called **interjudge reliability,** also called inter-rater reliability. The consistency may be established through statistical correlation or percentage of agreement among two or more observers. The correlation is more

> If two different administrators give the same child the same test on two different occasions, and the scores are reasonably the same, what two types of reliability are established?

often used with standardized test scores and percentage of agreement with child- or client-specific measures.

Intrajudge reliability. Consistency of scores when the same clinician administers the same test to the same person a second time with a reasonable interval between the two administrations is called **intrajudge reliability**. This may also be an index of how well a clinician is trained to administer and score a test or measure the same phenomenon repeatedly and get similar scores. If well-trained clinicians get vastly different scores from the repeated administration of the same test, then the test is not reliable.

Alternate form reliability. Consistency of scores on parallel forms of the same test administered to the same individual is **alternative form reliability**. Also called parallel form reliability, this applies mostly to standardized tests, not to child-specific measures. Some standardized tests provide two forms of the same test. Their items are different, but they measure the same skill. If two forms of the same test give divergent results, then the test is not reliable.

Test–retest reliability. Consistency of scores obtained from repeated administration of the same test is **test–retest reliability**. The concept applies to child-specific measures as well. To be reliable, the same child-specific measures obtained two or more times should be consistent with each other.

Split-half reliability. Consistency of scores calculated separately for the two halves of a test is **split-half reliability**. Two scores from the same test may be derived either from splitting the test into the first and the second half, or by separating scores of the odd numbered items from even numbered ones (called odd–even reliability). This is a measure of internal consistency of a test. Tests of language skills are constructed to become progressively more difficult, so that the first half is at an entirely different level than the second half. Consequently, this type of reliability is of questionable value to many standardized tests of language skill. The odd–even method may be slightly more appropriate than the split-half method of establishing this type of reliability. Even then, split-half reliability generally overestimates reliability as it does not measure stability of test scores over time.

> Describe clinical activities and verbal stimuli that would provide **obligatory contexts** for production of: (1) present progressive *-ing*; (2) prepositional phrases (3) past tense *-ed*; and (4) pronouns.

Strengths of Standardized Tests

The most obvious advantage to standardized testing is that it is a socially accepted means of justifying clinical or special educational services to children. Another common advantage is that within their limitations, standardized tests help make clinical and educational decisions. Based on their scores for example, individuals may be classified as "normal" in skills tested or abnormal in the sense that the skills are outside (typically below) the normative range. Within educational institutions, standardized test scores help qualify children for various special educational services. Standardized tests bypass the need for developing individual assessment tools, a time-consuming process. Part of what makes a standardized test "standardized" is that it must be presented in the same way each time it is given. Therefore, there is no need to prepare verbal and pictorial stimulus items, instructions, prompts, or models, because all are provided in the test manual. Consequently, this type of testing is often convenient to clinicians who become adept at administering tests they have repeatedly given. They are especially convenient when large numbers of children have to be tested fairly quickly to make clinical or educational decisions. In spite of widespread criticisms of tests, organizations and institutions accept the validity of tests, encouraging clinicians and educators to use them.

The belief that standardized tests provide objective and quantitative data is deep-rooted because of the long-standing tradition of psychometric testing in the United States. For many clinicians, therefore, tests provide a means of fulfilling administrative policies regarding service delivery.

Limitations of Standardized Tests

In spite of their generally accepted strengths, norm-referenced standardized tests as diagnostic tools have many serious limitations. It is necessary to understand these limitations to use the tests in a prudent manner. For instance, norm-referenced standardized tests have limitations relative to:

- Assumptions of statistical normality
- Inadequate sampling of language behaviors
- Linguistic and ethnocultural biases
- Standardization based on the representative sample as against the "normal" sample

Assumptions of statistical normality. Standardized testing is based on the assumption that the mean (average) performance of a larger number of children of a particular age sets the norm for that age. A child's performance that falls below the mean established for the age group justifies the diagnosis of a disorder. Norms, by definition, then, are an average of performance of a sample of children drawn randomly from the population. The sample that represents the population of children is a double-edged sword. Typically, samples are small and local, hence they would not represent all children in the country or even a state. If the samples are large enough to represent the population of children at different age levels, then the performance of that large a sample will be so varied that the mean derived from it will not be meaningful to an individual child. Because norms are a statistical representation of the mean (average), individual performances may not be reflected accurately. Norms ignore the many differences social and cultural variables create, even within the same ethnocultural groups. Furthermore, in diverse societies such as that in the United States and many other countries, norms may be irrelevant to the assessment of individual language performance.

Norm-referenced testing of language skills includes a controversial assumption that all children acquire language skills in a relatively fixed sequence. Children's language acquisition may show a broad and variable pattern, but the claims of an invariable sequence of language acquisition across children (Brown, 1973; Chomsky, 1968) are not universally supported. Critical analysis of developmental sequence has shown that many environmental variables including parents' education, language expressions, and informal teaching efforts are related to variations in children's language learning (Moerk, 1983, 1992, 2000).

Experimental research has shown that the sequence of language acquisition can be changed if certain environmental variables are manipulated. For instance, children can be taught language structures out of their known sequences (Atherton & Hegde, 1996; Capelli, 1985; DeCesari, 1985; Nelson, 1977).

Inadequate sampling of language behaviors. Authors of standardized tests are chiefly concerned with sampling enough participants, not about adequately sampling the skill to be tested. Most if not all standardized tests test the skills in a cursory manner. For example, many tests provide only one or two opportunities to produce grammatic morphemes or sentences of particular structures, resulting in woefully inadequate data on a particular child. To make decisions about a child, that child's behaviors must be sampled adequately. That the test was based on a large number of children is not relevant to this task. In-depth sampling of skills is necessary to make valid judgments about a child. Instead of asking a child to name one set of objects to evoke plural -s, for example, the clinician needs to present multiple sets of objects.

Linguistic and ethnocultural biases. Norm-referenced standardized tests tend to be linguistically and ethnoculturally biased—a serious limitation examined in detail in Chapter 11. Many norm-referenced tests do not fully take into consideration the ethnocultural and linguistic diversity of children being tested, although many test developers are paying increasing attention to linguistic and ethnocultural diversity of samples on which tests are standardized (Brice, 2002; Laing & Kamhi, 2003; Washington & Craig, 1992).

Standardization based on the representative sample as against the "normal" sample. In drawing samples on which to standardize norm-referenced tests, test developers tend to exclude children with various kinds of disabilities (McFadden, 1996). For instance, a norm-referenced test of language skills in children may have been standardized exclusively on children who had normal language skills. The test developer in this case will have excluded not only children with language problems, but also children with other communication and intellectual disabilities. Such a "normal" sample would not represent the entire population of children, and the test based on the performance of only normal children may falsely identify many more language handicapped children than is justified.

Criterion-Referenced Assessment

An alternative to norm-referenced testing is **criterion-referenced assessment,** which is defined as a method of assessment whose results are interpreted not in relation to norms, but only in relation to a performance standard (American Educational Research Association, American Psychological Association, and National Council of Measurement in Education, 1985; Laing & Kamhi, 2003; McCauley, 1996). Instead of evaluating a child's performance against norms established on a sample of children, the criterion-reference assessment seeks to establish the level at which a child performs and whether this level is functional for the child. The clinician's main concern is to find out whether a skill is present, absent, mastered, not mastered yet, and so forth. The mastery criterion may be clinically established. For instance, instead of asking whether a 5-year-old boy's production of the plural morpheme is at or below the normative level for his age, the clinician will sample the production of that skill and find out that it is produced with 60 percent accuracy. The clinician will then judge whether the skill level is adequate to succeed in the classroom. To give another example, the clinician may find that a 10-year-old child's topic maintenance during conversation is only 10 percent and then conclude that this level is inadequate for social communication. In most cases, the clinician may use a criterion such as 80 or 90 percent accuracy as the target level of performance. Skills that do not meet this criterion level may be evaluated as deficient and targeted for treatment.

An adequate language sample and analysis of language skills exhibited at different mastery levels is a prime example of criterion-referenced assessment. In addition, the clinician may assess specific skills in greater depth by developing client-specific stimulus materials. For instance, a clinician may use 20 pictures that depict various kinds of actions (e.g., a boy walking, a girl reading, a dog jumping) to assess the production of the present progressive -*ing* and the auxiliary *is*. In selecting stimulus items, the clinician may pay particular attention to the child's ethnocultural and linguistic background. Because the production is evoked on multiple stimulus items, a percent correct response rate can be determined. Such percent correct response rates help establish the initial mastery levels that provide a basis for evaluating treatment progress.

Strengths of Criterion-Referenced Assessment

Criterion-referenced assessment approach was developed to avoid some of the major limitations of norm-referenced standardized testing. Its main goal is to assess a child in relation to performance standards that should be met. Therefore, the approach does avoid the problem of evaluating a child against the performance of a large sample of children, with its attending problems that were pointed out earlier. Criterion-referenced assessment is similar to child-specific assessment. Unlike norm-referenced tests, criterion-referenced measures may include sufficient number of opportunities for the child to produce language skills. The clinician may be free to develop stimulus materials that are appropriate for the child to sample language skills. Consequently, criterion-referenced assessment may observe skills in greater depth than norm-referenced standardized tests.

Criterion-referenced assessment tools are especially useful when the norm-referenced tests are either unavailable or inappropriate for a given client. Criterion-referenced tools are most appropriate when assessing the communication skills of children of varied ethnocultural and linguistic backgrounds who may be inadequately represented in the sample on which norm-referenced tests are developed. In most clinical situations, criterion-referenced assessment serves the purpose of continuously evaluating the progress clients make in meeting treatment objectives (e.g., a 80 or 90 percent accuracy criterion).

Limitations of Criterion-Referenced Assessment

Some clinicians believe that criterion-referenced measures do not completely avoid reference to developmental norms (Laing & Kamhi, 2003). To judge whether a skill level a child exhibits is appropriate or not, some clinicians may find it necessary to resort to developmental norms. If this is the case, the distinction between norm-referenced tests and criterion-referenced measures is blurred. It is, however, possible to interpret the child's performance level as adequate or inadequate in light of the social (and perhaps more effectively) academic demands made on the child. Such interpretations, however, demand in-depth observation of the child and a detailed analysis of academic demands placed on the child.

In assessing children with varied ethnocultural background, the criterion-referenced assessment may still require an extensive knowledge of a given child's linguistic and cultural background along with the family communication patterns. Differences in acceptable mastery levels of language skills, if they were to be present across different cultural groups, would pose clinical challenges. Finally, criterion-referenced assessment requires extensive preparatory work. The clinician may have to design stimulus materials for particular children.

Child-Specific Measurement

Child-specific measurement procedures (also known as client-specific measurement) are those that a clinician constructs to meet the specific needs of a child. They do not use norm-referenced standardized tests, and the results are not meant to compare a child's skill level to normative data; they are meant to make decisions specific to the individual child. The clinician uses a variety of means, including language sampling and procedures designed to measure specific aspects of communication. For instance, the clinician who needs to measure irregular plural productions in a given child can prepare a list of such words, find pictures for them, and ask the child to name them. The resulting data are specific to the child and to the particular behaviors the clinician wishes to assess. In this sense, child-specific assessment is similar to criterion-referenced assessment, except that the former places a greater emphasis on the child's current and unique situation, ethnocultural background, family communication, and specific communicative demands made on the child.

In addition to language sampling, child-specific assessment includes such procedures as (1) interviewing parents and other family members to assess the cultural and linguistic background of the child; (2) making a list of words from the child's home environment to assess the child's production and comprehension of words, phrases, and speech sounds; (3) preparing stimulus materials that are familiar to the child to assess morphologic and syntactic productions; (4) selecting stories and storybooks that reflect the child's cultural and home background to assess pragmatic language skills; (5) obtaining language samples from home; and (6) structuring multiple opportunities for the child to produce skills being measured.

Reliability and validity of child-specific measurement. Reliability and validity of child-specific measures are not statistical, but clinical and data-specific. In-depth assessment with multiple opportunities, repeated measures, and greater family involvement in structuring the assessment tasks and situations ensure clinical relevance and meaningfulness of assessment data. Validity is assured when the tasks are relevant to make clinical decisions. Reliability is assured by multiple and repeated assessment, as in repeated clinic language samples supplemented by home samples. When the production of a morphologic feature, such as the plural s, is measured not with one or two canned words but more than a dozen child-specific words, reliability is assured. Contrasted with standardized tests, child-specific measurement establishes reliability *every time* the method is used (Hegde, 1996b).

Clinicians establish reliability of data for an individual child chiefly through measuring language behaviors produced during repeated language sampling. For example, if the clinician observes during the initial language sample that the child omits plural -*s*, further language samples should be gathered during clinical activities that are designed to evoke many plural -*s* productions. The clinician might read a picture book about counting, asking the child, "What do you see here?" or play with a toy barn and animals, asking the child to describe what is in the pen, what is in the barn, and so forth. Such clinical activities provide **obligatory contexts** (Brown, 1973), situations in which the rules of language dictate the use of a particular language structure. The question "What do you see in the barn?" must be answered, "I see ducks!" if there is more than one duck in the barn. The clinician counts the number of times the child produces it, in each language sample and divides that number by the number of opportunities given to produce it, resulting in a percentage of accuracy for production of plural -*s*. If the percentages calculated for each language sample are reasonably close, then reliability of that measure is established. Because a percentage of accuracy is a suitable measure for the production of plural -*s*, it is a valid measure. In this manner, reliability and validity are established each time a child-specific method of measurement is employed.

> Identify the type of child-specific measure described when: (1) the clinician observes behaviors of the child during communicative exchanges with others; and (2) the clinician times how long the child can maintain a topic of conversation; and (3) the clinician counts the number of times a child produces an irregular plural form.

Types of child-specific measures.   There are several types of child-specific methods and measures, but we sample only a few here. An important and frequently used method results in a **frequency measure** of a skill, which is the number of times a behavior was exhibited under specified stimulus conditions. Frequency measures, most often expressed in terms of a percentage of accuracy, are a valid means of measuring the production of many language structures. Language samples and special assessment procedures the clinician designs (for example, a set of child-specific words to measure the plural -*s* productions) yield frequency measures (Hegde, 2003a).

Another child-specific measurement is durational measures. Unlike the frequency of language skills, **durational measures** specify time periods for which a skill was sustained. Durational measures are especially useful for assessing certain conversational skills. A clinician might need to know how long a child can sustain eye contact, maintain a topic of conversation, or attend to a task. Generally, a durational measure may be combined with a frequency measure. For example, the frequency with which eye contact is made and the duration for which it is sustained will give a comprehensive view of that skill. Durational measures are more difficult to take than frequency measures; they are often reported in terms of a range of measures, from shortest to longest duration (e.g., "Sally established eye contact six times during language sampling, with the duration of eye contact ranging from 1 to 10 seconds.").

Verbal interaction sampling, another child-specific procedure, is especially useful in measuring language skills exhibited during social dialogue (Hegde, 2003a). Often, clinicians observe and measure behaviors that occur during communicative exchanges between the child and parents, peers, teachers, or others. In verbal interaction sampling, behaviors of one or more individuals are measured during social communication. For example, the clinician may observe how a parent reads storybooks to a child. The clinician could ask the parent to read a storybook just as he or she typically would at home and observe the interaction. Does the parent require the child to sit still and be silent while being read to? Or does

> What kind of treatment is given for conditions for which there is no known cause?

the parent ask questions, invite the child to ask questions, or encourage comments? The measures obtained from verbal interaction sampling will vary, depending on the stimulus conditions, response characteristics, and the type of information the clinician is seeking. In the case of storybook reading, the clinician might count the number of times the parent asks the child questions (a frequency measure) or the length of time the child looks at the text while the story is read (a durational measure).

Limitations of child-specific measurement. The most obvious limitation of child-specific measurement is that it takes more time and effort than administering standardized tests. It requires the clinician to plan and devise valid means of child-specific measurement. Many institutions, especially schools, do not require it and do not support the additional time and effort the clinicians need to expend on it. Some of these limitations, especially the need to spend more time and effort and lack of institutional requirement and support are practical barriers to using them. None of these limitations raise questions of validity, reliability, meaningfulness, and clinical relevance of child-specific measures, however.

Strengths of child-specific measurement. Even though the child-specific measurement avoids standardized stimuli, it yields quantitative and objective data on a child's performance. Because it involves extensive and systematic observation of the child and the family, it also yields much qualitative data that are useful in making clinical decisions. A clinician who has completed child-specific assessment knows more about the child and the family than one who has just administered standardized tests. Additional advantages of child-specific measurement include an adequate sampling of behaviors, potential to tailor assessment procedures to the needs of the child, potential to make a child- and family-specific diagnosis and treatment plan, and relevance to a child's ethnocultural and linguistic background.

Diagnosis

Ideally, **diagnosis** is the determination of the cause of a disorder, although this ideal is rarely realized in most cases of language disorders. This ideal is not always realized even in medicine from which the term is borrowed. Diagnosis in speech-language pathology is the determination that there *is* (or is not) a disorder based on the results of valid and reliable measurement of relevant skills. Beyond that, the diagnosis may describe the nature and extent of a disorder, rather than its causes. Such a determination is always a matter of clinical judgment, but it is not entirely a subjective judgment. It is a well-informed judgment based on systematic observation of the child, case history information, and results of various diagnostic tests and child-specific measurement. A diagnosis can either be positive for the presence of a language disorder or negative, meaning no language disorder exists. In either case, the diagnosis made should be supported by data gathered through measurement of language behaviors exhibited during the assessment process.

Ideally once again, treatment is offered only when the cause of a disorder or disease is found. This does not always happen, neither in medicine nor in speech-language pathology. **Symptomatic treatment** (treatment of the symptoms with no clear understanding of the cause) is quite common in medicine. Effective treatment of language disorders without a clear cause is typical in speech-language pathology. In contrast to the medical model, it is frequently not possible to pinpoint the cause of a language disorder. This is not to argue that a specific knowledge of the cause or causes of disorders is unimportant. To the contrary, treatment of the causes can be more efficacious and efficient than symptomatic treatment. But it is not helpful to treat *hypothetical* causes.

Some children have a diagnosis other than language disorder. For instance, some children have a language disorder and either autism, traumatic brain injury, or developmental disability. It is necessary to understand these associated clinical conditions and their characteristics. It is not always possible, however, to precisely predict the language profile of children based on those associated clinical diagnoses. For example, some children with Down syndrome have only mild developmental disability and have functional speech and language skills. Other children with the same diagnosis may present with profound developmental disability, may be nonverbal, and despite the best efforts of early intervention professionals, may require 24-hour-a-day care during their entire lifespan. Clearly, the same diagnosis does not always indicate the same language profile.

> What is the first piece of information on a child the clinician typically receives?

Beyond the broad concepts of measurement and diagnosis, however, lies a myriad of specific procedures clinicians use to perform the clinical activities leading to diagnosis and treatment of language disorders in children. In the following sections, we describe those specific procedures, beginning with screening procedures, diagnostic methods, methods for interpreting assessment data, writing a diagnostic report, and ending with suggestions for sharing diagnostic findings with parents, teachers, and interested others.

An Initial Judgment: Screening

Because of demonstrated efficacy of early intervention, it is important to discover language disorders in children at as young an age as possible. **Screening procedures** are those that are designed to identify children who may face the risk of a language disorder. Children may be screened using a variety of commercially available tests (see Table 4.1) or through procedures that clinicians devise to quickly check a child's language skills. Screening procedures are designed to be quick checks of a child's expressive or receptive language skills, or both, and can be conducted by individuals with less training than SLPs. School districts, for example, commonly require screenings to be conducted of kindergarten and third grade children each year, and often these screenings are administered by registered or licensed speech aides or assistants rather than fully licensed and credentialed SLPs.

Screening procedures are cursory and yield data that are insufficient to support a diagnosis. Results of a screening do not indicate whether or not a language disorder exists or what the nature of that language disorder might be. Rather, failure to pass a screening indicates the need for a full assessment conducted by a qualified SLP who will then determine whether or not a language disorder is present.

Assessment and Measurement Procedures

When a child is referred for assessment of language skills, or is identified through a screening procedure to be in need of a more thorough assessment, the clinician performs

table 4.1

Screening Tests for Child Language

Test	Ages	Administration Time	Language Skills Tested
CSBS DP Infant-Toddler Checklist and Easy-Score Wetherby & Prizant (2003b)	6–24 months	5–10 minutes	Gestures, sounds, words, eye gaze, object use, other nonverbal communicative behaviors
CELF-4 Screening Test Semel, Wiig, & Secord (2004)	5 yrs through 21 yrs	15 minutes	Expressive and receptive language: vocabulary and syntax
Fluharty-2: Fluharty Preschool Speech and Language Screening Test Fluharty (2000)	3 yrs through 6 yrs, 11 mos	10 minutes	Expressive and receptive language: repeating sentences, answering questions, following directions, describing actions, sequencing events (also screens articulation)
Joliet 3-Minute Preschool Speech and Language Screen Kinzler (1993)	2 yrs through 4 yrs	3–5 minutes	Expressive and receptive language: syntax and vocabulary (also screens articulation)
Joliet 3-Minute Speech and Language Screen (Revised) Kinzler & Johnson (1992)	K, 2nd, and 5th graders	3–5 minutes	
Kindergarten Language Screening Test, Second Edition (KLST-S) Gauthier & Madison (1998).	3 yrs, 6 mos through 6 yrs, 11 mos	5 minutes	Expressive and receptive language: following directions, repeating sentences, making comparisons between common objects
Speech-Ease Screening Inventory (K–1) Speech-Ease (1985)	K through 1st grade	7–10 minutes	Expressive and receptive language: vocabulary, associations, auditory recall, basic concepts

various clinical activities leading to a diagnosis. Initial assessment of a child's language skills should include the following activities:

- Obtaining a case history
- Conducting interviews of the child, the child's parents, caregivers, teachers, and any other relevant persons in the child's environment
- Conducting an orofacial examination
- Screening hearing
- Selecting and administering standardized tests
- Making child-specific measurement, including an oral language sample
- Discussing the results of the assessment with parents, teachers, and interested others
- Making recommendations on intervention, suggesting possible target behaviors, and making referrals if necessary

History

History, or **case history,** is a detailed written account of information on the child and the family. The information that is supplied is necessary to understand the child, the family, and the problem the child has. This understanding is essential to both an accurate diagnosis and effective treatment.

The case history is obtained initially by having the family fill out a standard form. The case history form begins by supplying necessary identifying information, such as the child's name, names of parents or caregivers, date of birth, address, telephone number, grade level, school attended, and names of the child's teacher, physician, or any other referring professional. In short, the case history provides any identifying information the particular clinical or educational setting requires.

Questions the family answers on the case history form will give detailed information on the child, the communicative problem for which help is sought, the family, health, education, and other related matters that help the clinician understand the child and the possible nature of the child's difficulties with language. See Box 4.1 for examples of questions commonly asked on a case history form.

The case history rarely, if ever, provides all the information the clinician needs to begin assessing a child. The case history is only a starting point in getting important preassessment information. For example, the parents may only report that the child is having "academic difficulties." This statement is not useful until further information is obtained to understand the nature and extent of those difficulties. Clinicians obtain this information and take an important step toward establishing a productive, professional relationship with the child and family by conducting interviews.

> Reinforcement for good test-taking behavior rather than for correct answers is what type of reinforcement?

Interviewing the Family and Others

An **interview** is a face-to-face conversation with the child, the child's family, and any other relevant individuals in the child's environment, such as teachers. The purposes of the interview are to:

- Obtain additional information that may have been omitted from the case history form
- Clarify or expand information that was reported on the case history form
- Become familiarized with the child, the family, and their ethnocultural and linguistic background
- Make some initial observations of the child and family

Before starting an interview, the clinician should review the completed case history form, noting areas that need further attention during the interview. There may be some questions answered in the case history form that will be repeated during the interview; however, information the clinician deems to be sufficiently reported in the case history does not need to be revisited.

The clinician should note the child's ethnocultural background and primary language. Prior to the interview, the clinician may talk to the parents or other family members to gain an initial impression of family communicative interactions. This information will better prepare the clinician for a productive interview and accurate assessment. Also, when not proficient in the child's primary language, the clinician may seek the services of an interpreter during the interview. See Chapter 11 for more detailed information regarding ethnocultural considerations in diagnosing and treating childhood language disorders.

box 4.1   Questions Commonly Asked on a Child Case History Form

Identifying Information (e.g., name, date of birth, address, telephone number, etc.)

General Information

Does the child live with both parents? If no, with whom does the child live?

Who referred the child?

What other specialists have seen the child?

What were the other specialists' conclusions or recommendations?

What language(s) does the child speak?

How does the child usually communicate? Gestures? Single words? Short phrases? Sentences?

When was the problem first noticed?

Who first noticed the problem?

What do you think may have caused the problem?

Since you first noticed the problem, what changes have you observed in your child's language?

Is the child aware of the problem? If yes, how does he or she feel about it?

What have you done to help your child with the problem?

Are there any other speech, language, or hearing problems in the family?

Prenatal and Birth History

How was the mother's general health during pregnancy?

What was the length of the pregnancy? The length of the labor?

What was the child's weight and general condition at birth?

Were there any unusual conditions that may have affected the pregnancy or birth?

Medical History

How would you describe the child's general health?

List the child's current medications.

Describe any major accidents, surgeries, or hospitalizations the child has had.

Has the child had any of the following? (followed by a checklist of medical conditions)

Developmental History

Write the approximate age when the child began to do the following: (followed by a list of developmental milestones such as crawling, sitting, standing, etc.)

Does the child have any motor difficulty? (e.g., incoordination)

Does the child have any feeding problems? (e.g., problems with sucking, drooling, swallowing)

Do you suspect any problems with hearing? If so, why?

General Behavior

Does the child eat well? Sleep well?

How does the child interact with other family members?

How would you describe the child's level of activity? (e.g., extremely active, restless, etc.)

Does the child bang his or her head, rock, or spin? Play by him or herself?

How does the child interact with other children?

Educational History

Where does the child attend school? What grade and who is the teacher?

Does the child receive any special services?

Are there any academic concerns?

During the interview, the clinician should go over the case history form and ask questions about unclear information or what needs to be expanded. The clinician should listen carefully; most family members of children with language disorders have a story they want very badly to tell. Wise clinicians ask a few well-directed questions and then sit back and allow the family members to talk. If the clinician needs clarification, the family should be gently directed to retell a point, or the clinician can restate what the family member has said to check for understanding. When clarification is not needed, the clinician should, at most, offer comments to suggest that what is being said is understood and appreciated. Clinicians should not criticize or contradict what family members say, even when there may be obvious discrepancies between what is being said and what the clinician may be observing during the interview. Instead, the clinician should carefully note the family's observations, preferably by audio recording the family's responses so that there is a verbatim record of the interview. No specific advice should be given to families during the initial interview.

If done in a professional, thorough manner, the initial interview should also provide the basis for a productive working relationship with the child and the child's family. An efficient interview yields information that will be clinically useful in formulating an assessment plan specific to the needs of the child and the people in the child's environment. Additional procedures of assessment include orofacial examination, completing a hearing screening, and gathering a language sample.

Orofacial Examination

An **orofacial examination** is done to check the speech structures of the face and mouth to rule out any gross anatomic and physiologic deviations that may be associated with the speech or language disorder. During the orofacial examination, the clinician makes observations on the range of motion and strength of the tongue and lips, movement of the soft palate, and the overall structural integrity of the orofacial complex. Such obvious factors as facial paralysis and cleft palate are noted during this examination. Box 4.2 lists some tasks clinicians commonly use for various aspects of an orofacial examination.

---

box 4.2 | | | | **Tasks Commonly Performed during an Orofacial Examination**

Examine facial features for symmetry

Check for range of motion by modeling oral motor movements for the child to imitate, including:
- Opening and closing mouth ("Big and wide!" "Close it tight!")
- Retract lips ("Smile!")
- Purse lips ("Pucker up!")
- Protrude tongue ("Stick it WAY out!")
- Tongue tip up, down, to the left, to the right, and then rapidly back and forth (a tongue depressor can be used to provide tactile cues)

Check for labial and lingual strength:
- Ask the child to push against a tongue depressor with his lips and then with his tongue
- Ask the child to puff cheeks and hold in the air (press gently against the cheeks—"Don't let any air out!")

- Have the child push against the inside of his or her cheek with the tongue; press against the cheek ("Don't let me push it away!"); check both sides

Examine structures of the oral cavity:
- Check dentition: Are there any malocclusions? Cavities? Missing teeth?
- Examine the pharyngeal structures: Are tonsils normal, enlarged, or absent?
- Examine the hard palate: Is it of normal color? Height? Width? Note presence of rugae.
- Examine the soft palate: Is it symmetrical? Does the uvula deviate to one side or the other?
- Observe velopharyngeal closure while the child phonates "/a/, /a/, /a/"

Hearing Screening

All children and adults who are assessed for a disorder of communication must be given a **hearing screening test,** which is a quick measure of hearing done to rule out a hearing loss. Using a calibrated audiometer, pure tones at 500 Hz, 1,000 Hz, 2,000 Hz, and 4,000 Hz are introduced to each ear at a level of 20–25 dB in a "free field" outside an audiological booth. The child may be instructed to raise a hand when a sound is heard. The child must respond appropriately to each tone presented to each ear to pass the hearing screening. If the child fails the hearing screening, a referral is made to an audiologist for a complete audiological evaluation. A typical form used to screen hearing is shown in Box 4.3.

Measurement of Oral Language Skills

After studying the written case history, conducting more in-depth family interviews, and ruling out structural deficiencies or hearing loss in the child, the clinician is ready to observe and measure the child's language skills. Ideally, language samples repeated in different settings give the most reliable and comprehensive picture of a child's oral language skills. This is not always possible in the time allotted for assessment, however. Most clinicians record one language sample during the initial assessment. Briefer samples and baseline data gathered during the initial stages of treatment help establish the reliability of measured language skills. Home language samples the parents submit to the clinician later will offer more naturalistic data.

A talkative child makes it easier to gather a language sample. Of course, most children referred to speech-language pathologists for assessment of a possible language disorder are not talkative at all. Some may be minimally verbal or even nonverbal, and these children will be assessed differently than a child who is highly verbal. Therefore, the clinician needs to have a rough idea about the verbal level of the child even before selecting the assessment procedures.

As noted before, the interview and the initial telephone contacts with the family will help make certain preliminary judgments about the assessment procedures. The clinician might also observe the child's interactions with family members through a one-way window in an adjacent room. During these initial observations, the clinician should take note of the following:

- What does the case history suggest; a nonverbal child or a minimally verbal child, with single words and gestures only?
- How do the child and the parent(s) interact? Do they gesture to each other?
- Does the child use words, phrases, or sentences? Does the child seem to understand sentences or only words?
- How does the child interact with the clinician? Is the child spontaneously verbal? Does the child answer the clinician's questions? Is the child able to tell the clinician his or her name? How willing is the child to talk to the clinician?
- Is the child shy and withdrawn? Does the child appear to hide behind the parent?

Observations of this kind help clinicians determine the approximate verbal level of the child and possibly useful assessment strategies. Generally speaking, the verbal level of a child may vary between nonverbal and essentially normal with only a few advanced language

| box 4.3 | Hearing Screening Form for a Child |

Name: _____   Date of Birth: _____   Today's Date: _____

Address: _____

School: _____   Grade: _____

Please check all that apply to your child: Comments:

_____ Family history of hearing loss?   _____

_____ Ear infections?   _____

_____ Earaches?   _____

_____ Surgery?   _____

_____ Diseases related to hearing loss?   _____

_____ Ringing in the ears (tinnitus)?   _____

_____ Exposure to noise?   _____

_____ Hearing aids?   _____

_____ Head injury?   _____

Please list any medications your child is currently taking, with their dosages:

Any previous hearing evaluations? (Please supply date, place, and findings.)

RESULTS

X or + = Responded appropriately
O or − = No response
CNT   = Could not test (specify reason)

dB level: _____

	500 Hz	1,000 Hz	2,000 Hz	4,000 Hz
Right:	_____	_____	_____	_____
Left:	_____	_____	_____	_____

_____ Passed screen

_____ Failed screen

Recommendations:

features missing. Therefore, the language level of the child will suggest what language behaviors should be measured during assessment.

What to measure: language levels as guidelines. The following somewhat arbitrary
verbal levels are to be used only as rough and not necessarily comprehensive suggestions
for determining what language behaviors should be measured for each language level. The
behaviors the clinician plans to measure will differ according to whether the child: (1) is
nonverbal, (2) is minimally verbal, (3) has some connected speech, or (4) has essentially
normal language, with deficiencies in a few advanced aspects of oral language.

The nonverbal child is essentially speechless, although very few children are totally
speechless. This does not mean that the child's language, or perhaps more appropriately
called communication skills, cannot be assessed. There are many observations that can be
made regarding the communicative repertoire of a nonverbal child. The clinician should
plan to observe and measure:

- Gestures, signs, and symbols the child may be using
- Vocalization or imitation of nonspeech sounds
- Vocalization or imitation of any speech sounds
- Nonverbal responses to verbal stimuli including correct pointing, discriminating be-
  tween objects (comprehension)
- Imitations of simple words and phrases
- Spontaneous production of words
- Pragmatic language skills such as eye gaze and turn-taking

Even though the indications are that the child is essentially nonverbal, assessment always probes slightly higher levels to make sure. That is why imitation and spontaneous production of selected words are probed and, if successfully evoked, described and measured.

The lack of spontaneous speech and language is almost always accompanied by some
other diagnosis. If the child is a toddler (18–36 months of age), and the SLP is the first professional person the child has been brought to see, referrals should be made to other professionals or agencies for further assessment. It is not uncommon for SLPs to be the first to suspect
diagnoses such as developmental disability, autism, or hearing loss, but other professionals,
such as physicians, psychiatrists, psychologists, or audiologists are the ones who are fully qualified to make such diagnoses. In Part III of this book we will describe children with various
additional diagnoses along with suggestions for assessment procedures that should be modified, expanded, reduced, or even discarded altogether to meet the needs of these children.

The minimally verbal child produces isolated word responses and perhaps a few phrases,
but does not produce even simple sentence structures. In this case, the clinician should
plan to observe and measure:

- Everything mentioned under Level I
- Naming common objects, toys, family members, items of clothing and food
- Counting, reciting the alphabet, the days of the week, the months of the year
- Word combinations; production and imitation of simple phrases
- Production or comprehension of certain grammatic morphemes such as the present
  progressive -*ing* and the plural morphemes
- Production and comprehension of simple sentence structures

The child with some connected speech may on occasion produce simple sentence forms, making it possible to gather a simple conversational speech sample. In this case, the clinician should plan to observe and measure:

- Everything mentioned under Levels 1 and 2
- Answers to simple questions
- Production of various grammatic features, syntactic structures, sentence types
- The mean length of responses, the length of typical utterances, and so forth
- Comprehension of conversational speech

Assessment of a child who produces some connected speech places a greater emphasis on language samples. Also, those clinicians who wish to administer standardized tests will find many opportunities to do so with children at this level.

There are some children referred to SLPs who have apparently normal language, with deficiencies only in advanced aspects of language; their language problems are subtle. The child may have near-normal language performance, but a few advanced language concepts or structures may not be used or may be misused (e.g., lack of passive, compound, or complex sentence forms; no use or comprehension of figurative language; no use of dependent clauses, etc.). Clinicians should plan to:

- Assess mostly through conversational speech
- Use client-specific procedures to sample the particular behaviors of concern

These described levels of language are arbitrary—children do not typically neatly fall into one of the levels. Rather, the levels illustrate a range of verbal behaviors. The suggestions offered are meant to be used as guidelines, not rigid criteria, for the assessment of children with varying degrees of verbal output.

After determining *what* behaviors should be measured, through initial observation of the child's language level, the clinician must consider *how* to measure those behaviors. As previously discussed, clinicians measure language behaviors through two main methods: (1) through the administration of standardized tests and (2) through the use of child-specific measurement. We have discussed the conceptual bases for each of these methods and have argued that child-specific measurement is preferable to standardized testing. More detailed information regarding procedures and analysis of resulting data will be offered in the following sections.

Selection and Administration of Norm-Referenced Standardized Tests

Most clinicians, including those who opt for criterion-referenced or child-specific measures will use some norm-referenced tests for their previously described advantages. In selecting norm-referenced standardized tests, clinicians should take several steps to minimize the negative consequences of the tests when they are required to use them. First, they should select tests that have sampled children from the ethnocultural group to which the child to be tested belongs. Second, clinicians should not solely rely on a child's performance on norm-referenced standardized tests to diagnose a language disorder. They should take multiple measures of a child's language performance to make an accurate diagnosis. Third, multiple measures cannot be multiple tests; they should include child-specific procedures. A good language sample, obtained perhaps with the involvement of the parents or other primary caregivers, using relevant stimulus materials, is a good start. Fourth, the clinician should be cautious in interpreting the results of a test that is based entirely on a "normal" sample (McFadden, 1996). When available, a test based on a truly representative sample (which does not exclude children with limited language skills) may also be administered.

It is desirable to make child-specific decisions when selecting a standardized test (see Table 4.2 for commonly given tests). Besides examining the test-specific validity and reliability data, clinicians should also determine that:

- The test is suitable for the age level of the child
- The test will give clinically useful information on the child's language skills
- Instructions for administering and scoring the test are clearly given
- The normative sample includes children who represent the child's socioeconomic status; living environment (urban-rural); and cultural, linguistic, and ethnic background

Clinicians who are not familiar with a standardized test should practice its administration before giving it to a child. The test developer's instructions should be followed in administering the test and in interpreting the data. In most cases, clinicians should administer tests without giving any prompts or reinforcement for correct responses or corrective feedback for incorrect ones. Instead, the clinician can give the child noncontingent reinforcement for general behaviors to keep the child motivated (e.g., "I like the way you are sitting so nice and straight!" "You are working hard!" "You are doing just what I asked you to do!").

> Describe the differences between standardized and criterion-referenced tests.

The test manual will guide the clinician in interpreting the scores the child achieves. There are a variety of statistical analyses that can be made to compare the child's score to the scores of other children of the same age in the standardization sample on which the test was normed. See Box 4.4 for terms and types of statistical data relevant to standardized testing. Most school districts require a student to fall 1.5 standard deviations *below* the mean on language tests for the student to receive special education speech-language services.

Language samples.　Recording a child's conversational or naturalistic verbal interaction with the clinician, family member, or both is called a **language sample.** Obviously, the amount of language recorded will vary depending on the child's level of language skills as described earlier. The interaction is not entirely spontaneous or naturalistic as the clinician designs and guides it to make specific observations. Nonetheless, it is the most naturalistic of the assessment procedures, especially when the parent engages the child in play-oriented conversation.

> One disgruntled teacher was overheard on a school campus saying, "Oh, yes! A speech-language pathologist! Those are the ones that can't talk to a child without their picture cards!"

Structure the language sampling session.　A language sample is audio recorded during the initial assessment session. Audio recording helps the clinician to maintain interaction with the child. Clinicians should not rush the child or be so exuberant in their efforts to engage the child in conversation that the child is overwhelmed by the situation. The objective of the language sample is to get the *child* to talk; clinicians should therefore keep their own verbal output to a minimum, and let the child do most of the talking.

Based on the interview and case history information, the clinician should select toys, pictures, storybooks, games, and other objects that are familiar to the child. These stimu-

table 4.2

Standardized Tests for Assessment of Children's Language Skills

Test	Ages	Administration Time	Language Skills Tested
Clinical Evaluation of Language Fundamentals, Fourth Edition (CELF-4) Semel, Wiig, & Secord (2003)	5 yrs through 21 yrs	30–60 minutes	Expressive and receptive language: vocabulary and syntax
CELF—Preschool, Second Edition Semel, Secord, & Wiig (2004)	3 yrs through 6 yrs	30–45 minutes	Expressive and receptive language: includes pragmatic language skills
Comprehensive Receptive and Expressive Vocabulary Test-2 (CREVT-2) Wallace & Hammill (2002)	4 yrs through 17 yrs, 11 mos	20–30 minutes	Expressive and receptive language: defining words and pointing to pictures
Expressive Language Test (ELT) Huisingh, Bowers, LaGiudice, & Orman (1998)	5 yrs through 11 yrs, 11 mos	40–45 minutes	Expressive language: syntax, sequencing, categorizing, describing
Expressive One-Word Picture Vocabulary Test (EOWPVT) Brownell (2000a)	2 yrs through 10 yrs, 11 mos	20 minutes	Expressive language: one-word naming of pictured stimuli
Expressive Vocabulary Test (EVT) Williams (1997)	2 yrs, 6 mos through adult	20–30 minutes	Expressive language: labeling and synonyms
HELP Test—Elementary Lazzari (1996)	6 yrs through 11 yrs, 11 mos	25–30 minutes	Expressive language: vocabulary, syntax, definitions
Peabody Picture Vocabulary Test, Third Edition Dunn & Dunn (1997)	2 yrs, 6 mos through adult	25–30 minutes	Receptive language: point-to-picture task
Preschool Language Scale, Fourth Edition (PLS-4) Zimmerman, Steiner, & Evatt-Pond (2002a)	Birth through 6 yrs, 11 mos	20–45 minutes	Expressive and receptive language: vocabulary, basic concepts, morphology, syntax
Receptive One-Word Picture Vocabulary Test Brownell (2000b)	2 yrs, 11 mos through 12 yrs	20 minutes	Receptive language: point-to-picture task
Structured Photographic Expressive Language Test 3 (SPELT-3) Dawson & Stout (2003)	4 yrs through 9 yrs, 11 mos	15–20 minutes	Expressive language: morphological and syntactical forms (includes alternative responses for African American dialects)
Test for Auditory Comprehension of Language-3 (TACL-3) Carrow-Woolfolk (1999)	3 yrs through 9 yrs, 11 mos	15–25 minutes	Receptive language: vocabulary, grammatical morphemes, elaborated phrases and sentences
Test of Language Development—Primary (TOLD-P:3)	4 yrs through 8 yrs, 11 mos	40–45 minutes	Receptive and expressive language: vocabulary, syntax, sentence imitation
Test of Language Development—Intermediate (TOLD-I:3) Newcomer & Hammill (1997a, b)	8 yrs, 6 mos through 12 yrs, 11 mos	25–30 minutes	Sentence combining, vocabulary, syntax, abstract language, semantic absurdities
Test of Semantic Skills—Primary (TOSS-P) Bowers, Huisingh, LaGiudice, & Orman (2002)	4 yrs through 8 yrs, 11 mos		Expressive and expressive language: labels, categories, attributes, functions, definitions
Test of Semantic Skills—Intermediate Huisingh, Bowers, LaGiudice, & Orman (2003)	9 yrs through 13 yrs, 11 mos		
Token Test for Children DiSimoni (1978)	3 yrs through 12 yrs	10–15 minutes	Receptive language: temporal and spatial concepts

---

box 4.4 | | | **Terms, Scores, and Statistics Associated with Standardized Tests**

Basal: A specified number of consecutively correct answers a child must achieve before continuing with the remainder of the test; it is assumed all items below the basal are correct. Sometimes, a basal cannot be achieved.

Ceiling: The highest test item completed by the child; it is assumed that all items above the ceiling are incorrect. The test manual will specify how many incorrect responses must occur before the test is terminated.

Raw Score: The number of the ceiling item minus the number of errors the child made during testing.

Standard Score: The raw score is converted to a standard score; a derived score with which standardized comparisons can be made. The standard score uses as its base unit the standard deviation of the population on which the test was standardized.

Standard Deviation: The average difference of scores from the mean score; indicates how far from the mean score achieved by the sample population an individual score falls.

Most school districts require a child to fall at least 1.5 standard deviations (SDs) below the mean to qualify for special education services.

Standard Error of Measurement: A range of probable scores within which a child's "true" score probably falls. Calculated because human performance of the same task will vary.

Confidence Band: Represented by the range of scores determined by the standard error of measurement. If the confidence band is, for example ±7, and a child's standard score is 80, it is assumed the "true" score is somewhere between 73 and 87.

Percentile Rank: Indicates what portion of the sample population scored lower than the test taker. For example, if a child's standard score indicates a percentile rank of 30 percent, it means that 70 percent of the children in the sample population had higher scores.

---

lus materials should be appropriate for the child's family and linguistic and cultural background. It may be helpful to use stimulus items the child brings from home. Parents may be asked beforehand to bring the child's favorite toys, storybooks, or other objects the child might be eager to tell the clinician about.

Child-specific stimuli are effective in evoking language from a child, but it would be a mistake to present too many toys and pictures that may limit verbal interactions. Some children can get overly absorbed in play activities, and their language production may be inhibited. Another mistake is too much reliance on physical stimuli (especially toys) to evoke speech from children. Some student clinicians forget that they can simply talk to the child! In fact, the best language sample is obtained when the clinician engages the child in a naturalistic conversation. If the child proves to be talkative, this is often all that is necessary to gather an adequate language sample. In general, the less talkative the child, the more necessary it is to manipulate stimuli to evoke a language sample.

Evoke extended language productions. To evoke extended speech from a child, clinicians should ask open-ended questions rather than those that are answered *yes* or *no*. For

Why are open-ended questions preferred over close-ended questions during language sampling?

example, the clinician should ask, "What did you do this weekend?" instead of, "Did you see a movie this weekend?" If a close-ended question is used, it should be used only as a prelude to open-ended questions that will lead to more language. For example, "Did you see a movie this weekend?" may be a good question, if a *yes* answer leads to more questions such as, "Oh, good! Which one?" "I haven't seen that one; tell me about it!" or "What was your favorite part?" Through such questions, the clinician can introduce

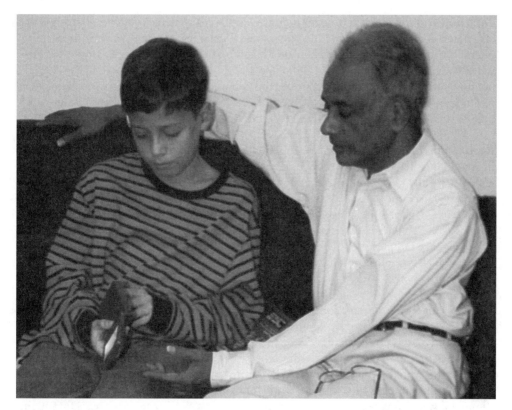

photo 4.1
Tell me about it!
Here, a clinician talks to an older child about his favorite video game.

a variety of topics including the child's school, leisure activities, favorite television shows, friends, birthday parties, vacations, siblings, grandparents, and so forth.

If pictures from storybooks are used, the clinician should ask such questions as, "What do you see here?" or "What is happening in this picture?" instead of "Is this a truck?" "Is he cooking in the kitchen?" and so forth. When the child seems to get lost in play, the clinician should gently move those toys away and begin a conversation or initiate an activity that encourages more talk from the child. An effective method of evoking extended language from children is to tell them a story and ask them to retell it. The clinician may read a brief and simple story aloud to the child and frequently ask questions about events and characters.

Vary the activities. During the language sample, the clinician should vary the activities and stimulus materials to keep the child interested and motivated. Clinicians may engage the child in conversation for a while and then move on to a play activity designed to evoke further language. A brief game activity that prompts the child to ask questions may help break the monotony. Reading aloud a story to the child will introduce variety and pique the child's interest. Clinician-induced activities may be interspersed with parent- or sibling-induced activities. When family members are asked to engage the child in play or conversation, the clinician has an opportunity to observe the child's more naturalistic interactions and verbal behaviors.

Take notes on the context of utterances. During verbal interactions, the clinician should take notes on the context of the child's utterances. Without such notes, some of the recorded utterances may be meaningless when later heard on the audiotape. For example, if a child is heard saying, "I see book" on an audiotape, the clinician may not know that the child did not produce the plural morpheme unless the note showed that the child was talking about multiple books. A single word utterance like "car" would not be later interpretable unless the notes say that the child actually wanted the car, but could not request it otherwise.

Record an adequate sample. Recommendations vary and some judgment is essential in concluding that enough is enough. Clinicians should gather a minimum of 50–100 utterances, ideally closer to the maximum. For most children, such a language sample can be gathered in about 30 minutes, but the duration depends on the individual child. Because a single language sample does not demonstrate reliability, clinicians need to obtain additional samples. This may be done when the child returns for the first treatment session. Brief language samples should be recorded during the first two or three treatment sessions. Also, language samples should be taken in a variety of settings, such as classrooms, playgrounds, or at home.

To check or not to check for stimulability. Although a language sample should assess the child's typical use of language, a traditional recommendation is to check for **stimulability**—the child's imitation of models provided. For example, a clinician who notices that a child has not produced any adjectives during the language sample may model some for the child to imitate (e.g., "Look, Johnny, it's a big, red ball, say 'big, red ball'!"). The child who imitates the clinician is said to be stimulable. Some clinicians assume that stimulability suggests good prognosis for treatment. But this is a tenuous basis for judging prognosis. A child who does not imitate certain kinds of responses still needs treatment and may be taught those responses through *shaping*, a procedure described in Chapter 6. Therefore, the value of the stimulability test is limited.

Arrange interaction to evoke conversational (pragmatic) skills. Most of the pragmatic language skills are indeed conversational skills (see Chapter 1 for details). The clinician should arrange the language sampling session to maximize the opportunities for such pragmatic skills as **topic initiation** (the skill of introducing new topics for conversation), **topic maintenance** (continuous conversation on the same topic without abrupt interruptions or introduction of new topics), **conversational turn-taking** (talking and listening, in alternative fashion), **conversational repair strategies** (verbal behaviors both listeners and speakers exhibit when there are breakdowns in communication), **narrative skills** (telling stories or personal experiences with sufficient details, temporal sequence, characterization, etc.), and **eye contact** (maintenance of mutual eye gaze during conversation). As described in Chapter 2, children with language disorders may have deficiencies in some or all of the pragmatic language skills.

The clinician can use a variety of stimuli to trigger topic initiation: objects, pictures, storybooks, topic cards (for children who can read), toys, and structured play situations using a play kitchen, a doll house, and so forth. The clinician should draw the child's attention to a stimulus item and then wait for the child to initiate conversation about that item. The conversational episode may be brief, but that the child initiated it is sufficient evidence of the skill. If the child does not initiate the topic, the clinician should direct the child to say something about the stimulus item. If the child still does not initiate a topic, the clinician can add a further cue, such as a sentence completion task (e.g., "This is a . . .").

To evoke topic maintenance, the child should be allowed to select topics of interest for talking. The clinician may prompt and suggest topics if necessary, but then should follow the child's lead once a topic is initiated. The clinician should respond as one normally would in conversation to keep it on the same topic. Comments like "I see!" "That's funny!" "I like your story!" "Tell me more!" "What happened next?" and so forth are appropriate. The clinician may start and stop a stopwatch to measure the duration (seconds or minutes) for which the child maintained the same topic of conversation. Topic maintenance should be measured for at least three topics.

Conversational turn-taking may be measured during the entire conversation. The clinician may right away notice that the child interrupts conversation by such extraneous or irrelevant comments as "You know what!" and "See my shoes!" in the middle of conversation on some other topic. After counting a few such interruptions, the clinician may tell the child to "Listen while I am talking" and after talking for a while, say "It is your turn to talk, now!" to judge the effects.

Requests for clarification, a conversational repair skill, may be evoked when the clinician makes ambiguous statements that require a request for clarification. For example, the clinician might say, "Give me the car," when several toy cars are displayed in front of the child, and wait for the child to ask for clarification. To check for stimulability of this skill, the clinician can model a request for clarification (e.g., "Ask me, 'What do you mean?' ") and wait for the child to imitate the request.

Clarification of one's statements, another conversational repair skill may be evoked when the clinician pretends or actually does not understand a child's statements and says so. The clinician can ask the child to repeat or may tell the child, "I don't understand" or "What do you mean?" Another technique is to negate a child's utterance so the child will clarify by assertion (e.g., "You're not 2 years old, are you?"; the child might answer, "No! I'm 4 years old!"). The clinician should wait a few seconds for the child to respond and should take note of whether the child makes no response, an inadequate response, or an adequate response to the request for clarification.

Eye contact may easily be noted during the entire period of assessment and conversation with the child. Lack of eye contact may be a culturally determined behavior, but the clinician should take note of it in assessment sessions as it may be a treatment target that culturally diverse families would still approve of as helpful for their child to learn.

Narrative skills may be evoked by asking the child to tell a story and by retelling a story just told. The clinician should have a few stories to tell children at different language levels. The clinician also may keep a collection of printed stories that are appropriate at different grade and language skill levels. The clinician then may read a brief story aloud and ask the child to retell it. If the child does not retell the story easily, the clinician may retell the same story to the child and pause before important phrases or critical story points to assess whether the child will supply them. A story can also be told with the help of pictures, and the child can be asked to retell the story while looking at the pictures. Even daily or occasional routines may be a means to evoke narrative skills. For example, the clinician may ask the child to describe such events as grocery shopping, eating in a restaurant, birthday parties, camping trips, vacations, playing certain games, and so forth.

Design and implement skill-specific tasks. Skill-specific tasks are an important aspect of child-specific (as well as criterion-referenced) assessment and measurement. Even an extended language sample may not provide opportunities for the child to produce many kinds of verbal skills. A clinician who fails to notice the absence of certain kinds of language responses and takes no steps to stimulate them during assessment will be frustrated during later analysis. It is true that not all missing language features may be identified during the initial assessment sessions, but to make the most of that session, the clinician needs to be diligent in observing the child's productions and to quickly identify needs for task-specific procedures to evoke as many different kinds of language responses as possible.

There are several skill-specific tasks that help examine a child's production of varied language responses. For example, if a child has not produced pronouns during a language sample, the clinician should present pronoun-specific tasks. Structured play activities using toys of identifiable gender might be used to evoke the production of pronouns *him, her, he, she, his,* and *hers.* For example, the clinician might ask, "Look! It's a hat! Whose hat is it?" to evoke *his* or *hers.* If the child did not produce some or any prepositions, the clinician can present preposition-specific tasks to evoke them. For example, the clinician may place an object or a toy on the table, under the table, in a box, behind a box, and so forth and ask, "Where is the___?" to evoke the production of prepositions. If the child did not produce the present progressive *-ing,* the clinician may demonstrate several actions (e.g., walking, drinking) and ask the child to describe the actions. See Table 4.3 for more examples of skill-specific tasks that help evoke some commonly assessed target behaviors.

table 4.3

Skill-Specific Tasks

Targeted Skill	Skill-Specific Task
Regular plurals	Ask the child to name pictures of, first, one object, and then, two of the same objects (e.g., show a picture of a ball and ask, "What is this?"; then show a picture of two balls and ask, "What are these?")
Irregular plurals	Ask the child to name pictures of multiple objects representing irregular plural nouns (e.g., *children, men, mice, feet, geese, sheep*)
Third person singular present tense (e.g., *talks, sleeps, eats, drinks*)	Show pictures depicting various actions, and ask the child, "What does she [he, they] do?" or, "Yesterday, he *talked*; today, he. . . ."
Regular past tense	Show pictures depicting various actions; use a sentence completion task (e.g., "Today, he cooks; yesterday, he . . . [*cooked*]")
Irregular past tense	Show pictures depicting irregular past tense verbs; use a sentence completion task (e.g., "Today, the baby sleeps; yesterday, the baby . . . [*slept*]")
Comparative *-er* and superlative *-est*	Using objects or pictures, give the child a sentence completion task (e.g., "The dog is big, but the horse is even . . . [*bigger*], and the elephant is the . . . [*biggest*]")
Adjectives	Show objects or pictures; use a sentence completion task (e.g., "This truck is . . . [*big*]"; "This flower is . . . [*pretty*]")
Adverbs	Demonstrate actions or show pictures depicting action; ask the child, "How am I running?" [*quickly* or *slowly*]; "How am I talking?" [*loudly* or *softly*], and so forth

Note: Always use multiple exemplars to ensure an adequate sample of the skill being observed.

If the child does not spontaneously produce the language behavior during these behavior-specific tasks, the clinician may prompt or model to see if the child would imitate (not to make inferences about prognosis, as in the case of stimulability). To continue with the example of toys of identifiable gender, if the child did not respond to the question, the clinician might give a further prompt, such as an indirect model (e.g., "I think it's *her* hat. What do you think?"). If the child still does not respond correctly, the clinician can give a full model: "It's *her* hat. Say, 'It's her hat.'" If the child responds correctly to these prompts, the clinician has gained good information about the types of prompts or models that are likely to be of help during treatment. In the assessment report, the clinician may report that the child does not produce certain responses, but does imitate them.

Check language understanding. So far, the emphasis has been on production of language responses. But it is necessary to assess whether the child has difficulty understanding spoken language (comprehension). Understanding or comprehension is assessed only by some action on the part of the child (or adult). Correct or relevant verbal or nonverbal responses during dialogue are a good indication of understanding. The clinician can give simple commands to see if the child performs the correct action. For instance, pointing to correct pictures or objects in a stimulus array is usually effective. The task may be made more or less complex, depending on the child's performance. Complex, multi-step commands (e.g., "First point to the truck and then to the cow"; "Point to the big red ball and the small blue car") are examples of more complex commands.

Unlike production of language, which may be scored (analyzed) from an audiotape, language understanding must be scored as the child performs the tasks during the assessment session. The clinician should take note of the number of mistakes the child makes in following commands. It is helpful to note the type of error the child makes. For instance, when the clinician requests, "Point to the big red ball and the small blue car," the child may forget the first part or the last part of the request. Also, the clinician should note the level at which the comprehension seems to break down. For instance, the child may follow correctly one- and two-step commands but fail at three-step commands.

Assess speech production in more or less detail. Children with language disorders typically have some speech-sound errors. Errors may be few in some and many in others. A child with a significant articulation disorder may be partly or mostly unintelligible. Therefore, an assessment of speech-sound production is essential for all children with language disorders. This assessment, however, may be more or less detailed, depending on the parental concerns and the extent of the errors the clinician notices during the initial stage of assessment. If the errors are few, the clinician can take note of them while talking with the child (language sampling). If the errors are many, the clinician may score them from the language sample. In some cases, the clinician may schedule another assessment session to administer articulation and phonological tests and to make a more detailed analysis of error patterns.

Assess nonverbal communicative behaviors. As noted earlier, some children being assessed may be mostly nonverbal. The case history, interview with the parents, and the initial observation of the child will suggest a need for nonverbal communication assessment. Instead of oral language skills, the targets of assessment will be gestures, pointing, grabbing the clinician's hand to get something, sign language, and other forms of nonverbal communication. Nonverbal communication and its assessment is an extensive topic that is discussed in more detail in Chapter 15.

Consider literacy skill assessment. In the public schools, language assessment and treatment are closely tied to academic performance of students. Speech-language pathologists are involved in literacy skill assessment and training. Often and perhaps ideally, literacy assessment is made after a language assessment has been completed. The clinician who integrates a few basic literacy procedures into language assessment can get some preliminary idea of a child's reading and writing skills, however. For instance, in assessing spoken word productions and understanding, the clinician may show a series of printed words to see if the child would point to the correct word, read named words correctly, name the letters of the alphabet, and say the sound a letter represents. To get a basic idea of the child's writing skills, the clinician may ask the child to print the letters of the alphabet, simple or complex words, phrases, and sentences, and so forth. When time is the critical element, however, the clinician may concentrate on oral language and communication skills and schedule a later time for assessing literacy skills in greater depth. See Chapter 10 for details on assessment of literacy.

Sample language in naturalistic settings. Ideally, a thorough assessment of a child's language skills includes observations of those skills in naturalistic settings. The home setting is particularly important to observe, and many school districts recognize this by sending early intervention teams out to the home to assess children referred for a possible language disorder. School speech-language pathologists should observe how school-aged children communicate in the classroom, on the playground, in the library, in the cafeteria, and so forth.

It is often best to wait until after the initial assessment session and subsequent language sample analysis to observe the child in other settings. If the clinician has a good idea about possible deficits in the child's language skills, those deficits can be specifically targeted for careful observation within more natural settings. At the end of the assessment session, the clinician should request a home language sample for analysis. As the parents will have observed and participated in the language sampling procedures, they may do this in an acceptable manner. The home sample is analyzed in the same manner as the clinic sample.

Although the clinician will be looking primarily for problems the child may have in communicating within various environments, it is also useful to look for strengths the child may exhibit. If a child is close to being nonverbal, for example, but appears to mand (request) through clearly defined nonverbal gestures, the clinician may base an initial treatment program on this strength. Many school districts require that a child's strengths as well as weaknesses be analyzed during assessment; documenting what a child *can* do is often as useful as documenting what a child *cannot* do.

Interview people who know the child. Observations in multiple settings should be supplemented by interviews with significant people in the child's various environments. While parents and other caregivers are the primary informants of children's behavior, siblings, peers, teachers, coaches, babysitters, and any one else who knows the child might offer useful information on the child's communication skills. Public school clinicians have excellent opportunities to talk to the peers, teachers, coaches, dining hall attendants, special education personnel, librarians, and so forth about a child's language and communication skills. Teachers can offer specific information on the types of language structures the child produces and the kinds of deficiencies the child typically exhibits in the classroom.

Analyze the language sample. The language sample should be transcribed, with notes showing the context in which the utterances were made. Each intelligible utterance should be transcribed on a separate line, and the number of unintelligible utterances should be noted. The transcription will help measure the frequency of various language skills, including the production and comprehension of words, sentence types (syntactic structures), morphologic productions, and conversational skills. In addition, most clinicians calculate a mean length of utterance and a type-token ratio. Box 4.5 shows a format that can be used for the transcription of language samples.

Calculate the mean length of utterance (MLU). A general measure of language development, the **mean length of utterance** is calculated by counting the total number of morphemes and dividing that number by the total number of utterances in a language sample:

$$\frac{\text{Total number of morphemes}}{\text{Total number of utterances}}$$

Box 4.6 provides some guidelines on counting morphemes. Roughly speaking, up to the age of 5, a child's MLU should be equivalent to chronological age, so that a 1-year-old child can be expected to be producing one-word utterances, a 2-year-old child is typically at the two-word level, and so forth (Brown, 1973). Certainly this is but a broad rule of thumb, and individual differences are more significant than this normative guideline. We have known typically developing 2-year-old children who produce two *paragraphs* at a time rather than two *words*!

Analyze word productions. The child's production and understanding of words (expressive and receptive vocabulary) should be analyzed. Clinicians should measure the frequency and accuracy of the following:

- Naming pictures, objects, and toys
- Naming objects by category (e.g. *food, toys, clothes*)
- Naming objects in a category (e.g., in response to the clinician's direction, "Tell me all the animals you know," was the child able to easily name a number of animals?)
- Naming actions depicted in pictures, acted out by the clinician, or performed by the child

The clinician should note any unusual word productions. Is there an evidence of overextension (e.g., use of the word *mother* to refer to all adult women or the use of the word *ball* to refer to all things round) or underextension (e.g., only the family pet is a cat and all other cats are not cats)? Did the child substitute vague, general terms for more specific terms (e.g., *stuff, thing, this, that*)?

The **type-token ratio** is a measure of word variety in a child's speech. It is calculated to find out the variety of *different* words a child produces. The clinician first counts all the words in the language sample. Then, the clinician counts each different word in the sample.

box 4.5 — Form for Language Sample Transcription

Name: _____   Clinician: _____

DOB: _____   Date of Sample: _____

Total number of morphemes: _____
  divided by
Total number of utterances: _____   =   Mean length of utterance: _____

Utterance	Context	Number of Morphemes

For example, if the word *house* is used three times, it is counted only once. The number of different words used is then divided by the total number of words used, as follows:

$$\frac{\text{Total number of different words}}{\text{Total number of words used}}$$

The TTR is typically about .45–.50 for children ages 3 to 8 (Templin, 1957). In other words, the number of different words spoken during a language sample is usually about half the number of total words spoken. A TTR that is significantly lower than .5 indicates a limited expressive vocabulary.

box 4.6   Guidelines for Counting Morphemes

Do Count:

- Each free morpheme as **one** (a word with no pre-fixes, suffixes, or grammatical markers)
- Each bound morpheme as **one** (e.g., *-ing, -ed,* plural *-s,* possessive *-s*)
- Contracted words as **two** (the word counts as one and the contractive morpheme as one, so a word such as *you're* is counted as two morphemes)
- Compound words as **one** (e.g., sidewalk, outdoors, birthday)
- Catenatives as **one** (e.g., *gonna, wanna, hafta*)
- Irregular plural forms as **one** (e.g., *feet, mice*)
- Irregular verb forms as **one** (e.g., *ate, threw, went*)
- Gerunds (verb forms that function as nouns, e.g., *"Running* is my favorite exercise!") as **one**
- Names of persons, places, or titles of books or movies as **one** (e.g., Aunt Mary, *Goldilocks and the Three Bears*, Peter Piper's Pizza Place)

Don't Count:

- Frequently used interjections such as *you know* or *um*
- Words used in false starts leading to revisions (*"I went to the*—Mom took me to the store.")
- Words that are repeated as dysfluencies; count only the final production (e.g., "I-I-I-I go to school" is counted as four, not seven)
- Words that are ritualistically repeated (e.g., *bye-bye* is counted as one)
- Utterances that are unintelligible
- Utterances that are imitations of adult models
- Utterances that are incomplete
- Rote utterances (e.g., recited nursery rhymes, dialogue from TV commercials)

Source: Compiled from Brown (1973), Owens (2004), and Shipley and McAfee (2004).

Analyze the sentence structures and types. The transcript affords a good chance for analyzing the child's production of various syntactic structures. The **frequency measure,** yielding the number of times a child produced a particular syntactic structure correctly, is a common measure. Clinicians should describe and measure production of such sentence types as:

- *Simple sentences (tacts).* An independent clause with no subordinate clause (e.g., "I laughed.")
- *Declarative sentences (tacts).* A construction that makes a statement (e.g., "This is my cat.")
- *Compound sentences.* A sentence with at least two independent clauses joined by a comma and a conjunction or with a semicolon; containing no subordinate clauses (e.g. "I went to the store, and then I went home.")
- *Complex sentences (tacts).* A sentence with one independent clause and one or more subordinate clauses (e.g., "I played with my doll while Mommy washed dishes.")
- *Questions, requests, and imperatives (mands).* Sentences that request more information (e.g., "What do you mean?" "Who is this?" or "Where is it?"), or request others to perform certain actions (e.g., "Please give me some milk"; "Tell me more"; "I want that."), or require a *yes/no* answer (e.g., "Is this a boy?" or "Is that a balloon?"), or direct commands (e.g., "Sit down!" or "Give me that!")
- *Negatives (tacts).* Sentences that reject or deny an affirmation (e.g., "That's not his ball, it's mine!")

In addition to the different types of sentences produced, the clinician should describe the kinds of grammatic words in the sentences. Did the child produce adjectives, prepositions, conjunctions, articles, pronouns, and so forth? Did the child combine words into noun phrases, using a noun with one or more modifiers preceding it (e.g., *pretty ball, my pink shoes*)? Did the child combine words into verb phrases, using auxiliary and copular verbs as well (e.g., auxiliary: "He *is eating*"; copular: "She *is* nice)? Did the child combine words into prepositional phrases (e.g., "The dog is *in the house.*")? Did the child use subject-verb-direct object construction (e.g., "He hit the ball.")?

Analyze morphologic productions. The child's production of morphologic features (both bound and free morphemes) may be measured for frequency. The frequency count may be used to calculate the percent correct production of most grammatic morphemes, especially the bound morphemes (such as the plural and possessive inflections, the present progressive, and the regular past tense inflections). The following formula is used to calculate the percent correct production:

$$\frac{\text{The number of correct production}}{\text{The number of obligatory contexts}} \times 100$$

Recall that an obligatory context is an occasion in which a certain morpheme must be included. For example, the child production, "Two hats," is an obligatory context for the plural morpheme *-s*. If it is missing, it is an error. As an example: If there were 20 occasions (obligatory contexts) for the child to produce the plural *s* morpheme, and the child produced it in only 10 of them, the correct plural morpheme production would be 50 percent (10 divided by 20 and multiplied by 100). Such percentages of correct production may be calculated for:

- Regular plurals (e.g., *cats, dogs*)
- Irregular plurals (e.g., *feet, mice*)
- Grammatical markers for verb tense (e.g., present tense *-s*, "He talks"; present progressive *-ing*, "He is walking"; past tense *-ed*, "He walked.")
- Irregular past tense verbs (e.g., *ran, ate*)
- Comparative and superlative forms (e.g., *big, bigger, biggest*)
- Possessive *-s* (e.g., *baby's bottle*)
- Pronoun forms (e.g., subjective or nominative case: "He went home"; possessive case: "It's her book"; objective case: "Give it to him.")
- Prepositions (e.g., *in, on, under*)
- Articles (*the, a, an*)
- Copulas and auxiliaries (e.g., *is, are, was, were*)
- Conjunctions (e.g., *and, but*)
- Adjectives (e.g., *big, small, pretty*)

The clinician may compare a child's production of morphologic and syntactic structures to typical sequences of language acquisition various researchers have described. See Table 4.4 for a description of the sequence in which children typically acquire various syntactic and morphological language structures, as well as semantic concepts.

Analyze conversational (pragmatic) language skills. For a child who exhibits even rudimentary language skills, certain pragmatic skills can be measured. Generally, the higher

table 4.4

Typical Sequence of Acquisition of Syntactic and Morphologic Structures and Semantic Concepts

Age	Syntactic Structures	Morphologic Structures	Semantic Concepts
1–2 yrs	One-word utterances; around 18 months, two-word utterances appear	Present progressive -ing and plural -s may appear at 24 months	Same one-word utterance can convey a variety of meaning; At 18 months, produces around 50 words and understands around 200 words; Follows one-step commands accompanied with gestures
2–3 yrs	MLU is 2.0–4.0; Telegraphic speech; Sentence forms include object-verb ("Baby eat"), verb-object ("Go car"), and subject-verb-direct object ("Mommy read book"); Wh- question forms ("What that?"); Expresses negation using no or not in front of verbs ("Not go!" "No eat!")	Regular past tense -ed (may overgeneralize, e.g., catched, blowed); Some irregular past tense verbs emerge (went); Prepositions in and on; Present progressive -ing; Plural -s; Overgeneralizes regular plural -s (mouses); Possessive -s	Comprehension at 36 months is approximately 3,600 words; Expressive vocabulary of 200–600 words; Answers simple wh- questions; Identifies some body parts; Follows one- and two-part commands; At 36 months, can tell a simple story
3–4 yrs	MLU is 3.0–5.0; Complex and compound sentences ("I jump and play!"); Embedded clauses ("That dog over there is big."); Passive voice ("Mommy was kissed by Daddy."); Negative sentences ("I can't do it!")	Irregular plural forms (children, feet); Third-person singular present tense (she talks); Past and present progressive tense (was running; is walking); Reflexive pronouns (myself, himself)	Comprehends 4,200–5,600 words; Produces 800–1,500 words; Asks how, why, and when questions; Understands common opposites (night/day; big/little); Has labels for most things in the environment; Relates personal experiences; tells about activities in sequential order
4–5 yrs	MLU is 4.5–7.0; Complete sentences; Future verb tense constructions ("I will go with Grandpa."); If . . . so construction ("If I am good, I get ice cream!" or "I am good, so I get ice cream!")	Comparatives (bigger, shorter); More consistent production of irregular plurals; Production of most pronouns, including possessives (mine, his, hers)	Names items in a category (animals, clothes, toys); Defines common words; Tells longer stories with accuracy; Identifies objects by function and attribute ("Show me the one that is round"; "Show me the one you write with."); Frequent use of why questions
5–6 yrs	MLU is 6.0–8.0; Present, past, and future tense constructions; Sentence forms become more complex; grammatical errors decrease; Language form approaches adult level	Indefinite pronouns (nobody, something, all, nothing); Superlative -est (nicest, tallest); Adverbial word ending -ly (slowly, quickly)	Understands and expresses spatial relations and prepositions (on top, in front of, behind); Describes similarities and differences in objects; Names positions of objects (first, second, third, last)
6–7 yrs	MLU averages 7.3; Perfect tense forms ("I have had enough"; "I will have eaten by then."); More frequent embedded clauses	Produces most morphological markers correctly; Irregular comparatives (good, better, best; bad, worse, worst); Gerunds ("I like to go fishing.")	Understands time concepts; seasons of the year, daily schedules; Can recite the alphabet, name capital letters, match lowercase to uppercase letters; Counts to 100
7–8 yrs	MLU 7.0–9.0; Complex sentence forms predominate expressive language	Produces most irregular verb forms correctly	Takes jokes and riddles literally; Produces some figurative language; Describes objects in detail; Retells a story in correct sequence

Source: Compiled from Roseberry-McKibbin and Hegde (2005) and Paul (2001).

the language skill level of the child, the greater the opportunities there are to measure conversational language skills. Skills that should be measured include:

- *Topic initiation.* The number of times the child initiated a new topic for conversation
- *Topic maintenance.* The duration for which the child continued to talk on a given topic
- *Conversational turn-taking.* The number of interrupting comments, the frequency of appropriate switching of listener and speaker roles
- *Conversational repair.* The frequency with which the child asked questions when something was not clear, the frequency with which the child correctly responded when requested to clarify his or her own productions
- *Eye contact.* The frequency or durations for which the child maintained eye contact during conversation
- *Narrative skills.* Accuracy and adequacy of story telling with a proper temporal sequence of events, character descriptions, correct story settings, without missing details, good beginning and ending, and so forth

Although most of the conversational skills may be measured from a written transcript (or audiotapes), eye contact must be measured during the assessment session. An alternative method would be to videotape the child during assessment and examine the videotape to observe eye contact later. The clinician may take note of the frequency or duration for which the child maintained eye contact during assessment. It is probably most efficient to take note of the presence or absence of all conversational skills during assessment, instead of measuring them off of transcripts or audiotapes. With some experience, the clinician can make quick notes on the number of times the child failed to initiate a new topic, interrupted the clinician (wrong turn-taking), switched topics abruptly (failure to maintain topics), failed to clarify unclear statements when requested, did not request clarification when the clinician made unclear statements, told stories in sparse language and with wrong temporal sequence, and so forth. For most of these skills, the clinician can calculate a percent correct response rate. For instance, the number of acceptable requests for clarification the child made may be divided by the total number of ambiguous statements the clinician made, and the result multiplied by 100 to calculate a percentage for correct requests for clarification.

Judge other aspects of speech. Although the child is referred for a language disorder, it is necessary to make an informal evaluation of other aspects of the child's verbal behavior. We noted earlier the need to assess articulation skills in children with language disorders. The clinician can analyze the language sample for speech sound errors. Furthermore, the clinician should make observations on such other aspects as voice and fluency. From what they hear during assessment, most clinicians note whether the child's fluency and voice characteristics are within normal limits. A clinician in doubt may count the number of dysfluencies for a segment of the speech sample to make a judgment. The clinician should note vocal intensity (loudness), frequency (pitch of voice), voice quality deviations (hoarseness, harshness, and breathiness of voice), and resonance characteristics (hyper- or hyponasality).

Analyze nonverbal communicative behaviors. Most children with language disorders are still verbal communicators. During verbal communication, children may use gestures, facial expressions, manual guidance of caregivers (e.g., taking the mother's hand and directing it to a desired object), pointing, and so forth. The clinician should take note of these nonverbal communicative behaviors during assessment. If the child is mostly nonverbal, a more detailed assessment must be made. The assessment procedures for analysis of nonverbal communication are described in Chapter 15.

Make preliminary observations on literacy skills. As noted before, a few simple procedures may have been used to get a basic idea of the child's reading and writing skills. To the extent literacy skills were assessed, the clinician may analyze the results and make some preliminary comments.

Making a Diagnosis

The case history information, combined with an analysis of the assessment results will provide the bulk of the information needed to make a diagnosis of a language disorder, describe the speech and language deficiencies, and write a diagnostic report. The report will contain recommendations and a statement of prognosis for improvement under treatment.

At the end of the assessment session, the clinician makes a tentative diagnosis and discusses it with the parents or other informants who have brought the child to the clinic. The final diagnosis is made only when all the assessment data, interview information, case history, and information obtained from other professionals are analyzed and integrated, and conclusions are drawn about the child's speech, language, and communication skills.

As noted earlier, measurement of the child's language skills should support the diagnosis. If the language skills are judged deficient; if the child's communicative needs and demands are not met; if the child's academic and social success is in jeopardy; a diagnosis of a language disorder is justified. Clinicians who have to follow the guidelines of their professional settings will do so in making this diagnosis. For instance, school clinicians may follow such guidelines as skills falling below a certain level (e.g., 1.5 standard deviations below the mean) to diagnose a language disorder and qualify the child for treatment.

Recommendations: Talking with Family Members

In private or hospital settings, the assessment session ends with a conversation with the family members or guardians who have brought the child to the clinic. In most cases, even without the final analysis and integration of data, the clinician will have enough information to make a tentative diagnosis of a language disorder or to rule it out. The clinician should emphasize that the initial impressions are entirely preliminary, and a final diagnosis will have to wait for a complete analysis of all the information gathered. A written report will convey this final diagnosis to the parents.

Avoiding professional jargon, the clinician should discuss the assessment findings and clinical impressions with the parents. For example, the clinician should talk about "the number of words Johnny uses at one time" or "the length of Johnny's sentences" instead of "mean length of utterance." The clinician may summarize the kinds of difficulties the child has in understanding and producing words, speaking in grammatically complete sentences, talking on a topic for an extended time, and so forth. Avoiding euphemisms, the clinician should give the information in a straightforward, professional manner, but in simple language. The clinician should answer any questions the parents or others might have. The clinician may suggest further referrals to other professionals, further assessment at the same facility, or language treatment for the child.

Writing a Diagnostic Report

By the time a thorough assessment of a child has been completed, the clinician has accumulated a good deal of information regarding the child's language skills, the child's family communication patterns, and the social and academic demands the child faces. Integrating all this information, the clinician writes a diagnostic report. It is best to invite the family back to the clinic so the clinician can sit down with the family and go over the report with them, rather than sending it through the mail. The clinician should answer any questions family members might have and observe the family's reactions to information contained in the report. The report may be mailed to the referring professionals (e.g., teachers or pediatricians).

The length and the format of the diagnostic report will vary across clinical settings. Generally, the report summarizes the family background; physical, language, and social development of the child; academic performance and demands; and the results of various

photo 4.2
The clinician should personally go over the information contained in the diagnostic report with the parents or caregivers.

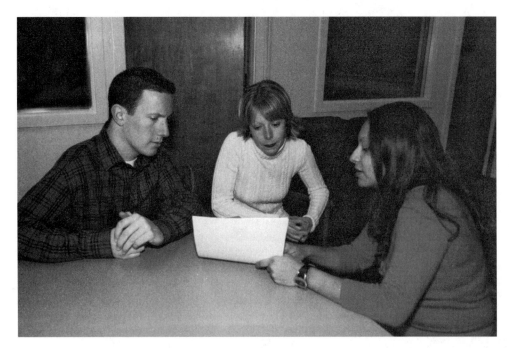

assessment procedures (e.g., orofacial examination, hearing screening, speech-language samples, client-specific measurement, interviews, etc.). The report usually ends with recommendations and a statement of prognosis. A **prognostic statement** is a considered, professional judgment regarding the course of the disorder under given conditions. For instance, the clinician may state that, "if the child receives treatment twice a week for 9 months, significant improvement in language skills may be expected." There is little or no research on the validity of prognostic statements speech-language pathologists make. Therefore, such statements should be treated strictly as professional opinion. A typical diagnostic report format is shown in Box 4.7. See Hegde (2003b) for a variety of examples of well-written diagnostic reports.

An assessment of a child's language that results in a diagnosis of a language disorder is but the beginning of the therapeutic process. If the clinician has done a thorough job of assessing the child's language skills, there should be clear indications as to what language behaviors need to be taught or increased. The clinician should have a good idea as to what undesirable language behaviors need to be decreased, as well. A good assessment, in other words, should make the transition to intervention a smooth one. The next chapters will set forth a basic framework for the treatment of language disorders along with specific techniques and variations that may be adapted as necessary to meet the needs of individual clients.

Chapter Summary

Assessment is a prerequisite for treatment and includes measurement of clinically relevant skills. Clinical measurements should be both reliable (consistent across measures) and valid (measure what the procedure intends to measure). Interjudge, intrajudge, alternate form, test–retest, and split-half are the five common types of reliability. Content, construct, concurrent, and predictive validity are the four common types of validity.

Norm-referenced standardized testing is a common method of measuring a child's speech and language skills because of its ease of use and the opportunity it offers to make comparisons across children. The limitations of norm-referenced tests include inadequate sampling of varied segments of a population, limited sampling of individual skills, and difficulty in predicting individual child's skill level based on norms. Criterion-referenced tests, which do not give norms but provide for mastery levels of specific skills, are an alternative to standardized tests. Child-specific measures, similar to criterion-referenced measures, are clinician-constructed stimulus materials that help measure a given child's skills in greater depth.

Initially, children may be screened to see if assessment is warranted. A complete assessment includes taking a case history; interviewing the parents; conducting an orofacial examination; screening the child's hearing; administering standardized tests, criterion-referenced tests, or both; making child-specific measurements of language skills; evaluating pragmatic language skills through conversational speech and narratives; and analyzing the results to make a diagnosis. Subsequently, clinical measures may be supplemented with language samples from home.

box 4.7 **A Typical Format for a Diagnostic Report**

LANGUAGE, SPEECH, AND HEARING CLINIC
1234 W. Main Street
Anytown, U.S.A. 54321
(123) 456-7890

DIAGNOSTIC REPORT

CLIENT:	BIRTH DATE:
ADDRESS:	CLINIC FILE NO.:
CITY:	DIAGNOSIS:
TELEPHONE:	REFERRED BY:
ASSESSMENT DATE:	CLINICIAN:

BACKGROUND AND REASONS FOR REFERRAL
HISTORY

Medical History

Family, Social, and Educational History

OBSERVATIONS AND ASSESSMENT RESULTS

Hearing Screening

Orofacial Examination

Language Production and Comprehension

Speech Production and Intelligibility

Voice and Fluency

DIAGNOSTIC SUMMARY AND RECOMMENDATIONS

Signed: _____
        Jane Doe, M.A., CCC-SLP

Study Guide

1. Discuss how assessment, measurement, and diagnosis are interrelated scientific and clinical activities. Define all the technical terms you use and justify the statement that "measurement is key to proper diagnosis."

2. During your first semester of clinical practice, your supervisor assigns you a 6-year-old child who has been referred to the clinic for language assessment. You learn that the child is English–Spanish bilingual. The supervisor has asked you to give her a list of assessment tools or procedures that you would use during assessment. In selecting the tools and procedures, what criteria would you use? Justify your answer.

3. Discuss the strengths and limitations of norm-referenced standardized tests versus criterion-referenced tests. Who are the most appropriate candidates for each test and why?

4. The author of a new test of language skills reported that she administered not only her new test to a randomly sampled group of children, but also administered a well-established test. She then correlated the children's scores on the two tests. Why did she do this?

5. Describe all the steps and procedures needed to make a complete assessment of a child. Address issues related to children of varied ethnocultural backgrounds. Specify the relative roles standardized tests and language samples play in a total assessment format.

6. How would you record and analyze a language sample? What specifics outcomes would you seek from your analysis? How does the results of your analysis help make a diagnosis?

chapter 5

Treatment of Language Disorders: An Evidence-Based Framework

outline

In this chapter we describe a framework for treatment, based on child language treatment research. What is a framework? It is an outline that needs to be filled in, expanded, and strengthened. We will have some suggestions on how to do this in subsequent chapters, but much will depend on the child, his or her family, and, of course, the clinician working with them. Ultimately, the success of a treatment program depends on the clinician, the client, and the family. A treatment that accomplishes its goals is the results of a carefully engineered partnership between the clinicians, their clients, and the families. The reader will find this viewpoint fully expanded in Chapter 8 on maintaining language skills of clinically treated children in naturalistic settings.

Our goal in this chapter is to offer a loose and flexible structure within which the clinicians, the clients, and their families form a partnership to make language treatment a success for all involved. The framework is loose and flexible because it offers the maximum latitude for clinical judgment, expertise, and modifications dictated by the special circumstances of the family and the uniqueness of the child. We often think that effective and functional treatment is an accomplishment for the clients and their families. Certainly, so it is. But effective and functional treatment is also a very satisfying accomplishment for the clinician. We expect that student clinicians who are about to enter clinical practice or those who already are in the process, will find the framework useful in achieving a satisfactory outcome for themselves, as well as for the families they serve.

It is our goal, as well, to help clinicians make their clinical judgments based on treatment research evidence. To address that goal, we start with the concept of evidence-based practice in medicine, other human service professions, and speech-language pathology.

What Is Evidence-Based Practice?

There is a myriad of suggested language treatment methods. Unfortunately, many of these treatment procedures have not been put to experimental test, and some are supported solely by expert advocacy. Professionals are now keenly aware that treatment methods should be evidence-based. Strictly defined from a scientific standpoint, **evidence-based practice** means the use of only those treatment methods that are supported by controlled and replicated research evidence (Hegde, 2003a). In this strictest sense of the term, evidence is experimentally demonstrated effectiveness of treatment procedures. More broadly defined, evidence-based practice requires an integration of best evidence for diagnostic and treatment methods with sound clinical expertise and judgment. Furthermore, evidence-based practice takes into consideration what is best for an individual patient and his or her preferences (Sackett et al., 1996; Sackett et al., 2000). A method supported by evidence may be unacceptable to clients, their families, or both. Evidence-based practice also implies that the clinicians delay the adoption of unproven methods and prevent the use of ineffective methods (Lohr, Eleazer, & Mauskopf, 1998). To use evidence-based methods, both student clinicians and professionals should critically analyze the quantity and quality of evidence supporting the use of advocated treatment techniques and consider the characteristics of the individual client seeking the services.

In the current age of freely and easily accessed information on the Internet, clients, parents, and other concerned individuals tend to demand that SLPs try out certain techniques. For example, consumers may demand that they receive such techniques as sensory integration training, facilitated communication, floortime, auditory integration training, or oral motor exercises, believing the techniques are effective, perhaps because they are new or vigorously promoted. Furthermore, experts, too, offer "new and revolutionary" treatment techniques to clinicians, strongly advocating their use. When faced with such consumer requests and expert advocacy, SLPs should critically evaluate the efficacy data on treatment procedures and discuss the evidence with their clients and their families to make a final selection with their participation and approval. To evaluate treatment efficacy data, clinicians should have knowledge of research methods used to generate such data and a standard framework they can apply to evaluate the evidence.

An Overview of Treatment Research

Generally speaking, treatment methods should (1) be effective and (2) have demonstrated functional outcome. This means that the treatment is better than no treatment (i.e., effective) and that it results in new communicative behaviors that are useful (i.e., functional) to the client in natural settings (American Speech-Language-Hearing Association, 1997–2003; Frattali, 1998; Hegde, 2003a; Warren & Rogers-Warren, 1985). Treatment methods should not be accepted based on anecdotal evidence or because of such subjective factors as the ease with which they are applied, the attractiveness of the materials they use, the appeal they may hold for clinicians, or the authority of the experts who advocate them.

SLPs instead need to ask themselves three questions when considering the selection of a particular treatment method: (1) Is the technique capable of producing improvement in clients? (2) Is the technique effective? (3) Does the technique have generality across settings, clinicians, and clients, including clients of different ethnocultural backgrounds? Unfortunately, these three questions cannot simply be answered *yes* or *no* in evaluating a given technique. Treatment research evidence is rarely categorical; evidence continuously evolves as research moves from one level to the next. To understand the levels of evidence, it is necessary to understand the different kinds of treatment research (Barlow, Hayes, & Nelson, 1984; Barlow & Hersen, 1984; Johnston & Pennypacker, 1993; Hegde, 2003a; Kazdin, 1982; Portney & Watkins, 2000), especially uncontrolled, controlled, directly replicated, and systematically replicated treatment research.

The single-subject designs are practical in evaluating the effects of treatment. The design in which skill is baserated, treatment offered, withdrawn, and reinstated is called the ABAB design. The initial A is the baserate condition, the first B is treatment, the second A is withdrawal, and the second B is the reinstatement of treatment. Other design options include the multiple baseline across subjects. In this design, participants receive treatment in a staggered fashion. After baserating the skill in all of the subjects, the clinician treats one of them; baserates the skills in remaining participants; treats the second participant; repeats baserates on not-yet-treated participants, and so forth. The design can show that only those who received treatment changed and those who did not remained unchanged.

Uncontrolled and Controlled Treatment Research

Treatment research may be uncontrolled or controlled. *Uncontrolled treatment research* does not compare treatment to no treatment. In the form of a case history, it reports that clients who received a treatment benefited from it. This only means that the treatment is associated with improvement, but because of lack of control (e.g., the absence of a control group that does not receive treatment or such control conditions as treatment withdrawal), no effect can be claimed for the procedure. The clients may have improved for other reasons. For example, children who receive language treatment may have improved because of maturation, a teacher's language stimulation program, or a parent's storybook reading. Routine clinical practice is uncontrolled in that it does not rule out factors other than treatment that may contribute to improvement. The clinician can claim improvement in the client behaviors, but not effectiveness for the procedure used.

In **controlled research,** treatment is compared against no treatment and may involve either a group experimental design or a single-subject experimental design. In the group design approach, one group that receives treatment (experimental group) is compared against another comparable group (control group) that does not. If the skill levels in the experimental and control groups were comparable to begin with, but only the skills of the former group improved significantly when measured at the end of the experimental treatment, then the treatment was effective. In the single-subject approach, a few clients (not necessarily one client) are observed during baseline (no treatment) and when an experimental treatment is offered, withdrawn, and reinstated. If the skills in the participants were low to begin with, improved when the treatment was first offered, declined when it was withdrawn, and improved again when it was reinstated, the treatment was effective. In both the cases, treatment is compared against no treatment. While clinicians in routine work who document positive changes in their clients during treatment can always claim improvement, effectiveness can be claimed only when treatment is compared against no treatment either with the group design or the single-subject design strategy. Note also that controlled research is also known as *experimental research.* In essence, only experimental research can show that a treatment procedure is effective (Barlow, Hayes, & Nelson, 1984; Barlow & Hersen, 1984; Hegde, 2003a; Johnston & Pennypacker, 1993; Kazdin, 1982; Portney & Watkins, 2000).

> What are two broad categories of experimental design that may be used in controlled research?

> When can treatment effectiveness rightfully be claimed?

Unreplicated and Replicated Treatment Research

Treatment may be unreplicated or replicated, and both the varieties may be uncontrolled or controlled. **Unreplicated** is the first or the original study on a given procedure. If it is uncontrolled, it is the first case study on the procedure. If it is controlled, then it is the first experimental study on the technique (comparing treatment with no treatment). Treatment research is **replicated** when it is repeated by either the same researcher or other researchers. Replications are needed to establish the reliability of improvement or effectiveness of treatment procedures and their general applicability.

> What do we call the type of evidence produced by the original, or first, study done on a given procedure? What do we call it if the study is repeated by other researchers?

Replication may be direct or systematic. In **direct replication,** the same researcher repeats his or her own earlier study with little or no modification in the treatment procedure to see if the results are reliable. The major difference between the original study and a direct replication is that the latter will recruit new clients for participation. If the earlier study was uncontrolled, then the repeated study is uncontrolled directly replicated. If the earlier study was controlled, then the repeated study is controlled directly replicated. In either case, if the results of the original and the replicated studies are similar, the procedure is thought to produce a reliable outcome (Barlow, Hayes, & Nelson, 1984; Barlow & Hersen, 1984; Hegde, 2003a; Johnston & Pennypacker, 1993; Kazdin, 1982).

In **systematic replication** the study is repeated in different settings, by different researchers, using different clients to show that the technique will yield similar results under varied conditions and with different clinicians. Systematic replication, therefore, establishes generality of treatment procedures. **Generality** means the wider applicability of a treatment procedure. Depending on the type of study that is repeated, it may be an uncontrolled systematically replicated or controlled systematically replicated study. See Table 5.1 for a summary of these types of treatment research.

 Whether or not treatment procedures are effective for culturally diverse children is a question of ethnocultural generality. More research is needed to establish ethnocultural generality for commonly used treatment techniques.

These varieties of treatment research create different levels of treatment research evidence; the levels may be arranged in a hierarchy. There are roughly six levels or categories of treatment research evidence. To this we have added one more, which is truly not a level of evidence, but exemplifies a common practice in our profession that clinicians need to recognize for what it really is. Note that these levels are on a continuum; the hierarchical points on the continuum (levels or categories) help make judgments, but should not be thought of as discontinuous. In considering a treatment procedure, the clinician should evaluate and categorize the evidence accumulated on it. A given technique may then be accepted or rejected based on the hierarchical level the evidence has attained.

table 5.1

A Hierarchy of Treatment Efficacy Evidence: Guidelines for Selecting Treatment Procedures for Evidence-Based Practice

Level of Evidence	Research Method	Interpretation	Recommendation
Level 1 Expert Advocacy	None	No evidence to support the advocated technique	Reject it until positive evidence begins to emerge
Level 2 Uncontrolled Unreplicated Evidence	A case study; not a controlled experiment	A claim of only improvement, not effectiveness, can be accepted	Use a technique with this level of evidence only when no technique with a higher level of evidence is available
Level 3 Uncontrolled Directly Replicated Evidence	A case study that has been replicated by the same investigator	Reliability of the originally claimed improvement is shown	The same as for Level 2; the claimed improvement may be more reliable
Level 4 Uncontrolled Systematically Replicated Evidence	A case study that has been replicated by others in varied settings	Greater generality of improvement is established; excellent candidate for experimentation	The same as for Level 3; the claimed improvement may be realized in different settings with the same technique
Level 5 Controlled Unreplicated Evidence	An experimental design of the group or single-subject approach	The first level at which efficacy, not just improvement, is claimed; treatment compared against no treatment	Use the technique with caution; prefer a method with a higher level of evidence; watch for replications and contradictory evidence
Level 6 Controlled Directly Replicated Evidence	The same experimental design used in the original study, implemented by the same original investigator	Reliability of the originally claimed effectiveness is shown	Use the technique with greater confidence; prefer a method with Level 7 evidence; watch for replications and contradictory evidence
Level 7 Controlled Systematically Replicated Evidence	An experimental design implemented by different investigators in varied settings	Generality of the treatment's effectiveness well established; the highest level of evidence for effectiveness	The most preferred treatment procedure; recommended for general professional practice; supports truly evidence-based practice

Guidelines for Selection: A Hierarchy of Treatment Research Evidence

There are alternative guidelines to select treatment procedures. For instance, in medicine, levels of research evidence that guide selection of diagnostic and treatment procedures are based mostly on randomized clinical trials in which large numbers of patients are randomly selected and randomly split into two (or more) groups. Then, one group may receive the new treatment whose effects are being evaluated while the other group may receive a placebo or an established treatment. If the new treatment is safe and at least as effective as the old treatment and more effective than the fake medicine (placebo), then the new procedure is approved for general use. Levels of evidence popular in medicine and advocated by ASHA do not adequately recognize single-subject designs in which small numbers of individuals are selected for treatment evaluation. In speech-language pathology and behavioral sciences, single-subject treatment evaluation is much more common than randomized, large-group clinical trials. Much of the treatment efficacy evidence in language treatment ASHA's website lists has been generated by single-subject research (www.asha.org/members/research/NOMS2/childlanguage). Therefore, we propose that a treatment evidence hierarchy that includes both the randomized clinical trials and single-subject experimental studies will be more useful to clinicians in evaluating treatment evidence to select effective procedures.

Clinicians can use the following hierarchical framework to evaluate not only language treatment techniques but any treatment technique offered in speech-language pathology, medicine, and all human service professions. As this new hierarchy of evidence is described in detail elsewhere (Hegde, 2003a), we will summarize it here. To facilitate a comparison of what is proposed here, the levels of hierarchy based on large-group randomized clinical trials are described in Box 5.1.

Level 1. Expert Advocacy

A common practice in speech-language pathology is to describe and advocate "new" and "exciting" treatment procedures with no research data. The technique may be justified on the basis of rational theories, clinical experience, logic, intuition, and conviction that it *ought to work*. Clinicians who do not demand evidence for accepting treatment procedures do not recognize this level for what it is—only an expert's opinion touted as evidence. Expert advocacy is no basis to apply a technique in routine clinical settings because it is not based on uncontrolled, controlled, replicated, or even unreplicated evidence. Techniques or ideas expressed in expert advocacy may be worthy of treatment research, but their clinical application is unethical.

> The costly mistake of taking expert advocacy too seriously is well known, though the practice goes unchecked. When the whole language approach or facilitated communication (for children with autism; see Chapter 15) was widely practiced, there was no controlled experimental evidence to support either of them. That did not stop their widespread use. They are now shown to be ineffective, but some clinicians are unaware of this.

Level 2. Uncontrolled Unreplicated Evidence

Level 2 treatment evidence is reached when a treatment technique has been applied to some individuals and positive or negative results are reported. This type of evidence is produced by the first case study, hence it is uncontrolled and unreplicated. Although described

box 5.1   **Levels of Treatment Research Evidence, Based on Randomized Clinical Trials Involving Large Groups of Patients**

Often, the levels of evidence in medicine are classified into three major classes.

Class I Evidence. Considered the best evidence supporting a diagnostic or treatment method, Class I evidence is generated by randomized clinical trials. At least one, large, randomized clinical trial's results should support a procedure to be classified Class I. The treatment to be evaluated is compared against a standard treatment, no treatment, or a placebo. The new treatment should at least be as effective as the old treatment and should significantly surpass the placebo effect (the subjective feeling of improvement when patients think they are being treated, even though they are not).

Class II Evidence. The second best level, Class II evidence is generated by studies involving comparison groups that are not randomly selected and assigned to different groups. When patients are not randomly selected and divided into groups, there is no assurance that they were similar to begin with. Hence, any difference they show after treatment offered to one of the

groups may not entirely be due to treatment. Nonetheless, the evidence is based on systematic observation of patients in different groups. In essence, the results are less robust because of methodological weaknesses in treatment studies.

Class III Evidence. The least preferred, Class III evidence is based on expert opinion, case studies, and case studies with historic controls. Case studies show that individuals or groups of people improved when treated. There will be no control groups to compare, therefore, case studies are *uncontrolled* (see the text for details) and can claim improvement, but not effectiveness. Historic controls are used when a current group's improvement with a new procedure is compared with a past group's improvement with a different procedure.

As noted in the text, judgment of evidence should take into consideration the *quality* of research studies. American Speech-Language-Hearing Association offers information on evidence-based practice on its website: www.asha.org/members/slp/topics/ebp.htm.

as Level 2, this is the first level in which some evidence favoring a treatment emerges because the earlier level offers no evidence of any kind. Evidence from case studies is better than expert advocacy because treatment has been applied with positive (or negative) results. If the results are positive, improvement can be expected with its application, but the clinician should wait for replications to see if the positive results are reliable. It is critical to know that positive Level 2 evidence means that the technique is likely to produce improvement, but it does not mean that the technique is effective. Level 2 evidence is no basis to recommend widespread application of a technique, and clinicians should resist any such recommendation. The only condition under which a clinician might use a technique that is at Level 2 is the total absence of techniques that have reached higher levels of evidence. In most cases of communicative disorders, this is not the case. In language treatment for children, the evidence for certain methods is at higher levels, as will be discussed later.

Level 3. Uncontrolled Directly Replicated Evidence

Investigators who replicate their own previous case studies with new clients produce Level 3 evidence. Typically done in the original clinical setting, the results test the reliability of the original outcome. When the results are positive, the same improvement will have been documented a second time, thus documenting reliability. Nonetheless, this is still an uncontrolled, though directly replicated, case study. Only improvement, not effectiveness, can be claimed for the procedure. It is still possible that such extraneous factors as maturation or language stimulation activities of other persons produced the positive changes in children who received the treatment. It is, however, very likely that the procedure may produce effectiveness in a controlled study. The technique is now a good candidate for controlled (experimental) study. Once again, clinicians can use a technique at Level 3 only if a technique with a higher level of evidence is nonexistent, a case not true of children's language treatment.

Level 4. Uncontrolled Systematically Replicated Evidence

When treatment researchers replicate case studies of other researchers, Level 4 evidence emerges. This evidence is still uncontrolled and can support only the claim of improvement, not effectiveness, because it is still case study evidence. The evidence is much stronger than in previous levels because other research clinicians have replicated the findings in other clinical settings using other clients. The evidence at this stage can multiply with each additional replication done in different settings. Therefore, the evidence at this level may be progressively expanding. Systematic replications may also involve changes in the treatment to improve its outcome. Therefore, Level 4 offers the best case study evidence one could have for a technique. Controlled research on the technique at level 4 is highly likely to produce positive effects.

Level 5. Controlled Unreplicated Evidence

In Level 5, controlled research on a treatment technique produces the initial evidence for the effectiveness of a treatment procedure. This is the first level in which treatment is compared with no treatment either in a group design experiment or a single-subject experiment. Therefore, the evidence goes beyond demonstrating improvement in clients. The investigator can claim that the treatment, and no other factor, was responsible for the positive changes documented in the research participants. This claim is justified in a group design study when those who received the treatment improved while those who did not remained unchanged. The justification in a single-subject study is that the same clients showed improvement when the treatment was offered and deterioration when the treatment was withdrawn. Clinicians can use the technique thus researched with some level of confidence. Clinicians still need to be cautious, because the experiment has not been replicated; their application may not get the same results as reported in the experimental research. Other studies may fail to find the technique to be effective.

> Randomized clinical trials, often used in medicine, are examples of controlled treatment evaluation studies. Various single-subject designs also help establish treatment effectiveness.

Level 6. Controlled Directly Replicated Evidence

The same investigator who did the initial experimental study on a treatment replicates (repeats) the study to produce the Level 6 evidence. Using different clients and the same experimental procedures, the original investigator establishes the reliability of results realized from the previous study. If positive results are shown to be reliable, the technique may be used with a greater degree of confidence; however, clinicians should watch for contradictory evidence that may be subsequently published. Note that direct replications, too, should use experimental designs.

Level 7. Controlled Systematically Replicated Evidence

Level 7 is the highest level of treatment efficacy evidence for a treatment procedure. This is the level of evidence investigators conducting treatment research strive to achieve. Level 7 evidence is established when other researchers in other professional settings experimentally evaluate the technique by recruiting a variety of clients. If the results of these experiments are positive and replicate those of earlier studies on the same technique, the generality of the procedure will have been established. The technique is then recommended for general professional practice. Note again, that systematic replications, too, should use experimental designs. Routine clinical application of a technique does not produce controlled replicated evidence.

Clinicians need to acquire the skills to review treatment research, evaluate the research methods used, and categorize the evidence according to the levels specified. It may be noted that in practice, research on a treatment method does not necessarily move from Level 1 to Level 7 in a systematic progression. Clinical judgment in selecting treatment procedures is unavoidable. The judgment will be sound if based on knowledge of treatment research. Essentially, clinicians should have the knowledge to separate clinical case studies that can claim improvement (or lack thereof) from experimental studies that can claim effectiveness (or lack thereof). Expert advocacy without any kind of treatment evidence should be obvious to the clinician. Similarly, multiple experimental studies conducted in multiple research clinics, treating a variety of clients, also should be obvious.

Negative Evidence

Negative evidence, although infrequently published, is always very clear, even in case studies. When a case study fails to document positive changes when a treatment is applied,

> Do not use a treatment method that is shown to be ineffective even in a case study. No need to wait for controlled studies to show it is useless!

there is no need to wait for experimental studies to discredit the method. A method that fails in a case study is unlikely to succeed in an experimental study. Only the positive results in a case study are suspect: it cannot be known whether the documented improvement was due to treatment or some other factor. Negative results even in a case study send a conclusive and clear message: the method is useless. However, before such a message is accepted, the clinician should make sure that the treatment method was used correctly and the study methods were not flawed. Obviously, one would not accept negative or positive evidence stemming from poorly designed and implemented studies.

Treatment Research in Children's Language Disorders

Experimental research on treatment of child language disorders has been conducted over more than three decades. Much of this research has been done within the behavioral approach based on the assumption that verbal behavior (language) of children and adults is shaped and maintained by contingent consequences (Skinner, 1953, 1957). This is in contrast to another influential viewpoint, that of Chomsky (1957, 1965), who postulated that language is a mental system. Such a belief precluded applied clinical research because mental systems cannot be observed or experimentally manipulated. For example, *language competence* as a mental system cannot be directly observed, taught, or objectively measured. Clinicians can teach verbal skills, but not mental systems.

> Language skills, structures, or verbal behaviors? We will use the terms *language skills* and *verbal behaviors* interchangeably. Skills and behaviors are observable and teachable whereas *language structures* (as mental systems) are not.

The view that verbal behavior is learned and maintained because of the actions of people (contingent consequences) made it easier to see if changes in actions and reactions would change aspects of that behavior. Following this logic, behavioral scientists launched a series of experiments to demonstrate that contingent consequences can indeed change the topography and frequency of verbal behaviors in adults and children. Beginning with the earliest and now classic behavioral studies showing that infant vocalizations (e.g., babbling) may be experimentally increased with positive social reinforcement (Rheingold, Gewirtz, & Ross, 1959; Schumaker & Sherman, 1978; Todd & Palmer, 1968; Weisberg, 1961), research has well documented the effects of changed social interactions on language skills. Continued research in the 1970s and 1980s demonstrated the effectiveness of behavioral methods in teaching language skills to varied groups of children with language disorders (see Bricker, 1993 for a historical review of behavioral treatment research on child language disorders). Treatment research conducted since the late 1960s has shown that teaching morphologic, syntactic, and pragmatic verbal skills as well as nonverbal communication skills to children with language disorders can be accomplished by such behavioral techniques as modeling, prompting, shaping, positive reinforcement, differential reinforcement, corrective feedback, and other procedures. Research also has documented the effectiveness of behavioral instruction that trained parents implement at home (Crutcher, 1993; Goldstein, 2002; Goldstein & Hockenberger, 1991; Hegde, 1998a; Kaiser, 1993; Kaiser & Gray, 1993; Reichle & Wacker, 1993; Warren & Kaiser, 1986; Warren & Rogers-Warren, 1985).

Treatment efficacy evidence for behavioral methods of teaching language skills to children with language disorders has been widely and systematically replicated (Bricker, 1993; Kaiser & Gray, 1993; Goldstein, 2002; Hegde, 1998a, 2001b; Maurice, 1996; Reichle & Wacker, 1993; Warren & Rogers-Warren, 1985). In a variety of settings researchers have documented the effectiveness through controlled experimental methods for behavioral techniques that include structured discrete trial techniques or such naturalistic methods as incidental teaching, milieu teaching, and peer training. In the treatment of language disorders in children with autism or developmental disorders and in controlling problem behaviors through communication treatment, the systematically replicated controlled evidence supporting behavioral methods of intervention is surpassed by no other technique or approach (Carr et al., 1994; Goldstein, 2002; Hegde, 1998a; Maurice, 1996).

> See Bailey et al., n.d. and Vollmer et al., 2000, for an extensive and impressive collection of reprints of articles from the *Journal of Applied Behavior Analysis* demonstrating the effectiveness of behavioral methods in teaching not only language skills, but also many other kinds of skills to children with various kinds of disabilities.

The American Speech-Language-Hearing Association's bibliography published on its website on evidence-based practice in child language disorders lists more than 170 treatment research articles, most of which report experimental data on behavioral methods (www.asha.org/members/research/NOMS2/child_language.htm; retrieved 1/1/2004). Extensive as it is, this bibliography, which stops at 1996, lists only a small number of available research on behavioral methods of intervention. Consequently, the treatment approach taken in this book is based on evidence that has reached Level 7, the highest level.

From the Beginning to the End:
An Overview of Treatment

Treatment in communicative disorders is designed to change the way (1) children interact with their verbal community and (2) the verbal community interacts with children. Clinicians establish new language skills by changing the way children interact socially, albeit in limited, clinician-arranged social interactions in the clinic. Clinicians promote naturalistic maintenance of newly taught language skills by changing the communicative behaviors of people who typically interact with the treated children. To achieve the final outcomes of treatment, the clinician should design a treatment plan in partnership with the child's parents and other caregivers.

In this chapter we will set forth a basic evidence-based behavioral framework that gives an overview of treatment. The term *framework* implies that what will be described is a basic and flexible procedure that lends itself to revision and to the inclusion of additional procedures that can be specific to the needs of the individual child. In subsequent sections of this chapter we will expand on the components, defining the terms and describing the procedures involved with each step. In subsequent chapters we will describe the details of establishing, expanding, and maintaining language skills and supporting academic performance through language intervention in schools.

In treating language disorders within the behavioral framework, the clinician:

- *Selects target behaviors.* In the initial step, the clinician selects the target behaviors based on the principles of target behavior selection. Parents and other caregivers, along with teachers, should be partners in selecting the skills to be taught.
- *Establishes baselines.* In the next step, the clinician establishes the pretreatment levels of the selected target behaviors. This will help compare the progress the child makes (or fails to make) during treatment.
- *Begins treatment.* Typically, the clinician may initiate treatment on the target behaviors using the *discrete trial procedure.*
- *Probes for initial generalized production.* When the child reaches a predetermined criterion for correct response, the clinician may conduct an *intermixed probe* to determine the level of production of the target behavior in new contexts. Analysis of probe data will provide guidelines on the course of therapy.
- *Provides additional treatment.* If the intermixed probes suggest a need for continued treatment on the same skills, the clinician may alternate between treatment trials and probe procedure until the child's correct generalized production meets the set criterion level.
- *Conducts a pure probe.* When the clinician judges that the target behavior has been learned in the clinic, he or she may conduct repeated final probes to find out whether the target behavior occurs in the child's natural environment. An analysis of the results of the final probes will help evaluate whether or not the child should continue in therapy, or be dismissed.
- *Promotes maintenance.* It is desirable to build maintenance procedures into treatment from the beginning and train parents and others in supporting the behaviors at home and in other naturalistic settings.

- *Provides post-dismissal follow-up assessment.* Periodic assessment of children who have been dismissed from treatment to ascertain skill maintenance is the essence of follow-up assessment.
- *Provides booster treatment.* If the skills are not maintained during a follow-up assessment, the clinician may arrange for booster treatment. Booster treatment is any treatment offered subsequent to dismissal from the first round of treatment. Its goal is to help maintain the skills in natural settings. The clinician typically uses the same technique that was found to be effective before or a new procedure known to be better.

As noted before, this treatment plan is developed in cooperation with family members and teachers. The parents may offer suggestions for stimuli or activities that will be attractive to the child. They may suggest specific language skills that will be useful at home and school. Although the treatment procedure will be modified in light of the child's performance, the basic treatment, probe, and maintenance procedures should be clear from the beginning and supported by the parents. All the elements of this basic sequence of treatment should be described in a written treatment plan which is presented to the client's parents or caregivers and thoroughly discussed with them before finalizing the plan. There are many formats that may be used for writing the treatment plan, and each clinical setting will likely require a unique format. See Hegde (2003b) for various examples of treatment plans for childhood language disorders.

Principles of Target Behavior Selection

A **target behavior** is any verbal or nonverbal skill a clinician wishes to teach a child. A child with a language disorder lacks many verbal and nonverbal skills. It is not possible to teach all of them at once, however. Also, although all verbal skills are important, some are more important (i.e., more functional, more effective in social communication) than others. Therefore, the clinician needs to select target behaviors that will be the most effective in personal, social, and academic situations.

What is a target behavior?

The most effective target behaviors are not only effective and useful, they also are functional response classes. Skills that are independent of each other form **functional response classes.** Responses within a class are normally learned under the same conditions; responses across classes are learned under different conditions. Individual responses within a class may be topographically different, but may produce the same effect on the environment (Baldwin & Baldwin, 1998; Carr, 1988; Catania, 1998; Drasgow, Halle, & Ostrosky, 1998; Hegde, 1998a; Johnston & Pennypacker, 1993; Malott, Malott, & Trojan, 2000). Only a few of the responses within a class need to be taught; others within the same class are learned on the basis of generalization and maintained with others' assistance. Teaching responses within a class will have no effect on the production of responses that belong to other classes. Linguistic categories, unfortunately, are not the same as response classes (Hegde, 1980, 1998a, 1998b; Hegde & McConn, 1981; Warren, 1985) as the following descriptions make clear:

- Present progressive *-ing* is a response class. This means that teaching a few verbs inflected with *-ing* is sufficient to have the child produce other similar words without additional training; similar responses produced without additional training are done so on the basis of generalization. Generalized production, therefore, suggests a response class (Hegde & McConn, 1981; Hegde, Noll & Pecora, 1979).

- The regular plural, though forming a single linguistic category, contains three response classes: (1) regular plural words that end with /s/ (e.g., *cats*, *hats*); (2) words that end with /z/ (*bags*, *dogs*); and (3) words that end with /ez/ (e.g., *oranges*). Several words from each class must be taught to generate the regular plurals (Guess et al., 1968).

- Each irregular plural word in English is a response class unto itself. A single response constitutes a response class; each of the irregular plural words (e.g., *women*, *children*, *men*, *knives*, *fish*) must be taught separately; teaching one irregular plural word will not result in the generalized production of other irregular plural words (Hegde & McConn, 1981; Hegde, Noll & Pecora, 1979).

- Regular past tense words, although a single linguistic category, belong to different response classes depending on whether the inflection ends in phonetic [t] (e.g., *walked*, *talked*), [ed] (e.g., *bagged*, *mowed*), [ted] (*painted*, *corrected*), and [ded] (*nodded*, *added*). Words with each inflectional ending have to be taught separately as they belong to their own response class (Schumaker & Sherman, 1970). It is likely that other regular past tense words that end with phonetic blends (e.g., *nurtured*) form yet other response classes.

- Each irregular past tense verb in English is a response class unto itself. This is another exceptional response class that contains only a single response; each response must be taught separately because teaching such words as *ran*, *went*, and *read* will have no effect on the production of *flew*, *dug*, *fell*, or *ate* (Hegde & McConn, 1981; Hegde, Noll & Pecora, 1979).

- Certain forms of the English auxiliary and copula, though considered grammatically separate, form single-response classes. For instance, a child who learns to produce the auxiliary *is* (as in "The boy is running," "The girl is reading") will produce the copular form (as in "The mother is kind," "The man is nice") without additional training (Hegde, 1980).

- The English subject-noun phrases (e.g., *the boy*, *the girl*) and object-noun phrases (e.g., *the apple*, *the dress*), though separate grammatically, may belong to the same response class, as teaching the one form is sufficient to have the child produce both the forms (McReynolds & Engmann, 1974).

- All requests (mands) are a response class. Teaching some mands may be sufficient to have the child produce other mands (Skinner, 1957; Winokur, 1976).

- Each pronoun, though belonging to a single linguistic category, is a separate response class, each requiring separate treatment; for instance, teaching the pronoun *she* will have no effect on the pronoun *he* or the pronoun *it* (Hegde & Gierut, 1979).

- Different kinds of questions may form different response classes (e.g., "What is that?" is a different response class than "Where is that?"); each type of question needs to be taught separately (Williams, Perez-Gonzalez, & Vogt, 2003).

There are many functional response classes that commonly serve as target behaviors, depending on the needs of the child. Functional response classes are not limited to a particular structure; they may be words, phrases, or sentences. For instance, clinicians might teach the production of the word *walking*, the phrase *boy walking*, or the sentence, "The boy is walking." More complex syntactical structures such as the noun-verb-direct object (e.g., "The boy kicked the ball") or noun-copula-adjective (e.g., "The ball is blue.") also may be targeted. Although it is not clear if they are independent response classes, such conversational (pragmatic) language skills as topic maintenance, eye contact, turn-taking, and narrative skills may be suitable functional response classes for some children. Some clinicians may target such cognitive skills as attending to task or remembering names as independent response classes.

A word of caution is in order on the use of common treatment targets. Response classes must be experimentally demonstrated to be so; they cannot be based on structural linguistic analysis. An elegant method of selecting language target behaviors will use the functional units of verbal behavior, not features based on linguistic-structural analysis of language. Unfortunately, much language treatment research, including those the applied behavioral analysts have done, is based on structural properties of language. Consequently, most language targets have not been validated by an experimental analysis in which teaching of a few responses are shown to be sufficient to have the child produce other responses without further training. Clinically, a response class created by the same or similar contingencies are functionally, but not necessarily structurally, similar responses. To understand how response classes are established, see Box 5.2.

---

box 5.2 **How Are Response Classes Established? Through Experimental Clinical Research, Not Structural Linguistic Analysis**

The precise experimental method of establishing response classes requires that you (1) first teach a few exemplars of a presumed response class and probe to see if other similar exemplars are produced without training, and (2) reverse or eliminate the learning of the initially taught exemplars and see if the production of other exemplars are consequently wiped out. In an early study on response classes, McReynolds & Engmann (1974) demonstrated that a group of children who produced neither subject-noun phrases (e.g., *the boy*) nor object-noun phrases (e.g., *the apple*) began to produce both structures after being directly taught only the subject-noun phrases. When the subject-noun phrase production was reversed by reinforcing the children to omit the article (hence, to produce only the noun), the children lost the production of object-noun phrase as well.

Studies by Hegde (1980) and Hegde and McConn (1981) have shown that although linguists have asserted that verbal auxiliary and copula are structurally different, teaching either one is sufficient to have the child correctly produce the other without further training. Furthermore, eliminating the learning of one of them will eliminate the learning of the other, regardless of

which one is taught first. Finally, when the original production (either the auxiliary use or the copular use) is reinstated, the other production is also reinstated without reinstatement training.

An early clinical study (Guess & Baer, 1973) showed that regular plural, though structurally a single category, actually breaks into three response classes: the plural morphemes /s/, /z/, and /ez/. Similarly, the allomorphic variations of regular past tense inflection (e.g., /t/ as in *walked*, /ted/, as in *painted*) are separate response classes. It is noted in the text that each irregular form is a class unto itself. If the clinical research shows that a single structural category has more response classes in it, the clinician has more work than linguistic structure suggests. If on the other hand, two structures are the same functionally (as in the case of auxiliaries and copulas, and subject-noun and object-noun phrases), the work is less than what linguistic structure suggests. In either case, a pure structural analysis of target behaviors is misleading. These studies clearly show that, as Skinner (1957) asserted, true verbal behavior response classes may not correspond to the structural linguistic categories.

Behavioral Cusps? Bosch and Fuqua (2001) describe *behavioral cusps* as a model for selecting target behaviors for intervention. Although not specific to language skills, behavior cusps are target skills that (1) help gain access to new reinforcers and environments; (2) generate new responses from learned responses; (3) compete with inappropriate responses; (4) positively affect others who interact with the client; and (5) help meet the demands of the social community.

As the research on functional response classes still remains limited, it is best for the clinician to use a child-specific strategy that emphasizes the uniqueness of each child and takes into consideration the child's personal, social, cultural, and educational needs and demands in selecting target behaviors for treatment. It is much more useful for a child to request a *cookie* to eat, *juice* to drink, or tell that he or she is hurting than it is merely to label objects. When children learn communication skills that affect their listeners, their communicative attempts are intrinsically and powerfully reinforced. Such skills are much more likely to be maintained in natural settings. As stated by Warren and Rogers-Warren (1985), "The successful experience of controlling the environment may in itself be a reinforcing event" (p. 6). Target behaviors that emphasize functional language over syntactic forms or semantic complexity provide children with that experience. Target response classes (language skills) selected for treatment:

- *Should be ethnoculturally appropriate for the child.* See Chapter 11 for additional information on ethnocultural factors that affect assessment and treatment.
- *Should be useful to the child in natural settings.* Nouns that are a part of the child's life (including the names of family members, pets, etc.), requests that are naturally reinforced in everyday living, descriptive and narrative skills that are expected to address events in the child's life, are especially useful.
- *Should make an immediate and socially significant difference in the child's communicative skills.* For example, teaching simple words or phrases for a child who uses undifferentiated and unclear gestures will notably improve social communication, as would an organized nonvocal system (e.g., American Sign Language).
- *Should help build more complex skills to expand communicative performance in natural settings.* Words that can be more meaningfully expanded into phrases by adding additional, functional words and phrases that can be expanded to similarly functional sentences help build more complex skills.
- *Should help meet the academic and social demands the child faces.* An analysis of the academic demands being made on a school-age child will help select skills the child needs in the classroom. Selecting target skills directly from the child's curricula will be useful.
- *Should be those that the child can initially learn without undue difficulty.* The clinician may make judgments based on the assessment and baseline results and gradually increase response complexity as the child experiences success in treatment.

Sequence of Target Behaviors

Children with language disorders often need to learn multiple target behaviors because of their varied language deficiencies. Although more than one skill may be taught at a time, most children cannot learn several targets simultaneously. Therefore, target behaviors should be carefully sequenced as some skills need to be taught sooner than others. The sequence should be logical, cohesive, and specific to the child's needs.

There are two approaches to sequencing language skills for treatment. One is the popular normative approach and the other is the client-specific experimental approach.

The Normative Approach

To select target behaviors, many clinicians follow the developmental norms for language; hence, it is the **normative approach.** Clinicians who choose the normative approach sequence language targets according to the known typical sequence of language acquisition. Among the multiple skills the child lacks and needs to learn, the clinician will first teach skills that are normally mastered earlier than those that are mastered later. Therefore, clinicians sequence language skills for treatment according to published age-based norms. Clinicians assume that skills that are normally mastered earlier are easier to teach than those that are mastered later. They further assume that it is either not possible to teach language skills out of their normative sequence or that such an attempt will somehow be damaging. Linguists and normative researchers consider these assumptions inherently valid.

> Follow the norms and leave it to chance! That all kinds of teaching should follow normative sequence is mostly responsible for not advancing or enriching language skills in normally developing children. Parents and clinicians who are willing to violate the normative assumptions will be richly rewarded by advanced skills in children.

The normative sequence is based on a few other assumptions. For instance, the clinician who follows this approach must assume that (1) there are valid norms for most if not all language behaviors; (2) the norms predict an individual child's language skills; (3) there is a fixed sequence with which children learn language skills; and (4) children with language disorders have to learn language skills in the normative sequence. Each of these assumptions is open to question. These assumptions have been critically examined elsewhere (Hegde, 1998a), and the arguments, therefore, are summarized here.

Validity of language norms is limited. Norms are a double-edged sword: if they are based on small local or regional samples of children, the norms do not represent children at large. If they are based on large national or state samples, the variability of skills across age levels will be so great that the norms, being averages, do not mean much to an individual child. Furthermore, regardless of validity, while norms for some basic language skills and morphologic features exist, there are no norms for many advanced language skills, including most pragmatic language skills and abstract language use (McLaughlin, 1998). Finally, norms reported in many standardized tests are not relevant to children of varied ethnocultural backgrounds (Lahey, 1990; Laing & Kamhi, 2003).

Norms do not predict an individual child's language skills. Whether based on small or large samples, when the performances of many children at a given age level are averaged to derive norms for that age, the average may not reflect the performance of most children. It will not reflect the performance of a normally developing individual child. In essence, norms mask the natural variability and individual differences in children. Except for some gross generalizations, clinicians can hardly predict the language skills of an individual child with any level of precision needed for clinical practice. Yet that precision is much needed because individual differences are the central concerns in clinical intervention.

All children do not acquire language skills in a fixed sequence. That there is an invariant sequence with which children learn language skills has been an untested and widely accepted assumption. Intensive and longitudinal studies of children who acquire language have shown significant individual difference in language acquisition (Brown, 1973; McLaughlin, 1998). Not only the sequence, but also the rate of learning differs across children. Once again, knowledge of these differences is clinically more valuable than presumed uniformity.

Language skills need not be taught in a normative sequence. The skills need not be taught in any other presumed sequence, either. Sequencing language targets according to published norms is easy, convenient, and popular. Unfortunately, being neither innovative nor child-specific, the normative approach discourages clinical experimentation with different sequences. What is the best sequence of teaching language skills? Innovative clinicians ask that question and proceed to find out by experimentation. They do not assume that the known normative sequence is indeed the best, when they do not know that it is. It may be, but only experimental clinical research will demonstrate it; not research on normal language acquisition. When different sequences, including the normative sequence, are experimentally evaluated, clinicians will know which one is the best. That children with language disorders have not learned language in the typical manner is sufficient reason to consider alternative sequences for clinical training.

Client-Specific Experimental Approach

A useful approach to sequencing language targets is the **client-specific experimental approach,** in which the selected skills are specific to the child, and the sequence of teaching is experimentally determined. Formal experiments on different sequences should suggest relatively more efficient sequences. In the absence of such research, clinicians in routine practice may select client-specific targets and sequence them to meet the individual child's needs. The clinician may informally experiment with the sequence. What if the skills are taught outside the normative sequence? What if normatively more advanced and academ-

photo 5.1
A functional phrase such as "Bye-bye, Mommy!" may be more easily learned by a child than a single word.

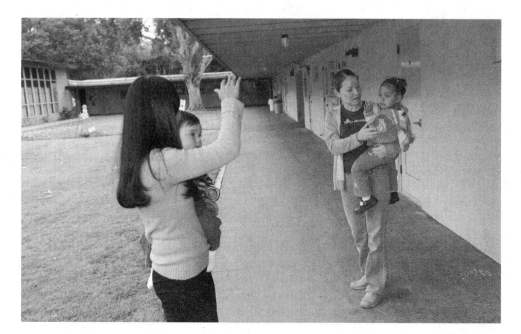

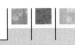

box 5.3 | Can We Enrich Children's Language Skills by Teaching Them Skills ahead of Their Normative Sequence? Yes, We Can Unshackle Children from the Normative Sequence

The sequence in which children learn language skills may be due to several factors, including genetic constraints, neurophysiological integrity, complexity of language, the hierarchical nature of that complexity, the relative richness of the environmental contingencies of stimulation and reinforcement, the degree of formal instruction, and other unknown variables. That normally children acquire language without too much explicit instruction does not mean that more systematic attempts to improve language skills in naturalistic settings are not beneficial. Obviously, a failure to typically acquire language necessitates systematic clinical teaching. Such systematic clinical teaching should be beneficial to children who are normally acquiring language and should lead to language enrichment beyond the normative expectations.

Following this kind of logic, Capelli (1985), DeCesari (1985), and Atherton and Hegde (1996) have demonstrated that typically developing children could be taught language skills ahead of their normative sequence. Using the well-researched behavioral methods of discrete trials, modeling, positive reinforcement and corrective feedback, Capelli (1985) and DeCesari (1985) taught the production of selected grammatic morphemes to preschoolers well ahead of their norma-

tive sequence. Using the experimental multiple baseline design across behaviors, the authors taught grammatic morphemes *out* of Brown's sequence of acquisition to six preschool children in the age range of 21 to 28 months. For example, children were trained to produce the uncontractible auxiliary (as in "The fish is swimming.")—which is ranked 12 in Brown's acquisition sequence (AC) before they were taught the third person irregular (as in "Mary eats.")—ranked 10 in AC, which was taught before the past regular (e.g., "Johnny yelled.")—ranked 9 in AC, which was in turn taught before the past irregular (e.g., "Daddy drove the car.")—ranked 5 in AC. In essence, the children were taught grammatic morphemes in the *opposite* order in which Brown found normally developing children to master them. All children mastered the morpheme productions in their reversed normative sequence and generalized their productions to nonclinical settings. Atherton and Hegde (1996) replicated the results of Capelli and DeCesari to demonstrate that the results are reliable. In addition, they also demonstrated that young children who have not mastered such pragmatic skills in turn-taking and topic maintenance in conversation also could be taught ahead of their normative expectations.

---

ically more useful skills are taught ahead of some normatively early but functionally less urgently needed skills? Experimental attempts to answer such questions will yield clinically useful data that will suggest flexible and variable sequences that may be more productive than the normative sequence. Is it possible to teach language skills out of their normative sequence? See Box 5.3 for some experiments and clinical data that not only give an affirmative answer to that question but also suggest exciting opportunities to advance children's language skills, even in children who are learning language typically.

A willingness to experiment and find out which sequence works the best for a given child is clinically beneficial as well as effective. For example, perhaps a child does not have any functional one-word productions, but articulates bilabial and velar consonants. A clinician who is using a normative sequence might automatically begin treatment on production of one-word utterances, incorporating bilabial and velar consonants. If this strategy has minimal success, treatment could be stuck at the one-word level for quite a while. A clinician who is using a client-specific approach, however, might decide to experiment with teaching the production of two-word or even three-word functional phrases and might discover that the child is actually more likely to produce utterances such as "Bye-bye mommy" or "Mommy go

> An experimental approach to selecting and sequencing treatment is self-corrective. That is, if a selected approach is not good, the clinician would know. The approach can then be changed.

bye-bye" when taught in a functional context. Individual children may benefit more from a sequence of treatment specific to their needs, but that sequence will never be discovered if clinicians are unwilling to deviate from the expected normative sequence in planning for treatment.

It is not argued here that the target behaviors selected on the basis of a client-specific experimental approach will always be different from those selected on the basis of the normative approach. In some cases, the behaviors may be the same, regardless of the approach. However, the client-specific experimental approach opens up possibilities that the normative approach shuts out. It is true that a treatment sequence is naturally suggested by most skills; certain language skills must be taught before certain other skills can be taught or be meaningful to teach. For example, the child needs to learn the main verbs before learning the present progressive -*ing*; nouns before plural inflections, verb plus -*ing* before the use of auxiliary *is*, and so forth. Common sense combined with a client-specific approach is the best formula for producing a cogent sequence of treatment.

Specifying Target Behaviors

Selected target behaviors should be clearly defined or described. A target behavior must be specific and defined operationally rather than constituently. A **constituent definition** defines terms with other terms, as does a dictionary. To understand a term constituently defined, the reader must look up other terms. An **operational definition** sets forth a target behavior in measurable and observable terms. When a behavior is measurable and observable, clinicians can directly document improvement in the client by first observing the level at which the desired behavior occurs prior to treatment and then carefully measuring the rate at which the behavior increases during treatment. *Any* behavior the clinician teaches children may be written operationally.

Poorly written target behaviors make it difficult to teach the behavior and then to judge whether the child has learned it or not. If the target behavior is not observable and measurable, the clinician will not know when to stop or continue the treatment, and it will be difficult to judge improvement or treatment effects. See Box 5.4 for examples of poorly written target skills contrasted with operationally written targets.

How do operational definitions describe target behaviors?

Operationally defined target behaviors contain the following components:

- *Topographic aspects of the target behavior.* Specify the skill in measurable terms. When exhibited, all target skills—including those that presumably involve some abstract or unobservable mental process—should still be obvious to any observer. For instance, the clinician who asks a boy to define a word and gets a wrong response may presume that the child lacks a cognitive structure of meaning in his head, but what is observed, measured, and recorded is a wrong definition or a total lack of a response. The following top the list of troublesome words: *process* (cognitive, auditory, linguistic), *ability*, *inability*, and *competence*. The general term *language* is equally troublesome because it is too broad. Avoid them in writing target behavior descriptions. Instead, substitute them with language skills that presumably index a *process, ability, competence,* or broadly defined *language*. For instance:

—Following verbal directions (e.g., "Touch your nose," "Sit down")

box 5.4 | How Should Target Language Skills Be Specified? Some Good and Poor Examples

Theoretically based, presumed, unobservable, and unmeasurable processes are prime candidates for poorly written target skills. What appear to be visible skills, too, can be couched in certain terms that render the description unsuitable for measurement. Measurement is the key to operational definitions. Contrast the following measurable and vague descriptions of target skills.

Vague, Unobserved, Unmeasurable

A clinician in a public school wrote the following as the target behavior for a girl in kindergarten: *The treatment target is increased auditory processing skills during classroom instruction.* In all likelihood, the clinician who wrote that target behavior instruction did so because of some observed behavior. Perhaps the girl would not promptly respond to questions. Perhaps she appeared to be confused when complex directions were given. Perhaps the girl had difficulty answering questions about what was read aloud to her. Maybe the child had scored low on a standardized test of auditory processing. Nonetheless, instead of targeting observable behaviors for treatment, the clinician specified an unobservable process inferred to take place in the child's head.

Concrete, Observable, Measurable

For the same girl, the clinician might well have specified the following specific target skills: *The treatment target is at least 90 percent correct verbal or nonverbal responses given to a minimum of 10 questions asked during typical classroom interactions.* (The clinician may give some examples of such questions.)

The treatment target is at least 90 percent correct verbal or nonverbal responses given to a minimum of 10 single-element directions given to the child. (The clinician may give some examples of such directions.)

The treatment target is at least 90 percent correct verbal or nonverbal responses given to a minimum of 10 questions on a story read aloud to the child. (The clinician may give examples of stories and questions to be asked.)

How would you rewrite such vague target behavior descriptions as the following?

The target is to increase expressive linguistic communication.

The goal is to increase the client's short-term memory.

The target is increased communicative competence.

The target is improved grammatic competence.

In rewriting them, think of actions or behaviors that indicate that the target has been accomplished.

—Production of the plural morpheme *-s*
—Asking 10 *wh-* questions
—Making five requests for food items
—Maintenance of topic of conversation for 3 minutes
—Correct interpretation of five common proverbs
—Correct responses given to six questions asked about a story the child has read silently
—Correct printing of 10 words
(Note that the descriptions are not yet complete; they only specify the skill.)

- *The topographic level at which the target behavior will be taught.* In the target behavior description, include the topographic (structural) level at which you plan to teach the skill. Specify multiple levels in the same description or write separate descriptions for different levels of teaching. For instance:

 —Following verbal one-step directions (e.g., "Touch your nose" or "Sit down.")
 —Production of the plural morpheme *-s* in 20 words

—Production of the plural morpheme -*s* in 20 phrases (alternatively, Production of the plural morpheme s in 20 words and phrases)

—Asking 10 *wh-* questions with three or four words

—Making five requests for food items in complete sentences

—Maintenance of topic of conversation for 3 minutes (this one already specifies topography: conversational speech)

—Correct interpretation of five common proverbs in complete sentences

—Correct responses in complete sentences given to six questions asked about a story the child has read silently

—Correct printing of 10 words

- *The accuracy criterion.* When is a skill learned? A specification of this is an accuracy criterion. For instance:

—Following verbal one-step directions with 90 percent accuracy (e.g., "Touch your nose" or "Sit down")

—Production of the plural morpheme -*s* in 20 words with 90 percent accuracy

—Production of the plural morpheme -*s* in 20 phrases with 90 percent accuracy

—Asking 10 *wh-* questions with three or four words with 90 percent accuracy

—Making five requests for food items in complete sentences with 90 percent accuracy

—Maintenance of topic of conversation for 3 minutes with 100 percent accuracy

—Correct interpretation of five common proverbs in complete sentences with 100 percent accuracy

—Correct responses, in complete sentences given to six questions asked about a story the child has read silently with 90 percent accuracy

—Correct printing of 10 words with 90 percent accuracy

- *Treatment stimuli to be used.* Various stimuli, some common and some special, need to be used during treatment. Target behavior description should include the stimuli at given levels of training. Stimuli change as treatment moves from one stage to the next. For instance:

—Following verbal one-step directions with 90 percent accuracy (e.g., "Touch your nose" or "Sit down") when given by the clinician

—Production of the plural morpheme -*s* in 20 words with 90 percent accuracy when shown pictures of plural objects and the question "What are these?" is asked (note that both the picture and the question are stimuli)

—Production of the auxiliary *is* in sentences with 90 percent accuracy when the pictures are shown, a question is asked, and the response is modeled (note, a complex set of stimuli—picture, question, and modeling—is used to get an imitative response)

—Asking 10 *wh-* questions with three or four words with 90 percent accuracy when presented with verbal contexts and prompts

—Making five requests for food items in complete sentences with 90 percent accuracy when asked, "What do you want?"

—Maintenance of topic of conversation for 3 minutes when the clinician initiates a topic with 100 percent accuracy

—Correct interpretation of five common proverbs in complete sentences, when the proverbs are orally stated, with 100 percent accuracy

— Correct responses in complete sentences with 90 percent accuracy given to six questions asked about a story the child has read silently (silent reading is the stimulus condition)

— Correct printing of 10 words when dictated with 90 percent accuracy

- *The setting in which the target behavior will be learned and sustained.* The initial setting for target behaviors is typically the clinic where they are initially established. Eventually, the setting used may be more naturalistic, including the home, the classroom, shopping centers, restaurants, and so forth where the target behaviors are sustained. For instance:

— Following verbal one-step directions with 90 percent accuracy (e.g., "Touch your nose" or "Sit down") when given by the clinician in the clinic setting

— Production of the plural morpheme -s in 20 words with 90 percent accuracy when shown pictures of plural objects and the question "What are these?" is asked in the clinic setting

— Production of the auxiliary *is* in sentences with 90 percent accuracy when the pictures are shown, a question is asked, and the response is modeled in the treatment room

— Asking 10 *wh-* questions with three or four words with 90 percent accuracy when presented with verbal contexts and prompts in the classroom

— Making five requests for food items in complete sentences with 90 percent accuracy when asked, "What do you want?" in the home setting

— Maintenance of topic of conversation for 3 minutes with 100 percent accuracy when the clinician initiates a topic in a social situation outside the clinic

— Correct interpretation of five common proverbs with 100 percent accuracy in complete sentences when the proverbs are orally stated by the teacher in the classroom

— Correct responses in complete sentences with 90 percent accuracy given to six questions asked about a story the child has read silently in the home setting

— Correct printing of 10 words with 90 percent accuracy when dictated in the classroom

Note that the target behavior specification does not say that "the child will produce. . . ." It is prudent to avoid this common practice because whether the child will or will not produce the target behaviors will depend on many variables. In the schools, the date by which the target skills will be learned is sometimes specified. If so, then the statement implies a promise that the child will produce the plural -s with 90 percent accuracy within a certain date; this promise may or may not be fulfilled. The target behavior examples given here avoid this inherent promise.

> What are the components of an operationally defined target behavior?

■ | ■ Principles of Treatment Sequencing

Clinicians structure treatment in a hierarchical fashion. This hierarchy is based on factors that affect treatment implementation. Whether skills are functional or normative, they vary in their topographic complexity. For example, a child can request milk with one word, a two-word phrase (*milk, Mommy!*), or a whole sentence ("I want some milk."); all are requests, all are functional, but teaching may have to move from the simpler word or phrase to the more complex sentence. This kind of treatment sequence is suggested by clinical data; the sequence, however, is by no means rigid. The other reasons for following a clinical sequence are that treatment procedures and treatment settings move through certain stages. Therefore, generally, treatment sequences are based on response topography, treatment procedures, and treatment settings as follows.

- Sequence based on response topography:
  - simple and basic skills to progressively more advanced and complex skills (e.g., from words to phrases, and then to sentences; and finally to conversation; following one-step directions to following two- and three-step directions; producing noun + verb sentence structures to producing noun + verb + direct object sentence structures)
- Sequence based on treatment variables:
  - from imitative productions to prompted productions
  - from prompted productions to spontaneous productions
  - from continuous reinforcement to intermittent reinforcement (see Chapter 6 for information on reinforcement schedules)
- Sequence based on settings:
  - from language skills evoked in highly structured, clinician-controlled stimulus contexts to skills produced under less structured, more spontaneous clinical contexts
  - from language produced in the clinic, with planned clinician-evocation to that produced in natural settings, evoked by everyday stimuli the child encounters in social situations
  - from establishment of skills in the clinic to maintenance of those skills in the natural environment

The commonly used sequences are also better subjected to informal experimentation because skipping a level may not negatively affect a child's learning. For instance, after establishing the production of selected grammatic morphemes at the word level, the clinician may offer a few trials at the sentence level, skipping the phrase level training. If the child continues to make progress at a higher level, training time and effort will have been saved. If not, the clinician can always drop down to a lower level.

Judging Improvement: Need for Baselines

Before initiating treatment, the target behaviors should be baserated. A **baseline** is a measure of response rates in the absence of treatment. It represents the typical, habitual level of response of the client *prior* to treatment and is usually expressed as a percentage of correct response.

Any behavior can be baserated to determine its natural occurrence, and subsequently, to claim or not claim improvement under instruction. Perhaps a nontechnical example can add to an understanding of this concept. Let us say that you are being paid to teach a 5-year-old girl to kick soccer goals—a girl who has never received formal instruction. During the first session, you discover to your pleasant surprise that she is a "natural"—without any instruction from you, she

A matter of terms. The term *baserate* is used as a verb (e.g., "She baserated the plurals.") as well as a noun (e.g., "She established the baserates."); the term *baseline* is used only as a noun (e.g., "I established baselines," not "I baselined.").

kicks the ball into the net 8 out of 10 attempts. Her baseline for kicking the ball into the net is 80 percent and any instruction may only yield small gains. If you continue teaching her to kick goals, people might be impressed with the "results" of your instruction, but she is unlikely to get much better than 80 percent accurate. Your instruction therefore cannot be said to have resulted in improvement in her goal-kicking ability, and it would be unethical for you to claim it had. If, on the other hand, during that first baseline session, she makes only 2 out of 10 attempts to kick the ball into the net (a baseline of 20 percent), there is much room for improvement and a justification for instruction.

Pretreatment baselines of language skills are necessary to:

- Establish the *need for treatment* by showing that the language skills did not exist or existed only at a low (inadequate) level. This will prevent offering unnecessary treatment and will help track improvement during treatment.
- *Claim improvement* in the child's language skills during the course of treatment. When the skills increase during treatment over the rates established in baselines, the clinician can document and claim improvement.
- *Make treatment modifications* in case of lack of improvement. If the skills do not improve over the baserates, the clinician can begin to analyze potential reasons for failure and modify the treatment being implemented. Perhaps the stimuli being used—line drawings, for example, to evoke target skills—are ineffective; pictures may do better. Perhaps the reinforcing stimuli used are not working; a different consequent event is needed. Maybe the procedure should be completely abandoned in favor of another.

To establish the need for treatment, baseline data should show that the production of the target behavior is either nonexistent or too low to be acceptable. A skill with 85 percent baseline accuracy is not a treatment target. Fey (1986) suggested that a 10–50 percent correct baseline response rate justifies treatment. Baseline percentages of 50 to 90 indicate an emerging skill, and, according to Fey (1986), a lower priority for direct intervention. Opinions may differ on skills at zero percent baseline response rates. It is recommended here that they be considered for trial therapy, because a response not being produced may be difficult to treat, but not always. If the skills prove difficult to treat, the clinician can always select other targets.

> Why is it necessary to take a baseline of a target behavior?

Baseline Procedures

Baseline procedures vary depending on the target behaviors. Advanced language skills including complex sentence forms, pragmatic skills, and abstract use of language require a different baseline procedure than words, morphologic use, basic syntactic structures, and so forth. Teaching more basic skills in the earlier stages, the clinician teaches more advanced skills in later stages of treatment. We will first describe procedures to establish baselines of basic skills, followed by procedures for advanced language skills.

In establishing baselines of language skills, the following steps are involved:

- *Writing exemplars to teach operationally defined target behaviors.* To begin with, one, two, or just a few target skills may be taught; the child's performance in the initial treatment sessions will serve as a guide. Some 20 exemplars of target behaviors are needed for at least three skills (e.g., basic words, plural -*s*, and the present progressive -*ing* in words). In the case of basic words, each of the 20 words is an exemplar. In the case of plural -*s* (e.g., *cups*, *hats*) and the -*ing* (e.g., *eating*, *walking*) each word that contains the inflection is an exemplar. The clinician can expand each of the exemplars into phrases (e.g., *two cups*; *boy eating*) or simple sentences ("I see two big cups" or "The girl is walking.") if the treatment is to be started at that level. Exemplars that will be taught later in the treatment sequence need not be written at this time as they will be baserated only just before starting treatment. See Hegde (1998c) for prepared multiple exemplars for a variety of language targets.

- *Preparing the stimulus items for target exemplars.* Carefully selected treatment stimuli help evoke the target responses efficiently.

  —*Physical* stimuli are needed to evoke each of the exemplars written. Physical stimuli usually consist of pictures and objects. For preschoolers or those with cognitive deficits, objects may be more effective than pictures in evoking responses. Objects from the child's home environment, such as favorite books, toys, stuffed animals, or other objects, are particularly useful. Pictures or photographs that are colorful, unambiguous, and attractive to the child, instead of line drawings or cartoon-like drawings will be especially effective. Selected stimulus items should be appropriate for the child's ethnocultural and socioeconomic background. If the client is a recent immigrant boy from Saudi Arabia, for example, pictures depicting snow scenes might puzzle him.

  —*Verbal* stimuli are needed to evoke the target exemplars. In the early stages of treatment, the clinician presents physical and verbal stimuli simultaneously. Verbal stimuli consist of the words, phrases, questions, sentences, and so forth that help evoke the target response. Verbal stimuli may be as simple as asking, "What is this?" for the target behavior of labeling common objects shown to the child, or "What is he doing?" for production of verbs. Other target behaviors will require more complex verbal stimuli. For example, to evoke past tense -*ed*, the physical stimulus might consist of a picture of a person performing an action coupled with a sentence completion task for the verbal stimulus, such as, "Today he walks, yesterday he _____."

- *Preparing a recording sheet.* Because the baselines are precisely measured rates of behaviors, a sheet on which every occurrence of the target skill is recorded needs to be prepared. The recording format will vary depending on the skill level; skills measured in conversational speech require a flexible format. Table 5.2 shows a typical recording sheet for basic skills.

- *Administering baseline trials.* Baselines of basic skills are established on **discrete trials.** A discrete trial is one structured opportunity to produce a given target response; it is discrete because trials are separated from each other by a short period of time. For each exemplar, the clinician administers one evoked and one modeled trial as shown in Table 5.2. For reasons explained later, all evoked trials should be administered before all the modeled trials. Evoked trials help establish the skill level under more naturalistic stimulus conditions (e.g., the child is presented with a physical stimulus, asked a question about it, and is expected to respond, much as he or she would be in the natural environment). Modeled trials help evaluate whether the child who cannot

table 5.2

Baseline Recording Sheet

Name:	Date:	Session #:
Age:	Therapist:	
Disorder:	Language	
Target Behavior:	Production of Possessive -*s* in phrases	
Reinforcement:	Noncontingent (Baseline trials)	

Target Exemplars	Trials	
	Evoked	Modeled
1. Mommy's hat		
2. Matt's socks		
3. Jenny's shoes		
4. Cat's mat		
5. Pat's bike		
6. Kate's ring		
7. Dad's jacket		
8. The rabbit's carrot		
9. The boy's books		
10. The girl's bag		
11. The dog's tail		
12. Kate's ring		
13. Teacher's chair		
14. Doctor's office		
15. Elephant's nose		
16. Bunny's house		
17. Pam's car		
18. Kitty's bowl		
19. Bird's feathers		
20. Beth's pencil		
Total Percent Correct		

Note: + = Correct response; − = Incorrect response; 0 = no response.

produce a response spontaneously can imitate when a model is given. Typically, the correct response rate is slightly higher on modeled trials than on evoked.

To administer an evoked trial, the clinician:

— Places one of the physical stimulus items in front of the child (e.g., a picture, one or more objects)
— Asks a question (e.g., "What are these?"), makes a request (e.g., "Tell me what the boy is doing"), or gives other verbal stimuli to help evoke the target response
— Waits a few seconds for the child to respond
— Records the response on the recording sheet (see Table 5.2)
— Removes the physical stimulus item from the child's view
— Waits for 2 or 3 seconds to mark the end of the trial
— Re-presents the stimuli to begin the next trial

To administer a modeled trial, the clinician:

— Adds an additional step of modeling soon after asking the question or making the request. For instance, after having placed the stimulus picture of two cats, and asking the question, "What do you see?" the clinician immediately models the target response, "Johnny, say, 'two cats.'" The clinician then records the response, removes the physical stimulus for a few seconds, and re-presents the physical and the verbal stimuli to begin the next trial.

An important feature of baserating is that *no feedback* of any sort is given for correct, incorrect, or lack of responses. Response-specific feedback is treatment, and baselines are response rates *without* treatment. Another notable feature is that all evoked trails are administered before any modeled trials. This is because modeling is an unusual stimulus, usually a part of treatment. Therefore, alternating evoked and modeled trials will invalidate baselines. Nonetheless, to keep the child interested in responding, the clinician may reinforce the child for "sitting quietly," "doing a good job," "being cooperative," "being so nice," and so forth. This type of reinforcement is not contingent (dependent) on the responses given to the baseline trials.

• *Analyzing baseline data.* The clinician calculates the percentages separately for evoked trials and for modeled trials as shown in Table 5.2. The following formula may be used to calculate the percent correct baseline response rate:

$$\frac{\text{\# of correct responses}}{\text{\# of total responses}} \times 100 = \text{percent correct}$$

Baselines in Conversational Language Samples

The discrete trial baselines should be supplemented with a language sample designed especially to evoke the skills immediately targeted for treatment. This would be the second sample, the first being taken during assessment. The language sampling should be structured such that the child is given plenty of opportunities to produce the target skills that were baserated. For instance, many plural objects may be used to evoke descriptions that are likely to contain the regular plural morpheme. To baserate production of prepositional phrases, structured activities giving the child many opportunities to describe objects' loca-

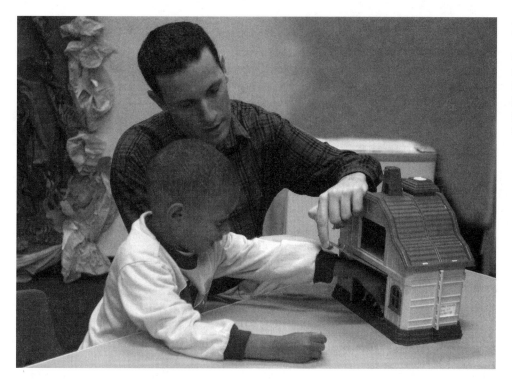

photo 5.2

Where are the cows? A clinician gives a child many opportunities to produce prepositional phrases during structured activities.

tions may be presented (see Photo 5.2 for an example of a structured activity). Many action scenes in children's storybooks may be presented to evoke verb and verb + *ing* productions. Results of the language sample analysis should be consistent with those of discrete trial baseline procedures.

Treatment Principles

Experimentally supported **behavioral treatment** may be defined as the management of an interdependent relationship between antecedent events, specified language skills, and consequences in the form of listener reactions. Language, being a social skill, gets established or fails to get established under varied social conditions when certain listener reactions either follow or fail to follow. **Antecedent events** are certain aspects of that social situation—isolated or simplified—to serve as specific stimuli that are systematically presented to the child during treatment. The antecedent stimulus events include pictures, objects, or events the clinician prepares for treatment.

The specified language skills are the functional verbal response classes, to the extent they are experimentally supported. When they are not, the clinician has to either guess or use topographically (linguistically) described response classes. Although unsatisfactory (see Box 5.2), this practice is common, and often without a choice. Consequently, language skills are typically described in terms of their topographic aspects or the form (shape) of the response. Words, phrases, and sentences, for example, have different topographic dimensions and serve as different target language skills.

Listener reactions shape and sustain language skills in social contexts. Therefore, the clinician carefully reacts to the child's attempts and productions so that the desirable skills are selected and strengthened. Such reactions from the clinicians are technically known as contingent consequences. Simply stated, how the clinician reacts *immediately* when the child gives a correct response, an incorrect response, or no response is the contingent consequence. The clinician reacts differently, depending on the child's response. There is no learning without such differential clinical reaction. Technically, the contingent consequence the clinician delivers will either reinforce and increase correct responses or weaken and reduce incorrect responses. The overall **behavioral contingency** is an abstract relationship between antecedent stimulus events that set the stage for communication, communicative behaviors themselves, and the consequences that follow, usually in the form of listener reactions. The clinician needs to manage this contingency in treatment. During treatment, the clinician repeatedly reenacts the basic chain of events (stimulus-response-consequence) that is inherent in that contingency.

Structure of Treatment Sessions

Clinicians sometime wonder whether to structure the sessions tightly or loosely. In tightly structured sessions, the clinician explicitly controls stimuli and the production of specific target behaviors, and gives specific and regular feedback on the accuracy of responses. Tightly structured sessions tend to use the discrete trial procedure, described in the next section. In loosely structured sessions, the clinician and the client engage in more naturalistic interactions with less specific direction and control from the clinician; such sessions do not involve discrete trials on which specific responses are evoked. The issue of loose or tight structure has been debated in the past, but it is a pseudo issue. Treatment structure is dynamic; tight and loose structures are two ends of an evolving, changing treatment setup. The structure changes as the needs of the child change. Tight structure is more efficient than loose structure in establishing target behaviors, especially at basic topographic levels (e.g., the word or phrase level). However, tight structure is weak in promoting generalization and maintenance and in teaching conversational speech. While being inefficient in establishing basic language skills, the loose format is efficient in teaching more complex and spontaneous language skills (e.g., conversation and narrative skills) and in promoting skill generalization and maintenance (Campbell & Stremel-Campbell, 1982; Hart, 1985).

> What is the basic chain of treatment, repeated many, many times? (Hint: Recall "S-R-C")

Furthermore, the degree of structure is selected to suit the individual child's needs. As we shall see in future chapters, children who are minimally verbal, or who have developmental disability, autism, traumatic brain injury, or attention deficits, are most likely to benefit from more structured treatment sessions than are children whose disability is limited to language disorders (e.g., children with specific language impairment). In addition, children with relatively better language skills may benefit from loosely structured, more naturalistic sessions from the very beginning (Campbell & Stremel-Campbell, 1982; Hart, 1985).

Therefore, the degree of treatment structure is not a matter of the clinician's subjective preference; it is a matter of treatment sequence and client characteristics.

Language treatment for many children, especially for those with more serious disorders and associated conditions, may start with relatively tight structure and move on to loose (and naturalistic) structure. As the child masters the initial skills, and as the treatment progresses to more complex skill levels, the clinician may gradually reduce the structure of treatment sessions to eventually resemble more naturalistic communication. Thus, in all cases, regardless of the degree of initial structure, latter stages of treatment will use progressively less structure. In the very final stage, in which naturalistic conversation is the treatment target, there should be no more structure than what is normal in such interactions.

■ | ■ Treatment Trials

With one important difference, the same discrete trial procedure used to establish baselines will be used to teach the basic skills in the initial stages of treatment: instead of *not* reacting promptly to the correct, incorrect, or lack of responses from the child, the clinician will react promptly and discriminatively. Technically, the differential feedback will be contingent on correct production of language skills, error responses, and lack of responses. The clinician will praise (and reinforce otherwise) the child for correct responses and will give corrective feedback for incorrect responses or lack of responses.

To begin treatment with *modeled discrete trials*, the clinician:

1. Places the stimulus picture or object in front of the child; acts out an event or demonstrates an action that will serve as the stimulus.
2. Delivers the prepared verbal stimulus and models immediately ("What are these? Johnny, say, 'cats.' ").
3. Gives the child a few seconds to respond.
4. Immediately praises the child for correctly imitating the modeled response ("Good! I heard the -s at the end of your word!"), reinforces in other ways (e.g., a token the child will exchange for a small gift at the end of the session), or both. If the response is incorrect, immediately gives corrective feedback ("Uh-oh! I didn't hear the -s that time.")
5. Records the response on the recording sheet of the kind shown in Table 5.3
6. Removes the picture or object for a few seconds to show that a trial has ended; introduces the next trial.

It is best to present the same stimulus item for repeated trials unless errors persist, in which case a new stimulus item should be presented. The goal is to give the child positive practice on a stimulus item to which a child has been successfully responding. This is especially important if the child has struggled to imitate the clinician's model. When the child finally begins to imitate the model, the clinician should not lose the momentum of the child's increased correct response rate by immediately shifting to another stimulus item.

An advantage of highly structured discrete trial training is that it provides many opportunities for the child to produce the target behavior in one treatment session. It is not unusual for clinicians to gather data on literally hundreds of responses from a child during a

■■■   **table 5.3**

Treatment Recording Sheet

Name:	Date:	Session #:
Age:	Clinician:	
Disorder: Language	Target Behavior:	
Criterion: 90% correct	Reinforcement:	

Target Responses	Blocks of 10 Training Trials									
	1	2	3	4	5	6	7	8	9	10
1.										
2.										
3.										
4.										
5.										
6.										

Note: + = Correct response; – = Incorrect response; 0 = no responses; m = Modeled trial; e = Evoked trial (no modeling).

30-minute session. The increased opportunity to produce the target behavior is one reason discrete trial training is efficient and effective in initially establishing the target behaviors.

The clinician designs treatment trials to establish the basic skills in the clinic. The child will eventually produce the target skill reliably when the clinician presents the treatment stimuli. The goal of treatment, however, is the production of the skill when the child encounters stimuli not used in treatment. If this does not happen, treatment will have failed. When the child encounters objects and events in social situations, including the home and school, the skill may disappear. Therefore, periodic assessment of whether the child will respond to stimuli that are not used in treatment is part of the treatment process. Such an assessment is called a probe.

▨ ▥ Probes for Generalized Productions

A **probe** is an assessment of generalized production, based on treatment. **Generalized productions** are those that are given to stimuli not used in training. Although initially shaky and tentative, generalized production demonstrates the spread of learning from the old stimuli (trained) to new stimuli (untrained). Typically based on stimulus similarity, generalized production will not be sustained until that too is reinforced in natural settings; we will return to this issue in Chapter 8 on maintenance of language skills. Though initially unstable, generalized productions are a boon both to the clinician and the child. It is the generalized production that makes an infinite amount of training unnecessary. For instance, learning a few exemplars of the plural morpheme -s in selected words may be sufficient to use that morpheme in many words that take that morpheme with no additional treatment effort for the clinician or learning effort for the child. When linguists say that language is generative, clinical scientists who document generalized production say that it is the spread of learning from the old to the new.

The sooner the clinician catches the beginnings of generalized production in the child, the greater the efficiency of treatment. Therefore, it is helpful to periodically take a break from treatment to assess whether generalized production emerges. When it does, the clinician can move on to higher levels of training. When it does not, the need for additional training on the same skill is evident. This additional training may be continued until the generalized production emerges. In essence, generalized production and eventual maintenance of the skill in natural settings is the final test of success of language treatment.

There are three types of probes: intermixed probes, pure probes, and final conversational probes. The first two are administered on discrete trials and the last, as the name implies, is a probe of skills in naturalistic conversation. **Intermixed probes** are so called because both trained and untrained stimulus items are alternated in assessing generalized production during the initial stages of treatment. **Pure probes** are so called because only untrained items are presented (no mixing of trained and untrained stimuli). The clinician administers pure probes when the child has met the criterion for intermixed probes. Before the child is dismissed from treatment, the clinician administers repeated **final conversational probes,** both in the clinic and in natural environments. Analysis of probe data will guide the course of treatment.

The distinguishing feature of all probes is that treatment is withheld for responses given to new (untrained) stimuli presented to the children. That is, the clinician will give no feedback—positive or corrective—to responses given to novel stimuli. In intermixed probes, however, the child receives feedback for responses given to the trained stimuli. On pure probes, there is no feedback because they do not contain trained stimuli, as any feedback given on probes is contingent only on already trained responses.

Probes, especially the pure probes, are similar to baseline trials. Nonetheless, probes should not be confused with baselines. Differences between probes and baselines become apparent when one understands why and when they are administered. Probes help assess the production of the newly taught target behavior in new contexts and are administered *during* or *after* treatment. Baselines help assess the pretreatment levels of target behaviors and are administered *before* treatment begins. Also, the clinician uses the data generated by

▨ Name and describe three kinds of probes used in treatment.

these two procedures differently. Baseline data mainly help document improvement that may be due to treatment, whereas probe data document generalized production of clinically established skills and guide the course of treatment.

Intermixed Probe Procedure

To administer an intermixed probe in the beginning stages of treatment, the clinician:

- Prepares a probe data recording sheet of the kind shown in Table 5.4. Notice that in the table, trained and untrained stimuli are alternated; this is what makes this probe intermixed. Trained stimuli are those that have been used in treatment to which correct responses have reached an initial training criterion (described later). Untrained stimuli are those that may have been used in baserating, but have not yet been used in training. Assume that a clinician administers the first intermixed probe when the child has just met an initial training criterion on four exemplars (e.g., 90 percent accuracy on *cats*, *hats*, *cups*, and *boots* in the training of plural -*s*). The clinician will have baserated on 20 exemplars (words with plural -*s*) and has just trained 4 of those 20, leaving 16 untrained stimuli. These trained and untrained stimuli are intermixed and written on the recording sheet. The clinician will recycle (reuse) the trained stimuli as they are fewer than the untrained. In our example, the four trained stimuli will be used as many times as they are needed to alternate with the 16 untrained stimuli.
- Administers the probe, using the evoked discrete trial procedure, presenting first a trained stimulus and then an untrained one. The clinician may continue to alternate between trained and untrained stimuli throughout the probe procedure.
- Provides consequences (reinforcers or corrective feedback) to correct or incorrect responses given to trained stimuli used during training. The clinician provides no consequences to responses given to untrained stimulus items.
- Scores each response as correct or incorrect and records it on the data recording sheet; if a child gives no response, the clinician counts it as incorrect.
- Calculates the percent correct probe response rate. Disregarding the responses given to trained stimuli, the clinician counts the correct and incorrect responses given only to the probe stimuli to calculate the percent correct probe response rate. If the probe response rate is at least 90 percent correct, the clinician moves on to other levels of training; if not, gives training on additional exemplars, as described in a later section.

Procedure for Conducting a Pure Probe

Pure probes are used in the later stages of treatment when the responses have been clearly established, as indicated by stable and acceptable intermixed probe rates (e.g., 90 percent correct). Pure probes are unnecessary at the word and phrase levels of training; intermixed probes will suffice to shift training to higher levels. Discrete trial pure probes may be conducted at the level of controlled sentence productions. When the child meets the pure probe criterion in sentences, the treatment may be advanced to conversational speech. Because only untrained items are presented on pure probes, *all* responses are used to calculate the pure probe response rate. The format of Table 5.4 can be used to record pure probe response rates, except that only *untrained* stimuli will be listed on it.

table 5.4

Intermixed Probe Recording Sheet

Name:	Date:	Session #:
Age:	Clinician:	
Disorder:	Target Behavior:	
Criterion:	Reinforcement: FR2 (responses given to the trained stimuli only)	

Target Responses	Stimuli	Score
1.	Trained	
2.	Untrained	
3.	Trained	
4.	Untrained	
5.	Trained	
6.	Untrained	
7.	Trained	
8.	Untrained	
9.	Trained	
10.	Untrained	
11.	Trained	
12.	Untrained	
13.	Trained	
14.	Untrained	
15.	Trained	
16.	Untrained	
17.	Trained	
18.	Untrained	
19.	Trained	
20.	Untrained	
21.	Trained	
22.	Untrained	
23.	Trained	
24.	Untrained	
25.	Trained	
26.	Untrained	
27.	Trained	
28.	Untrained	

Procedure for Conducting Final Conversational Probes

A final probe consists of a conversational language sample taken in the clinic and in such natural environments as home, school, or community settings. Therefore, there may be several final probes for each child. The clinician may collect language samples through direct observation of the child in various settings. Alternatively, the clinician may request from the parents tape recorded samples of conversations at home and other settings.

An analysis of these conversational language samples will show how well the child is using the newly learned target behaviors in natural settings. If the final probe indicates that the child has not achieved the probe criterion level, additional training at the conversational level may be necessary. Parent and sibling training in maintaining the skills in conversations also may be necessary.

Repeated discrete trials on which a single or a few target responses are trained need decision criteria: When do clinicians stop modeling the correct response? When do clinicians stop training the first exemplar (e.g., *two cups*, "The boy is walking," *Mommy's hat*) so they can move on to other exemplars? When do clinicians consider the target skill (e.g., the production of plural *-s* or verb + *ing*) learned? These are the matters of clinical decision that need some criteria to be followed.

Criteria for Clinical Decisions

Clinical decisions that help move the child through the course of treatment should be based on quantitative measures of the child's performance. What follows is a series of suggested criteria that should be applied with flexibility, good clinical judgment, and in light of the clinical data (client's performance measures). Most of the suggested criteria have been used in many child language treatment studies mentioned earlier in the chapter, so the criteria are empirically supported. Ultimately, clinical judgments based on client performance help shape criteria for decisions. Therefore, clinicians are free to discard or modify suggested criteria; they may invent new criteria. It will be helpful if the clinician specifies data-based reasons for such actions.

Criterion to Discontinue Modeling

Because treatment trials begin with modeling, when to stop using it is the first decision the clinician will have to make. As effective as it is in establishing target behaviors, modeling should not be overused. Modeling leads to imitative behaviors, but the clinician needs to move on to spontaneous (nonimitated) responses. Therefore, the clinician needs to stop modeling before imitative behavior is overly strengthened. But when? As a general rule:

> **Stop modeling when the child gives five consecutively correct imitated responses and introduce evoked trials with no modeling.**

Evoked trials will include all the treatment trial steps described before, except for modeling. By omitting modeling, evoked trials approximate natural contexts for language. For example, after presenting the picture of two cats, the clinician would ask the question "What are these?" and wait expectantly for the child's response ("Two cats"). A correct response would receive reinforcement and an incorrect response would receive corrective feedback.

Criterion to Reinstate Modeling

Children do not always maintain a correct response rate on evoked trials even after they have met the suggested criterion of five consecutively correct imitated responses on modeled trials. This raises another question—how many incorrect responses during evoked trials should suggest a return to modeled trials? As a general rule:

> **Reinstate modeled trials if the child gives incorrect responses on two consecutive evoked trials.**

A low criterion level for reinstating modeled trials is good, particularly at the beginning of treatment. Children should not be allowed to err on too many consecutive evoked trials; the child will unnecessarily receive too much corrective feedback. Reinstated modeling should continue until the child gives another set of five consecutively correct imitated responses. At that point, modeling is once again discontinued and the evoked trials are reintroduced.

As the child's correct response rate begins to stabilize, a more liberal criterion may be used to reintroduce modeling. As treatment progresses, perhaps four or five consecutively wrong responses on evoked trials may be noted before reinstating modeling. One or two wrong responses that interrupt several correct responses are no reason to reinstate modeling. Therefore, based on the child's performance, clinicians should be flexible in setting criterion levels for discontinuing and reinstating modeling.

Exemplar Training Criterion

When correct responses on evoked trials become more consistent, the clinician should decide when the child has learned the exemplar or exemplars under training. The suggested exemplar training criterion is as follows:

> **When the child gives 10 consecutively correct responses on evoked trials on an exemplar, move on to the next exemplar.**

An acceptable alternative criterion is 90 percent correct response rate on a block of at least 10 (or more) evoked trials. The clinician will have specified the criterion to be followed in the written treatment plan.

Note that the exemplar training criterion only says that a given exemplar, not the target behavior, is learned. That is, when a child meets the training criterion on an exemplar such as *cats*, in the case of plural -*s* at the word level, it only means that that specific utterance is learned; the feature of plural -*s* cannot be considered to have been mastered until the child meets other criteria to be described.

Probe Criteria

As noted earlier, probe criteria help assess generalized production of a skill so that training may move on. For all probes (initial intermixed, subsequent pure, and final conversational), a general criterion is as follows:

The probe criterion is a 90 percent correct probe response rate on the targeted language skill.

The same probe criterion may force different actions, depending on the kind of probe that was done. For instance:

- If the child meets an intermixed probe criterion (90 percent correct), it means the child has tentatively learned to use the feature at the level of training that was just completed. For instance, an intermixed probe conducted after training four to six exemplars of the present progressive -*ing* in words shows that the child can produce probed (untrained) verbs + *ing*. For a child who meets the intermixed probe criterion of at least 90 percent correct, the clinician may shift training to:
  - A higher level of response topography. For instance, if the grammatic feature was trained at the word level, training may be shifted to the phrase level (e.g., *boy walking* or *two cups*) and from the phrase level, to the sentence level (e.g., "The boy is walking" or "I see two cups.").
  - A different target skill. As training is shifted to the higher level of response topography on the first target, the clinician may add a second target to begin training at the basic (word or phrase) level. For instance, for a child who meets the intermixed probe criterion for plural -*s* at the word level, the clinician may shift training to the phrase level for this feature along with initiating training at a basic level for a new feature (e.g., preposition *in* or *on*).
- If the child's intermixed probe response rate is less than 70 percent correct, treatment may be continued with new exemplars. Teaching the production of three or four new exemplars before probing again with the intermixed procedure might be helpful.
- If the child's intermixed probe response rate is less than 90 percent but more than 70 percent, additional discrete trial training for already trained items is necessary; this may be sufficient to obtain a 90 percent correct response rate on the next probe.
- If the child's pure probe response rate is 90 percent or better for sentences (the first level at which the pure probe is conducted), the clinician may shift treatment to conversational speech. From then on, the clinician may:
  - Periodically conduct pure probes in conversation to see if the response rates are sustained with typical social reinforcement inherent to conversational speech (but no special reinforcement schedules).
  - Continue training if the child does not meet the pure probe criterion for conversational speech.
  - Request the family members to submit conversational speech samples from home when the child meets the pure probe response rate for conversational speech in the clinic. If practical, the clinician may obtain brief language samples from the classroom or playground in the school setting.
  - Consider the skill fully trained if at least three home or school samples meet the pure probe criterion. The clinician may also continue training at whatever the level necessary on other target skills that have not met the pure probe criterion.
  - Dismiss the child from therapy if the child meets the pure probe criterion for all the target skills. The clinician then puts the child on a schedule of follow-up and booster treatment.

Post-Dismissal Follow-Up and Booster Treatment

The need for follow-up assessment of dismissed clients and booster treatment is often neglected in speech-language pathology. Ideally, a child should not just be dismissed from treatment and then forgotten. It is helpful to see the child some 3 to 6 months after dismissal for a **follow-up assessment,** which is a pure probe of target language skills in conversational speech. Based on analysis of this pure probe sample, the clinician may judge whether or not the target language behaviors are being maintained in the absence of treatment.

If the target language behaviors are *not* being maintained, the child obviously needs **booster treatment,** which is treatment offered any time after an initial dismissal. Booster treatment is typically brief and may use the same procedure as before. If a new treatment is selected, it should be evidence-based. It helps reestablish or increase performance of a target behavior to a previously set criterion for accuracy. The need for booster treatment is not well researched in speech-language pathology; however, clinical experience suggests that many children may need booster treatment to maintain language skills.

Booster treatment is not the only strategy the clinician can use to help maintain target behaviors in natural settings and over time. Clinicians integrate additional maintenance strategies into treatment from its earliest stages, and they use such additional procedures as parent or teacher training to strengthen and sustain skills. Maintenance strategies will be discussed in Chapter 8.

What is missing from our description of the treatment framework are the many techniques clinicians may use to "fill in" the treatment framework in response to the needs of their clients—techniques for evoking correct responses, reinforcing correct responses, giving corrective feedback for incorrect responses, and reducing certain undesirable behaviors that may interfere with intervention. The next chapter will describe some of those techniques.

Chapter Summary

Because many language treatment techniques are advocated, clinicians should select procedures that are based on evidence, which is the hallmark of evidence-based practice. Treatments may be based on different kinds of research, although some are based on no research. Treatment research may be uncontrolled (case studies that demonstrate only improvement), controlled (experimental studies that demonstrate effectiveness), unreplicated (the first study with no known generality) directly replicated (the same investigator's repetition of a study), and systematically replicated (other investigators' repetition of a study).

A treatment may be based on evidence or its absence at seven levels: Level 1, expert advocacy (opinion touted as evidence); Level 2, uncontrolled and unreplicated evidence (the first case study on a treatment technique); Level 3, uncontrolled directly replicated (repetition of a case study by the same investigator); Level 4, uncontrolled systematically replicated (repetition of case studies by other investigators in different settings); Level 5, controlled unreplicated (the first experimental evaluation of a procedure); Level 6, controlled directly replicated (repetition of an experimental study by the original investigator); Level 7, controlled systematically replicated (repetition of an experimental study by other investigators in other settings). Behavioral methods of treatment are well supported by experimental research and most procedures have reached the Level 7 evidence. Clinicians should not select a procedure when another procedure for which a higher level of evidence is available.

Language treatment in children includes (1) selection of functional target behaviors; (2) baserating the initial target behaviors; (3) administering the discrete treatment trials; (4) probing for generalized productions; (5) promoting maintenance; (6) making follow-up assessments; and (7) offering booster treatments.

Selected functional skills may be taught in the normative or client-specific experimental sequence. There is no compelling reason not to use a sequence that does not necessarily follow the normative sequence.

Study Guide

1. Discuss the tenets of evidence-based practice. Describe varied views of evidence-based practice. How can student clinicians and professionals conduct evidence-based practice?

2. Describe the differences between uncontrolled research, controlled research, unreplicated research, directly replicated research, and systematically replicated research. What kind of research produces the highest level of evidence favoring a treatment procedure? Why?

3. Compare and contrast the different ways in which treatment research hierarchies have been proposed. Which one would you prefer and why?

4. Explore the different meanings of *treatment* in communicative disorders. How is treatment defined in this chapter? How do you critically evaluate it?

5. After completing the assessment of a 6-year-old child, you have diagnosed a severe language disorder requiring treatment. You have determined that the child qualifies for service according to the school guidelines you are expected to follow. Your assessment results indicate that the child has limited vocabulary, omits most grammatic features, speaks in short sentences, and has a variety of pragmatic deficits. For this child:

    a. Specify the target behavior selection approach or philosophy you would take; justify your selection

    b. Describe the initial and intermediate treatment targets you would select and define them in operational terms; give a brief justification for the selected targets

    c. Specify the initial treatment procedure

6. For the same child described in Question 5, describe the various ways in which treatment can be structured in a hierarchical fashion. Specify the sequence with which you would teach the selected target behaviors. Justify the approach you would take.

7. Distinguish between a baserate and probe. Do you give any kind of feedback for responses given during baserates or probes? Why or why not?

8. Discuss the debate over "loose" structure versus "tight" structure. What position would you take on this issue and why? What structure is typically used at the beginning of treatment and how is it modified as treatment progresses?

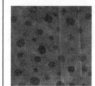

chapter

6

Evidence-Based Treatment Techniques

outline

In the previous chapter, we described an evidence-based framework for treating language disorders in children. We now need to fill in that framework with specific techniques of teaching basic language skills to children. The discrete trial procedure described in the previous chapter needs additional techniques to establish and strengthen language skills. This chapter will describe basic treatment procedures clinicians use in almost all treatment programs. In subsequent chapters, we will describe how basic language skills may be established, expanded, and maintained.

The techniques described in this chapter should be part of all clinicians' treatment repertoire. The techniques are effective not only in the treatment of language disorders in children, but also in the treatment of all disorders of communication in all age groups. In other words, they are generic treatment procedures that work across disorders of communication. Their effectiveness in treating language disorders has been well established through controlled clinical research. The techniques are also effective in shaping a variety of nonverbal skills and in reducing many undesirable behaviors children with disabilities exhibit (Baldwin & Baldwin, 1998; Barrera & Sulzar-Azaroff, 1983; Berg & Wacker, 1989; Camarata, 1993; Charlop & Walsh, 1986; Egel, Richman, & Koegel, 1981; Farmer-Dougan, 1994; Goldstein & Cisar, 1992; Goldstein & Ferrall, 1987; Goldstein & Mousetis, 1989; Goldstein & Wickstrom, 1986; Guess, 1969; Guess & Baer, 1973; Hart, 1985; Hegde, 1980; Hegde & McConn, 1981; Hegde, Noll, & Pecora, 1979; Laski, Charlop, & Schreibman, 1988; Lerman et al., 2004; Malott, Malott, & Trojan, 2000; Martin & Pear, 1999; Matson et al., 1993; Matson et al., 1990; Odom et al. 1992; Shabani et al., 2002; Taylor & Levin, 1998; Williams, Donley, & Keller, 2000; Zanoli & Daggett, 1998). The use of these techniques will be evidence-based practice. The techniques should be used in response to the child's needs, the child's responses under treatment, and parents' preferences. What works for one child in establishing a target behavior will not necessarily work for another. Clinicians should be flexible in applying procedures and be ready to modify them. Therefore, this chapter concludes with a section on modifying treatment procedures.

See Bailey et al., n.d., for a large collection of experimental intervention studies conducted from 1968 through 1985 and Vollmer et al., 2000, for another large collection of studies conducted from 1968 through 1999.

Starting with the Clinical and Moving to the Natural: Fading

A *social community* evokes and sustains verbal behaviors (language skills). People and aspects of physical and social environments (we will call these aspects *events* for the sake of brevity) serve as stimuli (antecedents) for verbal behavior. Unfortunately, for children with language disorders, people and events do not serve the stimulus function; people, events, objects, questions, requests, and so forth do not evoke expected verbal responses from them. Part of the clinician's job is to establish that stimulus function in children with language disorders, so they, too, like other children without a disorder, will verbally and socially respond appropriately.

Obviously, children with language disorders need special stimuli to respond, because language disorder is, in part, a failure to typically respond to natural stimuli. For example, the clinician may initially need to model a correct sentence for the child to imitate; such models are not typically and frequently used in everyday interactions. Therefore, clinicians are charged with arranging the clinical environment and providing special stimuli to help a child learn language skills. Those special stimuli include the techniques that will be discussed in this chapter.

> "I don't use anything but naturally occurring opportunities to evoke responses," some clinicians may state. But, such opportunities have not been sufficient to evoke language from children with language disorders. They need special stimuli arranged in ways not typically encountered in the "natural environment." After all, that is the essence of treatment.

The final goal in treating language disorders, however, is for the child to produce target language behaviors in natural settings, in response to naturally occurring consequences, without the need for the clinician-presented special stimuli. Therefore, while it is necessary to use special stimuli to establish a language behavior, those stimuli should be gradually withdrawn to maintain the correct response to naturally occurring social events. This process of gradual withdrawal of a special stimulus control is called **fading,** a technique in which the special stimulus control of target behaviors is gradually reduced until the child can produce them under typical social stimulus conditions (Baldwin & Baldwin, 1998; Malott, Malott, & Trojan, 2000; Martin & Pear, 1999). In most experimentally evaluated oral and sign language treatment programs as well as many social and academic skill training programs designed for children with various disabilities, special stimuli including modeling, prompting, and cueing have been initially used and later faded. Furthermore, studies have shown that parents, too, can be taught to use these techniques effectively (Barrera & Sulzar-Azaroff, 1983; Berg & Wacker, 1989; Charlop & Walsh, 1986; Egel, Richman, & Koegel, 1981; Goldstein & Cisar, 1992; Goldstein & Mousetis, 1989; Goldstein & Wickstrom, 1986; Hart, 1985; Kuhn, Lerman, & Vorndran, 2003; Laski, Charlop, & Schreibman, 1988; Matson et al., 1993; Matson et al., 1990; Odom et al., 1992; Shabani, et al., 2002; Taylor & Levin, 1998; Zanoli & Daggett, 1998).

When the child responds correctly to a special stimulus (such as modeling), the clinician reacts in a certain way to make that response more likely in the future. These clinical reactions that strengthen language skills are called reinforcers. Often, these reinforcers, too, are special (unusual), somewhat artificial, and more frequent than they are in the social environment. Therefore, reinforcers also should be gradually returned to a state typical of normal social interactions where they are infrequent and natural. This, too, is fading. Similarly, when the child gives incorrect responses or exhibits troublesome interfering behaviors (such as leaving the chair or not paying attention), the clinician reacts in a way to correct or stop them. This is called corrective feedback. This feedback also should be returned to a state typical of natural settings; this, too, is fading.

Every technique discussed in this chapter should be used sparingly, only to the extent necessary, and faded gradually, giving just enough support to help the child maintain the correct response without having the child become special cue- or stimulus-dependent, or unable to sustain skills without artificial reinforcers. Having the parents take part in the treatment of their children will help fade unusual stimuli into more natural events and interactions (see Box 6.1 for more on involving others in treatment).

How the fading is done depends on the specific stimuli used and the clinician actions (reinforcers and corrective feedback) that follow. Therefore, throughout our discussion of the various techniques clinicians use to evoke correct response, to reinforce correct responses, and to reduce undesirable behaviors, we will describe the manner in which those techniques can be faded.

| box 6.1 | | Fading the SLP—A Disappearing Act! |

The saying "fade into the wallpaper" describes what a clinician should eventually do in treating all clients. The most prominent special stimuli children encounter during language treatment are the clinicians themselves. Therefore, just like fading all special stimuli used in treatment, clinicians "fade" themselves, too. They fade themselves to some extent when they reduce the amount of modeling, prompting, instructions, manual guidance, and so forth. But the most important way in which the clinicians fade themselves is to get other people involved in treatment. The clinicians reduce their influence on the target skills when they bring other people as an audience into treatment sessions. When par-

ents, teachers, and others are taught to evoke and sustain target skills, clinicians will have taken additional and more powerful steps to fade themselves. When the child is nearing mastery of the target behavior, clinicians can literally fade themselves by standing in a corner (with or without wallpaper!) or even leaving the therapy room and observing the child's response rate in the presence of others.

Fading all special stimuli, including the clinician, is an important step in promoting maintenance of target behaviors in natural settings. See Chapter 9, Maintaining Language Skills, for details.

Putting the Child on the Right Path: Modeling

A **model** is the production of the target behavior by anyone who wants to teach a child an imitative response. Initially, it is the clinician who models the responses for the child to imitate. Soon, however, the clinician recruits others—teachers, parents or any other caregivers, and siblings to model the skills for the child. Modeling is an essential and effective technique in teaching a new skill (Baldwin & Baldwin, 1998; Malott, Malott, & Trojan, 2000; Martin & Pear, 1999). A majority of treatment research studies cited previously, including the classic studies done in the 1970s (e.g., Garcia, Guess, & Byrnes, 1973), have demonstrated the usefulness of modeling in teaching a variety of skills, including language skills, to children. Studies have shown that in addition to live modeling (e.g., Secan, Egel, & Tilley, 1989; Williams, Donley, & Keller, 2000), video modeling in which the desirable skills enacted by peers on a video can help teach language and other skills to children (Ballard & Crooks, 1984; Nikopoulos & Keenen, 2004).

> During clinic sessions, who provides the model? Who imitates?

The clinician models the expected skills soon after presenting one or more stimuli that would normally evoke the response but fail to do so, presumably because of the history of a language disorder. For example, the clinician may present the picture of a boy eating something and ask the question, "What is he doing?" This might evoke the response "eating" or "The boy is eating" from a typical child, but perhaps not from a child with a history of language disorders. Therefore, soon after presenting the picture and asking the question "What is he doing?" the clinician models, "Johnny, say, 'He is eating.'" The clinician then waits expectantly for the child to imitate the model. Note that the child's response that follows a clinician's model is called **imitation.** Therefore, modeling is a treatment procedure because it is the clinician's action; imitation is not, because it is the client's action.

Modeling is necessary when correct responses cannot simply be evoked, which is most common during the initial stages of therapy. Therefore, it is used frequently in treating communicative disorders. Modeling is, in fact, an indispensable procedure in speech and language training. Many treatment research studies cited earlier have demonstrated its effectiveness.

In treating childhood language disorders, modeling often is followed by a question that normally leads to a response. For example, when teaching production of the present progressive *-ing* at the sentence level, it is not desirable to show the child a picture of a person performing an action and provide only a model (e.g., "Say, 'The man is eating.'"). Rather, the clinician should first ask the typical question and then supply the model (e.g., "What is the man doing? Say, 'The man is eating.'"). If the model is consistently presented only after asking the question and faded as described later, the question alone may evoke the response—as questions normally do—when the model is discontinued.

> Children spontaneously imitate adult models in everyday situations. Modeling capitalizes on this tendency and takes it one step further by requiring the child to imitate.

Fading the Model

Modeling, frequently and consistently provided in the initial stages of treatment, should be faded as soon as possible. As treatment progresses, the need for modeling should be progressively less. The clinician—while training the skills in conversational speech—should model infrequently. In natural settings, parents and others should model only occasionally. Modeling leads to imitation. Both modeling and imitation should be faded because neither is excessively used in spontaneous conversation.

To fade modeling, clinicians can provide a partial model. A **partial model** provides only a portion of the correct response; just enough for the child to imitate the response. Using again the example of teaching present progressive *-ing* at the sentence level, the clinician would start with the full model (e.g., "What is the girl doing? Say, 'The girl is running.'"). If the child correctly and consecutively imitates the modeled response five times, the clinician should drop the model. If the child does not respond correctly to the question (without a model), the clinician might provide a partial model to evoke a correct response (e.g., "What is the girl doing? Say, 'The girl is run _____.'"). If the child responds correctly to the partial model, the clinician may progressively shorten the partial model until the question alone evokes the child's correct response.

Gradually decreasing the vocal intensity of modeling is another method of fading it. The clinician begins by presenting the model at a normal vocal intensity (loudness). On further discrete trials, the clinician progressively lowers the intensity of his or her voice until the modeled stimulus is faded out (no longer heard). If the child's correct response rate drops when the model has been totally faded out, the clinician may silently mouth as much of the model as is necessary to increase the child's correct responses.

Lowering the intensity of voice when presenting a modeled stimulus can also be used in a technique called **simultaneous speech,** in which the clinician and the client produce the target response at the same time. Before giving a model, the clinician says, "Please say it with me." For example, for teaching present progressive *-ing* at the word level, the clinician might present a stimulus card showing an action and give the verbal stimulus, "What is the girl doing? Say, 'running.' Say it with me; 'running.'" As the response is established, the clinician can then lower the intensity of her voice during simultaneous speech, first to the extent of only mouthing the words and then dropping the simultaneous speech altogether.

When a child imitates the clinician's model, very little else should be required to meet the desired criterion level for correct response rate. More often, children with severe language disorders may not imitate, or may do so only partially. If a child does not imitate a modeled response, the clinician must use shaping, an additional treatment method described later.

Giving a Hint: Prompting

A **prompt** is like a gentle hint; it is another special stimulus that is added or layered over other evoking or modeling stimuli. Prompting is a well-researched behavioral technique in teaching a variety of skills to children and adults (Baldwin & Baldwin, 1998; Malott, Malott, & Trojan, 2000; Martin & Pear, 1999). As noted before, prompts have been shown to be effective in many child language treatment research studies (e.g., Berg & Wacker, 1989; Goldstein & Wickstrom, 1986; Kuhn, Lerman, & Vorndran, 2003; Matson et al., 1990; Odom et al., 1992, among many others). Prompts may be verbal, textual, and nonverbal (Shabani et al., 2002).

Verbal Prompts

A **verbal prompt** is a special verbal stimulus designed to evoke a correct response. Partial models are verbal prompts. For instance, after having modeled the full response, "Say, 'I see two books'" on several trials, the clinician may give only a partial model: "Say, 'I see two. . . .'" The partial model may prompt the child to say "books" or "I see two books." These are clear verbal prompts. When the clinician varies the intensity of her voice, she is supplying a type of verbal prompt. Giving certain parts of a model vocal emphasis is also a verbal prompt (e.g., "Say, 'The boy is ea*ting*.'"). Clinicians often emphasize the target skill that is embedded in a chain of responses (Risley & Reynolds, 1970). In the example, the *-ing* is vocally emphasized.

What is the sentence completion task also called?

Another type of verbal prompt is the classic sentence completion method, or **cloze** method. In teaching the semantic concept of opposites, for example, a clinician might show a child two pictures, one of an elephant and one of a mouse, and, pointing to the appropriate pictures, supply a verbal prompt in the form of a sentence completion task. She might say, "This one is big, and this one is _____." The cloze prompt may evoke the response "little" from the child.

Verbal prompts do not necessarily have to contain any of the desired response. If a child appears hesitant to give a response, for example, the clinician might gently ask, "Can you remember?" or "What do you say?" This type of verbal prompt, although it does not contain any of the elements of the desired response, may help the child produce a correct response.

Textual Prompts

Textual prompts are printed cues that help evoke a target response. Textual prompts may be especially useful in integrating literacy skills with oral language training. For instance, in teaching the production of a set of functional words to children, clinicians typically use pictures of objects, persons, or actions as training stimuli. To integrate literacy skill training with such language treatment or to simply create an additional prompt or word productions, the clinician may print the relevant word under each picture. While modeling the word productions for the child, the clinician will point to both the picture and the word (e.g., "What is this? Say, 'cup'" while pointing to the picture of a cup as well as the printed word *cup*). Eventually, the clinician may ask the question ("What is this?") and, without modeling the word, point to the printed word as a prompt for the response. Even children who have not learned to read fully may learn to sight read and get a cue from the printed word. Eventually, to teach the child to read the words, the clinician may fade the picture stimuli and present only the printed words as a prompt (see Chapter 10 for more techniques to embed literacy training with language treatment).

Sometimes a clinician needs to keep telling the child "look at me" or "look at the picture" to maintain attention. While giving such verbal instructions, the clinician might also place on the table large cards on which the words are printed. The clinician can then point to the relevant printed message that prompts a specific response (e.g., "look at me," "look at the picture," "sit quietly," etc.).

Nonverbal Prompts

Nonverbal prompts can also be called physical prompts. **Nonverbal** or **physical prompts** are various signals or gestures the clinician gives to evoke the correct production of a target behavior. For example, in teaching a child to produce the present progressive *-ing*, the clinician might show the picture of a boy reading, ask "What is he doing?" and show the hand gesture of holding a book to evoke the verb *reading*. Similarly, after asking the question, the clinician may smile and point a finger to her smile to evoke the verb *smiling*. To evoke the preposition *on*, the clinician may tap *on* the table. To evoke the productions of adjectives *big* and *small*, the clinician may give alternating, contrasting hand signals to suggest bigness and smallness.

Tactile prompts are a special variety of nonverbal prompts known to be effective with some children, especially those with autism or developmental disability. A remotely controlled vibrating pager may be used to prompt verbal initiations from children on play grounds and such other natural settings (Shabani, et al., 2002; Taylor & Levin, 1998). A more common tactile prompt is a simple touch to prompt the child to produce a response.

In teaching narrative skills to children, sequenced photographs that show a series of activities or tell simple or complex stories also may be used as nonverbal prompts. After having told a story with the help of sequenced pictures, the clinician may use both verbal and nonverbal prompts (e.g., pointing to the pictures in sequence) to evoke narration of the story.

Some clinicians use hand motions associated with popular children's stories or finger plays to evoke language target behaviors from children. Others may find American Sign Language to be effective in helping children, particularly severely disabled children, learn a set of functional words. To cue (prompt) word order or syntactic structures, the clinician may use a form of manual (manually coded) English which uses rapidly executed hand gestures and finger spellings and follows the English syntax. In any case, all kinds of prompts used should be kept to the minimum required to evoke a correct response from a child.

Fading the Prompts

Verbal and nonverbal prompts may be faded the same way the modeling is faded. Partial models should become progressively shorter until they are faded altogether. Vocal intensity of a model (loudness) may be progressively lowered until the verbal prompt is no longer heard and rendered unnecessary. To fade nonverbal prompts, gestures and signals may be made progressively less conspicuous, until they are no longer needed for the child to produce a correct response. See Box 6.2 for a hierarchy of prompts.

Prompts will be easier to fade if the clinician uses the following guidelines, from Hegde and Davis (1999):

- Prompt more frequently in the initial stages of treatment. As correct responses become more stable, gradually reduce the frequency of prompts.
- Prefer a subtle or short prompt over a loud or lengthy prompt.
- Prefer a gestural prompt over a verbal prompt.
- Use partial modeling, whenever appropriate, rather than a full model as a prompt.
- Give prompts promptly, at the first sign of a hesitation or wrong response.
- Fade prompts by making them progressively more subtle or shorter.

---

box 6.2   **Using a Hierarchy of Prompting Techniques**

If clinicians use a variety of prompts, presented in a well-planned sequence, it will be easier to document what is working for the child and what is not. For example, if a child does not imitate a model, the clinician may add more vocal emphasis to the model, highlighting the missed portion. If the child still does not imitate correctly, the clinician might then add a physical prompt, such as a hand signal. The idea is to start with less obvious prompts, but be prepared to move to more obvious prompts, if necessary. Throughout this process, the clinician should use successive approximation, or shaping, reinforcing progressively better responses. Here is an example of a hierarchy of prompting techniques for evoking present progressive *-ing*.

Clinician: [showing a picture depicting action] What is he doing? Say, "He is running."
Child: He run.
Clinician: No, I didn't hear the whole sentence. [Removes the picture, records the incorrect response, and re-presents the picture] What is he doing? Say, "He *is* run*ning*." [adds vocal emphasis to the missed parts of the target response]
Child: He is run.

Clinician: That's better! [shaping by reinforcing a better response] But remember to say, "run*ning*." [removes the picture, records the incorrect response and re-presents the picture] What is he doing? Say, "He *is* run*ning*." [uses some arbitrary hand signal when modeling *running*; perhaps a line drawn by the index finger in the air]
Child: He is run . . . [hesitates, the clinician quickly provides the hand signal] ing.
Clinician: Very good! You got it! [records the correct response, noting that it was prompted]

Once the child has responded correctly, the clinician might fade cues by first deleting the hand signal and then the added vocal emphasis, until the child is responding only to the model. After five consecutively correctly imitated responses, the clinician should move to evoked trials.

In this brief example, the child produced one correct answer in three trials, for a percentage of 33 percent correct. If this ratio continued throughout the session, the clinician would record data by stating that the child was "33 percent accurate for modeled trials given with vocal emphasis and nonverbal prompts."

Building More Complex Skills: Shaping

Shaping, also called successive approximation, is a treatment procedure designed to teach more complex skills by building upon a series of simple skills. The classic clinical study on shaping involved a mute schizophrenic patient who was taught to say "gum, please" over a period of training (Isaacs, Thomas, & Goldiamond, 1960). Initially, small movements of the lips were reinforced while showing a piece of gum; in subsequent stages, an undifferentiated vocal response, a vocal response that barely resembled *gum* and eventually responses that better approximated that word production, and finally "gum, please" were reinforced. Since that classic study, shaping has been a part of effective language treatment techniques. Shaping has been shown to be effective in teaching children functional communication skills that replace self-injurious or aggressive behaviors often seen in autistic children (Maurice, 1996; Reichle & Wacker, 1993; Shirley et al., 1997).

> Most of our skills are shaped in everyday life. It is a technique in which people do what they *can* first. A small part of a skill is easier to learn than the total skill. We break all complex skills into smaller, manageable, easily learnable skills. We then put them all together.

> What is another term for *shaping*?

Shaping is needed when a child does not imitate a response or when a response is too complex for the child to learn as a whole, so it needs to be broken down into smaller skills or steps. In using shaping, the clinician describes a terminal (final) target behavior and identifies a chain of initial and intermediate skills that when combined will lead to its production (Baldwin & Baldwin, 1998; Malott, Malott, & Trojan, 2000; Martin & Pear, 1999; Hegde, 1998b). The clinician will then model the initial skill for the child to imitate and reinforce the imitative response. When the first skill is produced without a model, the clinician models and reinforces the second skill in the chain. Treatment continues in this manner until the child reaches the final step and produces the final (terminal) target behavior which integrates all the previous skills.

Shaping is especially useful in the case of children who are nonverbal or minimally verbal. Such children may not imitate even a single, simple word modeled for them. Treatment of such children should begin with the production of a few functional words (e.g., *Mommy, juice, cookie, bye-bye*) which they may not imitate. For example, in teaching the word *Mommy* to a child who does not imitate it, the clinician can reinforce an initial response that can be shaped into the target word. That initial and simple response might be simply putting the lips together in the articulatory posture for production of /m/, for which the child would receive reinforcement. Then, the clinician would "raise the bar" and move to the next step, which might be requiring the child to phonate with the lips together to produce the

> If clinicians insist at first on perfectly imitated productions of a target behavior, children may go for long periods of time receiving only corrective feedback and little, if any, reinforcement. To avoid this problem, clinicians should use the shaping procedure when the child does not initially fully imitate the clinician's model.

/m/ sound before receiving reinforcement. Out of these initial responses, the terminal response can be shaped by gradually adding more complex features of the terminal response. The /m/ sound can be shaped into *Ma*, which is then shaped into *Mom*, which is finally shaped into *Mommy*.

To shape a response when treating childhood language disorders:

- Define the target behavior
- Describe an initial response the child can imitate or produce with further cues (such as manual guidance, prompting, or instructions)

- Describe intermediate responses that should be shaped, leading to the production of the target behavior
- Begin treatment with the initial response, reinforcing the production of that response
- Move to the next intermediate response when the initial response is reliably produced
- Shift treatment to the next component of the terminal response each time one of the intermediate responses is reliably produced
- End treatment with the terminal response; provide more training on this
- Add additional language elements to shape phrases and sentences

The shaping procedure can incorporate other techniques that help evoke a correct response. If the child does not readily imitate even the initial response, the clinician may use manual guidance described in the next section.

Giving a Helping Hand: Manual Guidance

Some children, particularly those who are severely disabled, may need physical assistance to produce a response. **Manual guidance,** also called physical guidance, consists of the clinician providing gentle, but firm, physical assistance to help a child make a movement (Baldwin & Baldwin, 1998; Hegde, 1998b; Malott, Malott, & Trojan, 2000). For example, while shaping the production of the word *Mommy,* if the child does not imitate the initial response of pressing the lips together, the clinician might use her index finger and thumb to gently guide the child's lips into place, giving the child reinforcement as soon as the lips come into contact with each other.

Manual guidance is useful when teaching language comprehension as indexed by correct nonverbal responses given to verbal instructions or directions. For example, in teaching a child to follow one-step directions, the clinician may tell the child to "Put the ball in the box" and manually guide the child's hand to pick up the ball and put it in the box (see Photo 6.1 for an example of manual guidance).

Manual guidance can also be used to teach other kinds of nonverbal communication. Some children are so physically handicapped, cognitively impaired, or both, that verbal speech and language learning is an unrealistic goal, at the least as the initial treatment target. For those children, a system of augmentative and alternative communication (AAC) may give them a means to communicate. AAC is a specialized area of speech-language pathology and will be the subject of Chapter 15. Manual guidance can be used when teaching AAC systems in which the child needs to point to printed messages, pictures, signs, and symbols to communicate. Manual guidance will help a child who cannot point to correct messages. The clinician can use hand-over-hand manual guidance to point to a specific picture in a field of pictures. For example, with two pictures on the table, the clinician can instruct, "Point to the cup" and guide the child's finger to the picture of the cup.

Fading Manual Guidance

Manual guidance should be faded as soon as possible. The clinician can move from total hand-over-hand manipulation to gentle touches to no manual guidance at all when the child can perform the behavior independently.

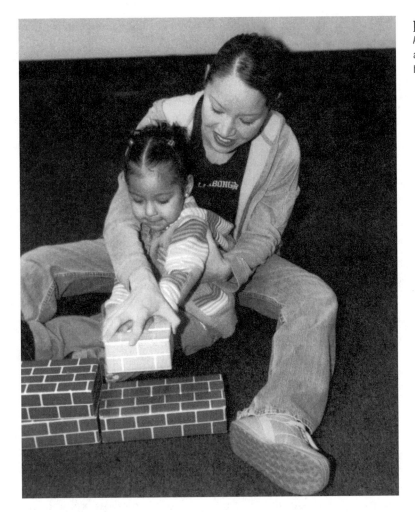

photo 6.1

A helping hand—a parent uses manual guidance to help a child put the yellow block *on* the blue block.

Fading in this manner can be accomplished in the case of all the previously cited examples. Manual guidance given for the production of the initial /m/ in the word *Mommy* may begin with the clinician gently but firmly pressing the child's lips together. As the child learns to make the /m/ sound, the clinician can gradually reduce the pressure with which the child's lips are held, then keep the fingers close to the lips but not touching them, and finally moving the fingers progressively farther from the lips until there is no longer manual guidance.

In the case of the boy learning to follow one-step directions, the clinician may fade total hand-over-hand assistance to "put the ball in the box," decreasing the physical manipulation to perhaps just a gentle shove toward the ball which is then completely withdrawn until the boy responds on his own. Similarly, in teaching to a severely disabled child the skill of pointing to messages, the clinician can fade the hand-over-hand assistance.

Manual guidance is perhaps the most intrusive technique discussed in this chapter. It should be used only when necessary, to as little an extent as possible, and then faded quickly.

This will help guard against the possibility of the child becoming dependent upon the clinician's manual guidance to produce correct responses.

▨❘▨ Just Telling Them: Instructions

The effectiveness of manual guidance, as well as the other techniques discussed in this chapter, may be enhanced if accompanied by the clinician's **instructions,** which are often verbal directions on how to perform an action. Instructions are typically combined with other kinds of behavioral contingencies, including modeling and positive or differential reinforcement (Baldwin & Baldwin, 1998; Ringdahl et al., 2002). Imagine what it would be like to simply receive a command immediately followed by manual guidance, as follows:

Clinician: [presents a picture of the child's mother] Who is this? Say, "Mommy" [reaches over and presses the child's lips together].

Contrast that scenario with the following:

Clinician: We need to put our lips together to say "Mommy." Watch me [demonstrates the production]. "Mommy." See how I put my lips together? Let's try it [presents a picture of the child's mother]. Who is this? Say, 'Mommy.' Now let me help you put your lips together" [reaches over and presses the child's lips together].

In the second scenario, the clinician gave instructions coupled with a demonstration. Instructions describe a skill to be learned. In the treatment of childhood language disorders, instructions can be used to describe the target behavior, specify under what conditions in natural settings the target behavior should be produced, and, when appropriate, how to produce it. See Table 6.1 for suggested instructions for common language target behaviors.

Although the second scenario presented may appeal more to the sensibilities of clinicians and clients, the effectiveness of instructions (alone or combined with other procedures) has rarely been experimentally evaluated. It is simply assumed that, because we refer to instructions to learn many basic skills in everyday situations, instructions should be incorporated into treatment sessions, perhaps even serving as the starting point in treatment.

Instructions may be more useful when coupled with demonstrations. A demonstration is similar to a model but is not expected to be imitated. A clinician only shows the client how to do something without requiring the client to imitate. In contrast, when using operant modeling (the type of modeling discussed in this and the previous chapter), the clinician requires an immediate imitation of the model. Another difference between demonstration and modeling is that demonstration is often accompanied by instructions that are much more detailed than the simple command the clinician gives preceding an operant model (e.g., "What do you see? Say, 'I see two cats.'").

> What is the difference between a demonstration and a model?

When giving instructions to a child for the production of a language target behavior, it is necessary to use simple, clear language the child can understand. Instructions should relate to experiences or concrete examples, never to linguistic rules. For example, for the production of plural -s, a clinician would not tell a child, "OK, Johnny, according to the

table 6.1

Instructions for Some Common Language Target Behaviors

Instructions should immediately be followed by presentation of discrete modeled trials.
Use vocal emphasis on the targeted behavior when giving instructions.

Target Behavior	Level	Suggested Instructions
Regular plural -s (e.g., /s/ in *ducks*, /z/ in *balls*, /ez/ in *houses*)	Word	When I show you one of these [show picture of one object, for example, a duck], you say, "duck." But when I show you two or more of these [show a picture of two or more ducks], you say, "ducks." Remember to make the /s/ sound at the end!
Irregular plurals (each one a separate target behavior)	Word	When I show you one of these [show picture of one object, for example, a foot], you say "foot." But when I show you two of these [show a picture of two feet], you say "feet."
Prepositions (e.g., in, on, under, over, behind, between, etc.)	Phrase	When the doll is here [demonstrating with a doll and chair] and I ask you where it is, you say, "*on* the chair." [demonstrate for each preposition being taught]
Present progressive -ing	Word	When someone is doing something right now, you say "ing" at the end of the word. So, if I show you a picture like this [show picture depicting action] and ask, "What is he doing?" you say, "runn*ing*."
Present progressive -ing with auxiliary *is*	Sentence	Look at this picture. She is doing something right now. She is reading. So, if I show you a picture like this and ask, "What is she doing?" you say, "She is reading." Remember to say the whole sentence!
Third person present tense -s (e.g., /s/ in *eats*, /z/ in *sings*, /ez/ in *washes*)	Word or Sentence	Look at this picture. The little girl does something. She sleeps. So, if I show you a picture like this and ask, "What does she do?" you say, "sleeps" [or, "She sleeps"].
Possessive -s (e.g., /s/ in *Jack's*, /z/ in *Daddy's*, /ez/ in *Maurice's*)	Word, phrase, or sentence	Here is a hat. It belongs to Mommy. So, if I ask you whose hat it is, you say, "Mommy*'s*" [or, Mommy*'s* hat, or, It's Mommy*'s* hat].
Regular past tense -d (e.g., /d/ in *cried*, /t/ in *walked*, /ted/ in *tasted*)	Word, phrase, or sentence	If you are laughing right now, you say, "I laugh!" But if you are finished laughing, you say, "I *laughed*."
Irregular past tense (each one a separate target behavior)	Word, phrase, or sentence	We will work on some special words that help you talk about things that happened some time ago—like yesterday. Look at this picture. Right now, he is eating pizza. Yesterday, he *ate* pizza.

rules of plural usage in the English language, when referring to more than one object, you need to add an *s* to regular plural words that end in an unvoiced phoneme." Rather, the clinician would describe the target behavior to the child in nontechnical terms, pointing out concrete everyday situations in which the plural -*s* would be used, illustrating instructions with picture stimuli, and demonstrating the production of the target form. The instructions given, then, may be something similar to the following:

Clinician: Johnny, when I show you one of these [showing Johnny a picture of a cat], you say, "cat." But, when I show you two of these [showing Johnny a picture of two cats], you say "cats."

Instructions may be most useful in establishing conversational skills (pragmatic language behaviors). Describing social conditions under which conversational skills are appropriate may be useful to the child. For example, if the clinician is teaching conversational repair, she might tell the child, "When you don't understand something someone is saying, ask, 'What did you say?'" In teaching social rituals, the clinician can describe the social situations and describe and demonstrate the ritual, such as, "When we meet someone for the first time, we look at the person, shake hands, and say, 'How do you do?'" Or, "If you have to walk in front of someone, you say, 'Excuse me.'" Such instructions need to be followed by modeling the behavior and reinforcing it.

The clinician should ask the child to repeat the instructions given. This will help assess the child's understanding of instructions and give a chance to repeat or expand the instructions if needed. In the case of children with receptive language difficulties, a quick assessment of comprehension of instructions is particularly important. Depending on the child's performance, instructions may need to be periodically repeated throughout the treatment sequence. Furthermore, new instructions should be given every time treatment is shifted to a new level.

To summarize, when giving instructions to children being treated for language disorders, clinicians should:

- Give instructions using simple, direct language
- Combine instructions with demonstrations
- Assess the child's understanding of the instructions given (e.g., ask the child to repeat the instructions)
- If necessary, repeat or clarify the instructions
- Periodically repeat instructions during the treatment sequence
- Give new instructions when treatment shifts to a new level of the same target behavior or to an entirely new target behavior
- Use instructions as a part of an overall treatment strategy

So far, we have described various techniques that can help evoke correct responses from a child with language disorders. In the stimulus-response-consequence treatment chain, these techniques are the *stimulus* links.

In the treatment process, if the *response* the child gives to the clinician-presented stimulus event is correct, the clinician should provide a *consequence* that will serve to increase the future likelihood of correct responses. If the response the child gives is incorrect, the clinician should provide a different consequence that will serve to decrease the future likelihood of that and similar incorrect responses. To accomplish these goals, the clinician needs two sets of techniques: (1) those that increase correct responses, and (2) those that decrease incorrect responses (including interfering behaviors—child behaviors that interrupt treatment). We will begin by discussing the first of these two types of consequences—techniques to increase correct responses.

Getting Them to Say More: Techniques to Increase Language Skills

Virtually all clinicians give feedback to children they work with; without such feedback children can hardly learn. When feedback is conceptualized technically, and used systematically, desirable skills can be increased and undesirable actions can be decreased. Technically, feedback is a *consequence* delivered soon after a response is given. Consequences can be delivered in varied ways to achieve differential results. Consequences, in turn, may be either reinforcing or corrective. Consequences that increase skills are reinforcing; those that decrease are corrective. The consequence the clinician delivers immediately following a child's correct response should reinforce that response (Baldwin & Baldwin, 1998; Hegde, 1998b; Malott, Malott, & Trojan, 2000; Martin & Pear, 1999).

> What two factors determine whether an event is a reinforcer?

To be called a **reinforcer** (e.g., a verbal praise, a token), the consequence should be delivered immediately after a response is made and should increase the correct response rate. If the correct response rate does not increase, the consequence is, in effect, not a reinforcer. Collecting data that document the course of the correct response rate will tell whether a consequence was a reinforcer. This is an objective, not a subjective, evaluation. The clinician and the child may feel good about what is being used for reinforcement, but if the correct response rate has not increased, there is actually no reinforcement going on to feel good about.

> Sally's school SLP allowed her to color a different part of a picture every time she gave a correct response. The correct response rate began to increase. Sally enjoyed the coloring. However, after three sessions, Sally's correct response rate stagnated. Even though the coloring activity looked like it should be reinforcing, and the child and the SLP felt good about the activity, it was not a reinforcer.

Whether or not a reinforcer is truly a reinforcer for a particular child, then, cannot be predicted before therapy starts. The clinician needs to experiment with different kinds of consequences before finding the best way to reinforce the child's correct responses. Before beginning treatment, the clinician might ask the child, or the child's parents or teacher, what the child's interests are to help assess what the child might find reinforcing.

A technique that is reinforcing to one child might not be reinforcing to another. An active child, for example, might work hard for the opportunity to play kickball with the clinician for the last five minutes of the therapy session. Another child may respond well when coloring a special picture or choosing a sticker to place on a book cover is the consequence of responding. Also, what works as a reinforcer for a child during one session might not work for a subsequent session. Clinicians cannot assume that a particular consequence will be consistently effective, even with the same child, over all treatment sessions. It is necessary to have a variety of consequences available and ready to be administered throughout all treatment sessions.

There are many types of reinforcers, which are all procedural examples of the principle of reinforcement. In treating childhood language disorders, the most commonly used procedure is *positive* reinforcement. Two broad categories of positive reinforcement are (1) primary reinforcement and (2) secondary reinforcement (Baldwin & Baldwin, 1998; Hegde, 1998b; Malott, Malott, & Trojan, 2000; Martin & Pear, 1999).

> What are the two main procedures of reinforcement?

Primary Reinforcement

Primary reinforcement is a method of increasing target skills by arranging consequences that have biological value to the recipients. Consequences that promote the biological survival of a species are called **primary reinforcers.** Food, drink, and shelter are examples of primary reinforcers. These are reinforcers whose effects do not have to be learned; human beings naturally seek out primary reinforcers. Even children who have learning difficulties, then, respond to primary reinforcers.

Food and drink are most useful in treating childhood language disorders. Clinicians may reinforce a child's correct response by immediately presenting a small amount of food, such as a piece of the child's favorite breakfast cereal or a small amount of juice. Presentation of food or drink does not have to be a "natural" consequence of the behavior. Primary reinforcement can be used to increase any language behavior, such as labeling nouns or producing adjectives. However, food and drink are both powerful and natural reinforcers when teaching children to mand or request. For instance, to teach such mands as "I want juice" or "May I have a cookie, please," the consequences the mands specify are the only reinforcers.

There are some disadvantages to using primary reinforcers in the clinic when treating childhood language disorders. First, primary reinforcers for language responses other than those that mand certain consequence (e.g., food and drink) are not natural. At home and school, children do not receive primary reinforcers for naming objects or sustaining a topic of conversation. The use of primary reinforcers to establish a language behavior in the clinic, then, may not promote generalization and maintenance of the behavior in the child's natural environment. To minimize this problem, clinicians should always pair the presentation of primary reinforcers with *social* reinforcers in the form of warm verbal praise (e.g., "Good!" "That was just right!" "I like that!" etc.). By combining primary reinforcers with social reinforcers, the clinician can gradually fade the primary reinforcers as the child learns to respond to verbal praise alone—a type of reinforcer the child is much more likely to encounter in natural environments.

Second, for a primary reinforcer to be effective, a child must have been at least slightly deprived of it. A school child is likely to work less hard for food in a session held soon after lunch than in a session held just before it. Therefore, the clinician should plan the timing of sessions right if primary reinforcers are expected to be used. There are, of course, ethical concerns over too stringently depriving a child of food or drink. Nonetheless, some restrictions may be acceptable to both the child and the family. For example, a parent could be gently dissuaded from giving a child a fast-food lunch of burgers, fries, and coke on the way to language therapy.

Third, even children who have been slightly deprived of food or drink prior to clinic sessions are subject to the satiation effect, another disadvantage to using primary reinforcers. It may be that a bite of breakfast cereal, for example, will work fine as a reinforcer at the beginning of a treatment session in increasing the child's correct responses. However, as the session progresses, the child may simply become full and no longer feel like "working for food." If the child is very full, the child may actually work to *avoid* presentation of food, with disastrous consequences to the correct response rate. The way to avoid this problem is for the clinician to give food for some but not all responses.

Fourth, there are some practical problems in using primary reinforcers in the clinic. Food or drink can be messy and difficult to present response contingently, which may result in a delay between the response and delivery of the reinforcer. Waiting for the child to ingest the food may waste valuable treatment time. Any clinician who has had to wait for the child to finish a gummy bear, for example, has experienced this problem. Some clinicians may give the child a cup to collect food reinforcers to eat after clinic. This may not be practical, however, for children with cognitive deficits, who are often the candidates for primary reinforcers.

Fifth, extreme caution is needed in the use of primary reinforcers with children who have swallowing difficulties because of neurological problems (see Chapter 14 for details). It may not be safe to use food as a reinforcer unless the clinician is also trained in the management of swallowing disorders. If the problem is mild and the child has been self-feeding with minimal assistance at home, foods that quickly dissolve may be preferred; parental guidance about foods the child eats safely and consultation with an expert on swallowing disorders will help select the safe reinforcers.

Sixth, child- and family-specific health considerations or food preferences may prevent the use of food as reinforcers. Before using any type of primary reinforcers, clinicians should ascertain from parents whether they approve the use of primary reinforcers. If the parents disapprove, food and drink should not be used. If they do approve, clinicians should further ascertain whether the child has any food allergies, is on any kind of special diet, or if the parents object to certain types of foods. Similar to swallowing disorders, allergies can be life-threatening and must be taken very seriously. Many children with disabilities or chronic diseases have special diets that restrict certain types of foods or limit them to certain kinds of foods. In any case, parental approval of, and preferences for, food items should always be obtained.

Despite these disadvantages, food or drink can be effective primary reinforcers, particularly for severely disabled children who are nonverbal, or minimally verbal, who do not readily respond to verbal praise. With some children, the clinician may find that presentation of food or drink is the only manner in which correct responses can be reinforced during beginning stages of treatment. Therefore, clinicians should not hesitate to use primary reinforcers to initially establish behaviors, with the intention of fading such reinforcers out as soon as possible.

Secondary Reinforcement

The use of social consequences to increase skills is called **secondary reinforcement.** Unlike primary reinforcers, the effects of social consequences depend on past learning; their reinforcing effects are due to past experiences (Baldwin & Baldwin, 1998; Hegde, 1998b; Malott, Malott, & Trojan, 2000; Martin & Pear, 1999). People learn to respond to secondary reinforcers as a result of their interactions with their social cultures and environments. There are many types of secondary reinforcement procedures clinicians can use to help increase children's correct response rates. These include social reinforcement, informative feedback, conditioned generalized reinforcement, and the use of high probability behaviors.

Social reinforcement. A form of secondary reinforcement, social reinforcement consists of socially mediated consequences. The warm verbal praise given to children we described earlier in this chapter shows how integral the use of a social reinforcer is to the treatment of language disorders. Verbal praise is not the only type of social reinforcer; giving a child attention, making face-to-face eye contact, smiling at the child, and a pat on the shoulder are all examples of social reinforcers.

In the initial stages of treatment, social reinforcers are more effective when paired with some other type of reinforcement. Both primary reinforcers (e.g., food or drink) and other types of secondary reinforcers (e.g., stickers or tokens, which will be described later in this section) may be combined with social reinforcers. The advantage of pairing social reinforcers with other kinds of reinforcers is that the latter can be faded first. When the response rate is maintained only with the use of social reinforcers for some time, they, too, can be gradually reduced to approximate social reinforcement inherent to everyday interactions. For example, an explicit verbal praise (e.g., "You did add the *s* to the word! I like that!") may be faded and only the more naturalistic smiles, eye contact, nodding, and so forth may be kept as reinforcers.

There are many other advantages to using social reinforcement. Children are much more likely to receive social reinforcement in the natural environment. It is easy to teach people in the child's environment to reinforce the child's new language behaviors by making statements such as, "Wow! You are really talking now!" or "Listen to you talk!" (see Box 6.3 for other suggested social reinforcers). Therefore, the use of social reinforcement may help promote maintenance of the child's newly learned language behaviors in natural settings.

Also, social reinforcers have some definite advantages over the use of primary reinforcers. Social reinforcers are not dependent upon deprivation, are not subject to the satiation effect, and do not interrupt the treatment sequence. As noted before, social reinforcement is also effective in fading out primary reinforcement.

In spite of its significant advantages, social reinforcers have some limitations. One limitation is that by themselves, social reinforcers may not be enough to motivate children who have very severe language disorders—children who are most likely to require the services

---

box 6.3   **Alternatives to Saying "Good Job!"**

Social reinforcement should be delivered with warmth, enthusiasm, and variety. Too many clinicians get into the routine of saying, "Good job!" repeatedly throughout the session. Here are some examples to help you vary your delivery of social reinforcement.

1. That's it!
2. You got it!
3. Way to go!
4. Just right!
5. So much better!
6. I like the way you're talking!
7. I knew you could say it!
8. You know just what to say!
9. I like to hear you talk!
10. Yes! High five!
11. Hey! You got it that time!
12. That was such a nice sentence!
13. Exactly right!
14. Good for you!
15. Great!
16. That's the way!
17. Perfect!
18. Excellent!
19. Hey, you remembered your words!
20. That's just the way to say it!
21. You really said it right!
22. You are so good at this!
23. You did it!
24. Better than ever!
25. That was your best one!
26. That was just super!
27. Good! Keep it up!
28. There you go!
29. Wow! That was just right!
30. You are really using your words!

of speech-language pathologists. Such children who have extremely limited verbal repertoire may not be reinforced with verbal praise. Even with children whose disabilities are not so severe, pairing social reinforcers with some other type of reinforcers is often more effective in establishing basic language skills during the initial stages of treatment. Another limitation is that explicit social reinforcers, which include such statements as "That was good talking!" "You did say 'cups,' instead of 'cup,'" and so forth are somewhat artificial; they interfere with the normal flow of conversational exchanges. Therefore, as suggested earlier, the clinician should fade explicit social (and verbal) reinforcers and keep only such implicit social reinforcers as smile, touch, nodding, agreement (e.g., "Yes!" or "I think so!"), and so forth to reinforce the child. Such implicit social reinforcers do not interrupt the flow of conversation, do not sound artificial, and are inherent to normal communication. Parents, too, may be asked to use explicit social reinforcers only initially, fade them out, and use implicit social reinforcers consistently.

> Has anyone heard of people getting tired of praise?

Informative feedback. Increasing behaviors by providing feedback on the progress a child is making in learning a skill is called **informative feedback** (Baldwin & Baldwin, 1998; Hegde, 1998b; Malott, Malott, & Trojan, 2000). For example, a clinician may help a child keep a sticker chart to keep track of correct responses. At the end of the clinic session, the clinician might point out to the child that correct responses increased over the previous session and say something like, "Look, Antonio! Yesterday, you only had 10 stars, and today you have 22 stars. Good for you!"

A clinician might also pair informative feedback with verbal praise immediately after the child has produced a correct response, letting the child know not only that the response was correct but also exactly what it was he or she did to make it correct. If the target behavior is correct production of plural *-s*, for example, the clinician might say, "Good! I heard the *-s* at the end of the word!"

Many computer software programs designed to teach language behaviors to children also use informative feedback. Although the use of such mechanical means to teach target behaviors and provide informative feedback to children via computer programs is widespread, there has been limited research on their efficacy. Research on the efficacy of informative feedback used alone also is limited. Therefore, until further efficacy research is conducted, clinicians should be cautious in using computerized language programs that provide only the informative feedback.

> Clinicians can always add praise and other reinforcers to informative feedback.

Conditioned generalized reinforcement. The method of increasing behaviors with the help of consequences that give access to a variety of reinforcers is called **conditioned generalized reinforcement** or simply, generalized reinforcement (Baldwin & Baldwin, 1998). Consequences that have a wide range of effects and do not depend on a state of deprivation are called **conditioned generalized reinforcers.** They are (1) *conditioned* because their reinforcing effects depend upon past experience, and (2) *generalized* because they can gain access to a wide variety of other reinforcers. The most commonly used conditioned generalized reinforcer in most societies is money. Without past experience, money is nothing but little pieces of paper. However, money is reinforcing to individuals in a society because it gives access to many other backup reinforcers, namely, all the goods and services that money can buy.

When working with children with language disorders (and other skill training), token systems of reinforcement are often used to increase correct response rates (Heward & Eachus, 1979; Kazdin, 2001; Kirby, Holborn, & Bushby, 1981; Odom et al., 1985). Tokens can consist of stickers, stamps, check marks on a chart, plastic chips, marbles, beads, or any small object given to the child as a consequence for a correct response. When the child has accumulated a predetermined number of tokens, the tokens can then be exchanged for the child's choice of a backup reinforcer, usually either small toys, pieces of candy, fancy pencils or pens, or any other desirable object. Tokens may also be exchanged for the opportunity to engage in some preferred activity, such as playing with a special toy, listening to music, taking a trip to the ice cream store, and so forth. Whatever backup reinforcers are used, clinicians should remember to use them. The conditioned generalized reinforcers (tokens) are not reinforcing in and of themselves. The efficacy of tokens depends upon the availability of a wide variety of appealing, desirable backup reinforcers the child may "purchase" with tokens earned during treatment.

> Why are conditioned generalized reinforcers called conditioned? Why are they called generalized?

Using a system of conditioned generalized reinforcement has many advantages. As there is always something a child will be willing to work toward, the method is not dependent upon a state of deprivation nor is it subject to the satiation effect. Tokens are easy to dispense during clinical treatment and therefore do not interrupt the treatment sequence—they are particularly suited for group therapy situations in which the clinician can quickly reinforce a child while moving on to the next. There is no limit to the variety of backup reinforcers the clinician may provide, and it is possible to offer a backup reinforcer of some value, such as a field trip to the zoo or lunch at a popular restaurant.

The main difficulty with conditioned generalized reinforcement is the expense involved in maintaining an adequate number of backup reinforcers the child will find appealing. In some settings, funding may not be available, and clinicians wishing to use conditioned generalized reinforcement may have to personally finance their own "treasure chest" of backup reinforcers.

> A teenager who wants cash, not another T-shirt, for a birthday gift, knows the power of conditioned generalized reinforcers.

Another problem with conditioned generalized reinforcement is the difficulty with which it is faded. Research has shown that correct response rates tend to decline rather suddenly when conditioned generalized reinforcement is withdrawn, although this problem is not unique to this particular type of reinforcement (Kazdin, 2001). Again, if social reinforcement is *always* used in conjunction with conditioned generalized reinforcement, the child will learn to respond to social reinforcement without the need for a token system of reinforcement.

High probability behaviors. A method of increasing desirable but infrequently exhibited behavior by making a more frequently exhibited behavior contingent on the former is called **high probability behavior** (Baldwin & Baldwin, 1998; Hegde, 1998b; Malott, Malott, & Trojan, 2000; Martin & Pear, 1999). It is an unusual form of reinforcement in which the same person's one behavior helps reinforce another. It is a method of secondary reinforcement that uses an existing high probability behavior to reinforce a low probability behavior. A high probability behavior is a behavior that a child is likely to perform because it has been reinforced in the past. A low probability behavior is exhibited less frequently, possibly because of lack of strong reinforcers. Language skills are treatment targets for a child because they are low probability behaviors; if they were highly probable, the child would not need treatment.

There are many everyday examples of how high probability behaviors can be used to reinforce low probability behaviors. An adolescent boy might have a high probability behavior of playing video games and a low probability behavior of mowing the yard. If his wise parents make video game playing contingent upon yard mowing, there will be much less need for them to hire a gardener! Children might be required to complete their homework (a low probability behavior) before being allowed to watch television (a high probability behavior). A man struggling to stay on a diet might promise himself a scoop of ice cream at the end of the week *if* he is faithful to the diet for the entire week.

In clinical practice, SLPs use this technique when they offer the opportunity for the child to engage in some desirable activity when a criterion for correct response has been reached. The activity might be something such as coloring a special picture, playing with a desirable toy, drawing on a chalkboard, or jumping on a small trampoline. The use of high probability behaviors as reinforcement can be coupled with a system of conditioned generalized reinforcement (e.g., "Jenny, if you get 10 stars on your chart today, you can play with Mr. Potato Head for 2 minutes.").

In some cases, the high probability behavior made contingent on treatment tasks being completed may be anything the child chooses to do during a free time that is made contingent on the treatment task. That is, the clinician may say, "When you get 10 check marks like this on the sheet [standing for 10 correct responses], you can enjoy 2 minutes of free time. You can play, talk to me, listen to music, or anything else." There is evidence that performance-contingent free-time can increase the production of target behaviors (Zarcone, Fisher, & Piazza, 1996).

High probability behaviors can serve as powerful reinforcers in the treatment of language disorders and may serve to "liven up" what might be a monotonous treatment session. However, there are some disadvantages to this technique. Obviously, this is a very time-consuming method of reinforcement. Opportunities to perform high probability behaviors cannot be offered on a contingent basis for every correct response received; it would take too much time. The solution to this problem is to give tokens (conditioned generalized reinforcers) which are exchanged for an opportunity to engage in a high probability behavior.

Another disadvantage of high probability behaviors is that they are presented either in total or not at all. If the child fails to achieve the required criterion level, there will not be an opportunity to engage in the desired behavior, and the child will go totally unreinforced for the entire session—this is not good for the child's learning. Therefore, when using this method, the criterion level for correct response should, at first, be set at a low level and then gradually raised as the child's correct response rate increases.

Multiple Contingencies

Throughout our discussion of types of reinforcement, we have suggested that the different techniques should be combined to increase their effectiveness. In other words, clinicians should use **multiple contingencies.** Thus, social reinforcement should always be used in conjunction with any other type of reinforcement, primary or secondary. High probability behaviors may be combined with conditioned generalized reinforcers (tokens), and each token should be coupled with social reinforcement. Each combination of multiple contingencies should be client-specific. The clinician should experiment with several types of reinforcement and their combinations to determine the most efficacious method of reinforcement for each child.

Strengthening the Language Skills: Varying the Consequences

A child may receive reinforcers for every correct response, for only a certain number of responses, or during only a certain time period. In other words, reinforcers may be delivered on a certain schedule. A **schedule of reinforcement** describes the relationship between a criterion level for correct response or responses and the delivery of a reinforcer (Baldwin & Baldwin, 1998; Hegde, 1998b; Malott, Malott, & Trojan, 2000; Martin & Pear, 1999). There are two main schedules of reinforcement: (1) the continuous schedule and (2) intermittent schedules.

The Continuous Schedule of Reinforcement

What are the two main schedules of reinforcement?

In a **continuous schedule of reinforcement,** the child receives a reinforcer for *every* correct response. The continuous is the densest schedule of reinforcement. It is most effective during the initial stages of treatment to establish new skills; however, the continuous schedule of reinforcement must be faded as soon as possible, so that the child's correct response does not become dependent on a dense form of reinforcement.

Intermittent Schedules of Reinforcement

To fade reinforcement, clinicians move from a continuous schedule of reinforcement to an **intermittent schedule of reinforcement.** Intermittent schedules allow reinforcers only for *some* of the correct responses; a certain number of responses go unreinforced. This is done systematically, not randomly, and clinicians may select one of two types of intermittent schedules of reinforcement: (1) ratio schedules of reinforcement and (2) interval schedules of reinforcement.

The SLP gave Tommy a piece of cereal and told him "Way to go!" each time he produced a correct response. What types of reinforcement was the SLP using? What schedule of reinforcement was used?

Ratio schedules of reinforcement describe a relationship between the number of correct responses the child makes and the delivery of the reinforcer. Ratio schedules of reinforcement are either fixed or variable. In **fixed ratio** (FR) **schedules,** a specific number of responses earn reinforcers. The continuous schedule of reinforcement is also a fixed ratio schedule in which every correct response is reinforced (*FR1*). Fading the continuous FR1 schedule, the clinician gradually increases the number of correct responses required before reinforcers are given. The first intermittent schedule used may be an FR2, in which every other correct response is reinforced, and then the clinician may switch to an FR4 schedule in which every fourth correct response is reinforced.

The clinician might also use a **variable ratio** (VR) **schedule** to fade reinforcement. In variable ratio schedules, the number of correct responses required to earn reinforcers is varied around an average. In a VR3 schedule of reinforcement, for example, the clinician may first reinforce the third correct response, then the second correct response, and finally the fourth correct response. In this example, reinforcers were given three times for a total of nine correct responses. Therefore, on the average, three responses were required to earn a reinforcer (3 + 2 + 4 = 9 correct responses divided by 3 reinforcers = 3).

Interval schedules of reinforcement describe the relationship between the amount of time that is allowed to lapse before an opportunity is given for the child to earn a reinforcer. Interval schedules, too, may be either fixed or variable.

In a **fixed interval schedule** (FI) of reinforcement, a fixed amount of time should elapse before the child is given an opportunity to earn a reinforcer. In a fixed interval of 5 minutes (FI 5-min), the first correct response given after the 5-minute interval is over will be reinforced. The interval starts from the previously reinforced response. Thus, reinforced correct responses are spaced by 5-minute intervals.

In **variable interval schedules** (VI) of reinforcement, the time duration allowed to elapse between opportunities to earn a reinforcer is varied around an average. For example, in a VI 5-min schedule, an opportunity to earn a reinforcer may be given, first, after 5 minutes have elapsed since the previously reinforced response, then after 3 minutes have elapsed, and then after 7 minutes have elapsed. In this example, opportunities to earn a reinforcer were given 3 times over a time period of 15 minutes, for an average of once every 5 minutes.

In an interval schedule of intermittent reinforcement, only the opportunity to earn a reinforcer is guaranteed after the scheduled time lapses. The actual delivery of the reinforcer is contingent upon the child's response; if the response is correct, the reinforcer is given, and if the response is incorrect, the reinforcer is withheld.

Although clinicians more commonly use ratio schedules of reinforcement, there are some target behaviors for which variations of an interval schedule of reinforcement are appropriate. For example, school SLPs often work with children who lack such conversational language skills as attending to task and maintaining a topic of conversation. In teaching such skills, the clinician may use a variation of the standard fixed interval schedule. The child may be positively reinforced with verbal praise for attending to an academic task for 5 minutes or for maintaining a topic of conversation for 3 minutes. Reinforcers may be given for each block of specified time during which the skill is maintained. In successive stages of treatment, verbal praise may be made contingent on longer time durations for which the skill is maintained. Again, note that the delivery of the reinforcing praise is contingent upon the child's attending behavior or topic maintenance. If the child becomes distracted right before the end of the required block of time, reinforcement would not be given, and the opportunity to receive reinforcement should not come again until another block of time has elapsed.

When using any intermittent schedule, the clinician should not fade reinforcement too quickly. Abrupt and large shifts in reinforcement schedules result in **ratio strain**—a condition in which the correct response rates decrease drastically. For example, if a clinician

An SLP gave Timmy a token first for three correct responses, then for seven correct responses, then for five correct responses, and repeated variations of this pattern throughout the session. If Johnny had 10 tokens at the end of the session, he was allowed to select a prize from the SLP's "treasure chest." What type of reinforcement was used? What schedule of reinforcement was used?

The SLP presented discrete trials to Sally for 3 minutes. As a consequence for the first correct response Sally made after that time period, the SLP said, "Great! You got it!" and worked with Sally for 3 minutes more before reinforcing the first correct response after that time period. What type of reinforcement was used? What schedule of reinforcement was used?

abruptly moves from a continuous schedule (FR1) to a fixed ratio schedule of FR10, the client's response rate may come under ratio strain. The clinician should keep data on the child's correct response rate in all treatment sessions. If the correct response rate drops, reinforcement should move back to a more generous schedule, perhaps even to a continuous schedule for a while to reestablish the response.

An observant clinician may notice that children seem to take a little break after being reinforced. Such breaks are mini resting periods after receiving a reinforcer. This resting period is called a **post-reinforcement pause,** which occurs after the ratio or interval requirements of the reinforcement schedule have been met and the reinforcer has been delivered. Clinicians may also notice that the length of the post-reinforcement pause varies, depending upon what reinforcement schedule is used. This is a phenomenon that is part of the patterns of response that are characteristic of each type of schedule of reinforcement. Scientists have experimentally demonstrated how response rates are affected by schedules of reinforcement. Refer to Table 6.2 for a more complete description of patterns of response associated with schedules of reinforcement.

table 6.2

Schedules of Reinforcement and Patterns of Response

Schedule of Reinforcement	Response Pattern	Post-Reinforcement Pause
Fixed ratio (FR)	• High response rate • Cyclical pattern of working hard and resting • Can result in children working hard for progressively less reinforcement • Increasing the ratio too abruptly results in ratio strain—a drop in the correct response rate	• Distinct; a marked post-reinforcement pause • The larger the ratio, the longer the pause
Variable ratio (VR)	• High response rate • More steady and consistent response rate than fixed ratio schedules	• No marked post-reinforcement pause
Fixed interval (FI)	• Response rates are lower and less consistent than those under FR schedules • Response rates increase as time passes • Concentrated response rate right before the end of the interval • Response rate slowly increases after delivery of the reinforcer	• Distinct; a marked post-reinforcement pause • Pauses are longer in duration than those associated with FR schedules
Variable interval (VI)	• Response rates are steady • Higher response rate under VI than under FI • The shorter the duration of the interval, the higher the response rate, and vice versa • A consistent, evenly spaced response rate that may be lower than that generated by VR schedules	• No marked post-reinforcement pause

In general, when considering schedules of reinforcement:

- Begin treatment with a continuous schedule of reinforcement
- Fade reinforcement by moving to an intermittent schedule of reinforcement
- Prefer ratio schedules of reinforcement over interval schedules of reinforcement for strengthening most language skills
- Prefer interval schedules of reinforcement to strengthen skills based on time duration (e.g., eye contact during conversation for a specified time, sitting quietly for a specified duration, etc.)
- Fade reinforcers, instead of withdrawing them abruptly; keep data to monitor the correct response rate and adjust schedules of reinforcement accordingly

Getting the Children's Cooperation: Decreasing the Troublesome Behaviors

In the preceding sections we have discussed techniques designed to evoke and increase the correct communicative behaviors clinicians seek to teach children with language disorders. At the same time, however, clinicians need to decrease two kinds of behaviors: incorrect or inappropriate language behaviors and several interfering behaviors that some children exhibit during language therapy. Therefore, clinicians need not only the procedures that help increase the target skills but also those that decrease undesirable behaviors (Baldwin & Baldwin, 1998; Hegde, 1998b; Malott, Malott, & Trojan, 2000; Martin & Pear, 1999). Most of the treatment research studies cited earlier in this chapter have included some kind of procedure to decrease undesirable behaviors, often a simple verbal response as "No" or "That is not right!"

> What are two broad categories of response-reduction techniques?

Children in language treatment may produce both incorrect or inappropriate language responses (e.g., saying "book" for *books* or switching topics of conversation inappropriately) and interfering behaviors (e.g., crying in treatment sessions, off-seat behaviors, and asking interrupting questions). The clinician needs procedures to reduce all of these behaviors. Behavioral response-reduction techniques fall into two broad categories: (1) direct response-reduction techniques and (2) indirect response-reduction techniques.

Direct Response-Reduction Techniques

In **direct response-reduction procedures,** a contingency is placed on the behavior that needs to be reduced. This means that as the response to be reduced is about to be produced or has just been produced, the clinician does something immediately to reduce it. Direct response-reduction techniques used during clinical treatment of childhood language disorders include: corrective feedback; withdrawal of reinforcement, using such techniques as response cost and time-out; and extinction. Each of these techniques can be used to either decrease incorrect responses or to decrease troublesome behaviors that interfere with therapy.

> What are four types of direct methods of response reduction?

Corrective feedback. The most commonly used technique to decrease incorrect responses during clinical treatment is **corrective feedback,** in which the child is told that the response just given was not correct. This kind of response from the clinician is often described as a punishment procedure (Baldwin & Baldwin, 1998; Malott, Malott, & Trojan, 2000; Martin & Pear, 1999), but corrective feedback is a more neutral and appropriate term (Hegde, 1998b). This feedback may also include information as to why it is not correct. A verbal "no" and "wrong" are examples of corrective feedback. However, more naturalistic feedback with added information may be helpful to children and sound less harsh. While teaching the production of plural -*s*, for example, a clinician might give corrective feedback by saying, "Oh, oh! I didn't hear the -*s* that time! Let's try again!" followed by another discrete trial. Such corrective feedback is a part of all treatment sessions. The clinician should give the corrective feedback immediately after the wrong response is produced. Also, the clinician should measure the frequency of target behaviors so that if one type of feedback is ineffective, another type may be selected.

Matching facial expression to verbal response is especially important when working with children with cognitive deficits. Saying "Oh-oh! That's not right!" with a broad and approving smile is confusing and not at all helpful to children with limited receptive language.

Corrective feedback can also be given nonverbally, as any parent who has learned to quell an unruly child's misbehavior with "the look" knows. In clinical treatment, nonverbal corrective feedback might consist of a raised hand to interrupt at the first sign of an incorrect response or a brief shake of the head indicating "no."

Corrective feedback should be delivered gently, but firmly, with a facial expression that matches the message. Clinicians do not need to look overly stern, but presenting a constantly smiling face whether delivering reinforcers or corrective feedback can be confusing to a child. It is more effective to use a neutral facial expression when delivering corrective feedback for incorrect responses and a warm smile when delivering reinforcement for correct responses.

Reinforcement withdrawal. Whether intended or unintended, unwanted behaviors, too, are maintained only because of some reinforcing consequences. **Reinforcement withdrawal** is weakening behaviors by removing consequences that sustain them. Experimental research has shown that withdrawing reinforcing consequences or states of affairs is an effective strategy to reduce unwanted behaviors (Hegde, 1998b). There are two variations of this basic procedure: (1) response cost and (2) time-out. Both have been extensively researched and shown to be effective.

Response cost. A procedure in which each incorrect response results in the loss of a reinforcer is called **response cost.** In this procedure, a reinforcer the child has earned is withdrawn every time an incorrect response is made. The incorrect response "costs" the child a reinforcer (Baldwin & Baldwin, 1998; Hegde, 1998b; Malott, Malott, & Trojan, 2000; Martin & Pear, 1999).

Some clinicians may not use response cost because they fear it will discourage the child. But, clever clinicians find ways to increase token award and decrease token withdrawal so that the child always receives the backup reinforcer at the end of the session. Instead of one, the clinicians may give two tokens for correct responses but withdraw only one for an incorrect response. Holding a just-withdrawn token in her hand, the clinician may say, "Come on, I know you can do it!" The child then has a chance to get it right back.

There are two varieties of response cost: (1) earn-and-lose and (2) lose-only. Both the methods need conditioned generalized reinforcers (tokens). Recall that, when using conditioned generalized reinforcement, the clinician reinforces correct responses with tokens, stickers, check marks, or other tangible items for correct responses. These items can then be exchanged for backup reinforcers when the child has accumulated the required number. When using earn-and-lose response cost, the clinician presents a token as a reinforcing consequence for a child's correct response and withdraws one as a consequence for an incorrect response.

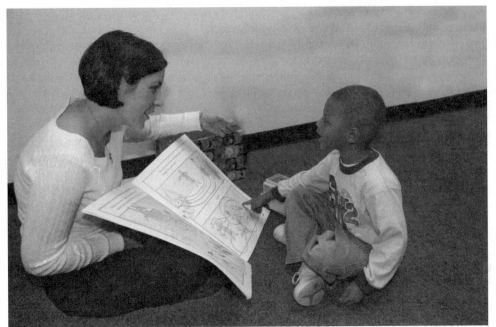

photo 6.2
"Come on, you
can do it!" This
clinician's facial
expression and pre-
sentation of a token
encourages the child
to work hard during
response-cost token
therapy.

The lose-only variation of response cost consists of presenting the child with a generous number of tokens at the beginning of the session, not depending on the production of
any desirable behaviors. When the child produces an incorrect response, a token is removed.
In essence, in the lose-only method, the tokens are not earned but given beforehand. They
are lost depending on each incorrect response.

There may be some disadvantages to using response cost during language therapy, especially in the beginning stages of treatment when the child's correct response rate is low,
and the incorrect response rate is high. Particularly with the lose-only variation, a child may
become emotional and frustrated over repeatedly losing tokens which offer the only access
to a desired reinforcer. To avoid such problems, some other method of decreasing incorrect response may be used until the child's correct rate of response begins to increase. Also,
the clinician may give two or three tokens for each correct response and withdraw only one
for each incorrect response. Consequently, the child will have an almost certain chance
of receiving the backup reinforcer at the end of the session—a much more desirable outcome than having the child leave the clinic room without having been reinforced at all for
correct responses (see Photo 6.2 for an example of the response cost method).

Time-out. In this procedure, the clinician terminates a reinforcing state of affairs. A **time-
out** is a period of nonreinforcement, imposed response contingently, resulting in the reduction of that response. It is a "time-out" from reinforcement, directly following an incorrect
response (Baldwin & Baldwin, 1998; Hegde, 1998b; Malott, Malott, & Trojan, 2000; Martin
& Pear, 1999).

Time-out can be used both for decreasing undesirable behaviors that interfere with
therapy (e.g., out-of-seat behavior, kicking the table, asking too many questions, etc.) and

for decreasing incorrect responses. There are three types of time-out, two of which are applicable to treatment for child language disorders.

The most extreme form of time-out, isolation time-out, is used in prison and institutions serving people with profound developmental disability or mental illness, or both. In isolation time-out, the person is removed from the environment and placed in a separate place, such as a barren room, in which the person has no access to any type of reinforcement. Parents who send misbehaving children to their rooms are attempting to practice a milder form of isolation time-out, although often the children's rooms are filled with reinforcing objects, such as toys, computers, or television sets. Consequently, such parental attempts at reducing undesirable behaviors may be ineffective.

What are the three types of time-out?

Isolation time-out is controversial even when applied to people with seriously aggressive, violent, or self-injurious behavior. It is therefore not suitable for use during the treatment of a child's language disorder. Isolation time-out is mentioned here only to supply a complete description of the time-out technique and to serve as a comparison to the other two types of time-out.

In exclusion time-out, the child is excluded from the activities going on in the environment. Teachers practice exclusion time-out when they require a misbehaving student to sit at a special desk that is placed beside the teacher's desk, or faced toward a wall, or even outside the classroom. During recess, teachers with yard duty may place unruly students against the fence, keeping them from playground equipment and activities.

Some clinicians use a brief period of exclusion time-out, perhaps turning a child to sit in his chair facing the clinic wall when the child has exhibited repeatedly a behavior that interferes with treatment. We believe that, if at all, this technique should be used infrequently. Treatment sessions are brief, and therefore, response-reduction techniques should not take up too much valuable therapy time.

Nonexclusion time-out is the third type, in which the child is not excluded from the normal flow of activity. Nonexclusion time-out involves imposing a very brief period of non-reinforcement upon the child—a "frozen moment" of time in which no reinforcing activity takes place. There is a substantial amount of controlled behavioral research that documents the effectiveness of nonexclusion time-out in reducing undesirable behaviors in children and adults (Brantner & Doherty, 1983). There is also research supporting the use of nonexclusion time-out in treating communicative disorders (Ahlander, 1999; Carter-Wagner, 1997; Costello, 1975; Hegde & Parson, 1990; James, 1981; Martin, Kuhl, & Haroldson, 1972; Onslow et al., 1997). In nonexclusion time-out, the clinician says, "Stop" as soon as a child makes a wrong response and turns his or her face away from the child for a few seconds (usually 5 seconds). Then the clinician reestablishes eye contact and continues the conversational speech or treatment trial presentation.

Sometimes, clinicians who apply the time-out procedure may discover that the technique appears to actually increase, rather than decrease, the targeted undesirable behavior. There are at least two possible reasons for this paradoxical effect. First, if the child finds treatment to be aversive (something to be avoided), the child may welcome the short break from therapy that application of the time-out procedure provides. Second, it may be that, instead of finding the technique to be aversive, the child may enjoy the attention the clinician is paying to the behavior. The undesirable behavior may be reinforced by this attention, and may therefore increase rather than decrease. A behavior, of course, may increase due to both of these reasons operating simultaneously; a child both enjoys the brief respite from therapy *and* the attention from the clinician. If the clinician suspects either or both of these factors are reinforcing to the targeted behavior, the procedure of extinction may be used to decrease, or even eliminate, the undesirable behavior.

Extinction. To simply terminate the reinforcer for a response while no attempt is made to stop it is called **extinction**. In the case of an undesirable behavior being maintained by the attention a clinician gives it, the reinforcer to be terminated is that attention. Extinction is the same as ignoring an undesirable behavior (Baldwin & Baldwin, 1998; Hegde, 1998b; Lerman & Iwata, 1996; Malott, Malott, & Trojan, 2000; Martin & Pear, 1999).

A child's crying behavior in treatment sessions may be a good candidate for extinction. If the child begins to cry during a treatment session, the clinician simply tells the child that "we can get back to work when you stop crying" and turns his or her back to the child and sits motionless. The clinician does not pay any attention to the child as long as he or she is crying. As soon as the crying stops, the clinician promptly turns toward the child, smiles, reinforces verbally or otherwise, and continues the treatment activity.

The clinician may notice that, when the procedure of extinction is first applied, the behavior may increase for a brief period of time. Called an extinction burst, this effect commonly occurs when extinction is applied to a behavior for the first time (Lerman & Iwata, 1996). For instance, the child's crying may intensify. The clinician should not "give in" to this extinction burst by responding to the child's undesirable behavior. Once the process of extinction has begun, it must be applied consistently or it will not be effective. If the clinician continues to ignore the child's undesirable behavior, it will eventually decrease and then cease altogether.

> Parents who apply extinction to their toddler's temper tantrums are well acquainted with extinction burst. Wise parents don't give in to the extinction burst, as long as the child is in no danger of harming himself or herself or others.

A behavior that has been successfully subjected to extinction may reappear at a later time. In such a case, extinction should once again be employed to eliminate the behavior. Research has shown that a behavior that has undergone the process of extinction before will respond more quickly to subsequent application of extinction (see Box 6.4 for more factors affecting extinction).

Indirect Response-Reduction Techniques

In techniques such as corrective feedback, response cost, and time-out, contingencies are directly applied to an undesirable behavior. It is possible to reduce behaviors without placing any contingencies on them, however. Procedures in which contingencies are placed only on desirable behaviors to reduce undesirable behaviors are called **indirect response-reduction techniques** (Hegde, 1998b). Indirect response-reduction techniques are a combination of the procedure of extinction applied to undesirable behaviors, resulting in the decrease

> What technique is used to simultaneously increase one behavior while decreasing another?

of those behaviors, and positive reinforcement applied to desirable behaviors, resulting in the increase of those behaviors. This process of reducing undesirable behaviors while simultaneously increasing desirable behaviors is called **differential reinforcement.** Much experimental research has been conducted regarding the efficacy of four types of differential reinforcement (Baldwin & Baldwin, 1998; Brown et al., 2000; Hegde, 1998b; Lerman & Vorndran, 2002; Malott, Malott, & Trojan, 2000; Martin & Pear, 1999; Reichle & Wacker,

box 6.4   **Factors Affecting the Extinction of Undesirable Behaviors**

The time it takes to extinguish an undesirable behavior is affected by:

- *Previous exposure to extinction.* Undesirable behaviors that are being extinguished for the first time will take longer to extinguish than behaviors that have previously undergone extinction and are making a reappearance.
- *Reinforcement schedule.* Undesirable behaviors that have received reinforcement under an intermittent schedule will take longer than behaviors that have been reinforced continuously (e.g., the behavior of a child who always gets his way when he whines will be easier to extinguish than the behavior of a child who only now and then gets his way when he whines).
- *Amount of past reinforcement.* A behavior that has been heavily reinforced will take longer to reinforce

than a behavior that has not been so heavily reinforced.
- *Duration for which the response has been reinforced.* A behavior that has been reinforced for a long period of time will take more time to extinguish than a behavior that has recently appeared.

In short, the behavior that is most difficult to extinguish is one that has never been extinguished before and has been heavily reinforced on an intermittent schedule of reinforcement for a long period of time. Conversely, the behavior that will be easiest to extinguish is one that has previously been extinguished and has been less heavily reinforced on a continuous schedule for a short period of time.

1993; Ringdahl et al., 2002): (1) differential reinforcement of other behavior (DRO), (2) differential reinforcement of incompatible behavior (DRI), (3) differential reinforcement of low rates of responding (DRL), and (4) differential reinforcement of alternative behavior (DRA). Clinicians treating children with language disorders may effectively use each of these indirect methods of response reduction.

Differential reinforcement of other behavior (DRO).

A technique in which a clinician tells a child that a particular undesirable behavior will not be reinforced is known as the **differential reinforcement of other behavior (DRO).** The clinician proceeds to ignore (or extinguish) that undesirable behavior while generously reinforcing any other desirable behavior. While the undesirable behavior targeted for extinction is specified, the desirable behaviors that receive reinforcement are many and unspecified.

For example, a clinician may use this technique to address a child's table-kicking behavior during therapy. The behavior, kicking the table, has therefore been targeted for reduction. The clinician then proceeds to ignore the table-kicking behavior and instead praises the child for every desirable behavior the child exhibits (e.g., "I like the way you are looking at my pictures!" "Your hands are so still!"). The clinician reinforces as many desirable behaviors as the child exhibits. Often, this approach will in itself result in the reduction of the undesirable behavior. Other times, it may be necessary to point out to the child the behavior that is undesirable and offer reinforcement for any other desirable behavior the child exhibits. The clinician might tell the child, "Jimmy, if you don't kick the table today, you can pick a prize from my treasure box," or offer some other type of reinforcement. The child in this case is reinforced for omitting the undesirable behavior. Sometimes, when one un-

What is another term used for *differential reinforcement of other behavior (DRO)*?

desirable decreases, another may emerge or increase. For instance, Jimmy may manage to make it through the session without kicking the table, but at the end of the session, may pinch the clinician. The clinician's new rule to earn reinforcers would then be, "No kicking *and* no pinching!"

Because desirable behaviors to be reinforced are many and unspecified in this approach, and the undesirable behavior is specified and needs to be omitted to receive reinforcement, this technique is sometimes called omission training. It is a well-researched procedure that has been shown to be effective in reducing undesirable behaviors in both clinical and educational settings (Carr, Robinson, & Palumbo, 1990; Rolider & Van Houten, 1990).

Differential reinforcement of incompatible behavior (DRI). Most undesirable behaviors have their counterparts that are desirable and incompatible with the former. A procedure that indirectly reduces undesirable responses by increasing a behavior that is incompatible with it is called the **differential reinforcement of incompatible behavior (DRI)**.

Suppose that, instead of reinforcing Jimmy for *any* desirable behavior and ignoring the behavior of kicking the table, the clinician notices that it is an infrequent behavior, waits until his feet are on the floor, and reinforces him with a comment such as "Your feet are nice and quiet—good for you!" In this case, the clinician does not reinforce Jimmy for just any desirable behavior; she reinforces him for a behavior that is incompatible with the targeted undesirable behavior.

There are many examples of desirable behaviors that are incompatible with undesirable behaviors. Keeping feet still is incompatible with kicking, keeping hands on the table is incompatible with pinching, looking at the clinician is incompatible with staring off into space, sitting in a chair is incompatible with running around the clinic room, and so forth.

As the previous examples suggest, the use of DRI is most effective when the behavior being reinforced is physically incompatible with the behavior being extinguished—the child simply cannot perform the undesirable behavior while performing the desirable behavior. The DRI technique, then, is differentiated from the DRO because behaviors reinforced with DRO are not necessarily incompatible with the undesirable behavior being reduced.

Differential reinforcement of low rates of responding (DRL). Suppose Jimmy kicks the table incessantly; during most of the treatment time, his foot is banging away on the table leg. In this case, the clinician may use the **differential reinforcement of low rates (DRL) of responding,** a method in which the child is reinforced for reducing the frequency of a troublesome behavior. The clinician, therefore, may reinforce Jimmy for kicking the table *less* often during the clinic session. She might let Jimmy know her plan, by saying something like, "Jimmy, if you can do a better job of keeping your feet still today, you can have some time to draw on the dry-erase board before you go home." If Jimmy's table-kicking behavior shows even a modest decrease, the clinician should reinforce that improvement. For subsequent sessions, the clinician should require progressively less table-kicking before reinforcing Jimmy—resulting in the "shaping down" of an undesirable behavior in much the same way a desirable behavior can be "shaped up" as previously described.

Some undesirable behaviors are so frequently exhibited that DRL may be the most likely technique to succeed in decreasing them. The major disadvantage to DRL is that the technique will result only in a reduction—not the elimination—of the behavior. After the behavior has been decreased to a notable extent through the use of DRL, another technique, such as the DRO, should be effective in eliminating the behavior.

Differential reinforcement of alternative behavior (DRA).

Replacing an undesirable behavior with a more acceptable, socially more desirable behavior is the **differential reinforcement of alternative behavior (DRA)**. The use of this technique requires a clinician to observe the reinforcing consequence that maintains an undesirable behavior. What if the child can receive the same consequence for a more desirable response? If the clinician arranges the consequence such that the child receives the same reinforcer for a desirable behavior, the undesirable behavior would decrease in frequency.

Often, children who have language disorders learn undesirable behaviors because the parents may have unwittingly reinforced such behaviors. A child who has not learned to ask for food or toys may grab an adult's hand and lead the adult to the desired object, scream or make other inappropriate verbalizations, fuss endlessly, or throw tantrums—all this while the adult tries to figure out what the child wants. By the trial-and-error method of eliminating the possibilities, the adult will eventually give something that will stop all the inappropriate behaviors. Unfortunately, the behavior thus stopped for the moment will have been positively reinforced. It will reappear with added force the next time.

SLPs can use DRA to eliminate inappropriate behaviors. The alternative behaviors in this case would be socially more appropriate communicative behaviors—requests for food and other items. The desirable alternative behaviors may be made to last by teaching the adults in the child's environment to respond only to the alternative behavior and to ignore the undesirable behavior being replaced. To the child who screams when she is hungry, for example, the clinician may teach the word *eat*, offering food as a primary reinforcer to establish that response. The clinician would then teach adults in the child's environment to ignore the screaming, evoke a production of the word *eat* from the child, and promptly reinforce that production by presenting the child with food.

In subsequent chapters, we will be discussing children who are nonverbal or minimally verbal. Many of these children exhibit undesirable behaviors that serve some communicative function. A nonverbal boy with autism, for example, may be self-sufficient and have good toileting skills when he is at home and knows where the bathroom is. When he is in an unfamiliar setting, however, he may indicate his need to use the bathroom by jumping up and down and screaming. If oral speech is not a realistic goal, an SLP might teach the child an approximation of the American Sign Language sign for *toilet*, thus eliminating the undesirable behavior (Carr et al., 1994).

> What is another term used for *differential reinforcement of alternative behavior (DRA)?*

Because the desirable behavior being taught serves the same function as the undesirable behavior being replaced, DRA is also referred to as functional equivalence training. The undesirable behavior and the desirable behavior are functionally equivalent; one is, however, more socially appropriate than the other.

Differentiating between DRO, DRI, DRL, and DRA.

All indirect methods of response reduction involve the process of differential reinforcement in which a desirable behavior is positively reinforced and increased while an undesirable behavior is reduced through extinction (ignoring). The types of indirect methods of response reduction can be differentiated from each other as follows:

- *Differential reinforcement of other behavior (DRO)*. In DRO, a specified undesirable behavior *will not* be reinforced; the clinician then reinforces *any other* desirable behavior while ignoring the undesirable behavior. Compared to the undesirable behavior being reduced, the behavior that is reinforced may not be a functionally equivalent alternative, nor a physically incompatible action.
- *Differential reinforcement of incompatible behavior (DRI)*. In DRI, the behavior increased and the behavior decreased are physically incompatible; both cannot be exhibited at the same time. This condition does not hold for the other methods of indirect response reduction.
- *Differential reinforcement of low rates of responding (DRL)*. In DRL, reinforcement is given when the client shows a reduction in the frequency of the behavior; a process of "shaping down" an undesirable behavior. Progressively lower frequency of a behavior is not a target of reinforcement in other methods.
- *Differential reinforcement of alternative behavior*. In DRA, an undesirable behavior that is serving a communicative function is replaced with a more desirable, socially acceptable behavior that serves the same function. In this method, the new desirable behavior and the old undesirable behavior are functionally equivalent. In the other methods, finding behaviors of functional equivalence is not the central concern.

Breaking the Rules: Modifying Procedures

No language treatment procedure is effective all the time with all children. What works for one child will not necessarily work for another child or even for the same child during a different treatment session. By keeping accurate records of the child's progress, the clinician may modify the procedures that do not produce the desired effects. These modifications may involve: (1) changing reinforcers and response-reduction techniques, (2) changing stimuli, and (3) modifying or changing entirely the target behavior.

Changing Reinforcers and Response-Reduction Techniques

An intrinsic feature of effective reinforcers and response-reduction techniques is that the data collected point to good progress and justify the treatment procedure. In other words, data should show that in the treatment sessions, the desired language skills are indeed increasing and the undesirable behaviors are decreasing.

Because there are no standard reinforcers or response-reduction techniques that are equally effective across time and clients, the clinician should continuously measure the child's performance in all treatment sessions. If the measures suggest that a procedure—response enhancing or reducing—did not have the expected effect, the clinician should find alternative methods. Failure of a particular consequence (response increasing or decreasing) is not the failure of the principles of reinforcement and corrective feedback. Within each set of techniques, alternatives that will be effective are always available. If verbal praise is ineffective, a token system might be. If verbal corrective feedback (e.g., saying "no") is ineffective, time-out might be.

Changing Stimuli

Poor stimuli used to evoke the target skill may retard learning during treatment. In some cases, children do not learn the target language skills because the physical stimuli are ambiguous or unattractive, or the verbal stimuli are confusing or inconsistent.

Pictures presented to a child should be attractive, colorful, and clearly representative of the concept they are meant to convey. A color photograph of a single common object or of a person performing one clearly depicted action, for example, is preferable over black-and-white line and cartoon-like drawings in which multiple things are depicted. If the clinician suspects that the pictured stimuli being used are ineffective in evoking the responses, those stimuli should be changed.

Sometimes, very young children or children with cognitive deficits may not respond well to pictured stimuli at all. In that case, real objects or acted-out actions may be more likely to evoke the target language skills from a child. Clinicians should experiment with different forms of stimuli to see their effects on the child's rate of correct responses.

A creative clinician constantly searches for better procedures and modifies established procedures to produce greater effects; it is always possible to improve the procedures. A clinician should not hesitate to change something when the response rates do not show improvement. Failures should be analyzed at the earliest stage, and ineffective procedures should be discontinued sooner rather than later. Therefore, the clinician must be doing one thing in all sessions: measuring the frequency of target skills. If clinicians do not do this, they will not know when to continue with the selected procedure, when to modify them, and when to abandon the procedure.

Modifying or Changing the Target Behaviors

In most cases, clinicians select initial target behaviors that teach words, grammatic morphemes in words or phrases, and pragmatic structures at simpler topographic levels. When the child meets the initial and tentative training criterion (a 90 percent or better probe response rate), clinicians move on to more complex levels of training. Also, clinicians initially select a small number of targets on which they work in every treatment session.

For example, a clinician might begin treatment with four grammatic morphemes. Sometimes the clinician may find out that the initial target behavior is too complex for the child, because the child cannot even imitate the behavior even when it is simplified within a shaping program. In this case, the clinician should drop to a lower level of response complexity. For example, if teaching certain morphological features at the phrase level proves to be too difficult, the clinician should teach them at the word level. If the feature is too difficult at any level even with the shaping technique, the clinician should switch to another feature, but return to the difficult feature later on.

In addition to a slow response rate, other behaviors of the child also may tell the clinician to change the target behavior. For example, boredom with the treatment, inattentiveness to treatment stimuli, attending to irrelevant stimuli, frequently asking interfering questions (e.g., "Are we done?" or "You know what?"), crawling under the table, and so forth suggest that the target behavior may be too difficult for the child. As noted before, the child may be exhibiting undesirable behavior to escape from the treatment that has become aversive to the child. The clinician in such cases should simplify the target skills, shape them, and find more powerful reinforcers.

A competent clinician moves the child quickly and efficiently through the various levels of response complexity to the level of conversational speech. It is at the level of social conversation that the final goal of language intervention is achieved—appropriate and sustained use of language skills in social settings. Therefore, Chapter 8 describes techniques to teach conversational skills, and Chapter 9 describes procedures to promote maintenance of language skills in natural settings. However, before we can address conversational skill training and maintenance in natural settings, we need to take a look at overall procedures that incorporate the techniques described in this chapter in establishing basic language skills. We address these procedures in the next chapter.

Chapter Summary

In treating children with language disorders, the clinician needs to arrange special stimuli and offer carefully arranged consequences that follow the child's attempts to produce the target skills. Because the final goal is for the child to produce target language behaviors in natural settings in response to naturally occurring consequences, the clinician should fade the special stimuli and reduce the explicit consequences.

The special stimuli clinicians use to trigger target language skills in children include pictures and other physical stimuli, instructions and demonstrations, verbal modeling (the clinician's production of the target behavior), prompts (hints that are less than a full model of the response), and manual guidance (e.g., taking the child's hand and pointing to a picture). Whenever a model is presented, the child is required to imitate the model. Modeling, manual guidance, and other special procedures may be faded by progressively reduced prompts. When children do not imitate modeled target responses, shaping, also called successive approximation, may help teach a nonimitated skill by breaking it down into simpler components and teaching the components separately and putting them all together.

The clinician can arrange reinforcing consequences for a child's correct responses to increase their frequency or offer corrective consequences for incorrect responses to decrease their frequency. Both reinforcers and corrective feedback are delivered immediately after the correct response is made to have the intended effect.

Reinforcers may be primary or secondary. Primary reinforcers(e.g., food, drink, shelter) promote the biological survival of a species; they are reinforcers whose effects do not have to be learned. Secondary reinforcers are those that are effective because of social conditioning and include social reinforcers (warm verbal praise, attention, smiles, etc.), conditioned generalized reinforcers (e.g., tokens), informative feedback (e.g., statements about the child's progress in meeting performance criteria), and high probability behaviors (frequently occurring behaviors that help increase less frequently occurring but highly desirable behaviors). Reinforcers may be given for every response (a continuous schedule) or only for certain responses (an intermittent schedule).

Clinicians decrease incorrect or inappropriate communicative behaviors and interfering (uncooperative) behaviors either through direct or indirect methods of response reduction. Direct response-reduction techniques include corrective feedback, response cost, time-out, and extinction. Indirect response-reduction techniques include various forms of differential reinforcement, which increase desirable behaviors while reducing undesirable behaviors as a consequence.

Because no language treatment procedure is effective all the time with all children, clinicians should monitor the progress a child makes in each session and if the data warrant, modify the treatment techniques. Such modifications may include changing reinforcers and response-reduction techniques, changing the treatment stimuli, and modifying or changing the target behavior.

 ## Study Guide

1. Justify the statement that "behavioral treatment of language disorders involves systematic stimulus manipulations." What kinds of stimulus manipulations are needed and why? Give a brief description of each of the treatment stimuli and point out their special relevance in teaching various language skills.

2. During your clinical practicum, you are asked to work with a child who is nearly nonverbal. The child typically produces only a few basic words (e.g., *mama, dada*). Your supervisor has asked you to develop an oral language program with an initial emphasis on teaching a set of basic, functional words. Design this initial treatment program. List a set of basic target words and describe how you would teach them. What specific treatment techniques would you be using and why?

3. Discuss the advantages and disadvantages of various kinds of positive reinforcement. Point out the particular kinds of children for whom certain kinds of reinforcers are especially needed or particularly effective. Specify the kind of reinforcers for which you should first obtain parental permission.

4. Describe at least three examples in which the frequency of a highly desirable everyday behavior that is exhibited at a low frequency is substantially increased with the help of a high frequency behavior of the same individuals. Specify how the procedure may be implemented.

5. During the very first treatment session, a 4-year old child begins to cry as soon as the mother leaves the treatment room. You bring the mother in, and the child stops crying. But the mother begins to interfere with treatment by frequently offering comments and suggestions which you believe are ineffective and actually disruptive. During the second session, you ask the mother to leave the treatment room, but the child begins to cry. You try to entertain the child with toys and games, and the child stops crying. You begin to show treatment stimuli, and the child again begins to cry. Your supervisor has told you that you need to use an effective technique to make the child stop crying during the session. How would you handle this child? Be specific about what went wrong during the first two sessions and what procedure you would use in the third session.

6. Describe the conditions under which treatment procedures need to be modified. What kinds of modifications are typically needed? How would you know that modifications are necessary? How do you show that the modifications have been successful?

chapter

7

Establishing Basic
Language Skills

outline

- Selecting Basic Language Skills
- Establishing Baselines
- Teaching Basic Language Skills
- Sequencing Treatment
- Preparing for the Next Stage
- Chapter Summary
- Study Guide

A n understanding of the evidenced-based treatment framework presented in Chapter 5 and treatment techniques described in Chapter 6 will prepare the clinician to establish basic language skills in children with language disorders (LD). The general approach taken in this book is not explicitly based on chronological ages and stages of language development in children; instead, the approach is skill based. Regardless of the ages and stages, certain language skills need to be taught to children. Sometimes, the age of a child may not be the most important consideration in teaching skills. For instance, a child with developmental disability may be taught a particular set of language skills at a chronologically older age than a child with specific language impairment (see Chapter 3 for details) with no cognitive deficiencies who is taught the same skills. Once the target language skills are selected for a child, the procedures described in Chapters 5 through 8 help establish and expand language skills. Chapter 9 will describe procedures to promote initial generalization and eventual maintenance of established language skills.

Typically learning younger children's language skills are different from those of similarly learning older children. In the most common conceptualization, language disorder is a phenomenon that violates expectation of typical language skills based on ages and stages. Clinicians cannot assume that older children with LD exhibit the same skills expected of typical younger children. At the same age levels, children with LD show different levels of skill deficits. In other words, language disorder does not follow a systematic stepwise *reversal* of typical acquisition patterns. For instance, not all 4-year-old children with language disorders are like 3- or 2-year-old typically learning children. A 6-year-old child with a severe language delay and intellectual deficits (developmental disability) may be more like a typically developing 2-year-old. This child may need to learn a set of basic, functional words. Another 6-year-old whose only problem is a mild or moderate specific language disorder may be more like a typically developing 4-year-old. This child may be more advanced in language skills and hence need to clinically learn grammatic morphemes, varied forms of sentences, and social use of language.

In essence, age and age-based norms may predict gross language skills of large groups of children, but they are an unreliable basis to select specific language targets for individual children. A useful clinical approach is to teach each child what he or she needs to learn, given the social, academic, family, and personal demands. Some younger children with LD may be taught relatively more advanced skills than some older children with LD. Therefore, the clinician who knows how to teach the different skills of language always can provide effective services to children of all ages, including infants and toddlers.

> Because the age-based norms are not a good basis to select target behaviors, we have advocated the client-specific approach to target behavior selection in Chapter 4.

Selecting Basic Language Skills

What are basic language skills? Clinicians may give somewhat different answers to this question. There is no universally accepted list of basic language skills; therefore, each clinician will make certain judgments. Judgments are fine if they are presented as such, and not as theoretical or personal dogma. The skills suggested as basic in this section are also a matter of judgment, and clinicians are free to eliminate or add skills to the description. This chapter provides a framework for making judgments—in both selecting and treating basic skills—with flexibility for clinical modifications. This judgment will be strongly influenced by the results of assessment that is specific to the child, his or her family, teachers, and others involved in the life of that child.

New treatment targets should not pose problems for a clinician who has mastered the basic treatment framework and procedures presented in Chapters 5 and 6. Clinicians can select and teach skills that they judge will result in improved family, social, and academic communication. Each child will need treatment for a pattern of skills that are unique to that child; ages and stages of language acquisition alone will not determine that unique pattern. Clinicians who use client-specific treatment targets will resist "canned" lists of communication skills that limit target selection to developmental norms. As the research base and the scope of practice of speech-language pathology expand, the target skills will change or expand. Addition of swallowing skills and literacy skills to the treatment targets is a case in point. Historically, language targets themselves were an addition to the list of treatment targets that were mostly limited to stuttering and articulation disorders.

Early Communicative Skills

Children may lack early communicative skills regardless of their chronological age. In the language acquisition literature, some of these skills are typically described as prelinguistic (Hulit & Howard, 2002; McLaughlin, 1998), because they do not have elaborate linguistic structures yet. Except for reflexive vocalizations, prelinguistic behaviors are communicative; therefore, the terms *early verbal skills* or *communication skills* describe them better than the term *prelinguistic skills*.

> What terms are preferred over the term *prelinguistic skills?*

Some early communicative skills the clinician may select for treatment include the following:

- *Early vocalizations.* Some early vocalizations in typically learning infants may be reflexive or devoid of communicative effects. Soon, however, they acquire communicative properties. A certain kind of vocalization that did not mean anything to the parent may soon mean that the infant is hungry or wet—this is what is meant by a vocalization acquiring communicative effect. The child's vocalization causes the parents to act (e.g., feed the infant or change the diaper). Children with profound intellectual and physical impairments and a few otherwise typical children who just do not vocalize much may need this target even at a relatively older age.

  > Recall that verbal behavior includes both oral and nonoral (sign) communication. The definition does not restrict communication to a particular form (oral, manual, or some other).

  Vocalizations include a variety of random and diffused behaviors that eventually get shaped into better organized speech-language behaviors (see Box 7.1 for typical development of early vocalizations). Early vocalizations are often not discrete behaviors that are easily observed and measured. The various sounds the infants make combine and create changing forms (Hulit & Howard, 2002; McLaughlin, 1998). Some 2-year-olds who are silent toddlers with no other complications (e.g., developmental disability, autism, or hearing loss) need to make reliable and discriminated (stimulus-specific) vocalizations. Therefore, vocalizations that may be treatment targets for young children and more profoundly impaired older children include the following:

  —Making cooing sounds (e.g., "oo" or "goo"), especially when speech is heard (typically a treatment target for infants and young children with language delay)

box 7.1 Early Vocalizations

Knowledge of how infants learn to vocalize is of some help in assessment and in suggesting possible target behaviors. Because the recommended approach is client-specific and skill-based, it is not necessary to follow rigidly the developmental order. Descriptions of the various stages differ according to various researchers. Oller et al. (1999) posited four stages of early vocalizations, described and expanded on below.

Stage	Age	Description of Vocalizations
Phonation	0–2 months	*Quasivowels:* Produced with speech-like phonation, differentiated from "vegetative" sounds (e.g., burping, sneezing) and "fixed signal" sounds (e.g., crying, laughing); phonated with vocal tract at rest.
Primitive Articulation	2–3 months	*Gooing (or cooing):* Beginning of articulating while phonating; production of soft velar sounds.
Expansion	3–6 months	Infants appear to "play" with the articulators; may blow raspberries, squeal, enjoy vocal play with adults; production of "marginal babbling" in which infants produce consonant-like sounds from a closed vocal tract to a full vowel.
Canonical Babbling	6–10 months	Production of well-formed consonant-vowel (CV) syllables; rapid transition from consonant to vowel sounds; adults in the environment assign meaning to these productions and thus shape first words (e.g., /baba/ assigned meaning as "bottle" or "blanket," /mama/ and /dada/ eagerly assigned meaning as "mommy" and "daddy"). Canonical babbling includes *reduplicated* babbling, in which the consonant sound does not change (e.g. /dadadada/) and *variegated* babbling, in which the consonant and vowel may change (e.g., /badidabu/.

Because most typically developing infants exhibit canonical babbling by the age of 10 months, absence of canonical babbling is thought to be an early indication of a speech disorder, a language disorder, or both.

Adults can enhance infants' vocalizations through modeling the sounds the infant makes, encouraging the infant to imitate, and then shaping by modeling different or more complex vocalizations.

Typically developing children begin canonical babbling (see Box 7.1) by 10 months. Lack of canonical babbling by that age could be an early sign of speech disorder, language disorder, or both.

—Babbling, including single-syllable vocalizations (e.g., "ba," "ga," "da," and similar sounds babies make); duplicated sounds (e.g., "bababa," "gagaga," "dadada," and similar vocalizations); and varied consonant-vowel combinations and changes (e.g., "badaga," "gabida," and similar vocalizations) (typically a treatment target for babies and young children with language delay and any child with a severe language impairment)

—Word approximations, including babbled sounds shaped into vocalizations that sound more like words (e.g., "ma" for *Mommy*, or "da" for *Daddy*) (these targets may be changed into progressively better approximations resulting in the next target)

• *Early eye contact.* This may include looking at the mother and shifting gaze in response to the mother's voice or to the source of speech sound. An established pattern of eye

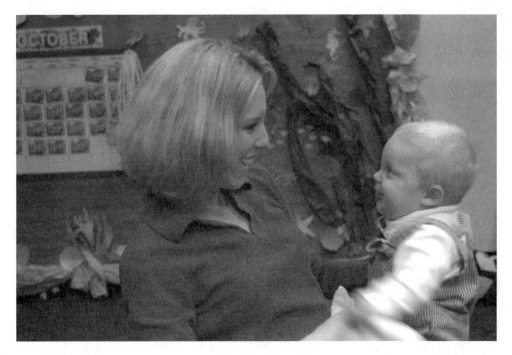

photo 7.1

photo 7.1
Eye gaze is established at a very early age; absence of eye gaze could be a sign of language or speech disorder, or both.

contact between the caregiver and the child is a part of social and communication development. This skill may be especially impaired in children with autism. Eye contact during conversation may be a later treatment target in children with pragmatic language impairments.

> Infants gaze into adults' faces and establish eye contact. Lack of eye contact may be an early sign of language disorder.

- *Pointing and gesturing.* Because they serve communicative functions, pointing and gesturing are appropriate targets if they are absent in babies and children. Such nonoral skills, when established, also may help teach oral skills.

The World of Words

Beyond vocalizations and gestures, words are the most well-organized target skills children with severe language impairments need to learn. As children and adults use them, words may mean just one thing or a world of things, with multiple, varied, and overlapping meanings. This suggests that pure linguistic structures (such as words, phrases, and sentences) are arbitrary divisions of language. Clinicians need to look at verbal productions as functional units. A single word may have the same effect as a phrase or a sentence as when a child says "Cookie!" with a certain intonation pattern that means, "I want a cookie!"

Target words selected for each child should be relevant to his or her family and social communication context and should emerge from the home environment, not from a standard list the clinician keeps. Although certain basic words will be common to most, if not all children, it is the unique words (names of family members, for example) that will make a difference in social communication.

Words are treatment targets not just for toddlers and young children with severe language delay, but also for school-age children with mild to moderate language deficits. For these children, academic curricula and teacher consultations will help supply the target words. Words may be treatment targets for children of any age and stage, but as children enter school, target words will be those that enhance social and academic communication.

The first few functional words as well as more advanced words are typical treatment targets for children with language disorders. Language acquisition literature describes the first 50 or so words children acquire (Gleason, 2001; McLaughlin, 1998). Targets that include the general and the child-specific words should be drawn from the following categories:

- Names of family members (including *Mommy* and *Daddy*), pets, the particular food items the child likes, the child's clothing items, favorite toys, objects around the house the child interacts with (e.g., *book, cup, bottle*), body parts, objects in the general living environment (e.g., *house, tree, snow, car, flower, chair, store*), literacy-related objects (e.g., *book, crayon, paper, pencil*), characters from children's TV shows that the child regularly watches, and characters or names from story books that are read to the child. Such general and child-specific words may be selected in consultation with parents or other caregivers.
- Action words that help describe activities typical to the child's home and play environment (e.g., *go, ride, up, down, sit, play, make, get, sing, walk, run, eat, drink, sleep, read, write, smile*), the majority of which may be later expanded to verb + *ing* (e.g., *going, riding, playing, eating, walking, smiling*).
- Descriptive and adjectival terms (e.g., *big, small, cold, hot, yucky, dirty, nice, allgone, smooth, round, red, blue*).
- Daily routine terms, some of which are often learned and produced as single-word units, even if they contain more than one word (e.g., *bye* or *bye-bye, night-night* or *good night, no, yes, peek-a-boo, please, thank you, see you, hi*).

Depending on the assessment results, the clinician may select more advanced words than early functional words. These words may include:

- Longer, full-formed words (e.g., *grandfather* versus *grandpa, good night* versus *night-night*)
- Abstract words (e.g., *good, bad, circle, this, that, food, clothes, clean*)
- Complex or less common words in the child's speech, including nouns (e.g., *table, chair, telephone, school, stove, desk, coat, dress*), verbs (e.g., *working, laughing, driving, mowing*), adjectives (e.g., *rough, soft, tall, sad, happy, high, low, thin, thick, yellow*), and words in other categories suggested by the child-specific information
- Academic and literacy-related words, selected on the basis of classroom teacher consultation and an analysis of the child's curricullum (e.g., *textbook, essay, add, subtract, history, math, drawing, compare*)

Clinicians who consult with classroom teachers will have a reliable source of more advanced and child-specific target words (e.g., scientific terms, geographic terms, literary concepts, etc.)

Words to Phrases

Basic language skill training moves on from words to phrases. Any word the child begins to reliably and appropriately produce may be expanded into phrases that contain two or more words. The phrases will always include the trained word; an additional word added may also be an already trained word or it may be new, in which case that word training takes place simultaneously. The clinician may start combining words into phrases when at least a dozen words drawn from different categories (e.g., nouns and verbs, nouns and adjectives) have reached the training criterion (e.g., 90 percent accuracy across three treatment sessions). Phrases then may be formed by combining words from the different categories as shown in the following:

- Combine trained nouns with trained verbs (e.g., *Mommy walk* or *Mommy walking, Daddy read* or *Daddy reading, Snoopy eat* or *Snoopy eating*)
- Combine trained descriptive terms or adjectives with trained nouns (e.g., *big book, small car, birdie all gone, smooth paper, blue crayon*)
- Create phrases that include daily routine terms (e.g., "Mommy say bye-bye," "Daddy say good night")

The clinician may also combine more advanced words into phrases as found appropriate. Once again, creating such phrases with already trained words will be helpful. Therefore, training of such phrases may be delayed until the child has learned a variety of words as in the following:

- Expand the longer and full-form words into phrases (e.g., "my grandfather," "Mommy say good night")
- Expand the relatively abstract words into phrases (e.g., *good cookie, bad dog, pretty kitty*)
- Expand the nouns that are more complex or less common into phrases (e.g., *dining table, my chair, hot stove*); verbs into phrases (e.g., *Mommy working, baby laughing, Tommy driving*); adjectives into phrases (e.g., *rough paper, soft ball, tall man, sad face*); and all words in other categories that were trained
- Expand academic and literacy-related words into phrases (e.g., *my textbook, writing an essay, adding numbers, drawing pictures*)

Early Morphologic Skills

Morphologic skills are essential to many functional response classes, both basic and advanced. Some phrases, and most sentences, involve one or more grammatic morphemes. Therefore, once the child has learned a set of basic and relatively advanced words, the production of morphologic features should be the treatment target. Brown's (1973) fourteen grammatic morphemes (see Table 7.1) provide a good starting point, although the clinicians need to consider the words the child has already learned and the functional targets that will be taught during the next stage of treatment.

Most grammatic morphemes can be trained at the word, phrase, and sentence levels. A few can be taught only at the basic sentence level. Depending on the words already taught, the clinician may select several grammatic morphemes, including the following (Hegde, 1998):

- *Present progressive -ing.* The clinician can teach these at the word (e.g., *walking, eating, jumping, smiling*), phrase (e.g., *Mommy walking, Daddy eating*), and sentence levels (e.g., "Mommy is walking"; "Daddy is eating").
- *Prepositions.* Prepositions (e.g., *in, on, under, behind*) may be selected for training. Prepositions are most meaningfully trained at the level of phrases (e.g., *on the table,*

table 7.1

Fourteen Grammatic Morphemes (Brown, 1973)

Morpheme	Age in Months	Examples of Morpheme
1. Present progressive *-ing* (with no auxiliary verb)	28–36	Doggie run*ning* Daddy eat*ing*
2. Preposition *in*	28–36	Dolly *in* house Daddy *in* car
3. Preposition *on*	28–36	Kitty *on* chair Hat *on* head
4. Regular plural *-s* and allomorphic forms: /s/, /z/, /ez/	28–36	Ducks go swim Stars in sky Mommy wash dish*es*
5. Irregular past tense	36–42	*Ate, saw, threw, went, came*
6. Possessive *'s -s*	36–42	Mommy*'s* hat Kitty*'s* ball
7. Verb form of *to be* as main verb (Uncontractible copula)	36–42	Daddy *is.* (answering question such as "Who's big?") *Is* Grandma sleeping?
8. Articles *a* and *the*	40–46	I see *a* baby. Daddy drive *the* car.
9. Regular past tense forms: /d/, /t/, /ed/	40–46	Baby cri*ed*. I walk*ed* home. I skat*ed* fast!
10. Regular third person verb form	40–46	Birdie sing*s*. Daddy eat*s*.
11. Irregular third person verb forms	42–52	He *has* it. She *does.* (answering question such as "Who's got the ball?")
12. Verb form of *to be* as auxiliary verb (uncontractible auxiliary)	42–52	*Is* Mommy coming? *Are* they going?
13. Contracted verb form of *to be* as the main verb in a sentence (Contractible copula)	42–52	They*'re* going home. I*'m* not here. She*'s* a dancer.
14. Contracted verb form of *to be* as an auxiliary verb in a sentence (Contractible auxiliary)	42–52	He*'s* eating a pizza. We*'re* playing a game. You*'re* making a mess!

Source: Brown, R. (1973).

in the box, behind the book) and simple sentences (e.g., "The ball is on the table"; "The car is in the box"; "The pencil is behind the book").

- *Regular plural inflection.* The three allomorphic variations of the regular plural *-s* (/s/, /z/, and /ez/) should be trained separately as they are independent response classes. They may be trained at the word (e.g., *cups, bags, oranges*), phrase (e.g., *two cups, five* *bags, many oranges*), and sentence levels (e.g., "I see two cups"; "Give me five bags"; "They are sweet oranges").

- *Irregular plurals.* Each irregular plural in English is a separate response class; each word has to be taught. Each feature can be taught at the word (e.g., *women, feet, teeth, mice*), phrase (e.g., *three women, two feet, many teeth, three mice*), and sentence levels (e.g., "I see three women"; "These are my two feet"; "I have many teeth"; "There are three mice").

Name some language forms that are described as single linguistic categories but are actually separate response classes.

- *Irregular past tense.* Each irregular past tense word is a separate response class; each has to be taught at the word (e.g., *ate, fell, flew*), phrase (e.g., *ate pizza, fell down, flew away*) and sentence levels (e.g., "I ate pizza"; "Suzie fell down"; "The bird flew away").

- *Regular past tense inflection.* Each of the three regular past tense inflections—/d/, /t/, and /ted/—form a separate response class. Exemplars from each class should be trained at the word (e.g., *climbed, kicked, painted*), phrase or short sentences (e.g., *she climbed, he kicked, man painted*) and complete sentence levels (e.g., "She climbed the stairs"; "He kicked the ball"; "The man painted yesterday"). Articles in these sentences, if not already trained, may be omitted.

- *Possessive inflection.* Three allomorphic variations of the English possessive -s, /z/, and /ez/ need to be trained separately as they form three response classes. They may be trained at the word (e.g., *cat's, baby's, horse's,*), phrase (e.g., *cat's tail, baby's bottle, horse's mouth*), and sentence levels (e.g., "It is the cat's tail"; "That is the baby's bottle"; "This is the horse's mouth"). Articles in these sentences may be treated as optional until they are separately trained.

- *Articles.* Though linguistically a single class, each article is a response class, although they are related in a contextual sense. All can be meaningfully trained only at the phrase (e.g., *a dog, the ball*) and sentence levels (e.g., "I see a dog"; "The ball is red"). The article *the*, being more specific than the article *a*, may be trained in a set of phrases that distinguish the general from the particular (specific). For instance, the clinician may teach "I saw a cat"; "the cat's name was Blanca"—showing the distinction between the two articles.

Name two language forms that are described as separate linguistic categories, but belong to a single response class.

- *Pronouns.* Multiple response classes, each needing separate training, are included in this structural category. Pronouns *he, she,* and *it* are good initial targets and may be trained at the word level (e.g., "Who is reading? Say "she"") or at the simple sentence level (e.g., "He is playing"; "She is nice"; "It is crawling"). Such other forms as possessive pronouns (e.g., *mine, ours*) or demonstrative pronouns (*this, that*) may be taught later.

- *Auxiliary.* Verbal auxiliary is a part of basic sentence structure that helps describe (tact) events and objects. The grammatic morpheme *is* or *was*, for example is a verbal auxiliary when it precedes a main verb (He *is* walking; She *was* sleeping). It may be contracted (as in He's walking) or uncontractible (as in She *was* sleeping); both the examples also show the present and the past forms of an auxiliary. They also have the singular and plural forms (*was/were; is/are*). Each form may belong to a response class needing separate treatment. Most can be trained only at the phrase (e.g., *he was, she is, they were*) or sentence level (e.g., "He was playing"; "She was running"; "They were jumping"), the latter being the most meaningful. The same is true of contractible forms (e.g., "She's hiding"; "He's throwing"). Note that if auxiliary is taught first, there may be no need to teach copula, as the two belong to the same response class; the clinician should probe copular production to make sure (see Box 7.2 for examples of auxiliary and copula).

- *Copula.* A copula takes the same form as an auxiliary, but it is used in sentences that describe a quality or a property of something or someone. The *is* in the sentence "She is smiling" is an auxiliary; the same *is* in the sentence "She is kind" is a copula. The many forms of copula need to be trained separately, but not if auxiliary is taught first. If copula is taught first, auxiliary may need no training; a probe will confirm that. Copula may be taught in both the contracted (e.g., "Clown's funny"; "She's nice") and uncontracted forms (e.g., "He was small"; "She was good"), again most meaningfully in sentences.

- *Conjunctions.* Because they help expand phrases and sentences, conjunctions are good early target skills. Conjunctions *and* and *but* are especially good early targets. Although the conjunction *and* may be taught at the phrase (e.g., *cat and mouse, milk and cookie*) and sentence level (e.g., "I see a cat and a mouse"; "I want milk and cookie"), the conjunction *but* may be taught only at the sentence level (e.g., "I like chocolate, but I can't eat it"; "Dan was sick, but he came to school").

- *Adjectives.* Adjectives are useful in early communication training as they help describe properties of objects and events. Each adjective is a response category unto itself, so each word has to be trained separately; there will be no generalized production. Adjectives can be trained as paired words with contrasting stimuli (e.g., *big/small,*

---

box 7.2   **Auxiliary versus Copula**

The verb *to be* is one of the most irregular verbs in the English language. Consider the conjugation of the verb *to be* in the present tense (and think of their past tense forms):

First person singular	I *am*
Second person singular	You *are*
Third person singular	He, she, or it *is*
First person plural	We *are*
Third person plural	They *are*

When a form of the verb *to be* is used as the main verb of a sentence, it is called a copula. Typically, a copula precedes a noun or a word that suggests a characteristic or quality. Examples include:

I *am* an attorney.
You *are* smart.
She *is* my mother
We *are* happy.
They *are* medical students.

When forms of the verb *to be* function as helper verbs, rather than as main verbs, they are called auxiliary verbs. Typically, auxiliaries precede a main verb. Present tense examples include (and, again, think of their past tense forms):

I *am going.*
You *are singing* sweetly.
He *is working* at the store.
We *are traveling* to China.
They *are sleeping* soundly.

Although copula and auxiliary forms are separate linguistic structures, the two have been experimentally demonstrated to belong to one response class. Teaching one is sufficient to have the other form produced on the basis of generalization.

tall/short, happy/sad), in phrases (e.g., *big house/small house; short man/tall man; happy woman/sad woman*), and in sentences (e.g., "This is a big house" and "This is a small house"; "He is short" and "He is tall"; "She is happy" and "She is sad").

- *Comparatives and superlatives.* Adjectives may be modified with *-er* or *-est* inflection to create comparatives and superlatives. They are mostly trained in sentences (e.g., "This is heavy," "This is heavier," "This is the heaviest"; "This dog is small," "This cat is smaller," "This mouse is the smallest"; "This car is big," "This van is bigger," "This bus is the biggest").

There are many other grammatic morphemes that clinicians will need to teach children with language disorders. The preceding lists offer only selected examples of morphologic target skills that may be taught to individual children.

Phrases into Basic Sentences

As suggested in the earlier section, some grammatic morphemes can only be taught in simple sentences. However, most functional words taught to children are expanded initially into phrases and then into sentences. This is true of both linguistic structures and behavioral response classes. A question may be a word ("Really?"), a phrase ("So what?") or a sentence ("What do you mean?"). A request (*mand*, a functional response class in the behavioral analysis) may be a word ("juice"), a phrase ("want juice"), or a sentence ("I want juice"). Clinicians should move the child as quickly as possible to the sentence level—a more elaborate form of the same response class—because the effect on the listener is more precise than that of the word or the phrase. Also, teaching sentence structures is essential to promote literacy in school-age children.

It is impractical to list all varieties of sentences that may be taught to children with language disorders. What follows are basic examples on which to build a series of more advanced language skills.

- *Sentences with targeted grammatic morphemes.* In establishing basic language skills, the clinician will target grammatic morphemes that help create a rich variety of sentences in children with language disorders. Sentences that include plurals, possessives, present progressive, auxiliary, copula, pronouns, articles, conjunctions, tense modifiers, adjectives, comparatives, and superlatives, as described in the previous section, will result in language skills that will make a difference in the child's social and academic life. Those skills will serve as a good foundation for building literacy skills in the school-age children. Going beyond sentences in which one or more grammatic morphemes were the targets, the clinician may teach additional sentence types to enrich basic language skills before embarking on conversational skill training, which involves significant elaboration of these basic skills.
- *Descriptive sentences* (tacts). Many verbal responses of everyday communication are sentences (again, they could be words or phrases) that describe or comment on events, people, and objects. Therefore, they would be highly useful targets to teach children with language disorders. From a structural linguistic standpoint, most active declarative sentences are descriptive. A child who learns to tact will have acquired significant language skills that will serve well in social communication and academic learning.

- *Negative sentences* (mostly mands). Children learn negative responses early, even if the response takes the form of "No!" or "Not that!" Negative sentences give the children some early verbal tools to affect the behavior of listeners; therefore, they are useful to a child who lacks language skills to affect the social world. Negative sentences may take several forms depending whether they include *no, not, do not, did not, is not, were not*, and so forth.
- *Mands* (questions and requests). Children who cannot ask questions and request help will experience a significant improvement in their social communication if they learn to mand. Children with severe language disorder need to learn these verbal skills. Mands are a large response class, varied in response topography, but they all specify what will reinforce them (e.g., the request "Water, please" specifies the reinforcer for it). The children may be taught varied forms of questions that start with *what, where, when, which, why*, and *how*. They may also be taught a variety of requests including those that seek information, help, and objects from others.

What do mands specify?

The words, phrases, and sentence varieties described so far form a rough sequence in which basic skills may be taught. Once the target skills are selected and described in operational terms (see Chapter 5), the clinician is ready to establish the baselines. Treatment will then follow.

Establishing Baselines

As noted in Chapter 5, baselines are pretreatment measures of target skills that help establish clinician accountability. When combined with treatment data, baselines show systematic improvement (or lack thereof) in language skills. Because they are measures of skills that exist before treatment, the clinician will give no feedback (positive or corrective) contingent on any of the responses produced during measurement. As noted in Chapter 6, reinforcers may be made contingent on general behaviors to keep the child interested in the activities that help evoke the target skills.

What type of reinforcement is given during baseline procedures?

Baselines go beyond the initial assessment, subsequent reassessment, and standardized tests; they are child-specific and clinician-designed to reliably sample target language skills. Without reliable baselines and continued measurement of target skills in treatment sessions, the clinician cannot judge improvement or make treatment modifications.

We described a basic discrete trial baseline procedure in Chapter 5. The same procedure, with needed modifications, may be used to baserate most of the basic language skills, including sentence productions. A naturalistic language sample will supplement the formal baseline results.

Baselines of Early Communication Skills

Early communicative behaviors may all be baserated in roughly the same manner. Both naturalistic observation and assessment-oriented manipulations (e.g., modeled discrete trials) will provide baseline data. Naturalistic observations are periods of time in which the occurrence of the behavior of interest is noted and its topography noted by precise transcription. This is a quantitative procedure that yields the frequency with which a behavior was exhibited during a specified time.

What do data collected during naturalistic observations describe?

Early vocalizations. All early vocalizations may be baserated by systematic observation of the infant or the child who needs treatment for vocalizations. Cooing, babbling, and other vocalizations of the child may be observed in a block of time when such behaviors have a high probability of occurrence. In the case of infants, the behaviors are likely when they are well fed, dry, physically comfortable, lying on their backs, playful by themselves, or playing with caregivers. For children who have passed the normal period of babbling and yet are nonverbal, early vocalizations are likely when they are similarly comfortable and are playing with toys or with caregivers.

Whether in the clinic or at the child's home, arranging playful and comfortable situations for the child and the mother (or another caregiver), observing for blocks of time, and recording the frequency of vocalizations will be necessary. The clinician may find, for example, that in a period of 3 minutes of observation, a child vocalized (cooing, babbling, word approximations, or some other vocal sound) five times. If vocalizations do occur, a 20-minute observational period, repeated three times on different days, will suffice. If the child did not make any, or made only limited vocalizations, the clinician should extend the observation or do it more frequently. In either case, the parental interview will help judge the reliability of the data. The clinician may ask the parents whether vocalizations observed in the clinic are representative of what the child does at home. Furthermore, the parents may be asked to audio- or videotape vocalization attempts at home and submit the records for analysis. Naturalistic observations of this kind will replace evoked discrete trials.

Modeled discrete trial observations may be made to supplement the naturalistic observations. The clinician should model various kinds of vocalizations (e.g., "aa," "oo," "baba") to the child and record the presence or absence of imitation or an approximation. Each modeled presentation of vocalization is treated as a discrete trial.

Early eye contact. Infants and babies look at the mother or turn toward the direction from which they hear human voice, especially the mother's voice. When spoken to, babies look at the face of the speaker and maintain eye contact. Naturalistic observations and discrete trials help baserate these early communicative behaviors. Interviewing the mother and directly observing the mother–child interactions will be sufficient to measure the frequency with which the child looks at the source of human voice and maintains eye contact during verbal interactions. Discrete trials on which the mother calls the child's name or produces other kinds of speech to observe the child's response will supplement the results of naturalistic observations.

Pointing and gesturing. Typically developing infants point and gesture. Children with severe language disorders may fail to point to the objects desired; instead they may cry or fuss. With children who have good motor mobility, the clinician can perform discrete trials to baserate pointing skills. The clinician should ask the child facing an array of objects to point to specific items. At least 20 opportunities to point to different objects will help establish a reliable baserate of pointing.

Naturalistic observations during play situations will supplement the discrete trial data on pointing and gesturing. By keeping certain objects and play materials, the clinician can measure the frequency with which the child points to the desired item. Also, if the child uses a gesture, the clinician complies with what the gesture seems to request or demand, and the child then seems to be reinforced (satisfied), those gestures should be noted as probably having communicative intent.

Children with severe physical disabilities may use subtle behaviors that are within their repertoire to communicate their wants and needs. For instance, a child turning toward an object, moving fingers or toes, or looking in the direction of an object may be trying to communicate. These behaviors also can be baserated with both naturalistic observations and some stimulus manipulations that approximate discrete trials.

> Toddlers point to things to establish joint reference, calling an adult's attention to an item of interest.

Baselines of Functional Words

It is neither useful nor necessary to baserate all potential target words at the beginning of treatment. At any one time, the clinician teaches only a few words—perhaps 5 to 20, depending on the child. The precise number of words presented in treatment sessions will be child-specific and will vary greatly across children. Therefore, the clinician should baserate only those words that are immediate treatment targets. Recall from Chapter 5 that stale baserates are invalid.

Immediate target words of any category described earlier (first few functional, more advanced, or academic and literacy-related) should be baserated on discrete trials. Up to 20 words may be selected and written down on a baserate recording form, shown in Chapter 5. For each word, a physical stimulus (preferably objects, if not pictures) should be selected. For the child with a severe language disorder, the basic words selected will be concrete, common in the child's environment, and evocable with objects. Each word may be presented on an evoked and a modeled trial. Presenting the stimulus object or picture, the clinician should ask questions (e.g., "What is this?" or "What do you see?") on all trials and model the response immediately during modeled trials. Analysis of the results will give separate baseline percentages correct for evoked and modeled trials. Naturalistic observations and parents' reports on the words they have heard the child produce at home will supplement discrete trial measures. Some words are better measured through naturalistic observations than discrete trials. For example, the child's productions of "hi" and "bye" should be noted during natural interactions.

Baselines of Phrases

Essentially, the same procedure designed for baserating target words will work for baserating phrases. The clinician should add another word to a trained word to create a phrase. Using the standard recording sheet to write the phrases, the clinician should administer evoked and modeled baserate trials.

Combined with naturalistic observations and parent information, the clinician can obtain a set of reliable data on the child's production of phrases at home and the clinic. For any phrase that is not meaningfully presented on discrete trials, the clinician should depend only on naturalistic observations and parent information.

Baselines of Early Morphologic Skills

All morphologic skills may be baserated on discrete trials as well as through naturalistic observation. A language sample may be obtained during play-oriented baserate procedures designed to evoke target morphologic features in naturalistic contexts. The clinician should set up the play-oriented sessions so that the opportunities for producing the target morphologic features are maximized. For instance, a variety of plural objects or pictures, multiple action pictures, or acted-out actions will help baserate the child's productions of plural nouns and verbs + *ing*.

Once again, morphologic targets are many and need not all be baserated at the beginning of treatment. At any one time, the clinician will teach a few features that should be baserated. Using the recording sheet shown in Chapter 5, the clinician should write about 20 exemplars for each target grammatic morpheme. The clinician then should baserate each exemplar on a set of evoked and another set of modeled discrete trials as described in the same chapter.

Initially, all morphologic features may be baserated in words or phrases, depending on the first level of training. For example, the present progressive -*ing* may be baserated in such phrases as *boy walking* and *girl dancing*, whereas the allomorphic variations of the plural morpheme may be baserated in such words as *books*, *bags*, and *oranges*. See Table 7.2 for examples of modeled and evoked trials of selected morphologic skills at the word or phrase level.

Baselines of Sentences

Sentences also should be baserated on discrete trials and in naturalistic language samples. Clinicians may structure the language samples to evoke a few sentence types that they will teach immediately. The clinician will then present each exemplar sentence on a set of discrete and modeled trials. By analyzing the language samples and the discrete trial responses, the clinician will obtain the separate baserates for imitated, evoked, and spontaneous sentence productions.

A language sample requested from parents will provide additional information on the naturalistic production of sentences at home. The clinician should describe the target behaviors of interest and offer suggestions to maximize the opportunities for the child to produce the target sentences. Encouraging the parents to watch as the clinician takes a language sample, and, better yet, asking the parent to participate in the sampling procedure in the clinic, will prepare them to take an adequate language sample at home. The clinician may expand on the words and phrases shown in Table 7.3 to create sentences for baserating and teaching. Table 7.3 shows a few examples of sentences expanded from those in Table 7.2, along with additional sentence types that may be used in baserating. The two boxes show only selected examples, but the clinician needs to write at least 20 exemplars for each sentence variety. See Hegde (1998b) for multiple exemplars for most of the language targets.

Descriptive sentences or tacts, as illustrated in Table 7.3 may be baserated by showing a variety of objects or pictures and modeling and evoking descriptive statements. Descriptive sentences are often baserated and trained in the context of several grammatic morphemes. For instance, the child who learns to say "I see two cups" (the plural -*s*), "The ball is big"

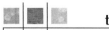

table 7.2

Grammatic Morpheme Exemplars and Their Baserating Procedures

Morphologic Feature	Evoked Trial	Modeled Trial
Present Progressive *-ing* Walking Running	**Using Pictured Stimuli** What is the boy doing? What is the girl doing?	**Using Pictured Stimuli** What is the boy doing? Say, "walking." What is the girl doing? Say, "running."
Irregular Plural Women Children	**Using Pictured Stimuli** Who are these? (Who are they?) Who are these? (Who are they?)	**Using Pictured Stimuli** Who are these? Say, "women." Who are they? Say, "children."
Prepositions On In	**Manipulating Objects** Where is the book? Where is the cat?	**Manipulating Objects** Where is the book? Say, "on the table." Where is the cat? Say, "in the hat."
Irregular Past Tense Ate Flew	**Using Pictured Stimuli** Jessie is eating pizza today. He ate pizza yesterday also. What did he do yesterday? Today, Susan is flying a kite. She flew a kite yesterday also. What did she do yesterday?	**Using Pictured Stimuli** Jessie is eating pizza today. He ate pizza yesterday also. What did he do yesterday? Say, "Jessie ate pizza." Today, Susan is flying a kite. She flew a kite yesterday also. What did she do yesterday? Say, "Susan flew a kite."
Regular Past Tense Hugged Kicked	**Using Verbal Stimuli and Objects** Today, Mommy hugs you. What did Mommy do yesterday? Today, you kick this ball. What did you do yesterday?	**Using Verbal Stimuli and Objects** Today Mommy hugs you. What did Mommy do yesterday? Say, "Hugged me." Today, you kick this ball. What did you do yesterday? Say, "I kicked."
Pronouns He She	**Using Pictured Stimuli** Who is playing? Who is writing?	**Using Pictured Stimuli** He is playing. Who is playing? Say, "He is." She is writing. Who is writing? Say, "She is."

(continued)

(adjective), "The man is nice" (copula), "The woman is running" (auxiliary and *-ing*), and so forth has learned to tact or describe aspects of the stimulating environment.

Negative sentences may take several forms depending on whether they include *no, not, do not, did not, is not, were not,* and so forth. It is important to baserate and teach them because they give the child access to deny, contradict, or request something other than what is offered, and so forth (this is why negative sentences are essentially mands—requests, demands, or commands). Table 7.3 gives some examples of negative sentences and procedures for baserating them.

Full-fledged or obvious mands in the form of requests are useful training targets that enhance the child's skills to affect people, produce results for themselves, and satisfy their motivational states (e.g., hunger, thirst). Many forms of questions also act as mands in that they imply a request or a command either for specific objects or consequences or for information. See Table 7.3 for examples of mands, including questions.

table 7.2 *(continued)*

Morphologic Feature	Evoked Trial	Modeled Trial
Auxiliary Verbs Is Are	**Using Pictured Stimuli** What is the boy doing? What are the girls doing?	**Using Pictured Stimuli** What is the boy doing? Say, "The boy is running." What are the girls doing? Say, "The girls are reading."

Copula
Is
Was
	Using Pictured Stimuli
	Look! It's a ball. Tell me something about the ball.
	Look! It's your teacher from last year in
	    kindergarten. Tell me something about her.
		Using Pictured Stimuli
		Look! It's a ball. Tell me something about the ball.
		    Say, "The ball is round."
		Look! It's your teacher from last year in kinder-
		    garten. Tell me something about her. Say, "My
		    teacher was nice!"

Conjunctions And	**Using Pictured Stimuli** What do you see?	**Using Pictured Stimuli** What do you see? Say, "cookies *and* milk."

Adjectives
Big
Small
	Using Objects
	Look at these two balls. [Pointing to the big one] Is
	    this big or small?
	Look at these two balls. [Pointing to the small one]
	    Is this small or big?
		Using Objects
		Look at these two balls. [Pointing to the big one]
		    Is this big or small? Say, "big."
		Look at these two balls. [Pointing to the small one]
		    Is this small or big? Say, "small."

Comparatives/
   Superlatives
Smaller
Smallest
	Using Objects
	This block is small. This block is _____?
	    [Pointing to the smaller block]
	This block is smaller than this one, but this one is
	    the _____? [Pointing to the smallest
	    block]
		Using Objects
		This block is small. This block is _____.
		    Say, "smaller." [Pointing to the smaller block]
		This block is smaller than this one, but this one
		    is the _____. Say, "smallest." [Pointing to
		    the smallest block]

Teaching Basic Language Skills

In most children, teaching basic skills through discrete trials is efficient. Once the basic skills are established, more naturalistic teaching in controlled play situations at the level of conversational speech will be productive. Although strong in promoting generalized production and maintenance of clinically established skills, more naturalistic approaches are less efficient in early stages of training because they do not allow massed trials to speed up the learning. Therefore, both modeled and evoked trials are recommended in establishing basic language skills.

The treatment of basic language skills will follow the general evidence-based framework described in Chapter 5. Specific treatment techniques described in Chapter 6 are all necessary to establish basic language skills. The following sections of this chapter will illustrate not only the methods of establishing basic language skills, but also the sequence and the overall framework of an evidence-based practice.

Teaching Early Communicative Skills

Most infants, toddlers, and young children with severe language delay need to be taught some early communicative skills before they can benefit from more advanced language

table 7.3

Sentence Type Exemplars and Their Baserating Procedures

Target Sentences	Evoked Trial	Modeled Trial
Present Progressive *-ing* Walking	**Using Pictured Stimuli** What is the boy doing?	**Using Pictured Stimuli** What is the boy doing? Say, "The boy is walking."
Irregular plural Women	**Using Pictured Stimuli** Who are these? (Who are they?)	**Using Pictured Stimuli** Who are these? Say, "These are women."
Prepositions On	**Manipulating Objects** Where is the book?	**Manipulating Objects** Where is the book? Say, "The book is *on the table*."
Descriptive sentences	**Using Pictured Stimuli** What do you see in this picture?	**Using Pictured Stimuli** What do you see in this picture? Say, "I see a man painting." What is here in this picture? Say, "Here is a big white cat."
Conjunctions But	**Using Pictured Stimuli** You like this coat. It's Sally's. What do you say?	**Using Pictured Stimuli** You like this coat. It's Sally's. What do you say? Say, "I like this coat, but it's Sally's."
Mands (requests)	**Manipulating Environmental Stimuli** When the child is looking at objects that cannot be reached, the clinician asks: What do you want? When the child is given a difficult puzzle and is having difficulty with it, the clinician asks: What do you want me to do?	**Manipulating Environmental Stimuli** When the child is looking at an object that cannot be reached, the clinician asks and models: What do you want? Say, "I want that car." When the child is given a difficult puzzle and is having difficulty with it, the clinician asks: What do you want me to do? Say, "Help me, please."
Questions	**Using Pictures, Objects, or Only Verbal Stimuli** Showing a strange object or picture to the child, the clinician asks: Do you know what this is? [The child says "No" or shakes head.] Ask me a question and I will tell you. When you don't see your Mom, what do you ask? Showing the picture of a woman, the clinician asks: You want to know who this woman is. Ask me a question. When you want to know how to play this game, what do you ask me?	**Using Pictures, Objects, or Only Verbal Stimuli** Showing a strange object or picture to the child, the clinician asks: Do you know what this is? Ask me a question and I will tell you. Ask me, "What is this?" When you don't see your Mom, what do you ask? Ask, "Where is Mom?" Showing a picture of a woman, the clinician asks: You want to know who this woman is. Ask me a question. Ask me, "Who is this woman?" When you want to know how to play this game, what do you ask me? Ask me, "How do I play this game?"
Negative Sentences	**Using Pictures or Only Verbal Stimuli** Showing a picture of a young boy, the clinician asks: Is he an old man? The clinician asks the child: Are you a baby? The clinician asks: Were you at the zoo this morning?	**Using Pictures or Only Verbal Stimuli** Showing a picture of a young boy, the clinician asks: Is he an old man? Say, "He is not an old man." The clinician asks the child: Are you a baby? Say, "I am not a baby." The clinician asks: Were you at the zoo this morning? Say, "I was not at the zoo this morning."

treatment. These children will be nearly nonverbal, and hence the training has to begin at the most basic level. A few general teaching strategies will help establish the early skills that provide a foundation for more complex skills.

Increasing early vocalization. Early vocalizations, which predominantly include cooing and babbling may be established by modeling and positive reinforcement. Some of the earliest language treatment studies were in fact done on increasing babbling and other infant vocalizations by positive reinforcement (Hegde, 1998a). To increase early vocalizations, the clinician should offer direct treatment as well as teach the caregivers to stimulate, reinforce, and sustain vocalizations. See Box 7.1 for the kinds of early vocalizations that may be targeted for treatment.

During direct treatment, the child's responses are recorded on a recording sheet. The parents also may be taught to record responses at home. The clinician should first apply the techniques that result in increased vocalizations, have the parents observe the treatment sessions, teach them to use the procedures at home, and monitor their home-based treatment. The following general strategies apply to both the clinician's work and that of the caregivers as treatment for increasing early vocalizations:

- Hold brief treatment sessions when the child is well fed, comfortable, and alert (note that the client may be an infant, a toddler, or an older child)
- Arrange treatment sessions with the child's favorite toys, picture storybooks, and common objects
- Play with the child, draw the child's attention to your face
- Keep talking to the child by describing the actions, pictures, objects, and the child's object manipulations
- Positively reinforce a vocalized response

  —In the case of babies, touch the cheeks, gently tickle, smile, or pick up the baby to reinforce vocalizations; if necessary, use such primary reinforcers as juice or milk
  —In the case of toddlers and older children, touch, smile, give a toy for play, offer juice or milk; to reinforce, add verbal praise ("good!" "nice job," etc.)

- Shape vocalizations in the absence of spontaneous responses

  —Stay close to the child and maintain eye contact
  —Frequently model early vocalization, especially babbled sounds
  —Model any vocalizations the child produces
  —Reinforce imitative responses, even if they are approximations
  —Model progressively more complex vocalizations (child's or expected)
  —Reinforce progressively better approximations and correct imitations
  —Shape vocalizations into syllables and words by modeling them
  —Fade modeling to have the child spontaneously produce words or as responses to questions

Increasing early eye contact. Eye contact during verbal interactions may be increased by instructions, modeling, positive reinforcement for imitated responses, and fading the modeling. Recording the correct and incorrect responses on a recording sheet, the clinician can maintain and reinforce eye contact while establishing early vocalizations through the following:

- Touch the baby, smile, say something endearing, or gently tickle whenever eye contact is established
- Move the face gently to reestablish eye contacts whenever that contact is lost; reinforce eye contact
- Give instructions (e.g., "look at me") to children who can understand them; reinforce the child for complying
- Give a nonverbal prompt (e.g., a hand movement that suggests "look at me") and reinforce the correct response
- Fade the prompt and continue to reinforce eye contact during verbal exchanges in all subsequent treatment sessions to maintain the skill

Increasing pointing and gesturing. The same procedures that help establish early vocalizations and eye contact will be effective in teaching pointing and gesturing. All correct and incorrect responses will be recorded on the recording sheet. Treatment strategies include the following:

- Teach pointing and gesturing as you teach early vocalizations as described
- Keep the desirable objects out of the child's reach
- When the child makes undifferentiated attempts to reach an object:
  - Ask the child, "Do you want this?" while pointing to the object; give manual assistance by taking the child's hand and pointing to the object
  - Immediately reinforce the child by giving the object
  - Hold something the child wants in your hand and ask, "Do you want this?"; prompt the child to extend the hand; give manual guidance if necessary; place the object in the child's hand
  - Prompt, manually guide, and reinforce all appropriate pointing and gesturing behaviors during verbal exchanges

Teaching Functional Words

Baserated functional words may be taught in discrete trials built into play-oriented treatment sessions (see Table 7.4) that become progressively more natural as the discrete trials are dropped. The same stimuli used to baserate the production of single words will be used in treatment sessions. All trials will be scored on a recording sheet. Strategies include the following:

- Teach the selected words initially in discrete trials during less formal, structured play sessions or more formal sessions in which the child is seated across you at a small table
  - Show an object or a picture during the session and ask the child, "What is this?"
  - Immediately model the correct response
  - Reinforce the child's correct imitation; provide corrective feedback for incorrect responses
  - Record the response, wait for a few seconds, and begin the next trial
  - Stop modeling when the child gives five consecutively imitated responses; initiate evoked trials on which you just ask the question and let the child respond; revert to modeling when you observe two or three incorrect responses

table 7.4

Play-Oriented Activities for Discrete Trial Training

Target Behavior	Play-Oriented Activities	Physical Stimuli	Verbal Stimuli for Evoked Trials	Verbal Stimuli for Modeled Trials
Production of functional words	Pretend activities based on daily routines at home, in school, or in the community	Toys or real objects taken from the child's home, school, or community	What is this? What do you need?	What is this? Say, "spoon." What do you need? Say, "pencil."
Production of present progressive -ing	Act out action words with the child (e.g., *running, jumping, singing, cooking*)	Those necessary to serve as props for acting out (e.g., a bowl and spoon for *stirring*)	What are we doing?	What are we doing? Say, "running."
Production of personal pronouns	Pretend activities using various toys	Popular toys, such as boy and girl dolls or other toys of identifiable gender	Whose _____ is this? Who is _____ing? Who did you give it to?	Whose _____ is this? Say, "his." Who is _____? Say, "she is." Who did you give it to? Say, "her."
	Board games	Any appealing board game appropriate for the child	Whose turn is it? Who rolled the dice? Who needs a turn?	Whose turn is it? Say, "my turn." Who rolled the dice? Say, "you did." Who needs a turn? Say, "he does."
Production of prepositions	Pretend activities with toy farms, dollhouses, play kitchens	Play sets for pretend play	Where is the _____? [dog, horse, cow, etc.] Where did you put the _____? [spoon, cup, bowl, etc.] Where does this one go?	Where is the ___? Say, "in the barn." Where did you put the cup? Say, "on the table." Where does this one go? Say, "under the sink."
Production of plural -s (/s/, /z/, /ez/)	Counting games, finger play (e.g., Five Little Monkeys), pretend activities	Multiple toy objects	Here is one ___. Here are two ____. How many are there? Who goes in the barn now?	Here is one *truck*. Here are two ___. Say, "trucks." How many are there? Say, "two trucks." Who goes in the barn now? Say, "two cows."

- Stop training a word when the child produces it correctly on 10 consecutive evoked trials (or attains 90 percent correct response rate on a block of trials)
- Conduct an intermixed probe in which trained stimuli are alternated with untrained stimuli that evoke the same word response (e.g., the picture of the same cup used in training, alternated with the picture of a cup that is different in color, size, style, etc.); retrain the words on which the child does not meet the probe criterion

Recall that a pure probe criterion is 80 or 90 percent correct responses when only the untrained (new) stimuli are shown.

- Conduct a pure probe on which you present only new stimuli that evoke the same target words; give additional training on trained words if the probe criterion of 90 percent correct is not met
- Stop teaching words that meet the pure probe criterion
- Begin phrase level training by combining the trained words into phrases

Teaching Phrases

Previously taught basic functional words or more advanced words may be combined with untrained words to create phrases. It may be noted that in all contexts, a trained target behavior has met the pure probe criterion. Trained nouns can be combined with adjectives (e.g., *big car*), or with personal pronouns (e.g., *my car*), trained verbs may be combined with nouns or pronouns (*house burning, she fell*), and so forth. As a treatment strategy, teach the phrases, using the same procedure you used to teach words.

- Show an object or a picture during the training sessions and ask the child, "What is this?" The child responds correctly with the trained word (e.g., "car").
- Model the phrase: "Whose car is it? It is your car, right? Say, "My car." The child imitates the phrase.
- Reinforce the child's correct imitation by verbal praise and a token (if preferred).

Review Chapter 5 for such clinical decision criteria as to when to stop modeling, when to probe, and so forth.

- Fade modeling, initiate evoked trials, continue this training, and alternate it with probes, as is done in training words.
- Stop teaching the phrases that meet the 90 percent correct probe criterion and begin teaching early morphologic skills, or alternatively, basic sentence structures.

Teaching Early Morphologic Skills

Morphologic skill training follows the same general strategy described so far. Grammatic morphemes may be taught in words, phrases, or simple sentences. Morphologic skill training is not locked into a particular topographic level (e.g., words or phrases). If the child can manage it, phrase-level training will be more efficient than word-level training, and training at the sentence level will be the most efficient. The clinician should design the entry level of training based on what the child can or cannot do, instead of following a rigid rule. The teaching strategy described for words will work well for training morphologic features that can be and need to be trained at the word level (e.g., *cups, walking, talked, bigger*, and so forth).

What turns a baseline trial into a treatment trial?

Morphologic features that can be trained at the phrase level will follow the procedures previously described for phrases. In all cases, clinicians will use the more or less structured discrete trials in which they will use modeling, evoking, prompting, fading, and probing. The clinician will use objects, pictures, events, and enacted events to stimulate the production of specific morphologic features. (Table 5.2 shows examples of baseline trials.) Adding positive reinforcement and corrective feedback to the responses will make them treatment trials. A few illustrations of morphologic features to be trained at the sentence level follow (see Hegde, 1998b, for multiple exemplars on treating several morphologic features):

- Teach the sentences, using the same procedure you used to teach phrases

- To teach irregular past tense words:
  - —Show a picture of a boy eating pizza.
  - —Say, "Jessie is eating pizza today. He ate pizza yesterday also. What did he do yesterday? Say, 'Jessie ate pizza yesterday.'"
  - —Emphasize the word *ate* (for more on emphasis as a prompt, see Chapter 4).
  - —Reinforce the child's correct imitation with verbal praise and a token if preferred.
  - —Give corrective feedback (e.g., "No, you said 'eat,'" I want you to say 'ate.'") for incorrect responses.
  - —Record the response and present the next trial.
  - —Fade the modeling according to the decision criteria (e.g., five consecutively correct imitated responses). Show the picture, and say, "Jessie is eating pizza today. He ate pizza yesterday also. What did he do yesterday?" Do not model the sentence, but reinforce or give corrective feedback.
  - —Reintroduce the modeling if necessary (e.g., two or more incorrect evoked responses).
  - —Probe according to the decision criteria (e.g., 10 consecutively correct evoked responses).
  - —Offer more training if the probe criteria are not met.

- To teach the regular past tense *-ed* inflection:
  - —Show a picture of a mother hugging a child; say, "Today Mommy is hugging her. Yesterday she did the same. What did Mommy do yesterday? Say, 'Mommy hugged her.'"
  - —Train other exemplars.
  - —Continue training and probing as described in the previous list on irregular past tense inflection.

- To teach comparatives/superlatives:
  - —Show pictures of two balls, one smaller and the other bigger.
  - —Say, "Look at these two balls [point to the bigger one]. Is this ball big or small? Say, 'This ball is big.'" [Emphasize *big*.]
  - —Reinforce or give corrective feedback.
  - —Say, "Look at this ball [point to the smaller one]. Is this ball big or small? Say, 'This ball is small.'"
  - —Reinforce or give corrective feedback.
  - —Train multiple exemplars.
  - —Follow the other procedures of training including fading the modeling, evoking, probing, and so forth according to the clinical decision criteria.

- To teach the possessive morpheme:
  - —Show a picture of a boy holding a toy car.
  - —Point to the picture and say, "This is Tommy. It is his car. Whose car is this? Say, 'This is Tommy's car.'"
  - —Reinforce or give corrective feedback.
  - —Train multiple exemplars.
  - —Follow the other procedures of training including fading the modeling, evoking, probing, and so forth according to the clinical decision criteria.

The examples given so far of morphologic training will serve as the model for teaching other grammatic morphemes. Note that when the training moves from one target to the other, treatment procedures stay constant with one exception: procedures evoking the target skill change. With each new target behavior, the clinician needs new evoking procedures. The physical stimuli and the evoking questions change, while the treatment procedures of modeling, fading, prompting, and response consequating (reinforcement or corrective feedback) remain the same. Therefore, the clinicians need not be concerned about finding new treatment procedures when new targets—including literacy skills—are selected for treatment.

Teaching Basic Sentences

The examples already given for morphologic training illustrate several sentence training strategies. The clinician may use those examples to create sentences for other language targets (Hegde, 1998b). By setting relevant stimulus conditions, the clinician can evoke, reinforce, and strengthen the following kinds of descriptive statements or sentences:

- To teach descriptive sentences (tacts):
  - Show a picture (e.g., a car) and ask, "What do you see?" Immediately model, "Say, 'I see a car.'"
  - Show a picture of a pencil, and ask, "What do you do with this?" Immediately model, "Say, 'I write with it.'"
  - Show something that is blue, and ask, "What color is it?" Immediately model, "Say, 'It is blue.'"
  - Put a hat on the child's head and ask, "What is on your head?" Immediately model, "Say, 'I have a hat on my head.'"
  - Reinforce or give corrective feedback. Follow the other procedures of treatment, including fading the model, probing, and alternating treatments and probes.
- To teach negative sentences, arrange situations that the child is forced to contradict:
  - Show a wrong picture (e.g., a cat) and ask, "Is this a dog?" Immediately model, "Say, 'No, it is a cat.'"
  - Show a white balloon, and say, "I think this balloon is blue. What do you think?" Immediately model, "Say, 'No, it is not blue, it is white.'"
  - Show a picture of a young boy and ask, "Is he an old man?" Immediately model, "Say, 'He is not an old man.'"
  - Ask a girl, "Are you a boy?" Immediately model, "Say, 'I am not a boy!'"
  - Hold two parts of a toy and ask, "Did you break this toy?" Immediately model, "Say, 'I did not!'"
  - Reinforce or give corrective feedback for responses. Follow the other procedures of treatment, including fading the model, probing, and alternating treatments and probes.
- To teach mands (questions and requests):
  - Place a few desirable items high on a shelf but in clear view of the child. Then pointing to an item (e.g., a toy car), ask, "Do you want that car on the shelf? I can get it for you if you say, 'I want that car, please.' Say, 'I want that car, please.'"

— Give the child a difficult puzzle to put together. When the child experiences difficulty, ask, "Do you need help? I can help you. Say, 'Help me, please.'"

— Create an imaginary situation. For instance, say, "You are very thirsty. You want a glass of water. What do you say? Say, 'I want water, please.'"

— Create another imaginary situation. For instance, say, "Your tummy is hurting. You want medicine from your Mom. What do you say? Ask, 'Can I have some medicine for my tummy ache, Mom?'"

— Create other stimulus conditions to evoke target requests.

— Reinforce or give corrective feedback for responses. Follow the other procedures of treatment, including fading the model, probing, and alternating treatments and probes.

Following the examples shown, the clinician can write additional target sentences and teach them within the general framework, using the evidence-based treatment techniques referred to in this chapter and described in detail in Chapter 5. Typically, the child is moved through modeling and evoking and probing and training.

Sequencing Treatment

The general guidelines of sequencing treatment at all stages have been described in Chapter 5. Treatment is sequenced for response topography: starting with the basic topography of words or phrases, the treatment moves through sentences and conversational speech. Treatment also moves through stimulus hierarchies: starting with modeling, the treatment moves through evoking, controlled conversation in the clinic, to spontaneous conversation in natural settings. Finally, treatment also moves through sequences based on response consequences: starting with a high density of reinforcement, it moves through stages of progressively lower density of reinforcement. Primary reinforcement, when used, will also create a sequence in which it is faded to better approximate the social reinforcement for language skills that is common in naturalistic settings.

These sequences are illustrated in the form of a case study. In this illustration, the child starts training at the word level and reaches the sentence level. Movement of treatment to more complex skill levels and more naturalistic settings will be described and illustrated in future chapters.

A Clinical Example of Treatment Sequence

Joe, a 4-year-old boy, had a severe language disorder. He spoke only a few words; he gestured and pointed instead of speaking. When he could not communicate, he also fussed and cried. There was no history of prior treatment for his language disorder. Treatment was recommended twice a week. The target skills were:

• Production of a set of functional words with 90 percent accuracy when asked to name pictures or objects in clinical and home situations across three measurement samples

• Production of a set of phrases with 90 percent accuracy when asked to name pictures or objects in clinical and home situations across three measurement samples

• Production of a set of basic sentences with 90 percent accuracy in at least three structured conversational speech samples recorded in clinical and home situations

table 7.5

An Illustrative List of Functional Words, as Described in the Case Study

Clothing Items	Toys	Food Items	Kinship Terms	Adjectives	Verbs
hat	ball	banana	Mommy	big	walking
socks	car	cake	Daddy	small	sleeping
shoes	train	juice	sister	happy	eating
shirt	doll	milk	brother	red	running
pants	bike	pizza	Grandma	smooth	playing

In consultation with Joe's parents, 30 functional words that could be expanded into phrases and sentences were selected for training. See Table 7.5 for examples of the words that may be expanded into different phrases and sentences. Pictures and objects were selected for stimuli. Each word was baserated on a set of evoked and modeled trials. Words Joe correctly produced on an evoked trial were replaced with new words he did not produce to maintain a 30-word list for training and probing. Therefore, the correct baserate for selected words was zero.

The training was initiated with a set of four words, two nouns and two adjectives: *ball*, *car*, *big*, and *small*. Note that a clinician might select more functional targets (e.g., mands *want* or *help*) than these descriptive terms (tacts), but mands are better taught in phrases or sentences (e.g., "Car, please"; "I want juice"). Children learn labels more easily than requests, which helps establish an initial success in treatment, increasing children's motivation. Of course, the clinician could teach such words as *Mommy*, *Daddy*, and names of family members. The training progressed as follows: first, the clinician taught the word *ball* with modeled discrete trials. She (the clinician) gave verbal praise and a token for each correct response. Joe exchanged the tokens for a gift of his choice at the end of each session. Within a few modeled trials, he gave five consecutively correctly imitated responses. The clinician then discontinued modeling. Presenting the object, she only asked the question, "What is this?" Joe's correct response rate dropped to zero on the first two evoked trials. Therefore, she reinstated modeling. After observing a second set of five consecutively correct imitated responses, the clinician again discontinued modeling. This time, Joe began to correctly say "ball" when the clinician showed the object and asked the question. When Joe gave 10 consecutively correct evoked responses, the clinician shifted training to the second and third words, *big* and *small*.

While teaching the words *big* and *small*, by contrasting stimulus objects (e.g., a *big* book and a *small* book) the clinician conducted intermixed probes to assess generalized production of the word *ball*. She presented balls of different size, shape, and color, and asked the same question ("What is this?"). She alternated the new stimuli with the trained object. If Joe did not give a correct response to a new stimulus, the clinician gave a few training trials involving that stimulus. When Joe correctly said "ball" for 4 out of 5 new stimuli (an 80 percent probe criterion acceptable at this level of training), she judged that the word *ball* was tentatively trained. She continued to teach the adjectives *big* and *small*. When Joe met the training criterion of 10 consecutively correct evoked responses on each adjective, she probed for generalized production of *big* and *small* by presenting objects that were different in size, color, and texture. When Joe correctly named 4 out of 5 untrained big objects and 4 out of 5 untrained small objects presented to him, the clinician shifted training to a new word (*car*) and the first phrase-level training. She created two phrases out of the three trained words: *big ball* and *small ball*.

The clinician then taught the word *car* and the two phrases *big ball* and *small ball*. She also taught other words and phrases created out of those trained words. Joe learned to produce about 30 words and 30 phrases and attained the probe criteria on all of them.

The clinician then began teaching a few grammatic morphemes (listed in Table 6.1). She taught each morpheme essentially the same way: by modeling, prompting with vocal emphasis on the target morpheme, fading the modeling, and probing. She gave additional training on new exemplars or already trained exemplars when Joe did not meet one of the probe criteria. When Joe met the pure probe criteria for the target morphemes when only untrained stimuli or objects were shown, the clinician moved on to sentences.

As the clinician had already taught a few sentences while teaching some grammatic morphemes, Joe was adept at learning additional sentences. The clinician taught a variety of sentences, some examples of which were shown in Table 7.3. She taught each sentence initially with modeling and prompting on discrete trials which she faded into evoked trials. She completed this level of training by teaching Joe a set of descriptive sentences, negative sentences, requests, and questions. For each sentence type Joe met the initial intermixed and the subsequent pure probe criteria.

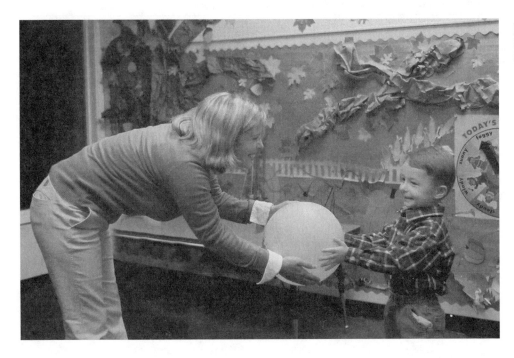

photo 7.2
Learning to say, "Big ball!"

Preparing for the Next Stage

For the child who has learned basic language skills, more complex targets, conversational speech, and maintenance of those skills at home and school become the next targets. While teaching complex language skills including conversational speech, the clinician should take steps to maintain the basic skills the child has learned.

Parent and classroom teacher training to promote maintenance of language skills is described in a later chapter. This does not imply that it is necessarily the last thing the clinician does. If the child does not maintain the basic skills, it will not be possible or meaningful to teach the more advanced skills. Therefore, to prepare the child for effective instruction in advanced language skills, the clinician should work with teachers, family members, and other caregivers in sustaining the language skills in naturalistic settings. The techniques are described in detail in Chapters 8 and 9, but a few initial steps the clinician should take from the beginning of treatment may be briefly noted here. The clinician should have the caregivers observe the treatment sessions. They should have a clear understanding of the target skills. A written list of target skills with examples should be given to the teachers and caregivers. A brief demonstration of treatment may be made in the presence of the teacher. As the child begins to learn the skills, teachers and caregivers should prompt and reinforce the production of language structures.

While working with the parents and the teacher of the child, the clinician should start planning the next level of treatment to expand the basic skills. We will address this level of treatment in the next chapter.

Chapter Summary

The approach taken in this book is *skill-based*—not explicitly based on chronological ages and stages of development. Each child with a language disorder needs to learn language skills that help meet social, academic, and personal demands. Clinicians must use their own judgment based on client-specific considerations of what basic skills the child needs to learn. For some children, early communicative skills (e.g., cooing and babbling) may be appropriate initial targets, whereas for others, advanced morphologic, syntactic, or pragmatic language skills may be the most useful initial targets.

The first few functional words that are taught initially should include the names of family members and labels for objects in the child's environment; action words; descriptive and adjectival terms; and daily-routine terms. Subsequently, progressively more complex and abstract words may be targets. Clinically established word productions should be expanded into phrases and sentences.

Early morphologic skills targeted for treatment include present progressive -*ing*; prepositions in phrases or sentences; regular plural inflections; irregular plurals; irregular past tense; regular past tense inflections; possessive inflections; articles; pronouns; auxiliary; copula; conjunctions; adjectives; and comparatives and superlatives.

Before the treatment is begun, the clinician establishes the baselines of target skills. Treatment typically begins with discrete trials in which each attempt to produce a target response is separated by a brief duration of time. Instructions, modeling, prompting, shaping, fading, positive reinforcement, and corrective feedback help establish target skills at levels of complexity. In the final stages of treatment, more naturalistic teaching with conversational interactions will help promote generalized productions and eventual maintenance.

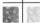

Study Guide

1. Compare and contrast the different approaches to selecting target behaviors for basic language skills. Discuss discrepancies between describing language forms as linguistic categories versus response classes. Give examples of response classes. How is treatment affected by response class?

2. Baselines are essential before starting treatment. What is the importance and necessity of baselines? Describe how you would baserate a set of words, phrases, and sentences. Specify each step involved in establishing baselines.

3. You have been assigned a 3-year-old child who can produce only a few two-word phrases. Your supervisor has asked you to write a comprehensive treatment program for this child. Detail the sequence with which you teach the following skills to this child; name all the techniques you need to establish the specific skills:

   - Increasing early vocalizations
   - Increasing early eye contact
   - Increasing pointing and gesturing
   - Teaching functional words
   - Teaching phrases
   - Teaching early morphologic skills
   - Teaching basic sentences

4. Once treatment is started, you face a variety of "crossroads" at which you have to make clinical decisions that determine what you do next and how the child will make progress. With the example of a child under treatment, specify the following clinical decision criteria:

   - The initial discontinuation of modeling
   - Reinstatement of modeling
   - Deciding that the child has learned a particular skill exemplar and moving on to the next exemplar
   - Deciding that the child has learned a particular skill (not just an exemplar)

chapter

8

Expanding Language Skills

outline

- Expanding Previously Learned Skills
- Teaching Varied Sentence Types
- Teaching Conversational Speech
- Teaching Narrative Skills
- Teaching Abstract Language Skills
- Integrating Conversational Skills:
  Putting It All Together
- Moving to Nonclinical Settings
- Chapter Summary
- Study Guide

238

In the previous chapter we described procedures to establish basic language skills with the help of techniques described in Chapters 5 and 6. To create an effective verbal repertoire in children, these basic skills should be expanded into more advanced language skills, including conversational speech, narrative skills, and various other skills that are described as pragmatic language skills. Finally, the children should be introduced to a few essential elements of abstract and academic language. This chapter will describe these target skills and strategies to teach them.

Expanding Previously Learned Skills

It was pointed out in Chapter 5 that initial target behaviors are selected, in part, because they are building blocks to more complex behaviors. Thus, the clinician may begin by teaching a child to label nouns (e.g., *ball, kitty, flower*) and then may build on that skill by adding adjectives (e.g., *big ball, pretty kitty, red flower*) and then verbs (e.g., *play big ball, hold pretty kitty, smell red flower*). Subsequently, the clinician may teach grammatically more complete productions that incorporate progressively more complex syntactic and morphologic forms. The clinician should move as quickly through these steps as possible, taking the child to more advanced levels of language skill training.

There is evidence that behavioral methods of teaching language skills can help promote more advanced social communication skills. Much of the research has been done with children who have autism or developmental disability. Such teaching programs as script fading (Krantz & McClanahan, 1998; Sarokoff, Taylor, & Poulson, 2001); video modeling (Charlop & Milstein, 1989; Nikopoulos & Keenan, 2004); time-delay (Charlop & Trasowech, 1991; Ingenmey & Van Houten, 1991); peer training and interaction (Goldstein et al., 1992; Kamps et al., 1992; Pierce & Schreibman, 1995); parent and sibling training (Kaiser, 1993; Neef, 1995; Schreibman, O'Neill, & Koegel, 1983); milieu teaching, which includes mand-model, delay, and incidental teaching by both clinicians and peers (McGee et al., 1992; McGee et al., 1983; McGee, Krantz, & McClanahan, 1985); and functional communication training (Duran, Berotti, & Weiner, 1993; Durand & Carr, 1992; Reichle & Wacker, 1993) have been shown to be effective in single-subject experimental research. These treatment programs have been effective in teaching social interactions including such specific skills as initiation of speech, spontaneous speech, conversational interactions, expansion of conversational topics, abstract language (idiom comprehension), spontaneous expression through sign language, and pragmatic language through alternative augmentative means (e.g., Carr & Kologinsky, 1983; Chandler, Lubeck, & Fowler, 1992; Charlop & Milstein, 1989; Charlop & Trasowech, 1991; Ezell & Goldstein, 1992; Goldstein & Cisar, 1992; Haring et al., 1986; Koegel & Frea, 1993; Matson et al., 1993; McGee, Krantz, & McClanahan, 1985; Pierce & Schreibman, 1994; Secan, Egel, & Tilley, 1989; Warren & Rogers-Warren, 1985, among many others). Results of these and other studies have been replicated across clinicians, settings, and participants. In all of these teaching programs, skills are established by such behavioral techniques as modeling, shaping, prompting, instructions, fading, positive reinforcement, differential reinforcement, delayed contingencies, and corrective feedback described in previous chapters. Therefore, the differences in programs are less striking than the

Controlled experimental research studies showing efficacy of treatment methods that have been replicated in different settings, by different researchers, with similar results are at what level of scientific evidence? (Hint: See Table 5.1.)

effective techniques they all share. A 1992 review of training, generalization, and maintenance of social skills in developmentally disabled individuals included 51 studies done between 1976 and 1990 and published in 21 journals (Chandler, Lubeck, & Fowler, 1992). The reviewers noted that a majority of studies produced either complete or partial generalization of treated social skills. Documented generalization is an indication of the success of the treatment offered.

Teaching Varied Sentence Types

As treatment progresses, the clinician should teach the child more varied and longer sentence types. Advanced target behaviors at the sentence level are most efficiently established by first using the discrete trials described in previous chapters. As the behaviors become more established, a looser structure of therapy should be used in which the target behaviors are evoked in more naturalistic contexts. When the shift from tight to loose structure is made, it may be necessary to begin by directly modeling the target behaviors and requiring imitations from the child during naturalistic activities. As the imitated responses get stabilized, the model can be faded until the child begins to produce the target behaviors spontaneously. In this section, we will first describe types of advanced target behaviors at the sentence level and then discuss variations on the basic treatment procedure to establish those target behaviors in more naturalistic contexts.

As always, selected target behaviors should be client-specific and relevant to the child's communicative needs and cultural background. Most often, such target behaviors are those that will allow a child to request, to make comments, to ask questions, and eventually to converse using more syntactically complex sentence forms.

Requests (Mands)

Requests (mands) specify their own reinforcers. When a child asks, "Can I have a cookie, Mom?" the mother knows what reinforces the request (a cookie). Therefore, the mands (that are reinforced) are highly likely to be maintained in a child's natural environment. A mand may request an object, make a command, or seek information. Mands are among the most effective forms of communication. Children who had deficient language skills will immensely benefit from mands, as they give children unprecedented control to affect their environment. Initially, mands may be established in two word phrases (e.g., "Want cookie!" or "Tell me!"). Subsequently, such requests should be expanded to grammatically more complete productions (e.g., "I want a cookie" or "Tell me a story"). Finally, elements of social politeness may be added to just-taught requests (e.g., "May I have a cookie, please?" or "Would you please tell me a story?").

> Mands specify their own reinforcers! "Want milk" (Milk is the reinforcer.); "Sit down, please," (Sitting down is the reinforcer.); "Tell me a story," (Telling a story is the reinforcer.); "Where is my doll?" (Telling where it is, is the reinforcer.). See Chapter 1 for details on mands.

Treatment may begin with discrete trials or semi-structured situations in which a variety of objects and activities are arranged for the child to get reinforced for mands. Asking a question, modeling the request, and complying with the request (which provides the reinforcement) is the typical training strategy. For instance, when the child is putting a puzzle together, the clinician may hold a crucial piece of the puzzle and ask, "What do you want? Say, 'I want that piece.' " When the child imitates the response, the clinician hands over the piece of the puzzle. Objects placed on a shelf the child cannot reach can help evoke requests that are then reinforced by giving the object. See Table 8.1 for verbal strategies to evoke requests during discrete trial therapy. For a child who cannot initially produce a full-form request, the shaping procedure may be used, in which progressively more complete responses are required before reinforcement is given. The initial request in such cases may even be a nonverbal response such as pointing, then a single word (e.g., *doll, gum*) which is expanded into more complete forms.

After the more complex mands are established in discrete trials, the clinician should evoke the responses in naturalistic communicative contexts. There are numerous activities clinicians can use during language therapy that will provide the child with many opportunities to produce targeted requesting sentences. See Table 8.2 for some suggestions; also see a later section on mand-model procedure. The clinician should not forget to evoke "thank you," if the child is being trained at more advanced levels!

Descriptions and Comments (Tacts)

Descriptions and comments—**tacts**—are integral to conversational speech. This class of verbal behaviors helps expand language skills to a great extent. Therefore, tacts are highly useful language targets. Academic performance of children with language disorders can be significantly improved with a good repertoire of tacts. Basic skills such as nouns and verb productions should be expanded quickly into phrases and then, on a more advanced level, into grammatically

See Chapter 1 for details on tacts.

table 8.1

Verbal Stimuli for Discrete Trial Training of Requesting Sentences (Mands)

Target Behavior	Modeled Sentences	Evoked Sentences
Production of *Give me . . .* requests	You want some milk. Say, "Give me some milk, please." You want the blue crayon. Say, "Give me the blue crayon, please."	You want some milk. What do you ask? You want the blue crayon. What do you ask?
Production of *I want . . .* requests	You want the yellow block. Say, "I want the yellow block, please." You want the doll house. Say, "I want the doll house, please." You want to play ball. Say, "I want to play ball, please."	You want the yellow block. What do you ask? You want to the doll house. What do you ask? You want to play ball. What do you ask?
Production of *May I have . . .* requests	You want another puzzle piece. Say, "May I have another puzzle piece, please?" You want some more glue. Say, "May I have more glue, please?" You want another turn. Say, "May I have another turn, please."	You want another puzzle piece. What do you ask? You want some more glue. What do you ask? You want another turn. What do you ask?

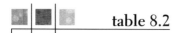

table 8.2

Clinical Activities for Establishing Requesting Sentences in More Naturalistic Contexts

Clinical Activity to Evoke Requesting Sentences	Possible Target Behavior
Board games	May I have a turn, please? Give me the dice, please. May we play another game?
Puzzles	May I have another piece, please? Help me, please.
Art activities	Give me the [scissors, glue, paper, glitter, stickers, etc.], please. Can you help me cut this, please? Give me the [specify color] crayon, please. May I have more [glue, glitter, paper, clay, paint, etc.], please?
Food preparation (e.g., making a peanut butter sandwich)	Give me the bread [peanut butter, jelly, spreader], please. Can you help me cut it, please? May I have a bite, please? May I have more, please?
Pretend play activities (e.g., playing tea party)	Give me the cup [saucer, tea, sugar, cream, spoon], please. Pour it in the cup, please. May I have more tea, please?
Children's games (e.g., Mother May I? and Go Fish.)	Mother, may I take one step? Give me your fives, please.

complete forms that describe events and comment on them. Possible target behaviors designed to teach a child to describe or comment include:

- Describing the characteristics of an object (e.g., "The ball is round and red."; "The kitty is white and fluffy.")
- Describing the parts of an object (e.g., "The car has tires, a hood, and a gas tank.")
- Describing how objects are used (e.g., "You use a comb to fix your hair."; "You use a pencil to write.")
- Using adverbs to describe action (e.g., "He runs fast!"; "She walked slowly.")
- Commenting on objects or events (e.g., "The flower is beautiful."; "This game is fun!")
- Using comments to describe action sequences (e.g., "He is walking to the store. Now he is shopping for groceries. Now he is paying for his groceries. Now he is walking home.")
- Expressing emotions (e.g., "I like this car!"; "I don't want to play that game.")

Object and picture stimuli can be used during discrete trial therapy to initially establish the just described sentence forms. See Table 8.3 for suggested strategies for establishing target behaviors for commenting. The clinician should move to a looser structure as the child learns each target behavior. Clinical activities that will evoke comments from a child include:

Describe how you would reinforce correct responses and give corrective feedback for incorrect responses for each of these tacts.

- Playing with toys that have parts to describe (e.g., toy farms, cars, trucks, trains) and evoking responses with such verbal stimuli as, "Tell me about this."; "What is this for?"; and "What's happening now?"
- Acting out verbs with the child and having the child describe the action and evoking responses with such verbal stimuli as "How are we running—quickly or slowly?" and "How are we singing—loudly or softly?"
- Completing art activities or cooking simple foods and evoking responses from the child by asking, "What do we do first?" "What are we doing now?" and "What do we need to do next?"

Some controlled treatment evidence suggests that it may be more effective to teach both mands (e.g., requesting a missing object) and tacts (naming) in the same session as against only the tacts (Arntzen & Almas, 2002; Carroll & Hess, 1987). Although these studies involved only simple labeling (tacts), it is possible that more complex tacts also may be better trained in conjunction with mands. On one trial, the child may describe an object

table 8.3

Stimuli for Discrete Trial Therapy for Establishing Comments (Tacts)

Target Behavior	Modeled Sentences	Evoked Sentences
Describing attributes (e.g., appearance, parts, and use) using object stimuli	Here is a comb. I want you to tell me about the comb. You may tell me what the comb looks like, what parts it has, what you use it for, or anything else you can think of. Say, "The comb is black; it has a handle; you use it to comb your hair."	Here is a comb. Tell me at least three things about the comb.
Producing adverbs using pictured stimuli	The girl sleeps soundly. How does the girl sleep? Say, "soundly." The rock star sings loudly. How does the rock star sing? Say, "loudly." The mother smiles warmly. How does the mother smile? Say, "warmly."	The girl sleeps soundly. How does the girl sleep? The rock star sings loudly. How does the rock star sing? The mother smiles warmly. How does the mother smile?
Commenting on action sequences using pictured stimuli	The puppy needs to be fed. What does his owner do first? Say, "Get the can of dog food." What does the owner do next? Say, "Open the can." What does the owner do next? Say, "Put the food in the dish." Then what happens? Say, "The owner gives the puppy the food." What happens last? Say, "The puppy eats the food."	The puppy needs to be fed. What does his owner do first? What does the owner do next? What does the owner do next? Then what happens? What happens last? Eventually, fade to: "The puppy needs to be fed. What happens?"

("This is a round, yellow ball.") and on the next trial, the child may request it ("May I have that round, yellow ball, please?").

Mands are often effective in reducing undesirable behaviors in children, because children who cannot make an oral or signed request may throw tantrums or exhibit aggressive behaviors (Reichle & Wacker, 1993). The results of studies that have reported on successful teaching of simple mands may be extended to complex mands (Winborn et al., 2002).

Asking Questions

When they learn to ask questions, children acquire a powerful tool in furthering their education. Children with language delays often need to be taught basic question forms through discrete trial therapy and then directly prompted to use them in naturalistic settings. Between the ages of 12 and 26 months, typically developing children begin by using one-word utterances with a rising intonation to ask yes/no questions (Justice & Ezell, 2002b). Refer to Table 8.4 for the developmental sequence of other question forms. It may be recalled from earlier chapters that we advocate a child-specific approach to intervention, and this developmental sequence should not be slavishly followed in writing target behaviors. If it is the clinician's judgment that learning to ask *how* questions will be most useful to a child in

table 8.4

Sequence of Development of Question-Asking

Age	Type of Question	Example of Production
1–2 yrs	*Yes/no* questions using rising intonation of voice	Go?
	Two-word *what* questions	What that?
	Two-word *where* questions	Where kitty?
2–3 yrs	Single-word *why* questions	Why?
	Three- to four-word:	
	what questions	What Grandma do(ing)?
	where questions	Where Daddy go(ing)?
	what questions using copula	What is that?
	where questions using copula	Where is ball?
	when questions	When go bye-bye?
3–4 yrs	*Yes/no* questions using auxiliary inversion	Is that my juice?
	Wh- and *how* questions using auxiliary inversion:	
	what	What are you making?
	where	Where is my dolly?
	when	When is my birthday?
	how	How is the baby?
	Do questions	Does he like baby?
	Tag questions	He is nice, isn't he?
	Modals	Would you read to me?
	Multiword *why* questions	Why is he crying?

Source: Compiled from Justice and Ezell (2002b), Paul (2001), and Roseberry-McKibbin and Hegde (2005).

the natural environment, then that should be the target behavior, even if the child has not acquired the earlier mastered question forms.

Initially, discrete trial therapy is useful in establishing question forms that are not in the child's repertoire. See Table 8.5 for suggested strategies for teaching question asking. The clinician should praise the child for correctly—even if imitatively—asking the question and then go ahead and answer the child's question as one would in naturalistic settings. The answer is also the naturalistic reinforcer for the child's question asking behavior:

Clinician [teaching *what* questions; using pictured stimulus]: You don't know what this is. Ask me, "What is this?"
Child: What is this?
Clinician: Excellent! You asked a good question! It is a computer.

When the child's question-asking behavior has been established in the clinic, questions may be evoked in more naturalistic contexts. Various structured activities can be used in which the clinician is careful to stimulate an adequate number of opportunities for the child to produce the target behavior. Possible clinical activities include:

- *Dialogic storybook reading* (see Chapter 10). This is an interactive style of reading to a child that encourages the child to ask questions and comment on the story.
- *Children's games.* Many can be adapted to evoke questions from a child (e.g., hide-and-seek using objects for *where* questions, guessing games for *what* and *who* questions, etc.).
- *Board games.* Children can be prompted to ask *how* to play the game, to ask *what* comes next, *who* takes a turn next, and so forth. (See Photo 8.1.)

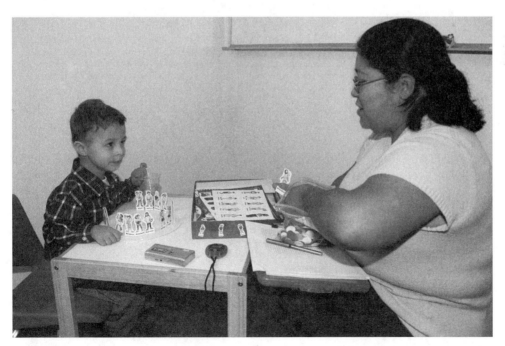

photo 8.1
Whose turn is it? Board games can be used during more advanced language training to evoke a number of target behaviors, such as pronouns.

table 8.5

Verbal Stimuli for Establishing Questions in Sentence Forms

Remember to reinforce directly (e.g., "Good question!" and by answering the child's question).

Target Behavior	Modeled Sentences	Evoked Sentences
Production of *what* questions Using only verbal stimuli	When you want to know something, you ask a question. If you want to know a person's name, you say, "What is your name?" You don't know my name. Say, "What is your name?"	You don't know my name. What do you say?
Using pictured stimuli	You don't know what this is. Say, "What is this?" You don't know what they are doing. Say, "What are they doing?"	You don't know what this is. What do you say? You don't know what they are doing. What do you say?
Production of *why* questions Using pictured stimuli	When you don't understand something, you ask, "Why?" Look at this picture. He looks mad. Ask me, "Why is he mad?" Look. The pig is dirty. You want to know why. Say, "Why is the pig dirty?" Look. The toy is broken. You want to know why. Say, "Why is the toy broken?"	Look at this picture. He looks mad. You want to know why. What do you say? Look. The pig is dirty. You want to know why. What do you say? Look. The toy is broken. You want to know why. What do you say?
Production of *when* questions Using only verbal stimuli	If you want to know what time something happens or is going to happen, you can ask a question that starts with the word *when*. So, pretend your mother says your family is going to the zoo. You want to know when. Say, "When are we going to the zoo?" Your friend tells you he is going to visit his grandmother. You want to know when. Say, "When are you going to visit your grandmother?" You want to know what time I go to bed. Say, "When do you go to bed?"	Your mother says your family is going to the zoo. You want to know when. What do you say? Your friend tells you he is going to visit his grandmother. You want to know when. What do you say? You want to know what time I go to bed. What do you say?

(continued)

- *Role-playing activities.* Pretending to order food in a restaurant ("What would you like today?"), to go grocery shopping ("Where is the [name food item]?"), to take a bus trip ("Where is my stop?"), and so forth.

Producing Syntactically More Complex Sentences

Treatment research on teaching syntactically complex sentences is limited. Although we need more controlled evidence than exists, there is no empirical reason to assume that complex sentence forms are immune to shaping, prompting, modeling, and differential reinforcement effects. Nonetheless, many complex sentence structures are expansions of basic structures. Children with language disorders may have difficulty advancing beyond the production of simple sentence forms. As they enter adolescence, they may continue to pro-

table 8.5   *(continued)*

Target Behavior	Modeled Sentences	Evoked Sentences
Production of *where* questions Using only verbal stimuli	When you don't know how to find someone or something, you ask a question that starts with *where*. So, let's pretend you don't know where your sister is. Ask me, "Where is my sister?" Pretend you are going to a birthday party, but you don't know where it is. Say, "Where is the birthday party?"	Pretend you don't know where your sister is. What do you say? Pretend you are going to a birthday party, but you don't know where it is. What do you say?
Production of *who* questions Using only verbal stimuli Using pictured stimuli	If you want to know which person did something, or you don't know someone, you ask a question that begins with *who*. Pretend someone cleaned up your room. You want to know who did it. Say, "Who cleaned up my room?" Pretend you have new neighbors. You don't know who they are. Say, "Who are the new neighbors?" Look at this picture. You don't know this boy. Say, "Who is that boy?"	Pretend someone cleaned up your room. You want to know who did it. What do you say? Pretend you have new neighbors. You don't know who they are. What do you say? Look at this picture. You don't know this boy. What do you say?
Production of *how* questions Using only verbal stimuli Using object stimuli	If you don't know the way to do something, you ask a question starting with *how*. Pretend you're hungry. You want a peanut butter sandwich, but you've never made one before. Say, "How do I make a peanut butter sandwich?" Here is a puzzle. Pretend you don't know the way to put it together. Ask, "How can I put this puzzle together?" Here is a new game you haven't played before. Ask me, "How do I play this game?"	Pretend you're hungry. You want a peanut butter sandwich, but you've never made one before. What do you say? Here is a puzzle. Pretend you don't know the way to put it together. What do you say? Here is a new game you haven't played before. What do you say?

duce syntactically less complex sentences than do their typically developing peers. Compared to their normally speaking peers, adolescents with language disorders characteristically produce fewer compound sentences (e.g., "He ate a pizza, *and* his wife ate a salad.), fewer dependent clauses (e.g., "*After I finish this paper*, I will go to bed."), and fewer embedded clauses (e.g., "The man *who was standing on the corner* waved to the taxi driver."). The production of syntactically more complex sentences may be taught, as any other target behavior can be, through discrete trial therapy. See Table 8.6 for suggested strategies for teaching advanced syntactical structures.

As responses become more established, the clinician should move as quickly as possible to the level of conversational speech in naturalistic settings. Direct prompts, including modeling when necessary, should be used to evoke complex sentences from the child. For example:

Clinician [after evoking the shorter productions]: You said your "daddy works hard." You said, "then he comes home." Can you say that in one big sentence? Say, "My daddy works hard, and then he comes home."

■ ■ | ■ | ■   **table 8.6**

Evoking Complex Sentence Structures

Target Behavior	Modeled Sentences	Evoked Sentences
Compound sentences (e.g., The man read a book, and his wife watched television.) using pictured stimuli	Here are two pictures of people doing things. We can make one big sentence about these pictures. Say, "The man read a book, and the woman watched television."	Make one big sentence about these two pictures.
	Here are two pictures. We can make one big sentence about these pictures. Say, "The elephant is big, and the mouse is little."	Make one big sentence about these two pictures.
	Expand further, using adverbs and compound adjectives	
Dependent clauses (many varieties; modify according to the specific target behavior)	The children will eat dinner first. Then, they will do their homework. We can make one big sentence about the children. Say, "After the children eat dinner, they will do their homework."	The children will eat dinner first. Then, they will do their homework. Make one big sentence about the children.
	The boy is happy. It is his birthday. We can make one big sentence about this boy. Say, "The boy is happy because it is his birthday."	The boy is happy. It is his birthday. Make one big sentence about the boy.
Embedded dependent clauses	The woman is my mother. She works in the cafeteria. We can make one big sentence about this woman. Say, "The woman who works in the cafeteria is my mother."	The woman is my mother. She works in the cafeteria. Make one big sentence about this woman.
	He borrowed my lawn mower yesterday. It is broken. We can make one big sentence about the lawn mower. Say, "The lawn mower he borrowed from me yesterday is broken."	He borrowed my lawn mower yesterday. It is broken. Make one big sentence about the lawn mower.

Child: My daddy works hard, and then he comes home.
Clinician: That's nice! You said it in one big sentence!

Subsequently, the clinician should fade the model. After first evoking shorter productions (e.g., "My sister goes to school every day" and "She does homework."), the clinician may ask the child to combine them.

Instruction in the use of syntactically more complex sentences can also be embedded in literacy instruction (see Chapter 10), because the written language mode is inherently more syntactically complex than conversational oral language. Complex sentence forms the child can produce in speech may be included in literacy instruction. Writing short stories based on pictured stimuli can be useful to teach writing longer sentences.

Milieu Teaching: A Treatment Variation

Throughout this discussion on establishing the use of longer and more complex sentence structures, we have advocated for the use of discrete trial therapy in initial stages and then various clinical activities to evoke the target behaviors in more natu-ralistic contexts. Such naturalistic clinical activities are similar to those used in milieu teaching—a treatment method that has been experi-mentally demonstrated to be effective. Milieu teaching and other sim-ilar methods are sometimes described under the umbrella term, *naturalistic language training techniques* (Hart, 1985).

> Parents who learn milieu teaching can be especially effective in teaching new language skills to their children. Parents have many op-portunities to embed language treatment into daily routines.

Milieu teaching embeds behavioral principles into naturalistic settings (Hancock & Kaiser, 2002). The overall goal of milieu teaching is to evoke and reinforce child-initiated communicative interactions in response to environmental stimuli; therefore, the method is child-centered. Its two main strengths are that it uses natural contexts of communication and uses the conversation format to teach skills. It is a collection of methods that has been most extensively researched with children who have severe language disorders, as in devel-opmental disability or autism. Results have generally been positive, with demonstrated gen-eralization of target behaviors across stimulus materials, settings, and individuals. Using controlled experimental methods, the effects of milieu teaching have been systematically replicated in different settings by different clinicians. Therefore, this procedure is recom-mended for general application (Kaiser & Hester, 1994; Warren, 1992; Warren et al., 1994; Warren et al., 1993; Yoder et al., 1994). Positive effects have also been shown on the lan-guage of children whose parents have received training in the use of various methods as-sociated with this approach (Hemmeter & Kaiser, 1994; Kaiser, Hancock, & Nietfeld, 2000; Yoder & Warren, 2002).

The milieu approach is not entirely new. The actual treatment techniques used in it are based on proven behavioral principles. Contingency management, described in previ-ous chapters, is the main treatment procedure, even in the milieu approach. The novel as-pect of the approach is its reliance on naturalistic contexts in which language responses are evoked and reinforced. Compared to discrete trials, the approach provides a looser struc-ture in which language targets are established. The advantage is that the skills established may generalize to natural settings more readily than those that are established through the discrete trial method.

Three specific methods used within a milieu teaching framework have been shown to have efficacy in evoking and expanding child language: (1) mand-model, (2) delay, and (3) incidental teaching. Hart (1985) provided detailed descriptions of these three methods, summarized in the following sections.

Mand-model. The objective of the **mand-model** technique is to establish joint attention as a cue for verbalization (Rogers-Warren & Warren, 1980). Parents using the mand-model technique observe the child approach a desired object and immediately prompt (or mand) the child to produce an utterance (e.g., "Tell me what you want."). If the child does not re-spond, or gives a minimal one-word response, the adult can then provide a model to ex-pand the child's utterance, as follows:

Adult (observing a child looking at a videotape): Tell me what you want.
Child: Movie
Adult: Tell me, "I want movie."
Child: I want movie.
Adult: Good! You said, "I want movie!" Here it is!

The mand-model procedure has been shown to be effective in teaching children to make requests (Mobayed et al., 2000; Rogers-Warren & Warren, 1980). The mand-model technique establishes instances of adult-directed moments of joint attention, although the overall goal of milieu teaching is child-initiated communicative interaction. It is a good step toward encouraging a child's initiations of communication, but, "what is needed (and what occurs in the natural environment) is for verbalization to come under the control of stimuli other than the attending presence of an adult" (Hart, 1985, p. 72). Additional techniques, such as *delay* and *incidental teaching* train a child to call an adult's attention to an object or event, which results in a child-initiated, rather than an adult-directed, communicative interaction.

> What is the overall goal of milieu teaching?

Delay. A technique used in the milieu approach to teach a child to respond to environmental stimuli other than listener attention as cues for verbalization is called **delay.** Rather than immediately prompt a child to produce an utterance, adults using the delay technique *wait*, with expectant facial expressions, for the child to initiate a communicative interaction. Halle, Marshall, and Spradlin (1981) outlined the following steps in using delay to spontaneously evoke language from a child:

1. An adult, perhaps displaying some appealing object, looks expectantly at the child.
2. When the child looks at the adult, the object, or both, the adult continues to look expectantly at the child and does not speak for at least 15 seconds.
3. If the child does not verbalize, the adult provides a prompt, and, if necessary, a full model, to evoke a verbalization. The adult repeats the prompt or model twice, each time waiting for up to 15 seconds for the child to speak.
4. After giving the child three models, the adult gives the child the desired object—whether or not the child has produced a verbalization.

The objective of the delay technique is to encourage the child to speak first—it is, however, a procedure that still requires the attending presence of an adult to present an opportunity for the child to initiate (See Photo 8.2 of a clinician using the delay technique). The goal of having the child independently initiate a communicative interaction with an adult is more likely to be realized using procedures of incidental teaching.

Incidental teaching. A technique that helps teach elaborated language productions to children who independently initiate a communicative interaction with an adult is called **incidental teaching.** In incidental teaching, the adult waits for the child to initiate a topic, prompts the child's elaboration of language, and then provides the reinforcer specified by the child's initiation (Hart & Risley, 1975). The method has been extended to teaching reading skills in children with autism (McGee et al., 1983; McGee, Krantz, & McClannahan, 1986). Steps involved in incidental teaching of oral communication skills include:

1. When a child initiates an interaction, the adult gives the child full attention, creating joint focus of attention on the child-initiated topic.
2. The adult asks for language elaboration (e.g., "What do you want?" or, whatever verbal stimulus will evoke an elaboration of the topic). The adult may provide a model prior to asking for elaboration (e.g., "You want a cookie! What do you want?").

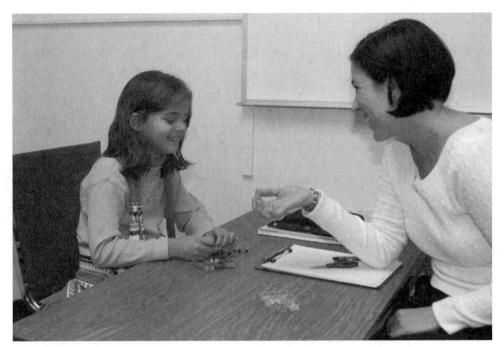

photo 8.2
This clinician is using a time-delay technique, waiting for the child to ask her for the glue with an expectant look on her face.

3. If the child does not elaborate, the adult provides a further prompt. If the expected response has not been previously observed in the child's language repertoire, the adult provides a full model of an appropriate elaboration for the child to imitate.
4. When the child provides a language elaboration, either spontaneously or in response to a prompt, the adult reinforces the utterance verbally or gives the child the desired object (e.g., "That's right—good for you! Here's your cookie!").

Parents, teachers, and clinicians using incidental teaching methods do not have to passively trust the "natural environment" to provide stimuli likely to evoke a child's initiation of a communicative interaction. Adults should arrange the environment with various stimuli that are likely to provide opportunities for the child to initiate. During crafts activities, for example, materials necessary to complete a project can be kept out of the child's reach, so that the child must ask an adult for them. Parents can be taught not to anticipate a child's needs by providing whatever it is they think the child wants, but to *wait* for the child to initiate the communicative interaction, prompting for more language when the child does so.

Teaching Conversational Speech

When previously learned skills have been expanded into varied sentence types, the child may be advanced to the conversational level. The treatment setting should become increasingly similar to typical environments to enhance generalization and maintenance of the target behaviors in natural settings. The final goal of language intervention is the maintenance of conversational skills in social situations. Target behaviors must be trained at the conversational level. Final conversational probes should be held in natural settings. A plan must also be in place to promote maintenance of conversational skills over time in natural settings (see Chapter 9 for details).

At this advanced stage of treatment, conversational skills should be taught in conjunction with previously trained target behaviors. Conversational skills are typically described as pragmatic aspects of language. Pragmatics is the study of social use of language. As such, any communicative attempt is pragmatic. Pragmatic skills may be taught in two dynamic stages: production of single words or phrases in socially meaningful situations, and the production of such conversational skills as initiating a social interaction, maintaining a topic of conversation, taking conversational turns, and using conversational repair strategies. Obviously, the first stage of pragmatic training involves less complex target skills than the second stage.

For some children, especially those with such associated clinical conditions as autism or developmental disability, a deficit in social communication may be either the only deficit or the most serious deficit. Furthermore, children with cognitive deficits who have received optimal language intervention may still exhibit significant difficulty producing their clinically acquired language in social situations. Children with developmental disability or a pervasive developmental disorder (particularly with Asperger's Syndrome), may need sustained treatment at the level of conversational speech. Characteristics of language disorders in children with associated clinical conditions, as well as modifications in assessment and treatment procedures to address those characteristics, will be discussed in future chapters.

When the words and phrases taught in the clinic are produced in natural environments to achieve the desired effects, those simpler target behaviors will have achieved their pragmatic goal. The conversational skills, which are more complex pragmatic skills, also need to be initially established in the clinic and then generalized and maintained in the natural environment.

The pragmatic approach does not replace semantic or grammatical training targets, nor does it require a different set of treatment procedures. All of the treatment procedures discussed in previous chapters are means of teaching conversational (pragmatic) skills. The basic treatment sequence, involving operationally defined target behaviors, reliable baserates of target behaviors, treatment using the principles of reinforcement and corrective feedback, and collection of data to monitor the child's progress, is useful in treating pragmatic language behaviors.

Assuming that the clinician has established the basic language skills and their generalized productions, we will concentrate on conversational skills in this section. Conversational skills build on semantic, morphologic, and syntactic targets the child has previously learned. This section will describe techniques to teach selected conversational skills. We will begin at the level of controlled conversation and then move to spontaneous conversation, incorporating specific conversational skills of topic initiation, topic maintenance, turn-taking, and conversational repair.

Controlled Conversation

For most children, controlled conversation is an intermediate skill that bridges the gap between sentence production on highly structured discrete trials and loosely structured spontaneous conversation. **Controlled conversation** is verbal interaction between the clinician and the child that is more directed than spontaneous conversation. To evoke a controlled conversation, the clinician should select activities that will encourage production of the target behavior during directed, prompted, hinted, conversational speech. For example, if the target behavior is production of pronouns such as *he* and *she*, the clinician may set up an activity using popular toys with identifiable genders. Storybooks with pictures of men and women or boys and girls also may serve the purpose. If the target behavior is production of prepositions, the clinician may use a toy farm in which animals can go *in* the barn or *out* of the corral, or a toy train that can go *on* the track and *over* and *under* the bridge. Conversation regarding the course of the activity should be kept as natural as possible. The clinician should let the child take the lead in talking about the objects, events, and imaginary stories the stimuli prompt. In the early stage of controlled conversation, however, the child may need a level of support and assistance that will vary across children. When the child's language production is limited, the clinician should ask questions about events, characters, stories, and activities as he or she would with any child. The clinician should prompt or hint only when necessary. It is only when prompts and hints fail to evoke conversation, does the clinician model sentences for the child to imitate.

There are countless activities a creative clinician can use to evoke target behaviors at the level of conversational speech in the clinic setting. The major requirement of such activities is that they are somewhat more structured and directed than are spontaneous conversational exchanges. The sessions are structured to give the child practice in producing the target behaviors in response to more naturalistic stimuli. Hints, prompts, and models make the exchange more directed than typical conversation. The clinician should avoid unplanned play activities that are conducted for the sake of making therapy "fun" without evoking the targeted behaviors. Such activities are a waste of valuable therapeutic time.

When treatment is shifted to the level of controlled conversation, the clinician may find that the child's correct response rates drop. To improve the response rates, the child may need extensive modeling. The clinician may continue to model for a while at this higher level and then fade it. If the need for modeling-imitation sequence persists, it may be necessary to drop to the level of controlled sentence production for a brief period of time.

Spontaneous Conversation

Spontaneous conversation is evoked by social and natural contexts and stimuli. These stimuli may be physical (e.g., another child's play activity being observed) or verbal (e.g., "Hi, how are you today?"). To promote spontaneous conversational speech, the clinician needs to fade the special stimuli provided throughout the treatment sequence. The child should produce the target behavior during conversation in the clinic setting that is evoked by stimuli inherent to the conversational topic and the natural interactions, with no prompting and certainly no modeling from the clinician. Treatment is conducted with a loose structure that closely approximates conditions encountered in the child's natural environment.

Some children may produce their newly acquired language behaviors socially and appropriately without the need for extensive training at the conversational speech levels. Other children may fail to produce their newly learned communicative behaviors in social contexts, or their productions may be inappropriate or irrelevant. Such children require instruction in the production of language response classes in the context of social communication.

Some children who have normally acquired basic language skills may be notably deficient in social communication. In such cases, it may be necessary to target social communication—mostly conversation—during treatment.

Conversational skills may be taught using the procedures described in previous chapters. Defining target behaviors operationally, baserating their pretreatment frequency, conducting treatment with reinforcement and corrective feedback, and collecting data to monitor the child's progress are all parts of conversational skill training. Discarding the discrete trial procedure will help promote conversational speech that is child-centered—the child's lead may be followed in picking a topic, and the child's interest will help direct spontaneous conversation. The training structure will be looser, within the context of natural discourse designed to evoke spontaneous speech. More natural consequences will replace any tangible or primary reinforcers used previously. Instead of giving explicit verbal praise, tokens, or primary reinforcers, the clinician will reinforce the child's production of language skills during conversation through such naturally occurring consequences as smiles, attention, agreement or negation, responses to questions, and so forth.

Any behavior can be baserated! Procedures will vary according to the type of behavior targeted.

Specific conversational skills targeted for intervention include:

- Eye contact
- Topic initiation
- Topic maintenance
- Turn-taking
- Conversational repair strategies

Eye Contact

The extent of eye contact children learn to maintain during conversational discourse is shaped in large part by the culture in which they are raised. In some cultures, such as many within Hispanic and Asian groups, children are not encouraged to maintain direct eye contact with adults, and a downcast expression is thought to be a sign of respect (Roseberry-McKibbin, 2002). If there is a possibility that a child's lack of eye contact may be the result of cultural influence, the clinician should consult with the child's parents and teachers before setting a goal for the establishment of that skill (see Chapter 11 for information regarding cultural differences).

In mainstream American culture, direct eye contact is valued as an important part of conversational discourse; it is a sign that listeners and speakers are engaged with each other and are attending to the topic of the conversation. Among adults, a person who avoids eye contact during conversation may be thought of as somewhat dishonest or evasive. Children who do not establish eye contact may be considered inattentive or disrespectful to adults. American parents often reprimand their young children by saying, "Look at me when I'm talking to you!" It should be noted, however, that while the listener is expected to maintain eye contact with the speaker, the speaker may occasionally look away from the listener.

Children with language disorders often need help in maintaining eye contact during conversation. As we shall learn in Chapter 13, a lack of eye contact is often the first sign of a serious language disorder associated with autism. Even children with less severe language disorders, however, may need direct intervention to learn how to maintain eye contact. The clinician should teach maintenance of eye contact with the following procedures, to be modified as found necessary to meet the needs of the individual child.

Baserate the frequency and duration of eye contact. To baserate eye contact before treatment, the clinician should engage the child in conversation with the help of toys, pictures, or activities as needed. The number of times the child makes any kind of eye contact should be counted, and the duration for which eye contact is maintained should be measured. Some children may give no eye contact at all during the treatment session, in which case the baseline measure is zero. Other children may give very fleeting eye contact, lasting only a second or less, two or three times a session. Measures of eye contact should be taken over at least two sessions to get accurate baseline data before beginning intervention for it.

After baseline data are established, the clinician should begin treatment. The frequency and duration of eye contact should be measured during all treatment sessions. For example, a clinician might document that a child maintained eye contact five times during a 30-minute session, and the duration of eye contact ranged from 1 second to 3 seconds (a range or a median figure is preferable to an average). Such measures help document increases in the frequency and duration of eye contact.

Give instructions on eye contact. The clinician may begin treatment by giving such instructions as the following: "Johnny, when people talk to each other, they *look* at each other. When I talk to you, I want you to look at me so I know you are listening to what I say." A school clinician might talk to a small child about how "we listen with our *whole body*; we listen with our *ears* open, our *eyes* on the teacher, and our *body* still."

Model eye contact during conversation. Just as they do for correct verbal behaviors, clinicians should model eye contact for the child to imitate. At all times during treatment, clinicians should keep their faces in the child's line of sight.

Prompt the child to maintain eye contact. Children can be prompted to maintain eye contact with a variety of cues. A child might benefit from such visual cues as a picture of two people looking into each other's eyes. Verbal cues might include such prompts as "Look at me" or "Where're you looking?" The clinician may give a nonverbal manual cue by pointing toward his or her own eyes to draw the child's visual attention. The clinician may give a tactile cue, perhaps getting the child's attention and subsequent eye gaze by lightly touching the child's hand. If the child still fails to make eye contact, the clinician should use manual guidance, by gently directing the child's head to a position in which eye contact can be made.

The prompts that have been described were arranged in order from less intrusive to more intrusive. The clinician should start with the least intrusive prompt necessary to evoke a correct response. If a child responds to initial instructions and modeling, no other cues should be offered. Other, more intrusive cues should be offered only when less intrusive cues fail to help maintain eye contact. As with any other target behavior, prompts for eye contact and other conversational skills should be kept to a minimum and faded as the child begins to maintain eye contact.

Reinforce the child for making eye contact. Reinforcement for eye contact, as is the case with all conversational skills, should consist of natural consequences that usually result during normal discourse. A clinician can, for example, immediately smile when the child makes eye contact, giving the child full and enthusiastic attention—a reinforcing event that is consistent with what typically happens in the natural environment when people make eye contact with each other.

What kind of reinforcement is used when tokens, to be exchanged for a small prize at the end of the session, are given for correct responses? (Hint: See Chapter 6.)

Based on the frequency and duration of eye contact measured during treatment, the clinician should judge whether the target skill is increasing. If there is no increase, the clinician may have to use other less naturalistic consequences. A token system backed up with small gifts may be effective.

Other kinds of consequences may be just as effective as a token system. For example, a child who gives virtually no eye contact may love to play with toy trains. The clinician may bring in a toy train and a track that must be put together. The clinician may then hold each piece of the track up to his or her face parallel to the eyes. Consequently, the child who looks for the stimulus also will look at the clinician's face. When eye contact is established, the clinician should reinforce the child by giving the object (in this case, the train track piece) and by such verbal reinforcers as "You looked at me—good for you!" "Great, you looked at me!" "Thank you for looking at me!" "I like it when you look at me!" and so forth. Such verbal praise is probably preferable to the semantically odd "Good looking!"

Shape longer durations of eye contact. If it is necessary to establish eye contact with less naturalistic reinforcement methods, it may also be necessary to shape gradually longer durations of eye contact. A child who has a baseline eye contact close to zero may need to be immediately reinforced for any kind of fleeting eye contact at all. If the verbal praise is effective, instances of child's fleeting eye contact should increase. The clinician should then "up the ante" by requiring gradually longer (just two or three seconds more at a time) durations of eye contact before reinforcing the child. As the child learns to maintain progressively longer durations of eye contact, any less naturalistic reinforcers used may be faded out, and the behavior can be maintained through more natural reinforcing consequences (e.g., the clinician's attending to the child's conversation, smiles, head nods, etc.).

Topic Initiation: Get It Going!

Topic initiation refers to a speaker's introduction of new conversational topics. In effect, it is the initiation of conversation. Of all the conversational skills, topic initiation is probably the most spontaneous (least under the control of explicit stimuli). Many children with language disorders either fail to initiate topics or introduce inappropriate topics at inappropriate times; hence, topic initiation is a treatment target.

Baserate topic initiation. To baserate topic initiation, the clinician should engage the child in a series of structured play activities. The number of times the child speaks first, initiating conversation on an appropriate topic *without* prompting from the clinician, should be counted. The baseline data should be taken over at least two sessions and recorded (e.g., "Johnny initiated conversation with the clinician once during the first session and not at all during the second," or, as is very likely with children with language disorders, "During two sessions, Johnny did not initiate conversation with the clinician."). Once the baseline data have been taken, treatment will begin. In each session, the clinician will record the frequency of topic initiation to document progress (e.g., "Today, Johnny initiated conversation three times with the clinician.").

Use a variety of stimuli. At this advanced stage of language treatment, it is not necessary or even desirable to limit the number and type of stimuli available to the child. To tempt the child to initiate conversation, it is best to have a variety of stimuli available to suggest new topics for conversation. Novel and interesting objects, pictures, storybooks, topic cards (for children who can read), toys and structured play situations (such as a toy kitchen) may help trigger conversation.

If the child is hesitant to initiate, the clinician can draw the child's attention to a manipulated object or an unusual stimulus. The clinician also may show the initial picture of a series of pictures that tell a story. After doing so, the clinician should wait a few seconds to give the child the opportunity to initiate conversation about the stimulus presented.

Prompt the child. Topic initiation may be prompted using verbal and visual cues. If the child is hesitant to speak, a gentle verbal prompt such as, "Tell me!" may be given. Sentence completion, or cloze, techniques can be used to give a partial model of initiating topic. The clinician may prompt the child to start a conversation or story telling (e.g., in reference to a picture showing a family riding their bicycles, "They are. . . ."). The clinician should deliver such verbal prompts with an expectant expression inviting the child's initiation of the topic.

Visual cues, such as picture cards, may also be used to suggest new topics of conversation. Picture cards should reflect situations, actions, or objects that the child is likely to encounter in the natural environment and should be relevant to the child's cultural background. Although this is generally a good recommendation, it is possible that unfamiliar stimuli or situations may provoke more conversation from a child. Therefore, the clinician should experiment with stimuli that include familiar and novel events, animals, objects, or people. If the child is reluctant to talk because of unfamiliar stimuli, the clinician may select more from the child's family and cultural background. If the child can read, topic cards with just a written description of a potential topic (e.g., "my birthday party") can be used. Children can be taught to use topic cards to cue themselves to initiate a new topic of conversation. As treatment progresses, the topic cards can be faded, and the clinician can ask the child to think of new topics to talk about.

> Sometimes showing a child an unfamiliar picture or scene may help provoke conversation and teach something new. A child from the inner city, for example, who has never seen the ocean, might be stimulated to ask good questions about a picture depicting a coastline scene.

Reinforce topic initiation. The give-and-take of conversational discourse is intrinsically reinforcing to typically developing children. Adults reinforce the topic initiation behavior of typically developing children by giving attention when their children initiate. For children with language disorders, however, it may be necessary to offer more concrete and less naturalistic reinforcement in the initial stages of treatment.

Verbal praise specifically directed toward the behavior of topic initiation, for example, can be given any time the child says anything without explicit prompts or models (e.g., "Oh, I am so happy you asked me about that!" or "Thank you for talking to me!" or "Yes, I want to talk about that, too!"). At first, the clinician should accept statements that are even remotely connected to the current topic, stimuli, or events. As the behavior of topic initiation becomes more established, the clinician should require more spontaneous comments before delivering reinforcement. To make topic initiation more spontaneous, the clinician should fade all prompts, cards, pictures, and any other special stimuli, and reinforcement.

Topic Maintenance: Keep It Going!

Topic maintenance refers to extended durations for which a speaker continues to talk on the same subject. The duration is variable and dependent on the individual conversational episode and social acceptance. A person who frequently inserts irrelevant comments or who abruptly switches conversational topics is lacking in topic maintenance skills.

Children who have language disorders often not only have trouble initiating conversation, they also have trouble keeping the conversation going; in other words, they tend to be deficient in topic maintenance skills. Therefore, topic maintenance is a frequently targeted conversational skill in language treatment.

Baserate topic maintenance. The topic maintenance skill should be baserated before treatment begins. To baserate topic maintenance, the clinician should measure the duration for which the child speaks about the same topic *without* prompting. There should at least be three independent baserate measures of topic maintenance. The range of measures should be summarized in the treatment plan (e.g., "Johnny remained on topic for a minimum of 10 seconds to a maximum of 1 minute.")

Let the child suggest and choose topics. The clinician should ask the child and the parents to write down a list of topics the child may want to talk about. The clinician also may offer various topics for conversation initially and ask the child to select one (e.g., "Do you want to talk about your summer vacation, about your pet dog, or about your last birthday party?"). Later on in treatment, as the child's topic maintenance skills improve, the child can be prompted to select a topic without the clinician's suggestions or without consulting a prepared list. Topic maintenance can thus be taught in conjunction with topic initiation; as the child becomes more proficient in initiating conversation, the clinician should follow the child's lead in introducing the topic.

The clinician should at first target a brief, realistic duration of time for which the child will be required to speak on the same topic. Alternatively, the clinician can set a target number of words to be produced on a topic. Using the shaping procedure, the clinician should gradually increase the targeted time duration or number of words as the child's topic maintenance skills improve.

Prompt the child to help maintain the topic. The clinician should use verbal prompts to help the child keep the conversation going on the same topic. To do this, the clinician can use phrases and questions, such as:

- Tell me more
- Say more
- Say it in long sentences
- What about that?
- What happened next?
- Who said what?
- Who did what?
- Where did it happen?
- When did it happen?
- How did it happen?
- How did it end?
- What do you like about it?
- What was funny [interesting, bad, sad] about it?

Such verbal prompts help stimulate more speech on the same topic.

Reinforcement and corrective feedback for topic maintenance. The clinician should reinforce the child for talking continuously on the same topic. Again, while typically developing children are naturally reinforced for topic maintenance through their enjoyment of the give-and-take of conversation, children with language disorders may initially need more explicit reinforcement. Also, corrective feedback may be necessary if the child strays off topic during the conversation.

Verbal praise can be effective with many children, and should be tried before using any other forms of reinforcement. The clinician might tell the child, "Good! Keep going!" or "I like the way you are still talking about . . ." (e.g., " . . . your new goldfish!"). Verbal corrective feedback can be given if the child makes an irrelevant comment or abruptly switches the topic. The clinician can say firmly, "Stop!" and then ask for more details or ask questions about the same topic to encourage the child to return to the topic. As the child's topic maintenance skills improve, the clinician should share the data with the child to offer informative feedback which also may act as a reinforcer. For instance, the clinician may show a bar graph and say, "See, you talked on the same topic for 2 minutes last time, but this time, you talked for 4 minutes! This is great!"

Probe for generalization. There are no norms on the duration of topic maintenance or word output on the same topic that the clinician can apply to children of different ages. Therefore, the clinician will have to make judgments about the adequacy of the skill. When the child has learned to talk for acceptable durations or produces a reasonable number of words on four to five topics, the clinician should probe with new topics that have not been used during treatment to see if the skill has generalized. If the child does not maintain new topics of conversation during the probe, the clinician should train a few additional topics. Treatment should then alternate between training using a few exemplar topics (adding new ones if necessary) and probing for generalization.

Turn-Taking Skill: I Talk, You Talk

Typically developing children learn turn-taking skills as infants, especially when the adults around them engage in "baby games" such as Patty-Cake or How Big Is Baby? Adults who bounce babies on their knees and then stop, waiting for the babies to indicate through a vocalization or body movement that they want more, are reinforcing the type of turn-taking skills that are important to the give-and-take of communication. Later on, adults typically teach the importance of turn-taking by discouraging inappropriate interruptions.

"Don't interrupt!" is a commonly heard command adults give to their children who have not learned turn-taking skills.

Turn-taking skills involve the speaker and listener exchanging roles at a socially acceptable rate during conversation. Deficiencies in turn-taking skills become apparent when a child interrupts a speaker or does not respond to cues to talk. Children with language disorders often do not take turns appropriately and may need direct intervention to learn turn-taking skills.

Baserate the child's turn-taking skills. To baserate turn-taking skills, the clinician should count the number of times during a session a child interrupts the clinician or does not take a cue to talk. Once again, minimally three independent measures should be recorded. In this case, the baseline data will show the frequency of a behavior the clinician wants to decrease (e.g., the interruptions) and will also show the frequency of a behavior the clinician wants to increase (e.g., responding to cues to talk). Three baseline data for 10-minute conversations with a child, for example, may show that the child interrupted the clinician 8 to 12 times and responded only to 2 of 20 cues to talk (or, responded to cues to talk with only 10 percent accuracy). The treatment goal then would be to decrease the number of interruptions and increase the number of times the child responds to cues to talk. If subsequent treatment data show that the child only interrupted the clinician 2 to 3 times during a 10-minute conversation and that the child responded to 6 out of 10 cues to talk (a response rate of 60 percent), the clinician will have documented improved turn taking skills (Atherton & Hegde, 1996).

Prompt the child to take turns. Verbal or nonverbal prompts are helpful in teaching a child to take turns. Verbal prompts might consist of telling a child, "Your turn!" when the child should talk. Nonverbal signals might include a hand gesture coupled with an expectant facial expression to let the child know it is time to talk. If a child begins to interrupt, a verbal cue such as "Stop!" or a nonverbal cue such as a finger on the lips can be used to interrupt the interruption.

Objects may also be used to prompt turn-taking skills. A real or toy microphone, for example, may be used as a discriminative stimulus to teach the role of a speaker. The clinician may exchange it with the child, teaching the child to speak only when holding the microphone and to listen when the clinician is holding it (Atherton & Hegde, 1996). When using such objects, clinicians should follow the same rules they impose on the child (i.e., talk only when holding the microphone and listen intently when the child is talking with microphone in hand).

Reinforce the child for correct turn-taking. Regardless of how the behavior is evoked, any turn-taking must be promptly reinforced. A child should be verbally praised for talking when the microphone is handed to him or her. The clinician might say, "Thank you for talking when I give you the microphone!" Similarly, the child should be praised for yielding the floor (as when the child hands the microphone to clinician without prompts). The clinician might say, "Thank you for letting me take my turn!"

The child might also be taught to play the clinician's role. The child will then decide whose turn it is to speak. The child may be reinforced for saying, "It's your turn now," for giving the clinician a nonverbal signal to speak, or for handing the microphone. Many times, children will find having such control over the course of the treatment session to be reinforcing.

Fade the prompts. When the child meets a predetermined performance criterion, as set forth in the treatment plan, (e.g., no errors of turn-taking in two consecutive conversational exchanges), all signals and other prompts used as special discriminative stimuli should be faded. A brief period of silence after talking for a while with an expectant facial expression will help fade the use of a microphone or the verbal prompts (e.g., "Your turn"). A hand gesture to speak will help fade other stimuli, which will then be faded into a brief silent interval and eye contact to suggest it is the child's turn to talk. Additional sessions using new activities and new topics of conversation should be held to probe for production of turn-taking skills without the use of signals or other special discriminative stimuli to prompt the child. The child may be required to meet a specified criterion (e.g., at least 90 percent accuracy in turn-taking while not receiving reinforcers) before moving on to other targets.

Conversational Repair: Get It Right!

Conversational repair strategies are verbal behaviors both listeners and speakers exhibit when there are breakdowns in communication. Listeners use conversational repair strategies when they ask for clarification (e.g., "I'm sorry, I didn't quite understand that. Can you repeat it?"). Speakers use conversational repair strategies when they respond to such requests for clarification by restating their point in a different way, giving more details, providing background information, speaking more clearly or more loudly, offering examples, and so forth. Such listener requests and speaker reactions help maintain clear communication.

> Good conversational repair skills are especially important to students who need clarification of teachers' instructions. Students who let teachers know they do not understand lessons or assignments may increase their chance of success.

Children with language disorders often do not know how to ask for clarification. This is understandable because even competent communicators, unless they are comfortable with their communication partners, are reluctant to admit that they did not understand something said. Children with language disorders often do not feel comfortable or secure in most communicative situations. These children, even when they know they did not understand the message, may do or say something that might be inappropriate. Also, when asked for clarification of their own messages, the children often do not know how to vary their productions to help the listener understand their message. Faced with requests for clarification, the children may repeat their ineffective productions. Therefore, conversational repair strategies are suitable target behaviors for intervention.

Baserate conversational repair strategies. Before beginning treatment, the clinician should baserate the frequency with which the child exhibits conversational repair strategies. Engaging the child in a variety of activities, the clinician should offer discrete (measurable) opportunities for the child to ask for clarification. In offering such opportunities, the clinician should make the message unclear to the child. The clinician might, for example, present a crafts project to the child and give the child instructions, but mumble some of those instructions softly to see if the child asks for clarification. The child also should be given opportunities to clarify his or her statements. To offer such opportunities, the clinician should ask the child such questions as "What do you mean?"; "I don't understand"; "I don't know what you are saying," and so forth. Each such question is a discrete and measurable opportunity for the child to clarify statements (Hegde, 1998a).

The clinician should count the number of times the child asked the clinician to clarify instructions or adequately responded to requests for clarification during a treatment session. These baseline data should be summarized (e.g., "During the session, Susie asked for clarification one time, but did not respond to requests for clarification at all."), thereby providing a starting point by which progress can be measured. Once again, three such measures should be obtained to establish reliable baserates of conversational repair strategies.

Teach the child to request clarification from a speaker. The strategy used in establishing baserates will also help teach requests for clarification from speakers. Essentially, the clinician makes ambiguous statements that force the child to request for clarification. For example, the clinician may display several toy cars and then make an ambiguous statement, such as, "Give me the car," and wait for the child to request clarification. If the child does not request clarification and responds anyway (such as picking up one of the cars), the clinician can say,

"No, not that one!" and then wait again for the child to ask what it is the clinician wants. If the child still does not request clarification, the clinician can give instructions and a model, such as, "When you are not sure, I want you to ask me, 'What do you mean?' OK?"

The clinician should then make another ambiguous statement and immediately model the request for clarification for the child (e.g., "Give me the car—say, 'What do you mean?'"). The clinician should reinforce the child for imitating the request for clarification (e.g., the child says, "What do you mean?") by smiling and providing the requested information (e.g., "I need the red car, thank you!"). The clinician may give the child a few more modeled trials, but as soon as possible, the model should be discontinued. If the child does not ask for clarification when the model is dropped, a verbal prompt may be used (e.g., "What do you ask me?"), without a model. If there is still no response from the child, the model should be reinstated for a few more trials and faded again. The clinician can work in this manner, setting up situations and making ambiguous statements, and giving the child whatever support the child needs to produce a request for clarification (e.g., just the stimulus itself, a verbal prompt, or a modeled production) until the behavior of requesting clarification has been established (Hegde, 1998).

Teach the child to clarify statements when requested.　To teach the child to respond effectively when listeners ask for clarification, the clinician may play the role of a listener who does not fully understand the expressions of the child. For example, the clinician may initiate a topic for the child to talk on, and then pretend not to understand the child's story. The clinician should then ask questions or make comments that force the child to clarify statements. For example, the clinician may ask, "What do you mean?" or "What are you trying to say?" The clinician may also make such statements as "I am not sure what you are saying," "I don't understand!" "Can you say it differently?" "Say it in some other words" and so forth.

The clinician might also purposefully negate a child's utterance, so the child will clarify by assertion (Hegde, 1998a). For example, while the child is talking about an outing to an amusement park, the clinician might say, "You did not go on the roller coaster 20 times, did you?" to which the child might reply, "No, I went on it 2 times!" If the child did not respond correctly, the clinician might try another kind of prompt, such as rephrasing the child's utterance into a question and saying it with a rising intonation and emphasis on the incorrect part (e.g., "You went on the roller coaster 20 times?").

If the child still does not respond with an appropriate repair strategy, the clinician should model different ways of saying the same thing. The child should be asked to imitate the clinician's modeled utterances. As the child's skill in conversational repair increases, the clinician should drop the model, prompt the child to rephrase, and continue the treatment evoking conversational speech. With smiles and such verbal phrases as "Oh! Now I understand! Thank you!," the clinician should reinforce the child for producing varied phrases or sentences, either in response to a model or spontaneously.

Teaching Narrative Skills

Narrating stories and personal experiences make conversations both effective and mutually reinforcing. Narration is a collection of specific skills, the most important of which is moving the story from beginning to end in a logically consistent, cohesive, and temporally correct sequence. An important consideration in teaching narrative skills is the child's cultural background.

> Although cultural variations in narrative skills are not diagnosed as language disorders, all children's academic and social performance may improve with enriched narrative skills.

Cultural Considerations

Narrative traditions differ across cultures. For example, among some Native Americans, telling stories is a privilege reserved for esteemed adults; children are not expected to produce narratives, and therefore, may not be good at narrative skills. Diverging from the main course of narratives, African American children tend to offer their comments on the actions and personal qualities of the characters (Roseberry-McKibbin, 2002). Asian American children may prefer a level of conciseness in narrative detail that may seem too restrictive to other ethnic groups (McCabe & Bliss, 2003).

Variations in narrative skills across children may apply to many children in specific ethnocultural groups. Individual children may or may not conform to the group's tendencies. The statements made previously are general and should not be applied indiscriminately to all members of these groups. However, clinicians should consider the possibility that a certain pattern of narration may be an indication of a cultural difference—*not* of deficient narrative skills.

Teaching Story-Telling Skills

Across cultures, many children with language disorders often have difficulties with narrative skill. While telling a story, children with language disorders confuse the sequence of events, omit important details of the story, skip important story elements, fail to describe the emotions and reactions of characters, or end the story abruptly. Because children with language disorders often have these difficulties, narrative skills are targets for intervention. The following general procedures help establish narrative skills in children with language disorders (McCabe & Bliss, 2003).

Baserate narrative skills. Telling the child a short story and asking the child to retell it is a simple way to baserate narrative skills. The child should be asked to retell at least three stories, each story baserated three times (once without any pictures or prompts, once with only pictures, and finally with pictures and prompts). The child's narration should be tape-recorded for later analysis. The clinician should first tell the child a short story without any pictures or prompts and ask the child to retell it. The clinician should then retell the story, perhaps with the use of pictures to see if the narrative skills improve. The child should then be asked to retell the story a third time with the help of pictures and verbal prompts (e.g., "What happened next?" "Who said that?" "What did she say?" "What did he do then?" etc.) to have the child narrate the story in its correct sequence. The child should receive no reinforcement or corrective feedback during baserating. The clinician should analyze the child's story for logical sequence of events, details of the story, description of the characters and their actions and reactions, temporal order of events, and the story conclusion. The transcripts of the child's narrative attempts should be kept on file to evaluate improvement during treatment.

> Baserating narrative skills under these three conditions will give the clinician information that will be useful in devising a treatment plan. What clinical implications are there if the child's production of narratives progressively improves with the addition of visual and verbal prompts?

Tell/retell as a treatment procedure. The same procedures used to collect baseline data are effective in teaching narrative skills. The clinician should use the baserated stories to initially teach the narrative skills. New stories may be selected for additional training and for conducting probes. As in the baseline sessions, the child's narration should be tape-recorded for later analysis. The clinician should tell the child a short story with the help of pictures. The child should then be asked to retell the story with the help of pictures and verbal prompts used in the baserating sessions. The child should be positively reinforced for acceptable story telling. If the child narrates with an improper sequence of events, misses an important element of the story, or fails to respond correctly to the prompts, the clinician should gently stop the child's narration and give additional prompts, ask questions that lead to corrections, or model expected responses to help the child continue correctly. For example, while using the story of *Goldilocks and the Three Bears*, the clinician might say something like, "Oh, oh, did Goldilocks sleep on the three bears' beds *before* she ate their porridge?" or "Wait! Didn't she sit on Papa Bear's chair, too?" If the child does not respond to questions like "What did she do next?" the clinician may model by saying, "She then . . . Now tell me, what did she do next?" The child should be warmly reinforced for appropriately correcting the story or for imitating the clinician's modeled response (e.g., "Oh, I see! What a good storyteller you are!").

As the child's narrative skills improve, the clinician should use different and progressively longer stories. Pictures and modeling should be faded when the child begins to accurately narrate a story without them. The use of prompts should be at a minimum.

Shift treatment to describing personal experiences. After establishing the narrative skills of story retelling, the clinician should shift treatment to description of personal experiences. The clinician may ask the child's parent or guardian to take a series of pictures showing the child engaged in a daily routine at home, such as getting ready for preschool, going to the doctor, or getting ready for bedtime. The parents may also supply pictures of a recent family vacation, the child's or a sibling's birthday party, or any such special occasion. The clinician should use the pictures as topics of personal narration, first for baseline procedures and then for treatment.

Before starting treatment, the clinician should baserate the narration of personal experiences. Various questions help evoke narration of personal experience (e.g., "What did you do for your birthday?" "What did you do this weekend?" "Where did you go for summer vacation?" etc.). At least three personal experience narratives should be baserated: once without any pictures or prompts, once with only pictures (provided by the family), and finally with pictures and prompts (e.g., "What happened next?" "What did he do then?" etc.). The child's narration should be tape-recorded for later analysis. The clinician should analyze the child's personal narrative for logical sequence of events, details of the story, temporal order of events, and conclusion. The child should receive no reinforcement or corrective feedback during baserating. The transcripts of the child's attempts to narrate personal experiences should be kept to document improvement made during treatment.

Treatment should begin with the verbal stimuli used to baserate the same personal experiences. Verbal prompts that are similar to those suggested for story telling may also be used to teach personal narratives. The clinician should use the pictures presented during baseline procedures to help the child to sequence personal narratives. The clinician should stop and prompt the child as necessary, being careful to fade prompting as the child's personal narratives become more established. Probes should be taken with new personal experiences.

There is some evidence that clinicians who narrate their own personal experiences in treatment sessions may prompt narratives from children. After narrating her or his own experiences, the clinician may ask or prompt the child to narrate similar experiences (McCabe & Bliss, 2003; McCabe & Rollins, 1994; Peterson & McCabe, 1983). The clinician, for example, might begin by saying, "Yesterday, I went to the doctor to get a shot that will help keep me from getting sick. She was a friendly doctor, but I was still a little scared. Do you ever go to the doctor?" Similarly, clinicians who describe their own vacation trips, birthday parties, and so forth may encourage similar narratives from children. Prompts to elaborate and stay with the correct

> It is our experience that children love to talk about their "owies"—how they got them and what was done to make them feel better. Another favorite topic seems to be how a sibling got into trouble!

sequence, corrective feedback for mistakes, and positive reinforcement for good narrative skills will help stabilize personal narratives. As always, prompts and modeling used in the initial stages of treatment should be faded.

Script therapy. An effective procedure to teach personal narratives along with conversations and social interactions is script therapy. Scripts are plans or descriptions of routine events, episodes, and personal experiences that are played out by participants. As used in language therapy, a plan for any kind of pretend or imaginative play or other organized activities that children engage in with other children or adults is a script. For instance, descriptions or enactments of the routines of playing house, playing doctor, shopping, baking a cake, visiting a carnival, selling and buying at an imaginary shop, completing art or science projects, and putting a puzzle together, are scripts.

Scripts in this sense are not typically written, although the clinician may follow a written script in treatment (Thiemann & Goldstein, 2001). Scripts specify the correct sequence or steps that are necessary to complete a task, enact a scene, or re-create an imaginary event. Scripts are typically described as mental or cognitive representations of events and experiences (Schank & Abelson, 1977). All such representations are presumed with no direct observable evidence, however. Scripts may suggest abstract knowledge

> *Scripts* are suitable for group language therapy that has been experimentally shown to be effective. School clinicians can therefore use this method with confidence.

of events, but such knowledge is acquired only through social experience and learning. Both the clinician and the child may provide scripts (suggest activities or events to be played out) although in most cases, the clinician's scripts will help get the treatment started.

There is controlled evidence, gathered through both single-subject and group experimental designs, to support the use of script therapy in teaching social interaction among children. The evidence is systematically replicated across clinicians, typically developing children, and diagnostic categories (e.g., children with autism and specific language impairment); therefore, the script procedure can be recommended for general use (Goldstein & Cisar, 1992; Gronna et al., 1999; Krantz & McClannahan, 1998; Robertson & Weismer, 1997; Sarokoff, Taylor, & Poulson, 2001; Thiemann & Goldstein, 2001, among others). Script therapy may be useful in teaching language skills, especially social interactions, conversational language, or narrative skills. In treatment studies, various classes of verbal behaviors including initiating speech, asking questions, making requests and comments, and producing polite social exchanges, have been taught through script therapy. Nonverbal communicative behaviors also have been taught (Goldstein & Cisar, 1992).

In using script therapy, the clinician begins by describing the sequence of a selected event (e.g., taking part in a birthday party or running an imaginary store). The clinician then assumes a role and assigns other roles (e.g., shopkeeper, customer, pizza delivery person, etc.) to the target child and others (e.g., guests, parents, siblings, etc.). Using props, the clinician and the child act out the event. Each child is taught to produce language that is appropriate for the role being played. For instance, among other verbal responses, the storekeeper may be taught to ask, "May I help you?" and the customer may be taught to say, "Do you have pencils for sale?" The clinician then repeats the event with roles reversed. The event may be repeated until the children are fully familiarized with the event and language expressions used. While acting out the scripts, the clinician requires the child to describe and comment on the actions being performed; ask and answer questions; request materials or information; describe feelings and thoughts of the characters assumed, and so forth. If necessary, the clinician can prompt specific responses (e.g., "What do you say when you want another piece of pizza?"), model correct responses ("Say, May I please have another piece?"), highlight particular language structures by emphasizing them, (e.g., "Please pick up that napkin—it is *in* the box."), and so forth. The clinician also may use the cloze procedure (sentence completion or partial modeling), in which the clinician pauses before important phrases or critical descriptions, waiting for a child to finish the utterance and to carry the script further (e.g., "You're ordering a pepperoni pizza. Tell the man on the phone, 'I want a _____.'"). In all instances, the clinician should positively reinforce the child for correct enactment of the scripts and correct production of targeted verbal behaviors. The clinician should give corrective feedback as found necessary.

The cloze procedure is also called a partial _____.

Once the child has correctly performed a few scripts while exhibiting targeted language skills, the clinician should fade not only the prompts but also the scripts themselves. The clinician should ask the child to narrate events and actions without enacting the scripts. Pictures may be used as an intermediate prompt if the child does not go straight from script therapy to spontaneous description of actions and events. Eventually, however, the children should describe events and narrate experiences without scripts or pictures. To probe for generalization, the children should be asked to narrate new events or experiences which have not been rehearsed or scripted (Nelson, 1993; Paul, 2001; Ripich & Creaghead, 1994; Thiemann & Goldstein, 2001).

Script therapy is especially well suited to teach verbal interactions in groups. Most experimental studies by Goldstein and his associates have used the group format in which children with and without disabilities have learned social interaction skills (Goldstein & Cisar, 1992; Thiemann & Goldstein, 2001). Other studies also support the use of group format using scripts in teaching various social skills to children with language disorders. (Gronna et al., 1999; Krantz & McClannahan, 1998).

Teaching Abstract Language Skills

Abstract language skills include comprehension and production of similes, metaphors, idioms, and proverbs. All these share a common characteristic: collectively, the phrases and sentences in them mean more than or different than what the individual words normally mean. Abstract language also includes comprehension and production of statements that are humorous, ironic, or sarcastic. Such expressions, too, carry words that mean something special or different in particular contexts. Research on these skills has been sparse and mostly descriptive in nature.

Nippold and her colleagues have conducted a series of such descriptive studies to measure children's understanding of idioms. The authors gave groups of typically developing children in grades 5, 8, and 11 such tasks as writing explanations for idioms or selecting the best description of an idiom from a field of four choices. Results indicated a developmental progression in understanding idioms, as performance improved over grade levels (Nippold, 1996, 1998; Nippold & Taylor, 1995; Nippold, Uhden, & Schwarz, 1997). These results were interpreted to support the hypothesis that increased language experience and exposure to abstract language enhances a children's understanding of idioms and other nonliteral expressions (Nippold & Taylor, 1995).

Although normative data on abstract and figurative language are limited, such language skills are academically and socially useful to the child. Some researchers have claimed that children do not understand such abstract language elements as proverbs until adolescent years. In contrast, Nippold (1998) has argued that younger children do not score well on tests of proverbs and other abstract language when the context is missing, as it is in many tests. Abstract language skills may be taught to children with instructions, explanations, multiple exemplars, and simulated real-life situations. Therefore, if abstract language skills are appropriate targets for a child, then they should be taught. The emphasis on literacy skills in school-age children supports this approach.

The same teaching strategies that are effective in teaching less abstract verbal skills may be effective in teaching more abstract verbal skills. Although there is a great need to produce experimental evidence on teaching abstract verbal skills, available evidence suggests that such abstract skills as understanding and producing idioms may be taught with behavioral intervention techniques. For instance, Ezel and Goldstein (1992) have shown that children with developmental disability may be taught to distinguish the idiomatic meanings from literal meanings of such expressions as *to hit the sack, break the ice, wet the whistle, kick the bucket, pull the leg, kill two birds,* and so forth. Using a multiple baseline design across subjects experimental design (Hegde, 2003a), Ezel and Goldstein (1992) experimentally demonstrated that idiom comprehension may be taught to children with developmental disability. They used such techniques as describing literal and idiomatic meanings depicted in pictures, asking the child to point to the correct idiomatic expressions as depicted in pictures (e.g., telling the child that if someone said *to let the cat out of the bag* it means to *tell someone a secret*), and reinforcing the child for correctly pointing to pictures that represented the idiomatic meanings (as against literal meanings). There is, however, a great need to research strategies for teaching the correct production of idioms and other forms of abstract language skills in spontaneous social situations. See Table 8.7 and Box 8.1 for selected figurative verbal skills and their training strategies.

Integrating Conversational Skills: Putting It All Together

Most of the pragmatic language skills discussed in this chapter may be taught as separate target behaviors. During the course of conversation in natural settings, however, people exhibit specific pragmatic language skills simultaneously. In social discourse, pragmatic skills are integrated with each other and with morphologic and syntactic skills. For

table 8.7

Figurative Language: Target Behaviors, Suggested Stimuli, and Consequences for Discrete Trial Therapy

Target Behavior	Stimuli for Modeled Responses	Stimuli for Evoked Responses	Suggested Consequences
Production of similes (or metaphors) in response to verbal stimuli; use repeated trials of several exemplars	For similes: This boy runs slowly. Can you think of anything that moves slowly? . . . Good! A snail moves slowly. Say, "The boy runs like a snail." For metaphors: She has bright, sparkling eyes. Can you think of anything else that is bright and sparkling? . . . Good! A star is bright and sparkling. Say, "Her eyes were two bright, sparkling stars."	This boy runs slowly. Can you think of anything that moves slowly? . . . Good! A snail moves slowly. Make a sentence about how the boy runs. She has bright, sparkling eyes. Can you think of anything else that is bright and sparkling? . . . Good! A star is bright and sparkling. Make a sentence about her eyes.	For correct response: Excellent! You made a good sentence comparing the boy to a snail! For incorrect response: Oh-oh! I didn't hear anything about how her eyes are like stars. Try again. [Provide additional cues if necessary; see Box 7.2.]
Production of commonly used idioms; use repeated trials of several exemplars, use a delayed model for modeled trials	When it is raining heavily, people say, "It's raining cats and dogs." What do you say when it's raining hard? When someone has to study hard for a test, he may say, "I have to hit the books." What do you say when you have to study hard?	It's raining heavily outside. What do you say? You have to study hard for a test. What do you say?	For correct response: Good! You said, "It's raining cats and dogs!" For incorrect response: No, say it the way we learned to say it. [Provide whatever additional cue is helpful; see Box 7.2.]
Description of the literal meaning of commonly used proverbs; have the student read (or read to the student) material such as Aesop's Fables or Benjamin Franklin's *Poor Richard's Almanac* to introduce each proverb; use a delayed model for modeled trials	So, the moral of the story is that it is best to take care of a small problem before it becomes a big problem. "A stitch in time saves nine." What does that mean? So, the moral of the story is that if you save some of the money you earn, you will end up with something to count on. "A penny saved is a penny earned." What does that mean?	So, the moral of the story is, "A stitch in time saves nine." What does that mean? The moral of the story is, "A penny saved is a penny earned." What does that mean?	For correct response: That's right! That's just what that saying means! For incorrect response: No, that's not it. Let's talk about it again. [Provide whatever additional cue is helpful; see Box 8.1.]

example, people take turns, maintain topics of conversation, and ask for clarification in grammatically acceptable verbal productions.

Clinically, though, skills taught separately may remain separate unless their integrated production is also reinforced. Therefore, children with language disorders who have been taught skills separately may need additional training to integrate all of the newly learned conversational skills. After teaching specific skills, the clinician should shift training to conversational episodes that include all previously taught skills. The following procedures may be used to teach a child conversational speech that includes newly learned pragmatic language skills.

box 8.1   Additional Prompts for Teaching Figurative Language

To prompt correct responses for producing metaphors or similes, producing idioms, and describing the meaning of proverbs:

1. Review previous stimuli

    - "Remember what else runs slowly?"
    - "Remember what people say when it's raining hard outside?"
    - "Remember what 'a stitch in time' really means?"

2. Use the cloze procedure

    - "The boy runs like a _____ [snail]."
    - "It's raining cats and _____ [dogs]."
    - "Take care of a small problem before it becomes a _____ _____ [big one]."

3. Use partial modeling, with fading

    - "The boy runs like a _____," then, "The boy runs _____," then, "The boy _____," and so forth
    - Use the same procedure for idioms and proverbs

4. Use phonemic cues

    - "The boy runs like a s—."
    - "It's raining c—."
    - "Take care of a small problem before it becomes a b—."

5. Provide a full model

    - "Say, 'The boy runs like a snail.'"
    - "Say, 'It's raining cats and dogs.'"
    - "Say, 'Take care of a small problem before it becomes a big problem.'"

Prompting and Reinforcing All Pragmatic Language Skills

Integrative training of conversational skills should start with a topic on which the clinician and the client talk. The clinician may wait a few seconds to see if a child will suggest a topic for conversation. If the child does not, the clinician should ask the child to suggest a topic for conversation (e.g., "What would you like to talk about today?"). If the child does not initiate, the clinician should suggest a conversational topic. If necessary, topic cards and pictures books can be used, but only when more natural means are not effective in initiating a topic of conversation.

Eventually, physical stimuli should be faded and naturalistic verbal stimuli should be sufficient to initiate conversation. A prompt like "You know what we should do before we start?" might stimulate the child to say, "We should have a topic to talk about." Such prompts help fade topic cards, picture books, and other direct stimuli in favor of more naturalistic verbal stimuli that lead to conversation.

The clinician should reinforce the child for appropriate use of all pragmatic language skills previously taught. For example, if topic initiation, maintaining eye contact, and turn taking were the previous treatment targets, they should all be prompted if necessary and reinforced with verbal praise. If, for example, the child is now maintaining eye contact, that behavior should be reinforced (e.g., "I like the way you are looking at me!").

The clinician can help the child maintain the topic by asking more questions about it, requesting the child to say more, and prompting subtopics to keep the child on the same topic for an extended period of time. The child should be reinforced for continuing to talk on a specific topic (e.g., "You have a lot to say on this topic!" "You are talking for a long time on the same topic!" and "I am really enjoying talking to you about this!").

If turn-taking was a newly established skill, the clinician may need to remind the child to take turns. The clinician can say, "No!" or "Stop!" when the child interrupts the clinician's turn inappropriately. The clinician may prompt the child to take turns by saying, "It is your turn!" If the child is showing good turn-taking skills, the clinician should reinforce the child (e.g., "You really know when it is my turn to speak!" and "I like the way you talk when it is your turn.").

To integrate conversational repair skills, the clinician should occasionally make an ambiguous statement to prompt the child to ask questions or request clarifications. Also, the clinician can look puzzled and ask, "What do you mean?" to prompt modifications in statements to clarify the meaning. The child should be reinforced for showing good conversational repair skills (e.g., "That was a good question!" or "Thank you! Now I understand!").

The clinician should also evoke narratives to strengthen this skill in conversation. Again, the child should be explicitly reinforced for good narrative skills (e.g., "Good story telling! I liked the way you started and ended the story," "You nicely said how the characters [naming them] felt about it," and "I really liked listening to your story!"). Narratives are good conversational contexts for encouraging the production of figurative language. The clinician should introduce similes, metaphors, or idioms during narratives. The clinician then should and ask and reinforce the child for producing figurative language skills correctly (e.g., "I like the way you described her hair as being 'black as coal,'" and "You're right! He did 'let the cat out of the bag!'").

Any other previously taught pragmatic language skill may be integrated into conversational discourse using these methods. As the child becomes progressively more proficient in pragmatic language skills, the need for prompts and explicit reinforcement will diminish until they are faded out altogether. The clinician would then shift treatment to conversational skills in naturalistic settings.

Although the emphasis in this section has been on conversational skill training and strengthening, the clinician should keep in perspective the previously taught syntactic and morphologic skills. A child's correct productions of grammatic morphemes, description of objects (tacts), and particular syntactic forms (e.g., complex sentences) should also be reinforced along with conversational skills.

Moving to Nonclinical Settings

The methods described under the previous section to teach integrated conversational skills will be effective in strengthening those skills in nonclinical settings. The clinician should engage the child in conversation outside the clinic, in places such as the library, the cafeteria, the classroom, and if possible, the home, and other community settings. The child should, at first, receive explicit reinforcement for production of conversational skills in nonclinical settings. As the behaviors become more established, however, all prompts and reinforcement techniques other than those that are intrinsic to the give-and-take of natural conversational speech should be faded.

The final step is to treat and monitor the child's production of the target behavior in home, community, and educational settings so that the target behaviors will be maintained. Maintenance of target skills in naturalistic settings needs not only the clinician's reinforcement of skills outside the clinic, but also parent education in response maintenance procedures. During treatment, the family members should be taught to pay attention to the clinically established language skills. The parents should learn to prompt, model, and reinforce those skills. Language treatment will be successful only when a good maintenance plan is in place. Therefore, maintenance of the target behaviors in natural settings is the final goal of language intervention. We will address this topic in the next chapter.

Chapter Summary

After establishing basic language skills, the clinician expands them into more complex and socially more useful language. Such skills as making requests, offering spontaneous comments, asking questions, and eventually holding social conversations are the commonly targeted advanced language skills. Such advanced skills may initially be taught with discrete trials and subsequently with more naturalistic methods, implemented in social contexts.

In teaching requests (mands), the clinician may withhold desired object and thus motivate the child to ask for it. In teaching the child to offer descriptions and comments (tacts) the clinician may have the child initially imitate modeled descriptive statements and fade modeling to promote more spontaneous responses. Expression of emotions and making comments may be similarly taught. A child may be taught to ask questions by withholding needed information followed by modeling.

A number of naturalistic teaching procedures help expand skills that are useful in social contexts. These procedures include milieu teaching, in which the overall goal is to evoke and reinforce child-initiated communicative interactions to environmental stimuli in natural settings. Milieu teaching includes such specific procedures as mand-model, delay, and incidental teaching. All use naturalistic contexts to teach social communication skills to children with language disorders.

Teaching pragmatic language skills is an important task in expanding communication skills of children with language disorders. Teaching such conversational skills as topic initiation, topic maintenance, turn-taking, maintained eye contact, and conversational repair should begin at the level of controlled conversation and then advance to the level of spontaneous conversation. Controlled conversation is verbal interaction that is more directed than spontaneous conversation; the clinician selects activities that will encourage conversational speech that is directed, prompted, and hinted. Spontaneous conversation is under the control of natural stimuli; therefore, most special stimuli the clinician provides should be faded to promote it. Social communication skills also are taught with the help of instructions, modeling, shaping, prompts, positive reinforcement, and fading of special stimuli used in treatment.

Narrative skills are an especially important and advanced language skill that may be taught by telling a short story to the child who then retells it. The clinician prompts and positive reinforcement will help the child give as much details as possible. Eventually, the child may be asked to narrate on personal experiences with little modeling or prompting. A method especially effective in teaching narrative skills is called script therapy. It includes plans or descriptions of routine events, episodes, and personal experiences that are played out by the participants; pretend or imaginative play that children engage with other children or with adults exemplify scripts.

Abstract language skills may be targeted in the final stages of skill expansion. Comprehension and production of similes, metaphors, idioms, and proverbs are essential to succeed academically. More research is needed to establish effective procedures for teaching abstract language skills.

Study Guide

1. You have taught the basic language skills specified in the previous chapter to a 4-year-old boy. The parents, however, complain that the child is not saying much on his own at home. You reassure the parents that you have plans on teaching expanded language skills that are socially more useful to the child and hence he is likely to produce them at home. Your supervisor has recommended that you use the three techniques of milieu teaching to expand the skills and to promote social communication. Design a treatment program in which you specify the language target skills and the milieu teaching methods. Describe in which order you would use the three techniques and justify the order.

2. While teaching advanced or expanded language skills to children with language disorders, what special kinds of stimulus situations should you have to arrange? Contrast them with the stimulus situations you may use in teaching basic language skills. Give examples of expanded language skills and the special kinds of stimulus conditions that must be arranged to evoke and reinforce them.

3. While teaching such skills as making a request and asking a question, can you use *only* the verbal praise (e.g., "You made a good request!") for producing the target skill as you possibly could while teaching most basic skills? Why or why not? What is different about such advanced language skills? In teaching a child to make requests or ask questions, how would you positively reinforce the child? Give specific clinical examples.

4. Your child client constantly interrupts you as you present the stimulus materials, give instructions, ask questions, model responses, and so forth. You then decide that you will teach the child turn-taking skills in conversation. Give a brief but clear description of how you teach this pragmatic language skill to your client. Specify the measurement procedure with which you document improvement in turn-taking skills.

5. Operationally distinguish between controlled conversation and spontaneous conversation. How would you baserate the two kinds of conversational skills? In treatment, you move from controlled conversation to spontaneous conversation. How do you achieve a smooth transition from controlled to spontaneous conversation in treatment sessions?

6. Is it possible to teach multiple pragmatic language skills (e.g., eye contact, topic initiation, and topic maintenance) simultaneously? If so, describe the procedure in which you would target all three skills at once.

7. Justify the statement that "conversational repair strategies involve the behavior of both the speaker and the listener." Give examples in which the same person will have to learn different skills to play the role of a speaker and that of a listener.

8. Write a birthday party script for a child who needs to learn social communication skills. Specify the target social skills that your script may help teach. Specify the roles (and skills) of the guests, the family members, and the child.

9. How did Ezell and Goldstein (1992) teach comprehension of idioms to children with language impairment? Can you extend the technique to teaching the correct production of selected idioms? Describe your procedure.

chapter

9

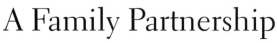

Maintaining Language Skills:
A Family Partnership

outline

No other issue illustrates the need for family partnership than the issue of mainte-nance of clinically established language skills in natural settings. Treatment is not over until the child's language skills are maintained over time and across natural settings. To accomplish this goal, the clinician needs to create a strong partnership with the family members, teachers, and individuals who spend a significant amount of time with the child. The task to promote maintenance is a shared responsibility between the clini-cian, the family, and often the teachers. The clinician can accomplish the task of establish-ing the target skills in the clinic with little or no help, but cannot accomplish maintenance without the help of others. It is the natural environment where the problem started (no causation implied here), and it is the natural environment, including the home and the school, where the problem needs to be solved for good.

Maintenance: Going beyond Clinical Treatment

For most children, typical home and extended social environment is sufficient to learn language skills. When it is not, children get referred to speech-language pathologists (SLPs). Obviously, children with language disorders have not benefited from the normal interactions that are sufficient for most children to learn and maintain language skills. Using the evidence-based treatment techniques described in previous chapters, clinicians effi-ciently establish language skills in the clinic. Clinicians systematically arrange stimulus con-ditions and provide consequences for children's communicative attempts that strengthen their language skills. The stimulus conditions and the response consequences may be some-what different from those found in the natural environment. Pictures and other clinical stimuli used to evoke responses and verbal praise for correct responses, though similar in principle to natural events, are different enough to create problems for the child. Moreover, target language skills are often initially established in offices, special classroom settings, or treatment rooms—all unusual settings. An exception and emerging trend to this common practice is home-based treatment, which we will address in a later section. Most school-age children who have language disorders, however, still learn new language skills in struc-tured clinical settings that bear little resemblance to typical social situations. Consequently, a child who consistently produces language skills in the clinic may not produce them at home and other natural environments. Also, clinically established target behaviors that are initially produced in more naturalistic settings may weaken over time.

An initial production of target behaviors in natural settings, called generalized produc-tion, may not assure the eventual success of treatment. Language skills should last in the child's natural environment. The skills should have positive effects on the child's academic and social life. Therefore, treatment should be considered complete only when children produce and maintain clinically established language skills at home, in the classroom, on the playground, and in other natural settings. There is yet another criterion of treatment success that is even more stringent: children should continue to expand their skills, learn new skills without much formal instruction, and build on what they learn at each stage of learning. Very few studies have documented that children who receive language treatment meet this stringent criterion.

Clinicians may find that promoting maintenance of language skills in natural environ-ments is more or less difficult, depending on the child who receives treatment. Certain diagnostic categories to which children belong can make a difference. For example, children who are autistic, developmentally disabled, brain injured, or who have a genetic syndrome may need special assistance in achieving generalized and maintained production of clinically established language skills. Studies have shown that language behaviors trained in children who are autistic or developmentally disabled are bound to the stimuli used in treatment. They may reliably give verbal responses to stimuli used in training, but may fail to produce the same response to similar, but untrained stimuli. This characteristic is described as (excessive) stimulus control or stimulus overselectivity (Alpert & Rogers-Warren, 1985; Bailey, 1981; Dube & McIlvane, 1999; Rincover & Koegel, 1975; Stremel-Campbell & Campbell, 1985). Among others, stimulus overselectivity is a reason for failure to generalize a trained skill to novel or naturalistic settings. Children with multiple handicaps who have severe language impairments also are slow to exhibit generalized language skills, although the reasons for this are not clear (Drasgow, Halle, & Ostrosky, 1998). Possibly, children with specific language impairment who are otherwise unimpaired may show better generalization; however, there is no firm evidence of this.

Although evidence for generalizability of clinically established language skills across specific diagnostic categories is limited, failure to obtain generalized productions with children with various disabilities is common. For instance, a review of 51 studies conducted from 1976 to 1990 on treatment of social skills, including language skills in children, pointed out that only 27 percent of studies reported complete or partial generalization of treated skills (Chandler, Lubeck, & Fowler, 1992). A majority of treatment studies, therefore, may not achieve the full goal of generalized and maintained skills. The reviewer also noted that the number of studies reporting better generalization had increased to 31 percent during the most recent 5 years of reporting (1985–1990). Presumably, this improvement is due to more attention being paid to produce generalized productions with special methods that we will describe later.

The difficult task of achieving maintenance of language skills in the natural environment has been complicated by some confused terms and inappropriate final goals sought for treatment. Therefore, in this chapter, we will address both conceptual and methodological problems, along with suggested solutions, to achieve the final goal of language treatment: an expanded and expanding skill base that is maintained over time.

Generalization: A Misunderstood Concept

Traditionally, clinicians have viewed the failure of children to produce target behaviors in natural settings as a failure to generalize responses learned in clinic settings to more typical environments. **Generalization** is a behavioral process in which learned responses are extended to new stimuli, new situations, and expanded into novel kinds of responses. That this may happen is well established in both clinical and laboratory studies (See Box 9.1). If generalization is a spread of old learning to new conditions, then it does look like the final goal of treatment. Clinicians reasoned that if a child who learns to name objects shown in the clinic begins to name similar objects encountered in the natural setting, treatment will have been successful. For example, a child who is taught to say "sock" when the picture of a particular sock is shown then goes on to produce the word when socks of different color and size are seen at home, the teaching has been successful.

Generalization is a technical term. *Carryover* is not. Nobody "carries" a skill or a behavior from one setting to the other.

box 9.1   Death of Generalized Responses

Unless intervention is provided, generalization—like language skills taught to children in clinics—is a behavioral process that does not last. Generalization was first observed in Pavlov's laboratory in conditioning salivary responses in dogs. Later, Skinner observed the same phenomenon in operant conditioning. Pavlov found that a response conditioned to one tone will be elicited by similar tones. Skinner found that an operant response such as bar press for reinforcement will generalize to bars of different shape, color, and location. Generalization was initially described as a spread of response to untrained stimuli. However, what is not typically understood is that both Pavlov and Skinner had reported that generalized responses are typically extinguished unless periodically reinforced. When Pavlov continued to present tones that differed progressively more from the conditioned tone, the salivary response was eventually extinguished. When Skinner let the rats press different kinds of bars with no reinforcement, bar pressing was eventually extinguished. Reinforcement for response given to a different tone or pressing bars of different shape would usually restore the response. This means generalized responses get extinguished unless reinforced.

To see if this would happen with children learning language, Cardoza and Hegde (1996) developed line drawings of geometric shapes. Each stimulus had variations in size, some progressively smaller and progressively larger. The variations at their extreme did not resemble the original shape. Children were taught an invented name for each of the original drawings (conditioned stimuli). When they could name each original stimulus reliably, the children were shown variations of the same stimulus. The results were that as the stimuli became progressively different from the original stimulus to which they were trained, the naming response dropped in accuracy. Eventually, when the stimulus looked much different from the conditioned stimulus, many children, failing to name them, simply shrugged their shoulders. In essence, a reliably learned response faded (extinguished) when the stimulus was different. This is precisely what happens when children, who learn to name objects in the clinic fail to respond when they encounter vastly different stimuli (of the same class) at home. They are more likely to respond to stimuli that are only slightly different from the conditioned stimuli. Even then, only reinforcement can sustain it. More importantly, if parents want to have the child respond to stimuli that are vastly different, they should reinforce the responses (and call it treatment, *not* a strategy to promote generalization).

Technically, if the child responds on the basis of similarities and ignores the obvious differences, generalization will have taken place. Therefore, clinicians often identify generalization, or "carryover," as the final goal of treatment. The behaviors learned in clinic are "carried over" into natural environments, and it is believed that if this happens, the child can be dismissed from treatment.

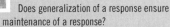
Does generalization of a response ensure maintenance of a response?

This is a common misconception resulting from an erroneous definition of the term *generalization*. Generalization refers only to an initial spread of response that may take place; it does not refer to maintenance of that response. In fact, generalized responses are not maintained unless reinforced, even if occasionally. Therefore, generalization should not be the final goal of clinical intervention. To better understand the issue, we need to examine two behavioral processes that are important in learning language both in natural settings and in the clinic.

Generalization and Discrimination

Verbal behavior (language as produced) is a vast and complex repertoire of skills. If all language skills have to be separately taught, the learning of language will be arduous.

Fortunately, each skill in that repertoire need not be taught. The vast collection of language skills are grouped as response classes. For instance, the plural *s* may be combined with many words in English, but for a child who does not produce it, the clinician need not separately teach all words that take that suffix. A child who is taught to produce a few exemplars of plural -*s* in words, will begin to use the morpheme correctly in many other words without additional training. For most elements of language, the clinician needs only to teach a few exemplars to have the child produce them in many untrained (novel) contexts. Such novel productions based on past learning, but without direct training, is generalization. In generalization, the child gives the same response to differing stimuli within a class (Baldwin & Baldwin, 1998; Malott, Malott, & Trojan, 2000). To give another example, the child who learns to say "cups" in the clinic when shown a cup of certain shape and color, may produce the same word at home, when shown cups of different shape and color.

Linguists pose a challenge to empirical scientists: how is it possible that children learn new and varied forms of language without explicit instruction? Linguists assume that if language is learned, all of the infinite variety of language productions need to be taught. This is not the case. New (creative) and varied learning without instruction is possible with generalization.

Generalization is the basis for a vast amount of new learning with little explicit instruction. Everyday situations evoke many generalized responses: a person who is fond of dogs, for example, reacts in similar ways (e.g., petting the dog, talking softly to the dog) in the presence of other, similar, dogs. Technically, generalization works within a concept; it works well when it is limited to responses within a class. For instance, as long as generalization takes places only to the words that do take the plural -*s*, it will be socially acceptable. If the plural -*s* generalizes to words that are irregular plurals, for instance, it is unacceptable generalization. While the plural -*s* is one concept, irregular plural is another concept. There should be generalization within, but not across, concepts.

Unacceptable generalization is limited by a process called discrimination. While generalization generates the same or similar responses to stimuli within a class, discrimination prevents the occurrence of same responses to stimuli belonging to other classes. **Discrimination** is the behavioral process of differentiating responses and concepts (Baldwin & Baldwin, 1998; Malott, Malott, & Trojan, 2000). It is through discrimination that people learn different responses (or concepts) to different classes of stimuli. Thus, the child learns to name "cups" as cups of varied shape and size based on generalization, and learns to name plates as "plates," not "cups," based on discrimination. Everyday situations evoke discriminative reactions: a person may warmly welcome a telephone call from a friend, but hang up on a telephone solicitor; a shopper may avoid a high-priced item and purchase a more reasonably priced item; a child may eagerly eat his spaghetti but pick at a green salad. See Box 9.2 for more on discriminative stimuli.

In essence, generalization is the opposite of discrimination. Discrimination occurs when different responses are given to different stimuli. Generalization occurs when different stimuli evoke the same response. Generalization is the lack of discrimination and vice versa.

When children acquire language, they may make errors as a result of overgeneralization, often called *overextension* by those who study child language acquisition (McLaughlin, 1998). A child who has learned the word *ball*, for example, may call all round objects *balls*, including the moon, a wad of gum, or an orange. Or, a child may initially call all men *daddy*. A child who learns such morphological features as plural -*s* or past tense -*ed*, may overgeneralize them, resulting in productions such as *feets* or *mouses* and *goed* or *drawed*.

box 9.2 | What Are Discriminative Stimuli?

We see and hear many things and many events unfold around us, but we do not respond to everything. We respond only to certain events, objects, persons, and so forth. Only those that we respond to are discriminative stimuli. People commonly say that we *choose* to ignore certain stimuli and that we *select* stimuli to respond to. We probably do neither. Both our responding or not responding are a function of past experience. We do not respond to certain stimuli because responses to them either have not been reinforced or have been punished in the past. We respond to certain stimuli because responses to such stimuli in the past have been reinforced. Stimuli, in the presence of which responses have been reinforced, acquire the power to evoke the same or similar responses in the future. Such stimuli are discriminative. All stimuli the clinician uses in treatment are discriminative because correct responses given to those stimuli will have been reinforced. When the child encounters those stimuli in the natural environment, the clinically established skills are more likely to be produced.

Children also tend to overdiscriminate, a process often called underextension in language acquisition literature (McLaughlin, 1998). A child may, for example, learn that the household pet is a *cat*, but not apply that label to any other cats. A child may learn to say "ball" when shown baseballs, but may not say that word when shown golf balls, footballs, soccer balls, and basketballs.

Children learn appropriate generalization and discrimination through the behavioral principle of differential reinforcement, in which desirable responses to a specific stimulus are reinforced and undesirable responses to the same stimulus are not reinforced. Parents are likely to positively reinforce a child for naming cups as "cups" and plates as "plates" but withhold reinforcement or express disapproval when the names are interchanged. To take another example, the child who calls the moon a "ball,"is told: "That's not a ball, it's the moon!" The child then may be praised for correctly naming the moon. In this way, the child learns to discriminate between balls and the moon through the process of differential reinforcement. Likewise, the child who overgeneralizes the morphological superlative form *-est*, resulting in productions such as *mostest* and *bestest*, similarly receives corrective feedback, weakening those responses, and approval for productions of *most* and *best*, strengthening those responses. Thus, both generalization within a class of stimuli and discrimination across them are established. Taken together, generalization and discrimination help establish different verbal concepts (verbal response classes).

During language treatment, clinicians establish discrimination by teaching them to respond appropriately to different stimulus conditions. For instance, the clinician may differentially reinforce the use of the suffix *-s* in producing the regular plural words (e.g., *cups* and *hats*) but give corrective feedback if the child generalizes it to irregular plural words (e.g., *mens* and *womens*). The clinician will positively reinforce the production of irregular plural words in relation to plural objects. Once the desirable behaviors are established in the clinic, the clinician's job is to promote an initial generalization and eventual maintenance of those behaviors in natural settings.

Generalization is nearly an automatic process based on physical properties of stimulus conditions and the functional properties of responses themselves. Although generalized behaviors can be changed, generalization is a behavioral law, not a purposive act. There are different kinds of generalization, all useful when they do occur. Although it will be shown later why generalization is not the final clinical goal, it helps when it does occur. Therefore, the clinician can take steps to promote generalization and eventual maintenance.

Stimulus generalization. The production of already learned responses in relation to novel but similar stimuli (not used in teaching) is called **stimulus generalization.** Stimulus generalization is based on the physical properties of stimuli; the phenomenon has been well researched in both basic and applied research (Baldwin & Baldwin, 1998; Malott, Malott, & Trojan, 2000). The example given of a dog lover's positive reaction to other, similar dogs is this type of generalization. In child language, children exhibit stimulus generalization when they learn a response in the presence of stimuli used during clinical training and then produce that same response in the presence of untrained stimuli of the same class. For example, a child may have learned to produce present progressive *-ing* in the presence of four picture stimulus items (e.g., "The boy is eating," "The boy is running," "The boy is sleeping," "The boy is laughing."), producing the correct response at the required criterion level. The clinician then conducts an intermixed probe to see if the response will generalize to other untrained stimulus items, sandwiching trained stimulus pictures in with untrained stimulus pictures (e.g., "The boy is reading," "The boy is walking," "The boy is jumping," "The boy is singing"). If the child's responses include the *-ing* in the untrained contexts, then stimulus generalization has occurred. Obviously, this is a highly desirable clinical outcome. Clinicians have to depend on stimulus generalization because they cannot possibly include all kinds of natural stimuli that evoke particular kinds of language behaviors.

Setting generalization. Production of responses learned in one setting in new settings that are not involved in training is called **setting generalization.** Treatment is successful when children who learn language skills in the clinic begin to produce them at home and other settings (Durand & Carr, 1991). A common clinical problem is presented when children learn to produce a response in the clinical setting, but fail to produce those responses in other settings. This occurs because clinical settings and natural settings are notably dissimilar. The treatment room (or clinic room or office) is furnished in a certain way, is isolated from natural settings, and is supplied with certain materials and equipment. This is necessary and desirable in initial stages of treatment, but can result in the child discriminating between the clinic setting and the natural setting. When a child discriminates between the clinic and all other natural settings, there is no generalized production of clinically established behaviors in those natural settings. Too often, the happy clinician in the school setting who has taught the production of /l/ to a child who substituted /w/ for it gets greeted by the same child on the playground with "Hewo, Mrs. Johnson!" Apparently, most clients who receive treatment say things one way in the clinic and another way in the real world. What has happened is setting discrimination instead of generalization. A major challenge for the clinician, then, is to promote setting generalization by lessening the distinction between the clinic room and the natural setting, using strategies that will be described in a following section of this chapter.

Conversational partner generalization. A special kind of generalization especially relevant to verbal skills is **conversational partner generalization,** which is the production of newly learned skills in relation to people who are not involved in treatment. Children who use the recently taught morphologic features or sentence types reliably when talking to the clinician may fail to do so when talking to the parents or siblings at home. While the clinician is the conditioned conversational partner for the skills, the family members are not. In fact, the family members are still the discriminative stimuli for the pretreatment, deficient skills. Therefore, the clinician's job, once again, is to promote the skills in relation to other people who typically interact with the child, including the family members and teachers.

Response generalization. While most forms of generalization that clinicians are concerned with are based on stimulus similarity (or dissimilarity), a useful form of generalization is based on the response properties themselves. Production of novel responses that are similar to those that were trained is called **response generalization.** For instance, a child who was just taught to use the possessive *s* in the context of a few words (e.g., *Mommy's hat, Daddy's coat*) may produce novel (untrained) responses that are longer or in some way different (e.g., "I see kitty's tail," "These are doggy's ears."). Response generalization contributes significantly to language expansion and its creative production.

> Clinically, the most useful forms of generalization are (1) stimulus generalization, (2) setting generalization, (3) conversational partner generalization, and (4) response generalization.

Obviously, it is helpful if a child exhibits generalized productions to new stimuli, settings, conversational partners, and responses. Most clinicians assume that if generalization is evident, the child is ready to be dismissed from treatment. In other words, clinicians assume that generalization is the final goal of treatment. Unfortunately, this is a mistaken assumption. When the concept of generalization is examined more carefully, however, it becomes readily apparent that it should not be considered the final goal of treatment.

A Clinical Problem

The popular idea that generalization should be the final goal of treatment is clinically problematic. As noted, when generalization occurs, it can serve as an intermediate step toward establishing behaviors in natural settings. However, the belief that it should be the final goal of treatment is based on a limited definition of generalization that does not take into account its nature and eventual course.

While novel responses are produced on the basis of generalization, generalized responses do not last without intervention. When intervention takes place, it is treatment, *not* generalization. It may be recalled that to reinforce is to treat (intervene) and generalization is what takes place when treatment ceases. Therefore, Hegde (1998b) has defined generalization as a declining rate of response when stimuli are changed and the reinforcement ceases. It may be recalled from Chapter 5 that when a target behavior reaches a certain criterion level during treatment, clinicians probe to see if the response is generalized to untrained stimuli. Using an intermixed probe, the clinician reinforces responses given to trained stimuli and withholds all feedback for responses given to untrained stimuli. The clinician does not reinforce correct responses to untrained stimuli because such reinforcement would be treatment, not an assessment of generalized production (unreinforced responses in the presence of new stimuli). However, if generalized responses continue to receive no reinforcement, they will diminish and eventually become extinguished—hardly a desirable outcome for treatment.

That the ultimate step in intervention is to *program generalization* is a view Stokes and Baer (1977) have helped popularize. However, their strategies to program generalization included reinforcement for skills that generalize. The assumption is that if the clinician reinforces correct behaviors, it is treatment. Implied in Stokes and Baer's recommendation is that if parents reinforce the same behaviors at home, it is a strategy to promote generalization. Surely, the clinician and parents would want to reinforce language skills that generalize, but this is not done to program generalization, but to make the skills last. Because generalized responses are unreinforced responses, and generalization eventually ends in extinction, the advocated strategy is confusing and contradictory; no clinician believes we should program a declining rate of response. As we will find soon, Stokes and Baer (1977) recommended a few steps that would promote generalized responses, and these present no conceptual or methodological problems. However, when generalized responses are reinforced, they are no longer generalized responses. Any reinforced response is taught, not generalized.

> To *reinforce* is to *treat*. It does not matter who reinforces. Parents' reinforcement is also treatment. When a physician gives a tablet, it is medicine. When the patient takes the same tablet at home, it still is medicine.

When a clinician asks parents and others in a child's environment to reinforce a generalized response, they are not being asked to promote generalization which has already taken place—they are being asked to conduct treatment in the child's natural environment to promote maintenance.

Maintenance of clinically established behaviors in natural settings is the final goal of treatment. Children must be able to use their newly learned language skills during typical conversations produced during the routine course of everyday life. Responses are maintained when they are reinforced. Reinforcement necessary to maintain responses in natural settings will not come from the clinician, but from the child's family, teachers, caregivers, and anyone else who has contact with the child on a regular basis. These significant individuals in the child's life must, in effect, be taught to conduct treatment in natural settings. The clinician's task, then, is to program maintenance, using various strategies which will be discussed in the following sections.

> What is the immediate goal of treatment? What is the final goal?

Maintenance: Skills That Last in Natural Settings

Maintenance is the continued production of clinically established skills across time and situations. Maintained skills last in varied settings and over time. It is necessary to program maintenance, because responses established in the clinic setting are often not maintained in more natural settings, even if they show an initial generalization. While generalization is prevented because of stimulus and setting dissimilarity, responses are not maintained because of lack of sustained positive reinforcement in the natural settings. In any setting, responses are maintained only because of sustained reinforcement (Skinner, 1953; Sulzer-Azaroff & Mayer, 1991).

In some cases, the clinician may well be the only person in a child's life who reinforces the child's correct responses. If the child's correct responses are ignored in the natural environment, they will be extinguished. Even worse, undesirable behaviors may be reinforced in natural settings, assuring an increase in those behaviors. For example, a minimally verbal child who has learned to say, "Help me, please," in the clinic may still whine and cry to communicate in the natural environment, because the adults reinforce those inappropriate behaviors by giving attention and assistance. In essence, within the natural setting, the child may continue to encounter old stimuli and consequences that may support ineffective and inappropriate methods of communication.

The clinician should program maintenance so that the natural setting—like the clinic—becomes a discriminative stimulus for the target behaviors the child is learning. This goal is more easily accomplished when treatment procedures used for maintenance in the natural setting are the same as those used for establishing the behavior in the clinical setting. People in the child's natural environment should reinforce the child's behavior in the same manner as the clinician does in the clinic room. Language skills are better maintained when family members, peers, and teachers become conversational partners with the child. The clinician should encourage these significant others to create positive and reinforcing opportunities for the child to communicate. People in the child's environment should let the child lead verbal interactions.

Bypassing the Problem: Home-Based Treatment of Children

One way of bypassing the problem of generalized productions at home is to teach children at home. When the teaching takes place at home, generalized productions are most likely, at least in the home environment. Maintenance is also more likely although it may need additional steps that will be described in the next section. Home-based treatments, especially for children in the age range of 0 to 3 years, are expanding as a result of increased interest in family-centered therapy. In family-centered therapies, parents and children take part in planning assessment and treatment. Clinicians in such programs include parent education and home-based treatment.

There is a growing body of experimental research to support the efficacy of home-based, parent-delivered treatment to language disordered children. For instance, using a multiple baseline across subjects research design, Derby et al. (1997) documented a decrease in problem behaviors and an increase in communicative behavior in four severely disabled language disordered children whose parents treated them at home. The parents had been taught to administer functional communication training (FCT; similar to differential reinforcement of alternative behavior discussed in Chapter 6) techniques, teaching their children appropriate communicative behaviors, such as signing *please* or *done*, or using the carrier phrase *I want* in place of undesirable behaviors.

Gibbard (1994) employed a group research design and documented increased expressive language skills in children whose mothers attended group parental language training sessions compared to a control group of children whose mothers had received no training. In a further experiment, they included three groups of children: (1) a group in which the mothers received parental language training; (2) a group in which the mothers received no training, but the children received direct therapy from a speech-language pathologist; and (3) a group in which mothers received parental training with an emphasis on general learning, rather than on teaching language skills. Results indicated the children in the first two groups showed significantly greater gains in expressive language than the children in the last group. Furthermore, there were no significant differences between the two groups

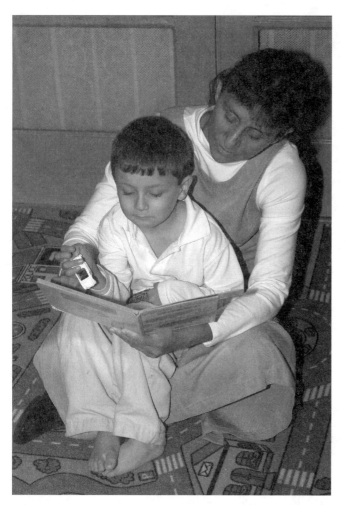

photo 9.1

Home-based treatment may result in greater progress for a language disordered child. This parent is at home, using storybook reading techniques taught to her by an SLP to encourage attending behavior in her autistic child.

with greater improvement, leading Gibbard (1994) to conclude that "parental training is as effective as individual speech and language therapy" (p. 131).

Various other studies have shown good results for a variety of home-based interventions (Eiserman, Weber, & McCoun, 1992; Howlin & Rutter, 1989; Miller & Sloane, 1976; Salzberg & Villani, 1983; Wulz, Hall, & Klein, 1983). Scientific validation of the efficacy of home-based methods, however, is incomplete. Studies evaluating the efficacy of parent education and home-based treatment programs have been plagued with methodological problems, including incomplete descriptions of the specific intervention offered, small sample size, lack of treatment fidelity, and short intervention periods (Goldstein, 2002). However, the generally good results obtained by the studies conducted indicate that home-based intervention is a promising treatment technique worthy of further scientific investigation. Certainly, the concept of teaching parents and caregivers to evoke, reinforce, and maintain target behaviors in the home setting is consistent with an emphasis on providing family-centered, collaborative therapy in natural environments.

Clinicians should therefore include in their treatment plans a substantial component of parent education. Parents should be encouraged to observe treatment sessions and then to learn to administer discrete trials as well as more naturalistic forms of therapy at home. Parents should learn all the techniques to establish language skills—modeling, prompting, reinforcing, and giving corrective feedback. The parents may initially learn these and other techniques through their observation of, and participation in, the clinic sessions. Subsequently, they get their techniques fine-tuned when the clinician visits their homes to observe home treatment and measure progress. As their children progress, parents can also be taught the techniques of *milieu teaching* (see Chapter 8), embedding language treatment in everyday routines. Parents are with their children so much more than are clinicians, who may only be with a child for two 40-minute clinic sessions a week. If parents can employ the more naturalistic techniques throughout the day, the child is likely to make faster progress and maintain the skills over time.

Bringing treatment to the child in natural settings, then, is a major strategy in promoting maintenance of skills learned in the clinic setting. The following sections describe other strategies the clinician can use to promote skill maintenance.

Strategies to Promote Skill Maintenance

Maintenance strategies are techniques that help extend treatment to natural settings. More research is needed before the problem of response maintenance in natural settings is solved. However, research has shown that various maintenance strategies are useful in extending treatment to naturalistic settings. One set of these strategies involves choices the clinician makes before, during, and after treatment; another set involves training significant people in the child's life to promote maintenance in natural settings. Both the sets require participation of the client, the family members or other caretakers, and the teachers in academic settings.

In devising a maintenance plan, the clinician's technical task is twofold: (1) diminishing the differences between the clinic and natural settings, and (2) teaching significant others in the child's environment to be the child's effective communication partners who evoke and reinforce new skills. The first task will help promote generalization *and* maintenance; the second task will more specifically target maintenance. Steps taken to promote generalization will help build a maintenance strategy. If the responses are initially generalized, it is easier for parents and others to take steps to prevent their deterioration over time. If the skills do not generalize to natural settings, parents and others will have to work a bit harder to have the skills first produced and then maintained.

Compared to generalization, maintenance has received little attention partly because clinicians have been typically concerned with establishing and increasing children's language skills. Maintenance requires that treatment include family members and others who are involved. As noted before, if people continue to behave toward the child the way they have before treatment, skills may not be maintained. This means that not the only the child, but the others in the child's life, should be changed. This change may be harder to achieve than the change in the child who interacts with a professionally competent clinician in a controlled clinical setting.

Clinicians should show family members, teachers, and others how to change existing interactional patterns; to act and react differently; and to set the stage for the child to use newly learned language skills. When the child exhibits those language skills, adults in the environment should give social approval and desirable natural consequences. Conversely, adults should discontinue support for the child's old, undesirable, and ineffective methods of communication. In essence, to implement a maintenance strategy, clinicians transfer antecedent and consequence control from the clinic setting to natural settings, and from themselves to the significant others in the child's environment.

> Some clinicians argue that it is unnatural to exert control over children's communication. But communication is always an interdependent social relationship between two or more persons. Control in this context means using procedures that are effective in changing patterns of communication. Without that control, neither the clinician nor the parents can promote good communication skills.

Maintenance strategies should be a part of the treatment plan—always developed and written with the participation of the child, the family members, and the teachers. Therefore, the clinician must think about the promotion of initial generalization and eventual maintenance of language skills from the very beginning of treatment, even when choosing target behaviors.

Maintenance strategies should be systematically programmed throughout the entire treatment process as well. Fortunately, the behavioral treatment techniques described in previous chapters do promote complete or partial generalization in a number of cases, although failures are not uncommon. For instance, in the previously described review of 51 treatment studies on social skills, Chandler, Lubeck, and Fowler (1992) found that such treatment techniques as prompting, positive reinforcement, instructions, corrective feedback, and modeling were used in studies that were successful in obtaining generalized production of trained skills. The review also showed that the same techniques, though successful in establishing the skills, may not lead to generalized production in many cases. More importantly, a majority of studies (73 percent) that were successful in obtaining generalized productions used one or more special techniques to promote it. Of the various strategies to promote generalization, selection of functional targets, using reinforcement schedules that approximated those in the everyday environment (indiscriminable contingencies), training loosely, selecting common stimuli from the environment, reinforcing generalized responses, and just giving additional training were more common in the studies. Therefore, the need to give special consideration to promote an initial generalization and subsequent maintenance is essential.

It may be recalled from Chapters 5 through 8 that in discrete trial therapy, the treatment chain consists of stimulus-response-consequence, with the clinician and significant others presenting a stimulus, the child responding, and the clinician and significant others providing a consequence designed to increase the correct response rate and decrease incorrect responses. Maintenance strategies relevant to each component of this treatment chain can be applied to increase the likelihood that the behavior will eventually be maintained in the natural environment. However, a pervasive factor is the structure of the treatment sessions themselves. Therefore, effective maintenance strategies include four kinds of operations: (1) structure and nature of treatment sessions, (2) management of stimuli, (3) management of responses, and (4) management of consequences (Durand, Berotti, & Weiner, 1993; Goldstein, 1993; Hegde, 2001b; Stremel-Campbell & Campbell, 1985).

Structure of Treatment Sessions

As pointed out in Chapter 4, the degree of structure used in treatment sessions will vary according to the stage of treatment and the characteristics of the child. In the initial stage of treatment, clinicians who use the discrete trial procedure to establish language skills will use structured treatment sessions. Relatively tight structure is needed for children who have severe language disorders and associated clinical conditions (e.g., autism or developmental disability). In all cases, once the basic language skills are established in the clinic with relatively tight structure, a loose, more naturalistic structure is useful in promoting generalized production and eventual maintenance of language skills (Campbell & Stremel-Campbell, 1982; Hart, 1985).

Tailoring the structure to suit the child. An assessment of child's strengths and weaknesses will help tailor the degree of structure of treatment sessions. If basic words and phrases need to be taught, the child's learning is likely to be efficient with discrete trial-based, tightly structured, treatment sessions. If the child needs training on more advanced language skills (including syntactic structures and pragmatic language skills), then the clinician should avoid a tightly structured format. More naturalistic, conversation-oriented treatment will not only be more useful even in the early stages, but actually needed. Children who begin their training at the conversational level and with naturalistic formats begin their treatment that promotes maintenance.

Fading the structure of treatment sessions. A tight structure, when used, should be faded into more naturalistic social exchange format. The clinician fades the structure as the child becomes more proficient in producing the language skills. Fading the structure involves moving away from discrete trials, using a more natural conversational exchange format. In this format, the clinician lets the child choose conversational topics, lead conversational exchanges, and generally assume a more active role in social exchanges than before. Fading the structure also involves changing the physical setting of treatment. We will return to this point in the next section, as it is a matter of physical stimulus manipulation.

Management of Treatment Stimuli

The stimulus items used during treatment will take on special status to the child as discriminative stimuli that evoke target responses. If the clinician chooses stimulus items arbitrarily, an opportunity to promote maintenance may be missed. Stimulus items used in treatment should help extend control over correct responses produced in the natural environment. Such control is more likely to be achieved if the clinician selects stimuli that include: (1) physical stimuli from the child's natural environment, (2) verbal stimuli the child is likely to encounter in natural settings, and (3) variations in conversational partners and physical setting.

Physical stimuli from the child's natural environment. Because it is convenient, clinicians too often select treatment stimuli from a dizzying array of commercially available stimulus materials—none of which may be particularly relevant to an individual child's past experience and cultural background. Response maintenance may be poor if the clinician uses stimulus items during treatment that the child is unlikely to encounter in natural settings. Stimuli selected from the child's own environment, however, will acquire discriminative value in evoking target behaviors from the child during clinical treatment. When the child comes into contact with those stimuli at home, in school, or in the community, target behaviors may be similarly evoked in those natural settings. Selection of stimulus items, then, should be child- and family-specific. Consultation with the child, the parents or caregivers, and the teachers of the child will help select the target behaviors for which they can suggest natural stimuli. Common, functional items, preferably objects, should be used; the child should be encouraged to bring toys or other favorite items from home to use during therapy sessions. A study has demonstrated that when compared to picture cards and photographs as stimuli, objects selected from the natural environment were more effective in producing generalized production of naming responses learned by children with developmental disability (Welch & Pear, 1980).

Pictures can be of value if they are realistic, unambiguous, and colorful. Pictures, compared to objects, are more portable, varied, and can help represent many kinds of events.

If practical, when pictures are used, they should be paired with real objects to promote better generalized productions (Welch & Pear, 1980). Nonetheless, objects are preferred over pictures, especially in the early stage of noun, verb, and morphologic training. Many commercially available line drawings are neither especially attractive nor particularly realistic. Further, objects can be manipulated to demonstrate events and concepts. For example, if a child brings toy trucks and cars from home into the clinic, they can be used to demonstrate verbs such as *go, stop, drive, dump, tow, pull, dig*; adverbs such as *fast* and *slow*; and adjectives such as *big* and *small*. All of these words may be expanded into phrases and sentences and incorporated into conversational training.

Whether pictures or objects, the clinical stimuli should be representative of items that are present in the child's natural environment. This is especially important when the child is from a diverse ethnocultural background or from a low socioeconomic household. For example, if pictures are being used, they should include pictures of people from the child's own ethnocultural group, although they need not exclude pictures from other groups. Culturally relevant objects may be brought from home to be used in initial stages of treatment. Also, clinicians should be sensitive to the possibility that children from low socioeconomic households may not encounter certain items of furniture or appliances, or have access to many toys or sporting goods in their natural environments. Stimulus items taken from the child's school settings will be appropriate for most children. Stimuli that are not familiar to the child may be used in later stages of treatment. In such cases, the names, functions, or uses of stimuli will have to be taught to the children. This is fine because the goal of language therapy is to expand the child's vocabulary and increase the child's exposure to unfamiliar objects or events.

> We do not suggest that stimuli that are unfamiliar to children should never be used in treatment. Sooner or later, children will come across novel stimuli. Familiar stimuli are perhaps the most effective in initial stages of treatment.

Verbal stimuli from natural settings. In the initial stages of treatment, it is necessary to provide uniform verbal stimuli and models. For example, a clinician may teach plural *-s* by showing the child two pictures, one representing a single object and the other, multiple objects. A verbal stimulus is then delivered, with the clinician saying, "Here is a picture of one cat. Here is a picture of two _____. Say, 'cats.'" The response may be efficiently established in this way (and may be necessary in some cases), but this verbal stimulus is not commonly used in the natural environment. The clinician may find that the response can just as effectively be established by showing the child a picture of two cats and asking, "What are these? Say, 'cats.'" When the model is eventually faded, the child will have learned to respond to a simple question adults are much more likely to ask in natural settings. Similarly, all other prompts the clinician may use to initially establish a response should be faded as soon as possible, so that more natural verbal stimuli (e.g., "Tell me about it," "What is happening?" "What is he doing?"; etc.) are used to evoke responses from the child. In other words, verbal stimuli should consist of questions or phrases that are commonly heard in the child's environment (e.g., "What's this?" instead of "Label this picture.").

Variations in conversational partners and physical setting. The clinician, who initially is the sole person reinforcing correct responses, and the clinic room, which is the sole setting in which responses are initially reinforced, can both become discriminative stimuli to a child. When this happens, the child may produce the desired response only in the presence of a particular clinician administering treatment in a specific room. To avoid this problem, the clinician should recruit different conversational partners and vary the physical settings in which the child is reinforced for producing the language skills.

To vary the conversational partners, the clinician may bring in other people to participate in treatment sessions. Initially, the clinician may invite the family members to observe the treatment sessions. However, they should soon take part in treatment. The family member, along with the clinician, should engage the child in conversational speech. This gives an opportunity to the clinician to demonstrate reinforcement and corrective feedback. In subsequent sessions, the clinician should teach the family members to evoke and reinforce correct responses from the child. In this way, family members will also quickly acquire status as discriminative stimuli, and the child will be more likely to produce correct responses in their presence. The clinician may recruit other conversational partners by inviting other clinicians, students, teachers, professional colleagues, or any other willing persons into the clinic room to observe and interact with the child, and reinforce the child's language skills.

> Having the family members observe, and then take part in, formal clinic sessions are the first steps toward educating family members to administer home-based treatment.

The physical setting should be varied in a similar manner. The clinic room can also become a discriminative stimulus for the child's correct responses, which will then be less likely to be produced in more natural settings. To vary the physical setting, treatment should be moved to more natural and less structured situations as the child's responses become more established in the clinic room. The clinician may begin by simply changing clinic rooms, occupying a different office for treatment sessions, or, in the school setting, conducting treatment in the classroom, embedded in regular classroom routines. Soon, the child should be taken out of the clinic room altogether, perhaps for a walk around the facility or a visit to the school library or classroom. The clinician can informally monitor the child's production of target behaviors in the playground, school cafeteria, classroom, hallway, shopping center, restaurant, and the child's home.

Informal treatment given in natural settings should involve mostly conversational speech. When working with children in non-clinical settings, target behaviors should be prompted in a subtle manner, perhaps by using facial expressions or hand signals. Similarly, reinforcement and corrective feedback should also be delivered in a subtle manner. Actually, by the time the child is being treated at the conversational level in natural settings, there should be minimal need for reinforcement or corrective feedback; those contingencies will increasingly be provided by natural consequences.

> Because the clinic setting is likely to be a discriminative stimulus, children should be told before the outing that they should use their "good talking" when they go outside the clinic.

Stimulus management—including stimuli from the child's natural environment; simple, common verbal stimuli; and varying conversational partners and physical setting—will facilitate maintenance of clinically established responses in natural settings. But clinicians should consider the problem of maintenance even before treatment begins by selecting target behaviors that are useful to the child and are likely to be produced and reinforced in natural settings.

Management of Responses

A significant part of maintenance strategy is to select appropriate target skills and manage them efficiently. Before selecting target behaviors, the clinician should consider their maintenance potential. Once those target behaviors have been selected, the clinician should

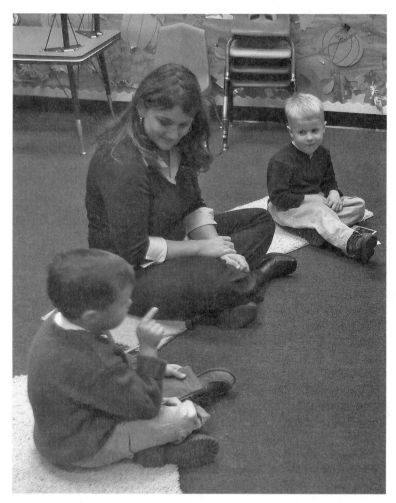

photo 9.2

It's your turn! Clinicians should join in to promote production of target behaviors in the classroom setting.

use multiple and varied exemplars to establish the skills in the child. Also, the clinician should give sufficient training on all levels of response topography, always ending with the conversational level. If responses are managed in this manner, maintenance of correct response in natural settings will be much more likely.

Selecting target behaviors. In Chapter 4 we discussed a child-specific procedure in selecting target behaviors. It was suggested that target behaviors should be suitable for the child's ethnocultural background and environment. Target behaviors should be useful to the child, including skills that will be relevant to the child's everyday life. Newly acquired language behaviors should make an immediate and socially significant difference in a child's communicative skills. Such target behaviors, often called functional to the child, have an effect on the listeners (Warren & Rogers-Warren, 1985). Of the 51 studies Chandler, Lubeck, and Fowler (1992) analyzed, 65 percent of studies that documented generalization of social skills had selected functional target behaviors for training. The clinician who has studied the academic and social demands placed on the child along with the child's cultural background can select target skills that will serve the child best. As discussed in Chapter 5, behaviors that can be expected to be produced at home, in the classroom, or both should be chosen as targets. When children learn communicative skills that allow them to have a powerful, positive effect on their environment, those skills are likely to be maintained.

Too often, clinicians select target behaviors based on what they or other adults may think are appropriate to the child's age level, according to developmental norms. For example, much valuable therapy time may be used teaching an essentially nonverbal child such target behaviors as naming colors, shapes, body parts, nonfunctional objects (e.g., sofa, carpet, wall) and counting objects. But what if the child lacks the

An exemplar is a specific example of a target skill that clinicians teach. *Two cups* and *four hats* are exemplars of the regular plural -*s*. How many such exemplars should be taught?

language skills necessary to ask for something to eat or drink, to ask for help, to go outside and play, or to greet a person and ask his or her name? Target behaviors based on such basic needs and social interactions are more likely to be produced in the child's home environment, in response to typical stimuli encountered in natural settings, than are those that are based on abstract concepts or normative information. For example, a child who learns to make such requests as "I want . . ." or "Please help me" will find that she or he now can produce significant effects on others. Furthermore, such requests name their own reinforcement (e.g., "I want a *cookie*."), which the adults in the environment are highly likely to provide.

Selecting multiple and varied exemplars. Generalization and maintenance failures may be due to insufficient training or training with just a few exemplars of target behaviors. A sufficient number of varied exemplars need to be taught to promote maintenance (Chandler, Lubeck, & Fowler, 1992; Hughes et al., 1995; Kreimeyer & Anita, 1988). The number of exemplars of a target behavior necessary to establish a behavior varies across children. The criterion that determines the number is the probe response rate, as described in Chapter 5. If results of intermixed probes indicate little or no generalization has taken place, training on additional exemplars will be necessary. In most cases, 6 to 10 exemplars may be needed to obtain an 80 to 90 percent correct probe response rate.

If exemplars are not varied, the child may become stimulus-bound, with the correct response becoming overly dependent on the presentation of the same stimuli. To avoid this problem, the clinician should teach multiple and varied exemplars of the target behavior. If the word *ball*, for example, is one of the target nouns to be taught, pictures of all kinds of balls—baseballs, basketballs, golf balls, soccer balls, and so forth—should be presented. If the sentence "The boy is running" is used as an exemplar for the present progressive *-ing*, then several pictures of different boys running under different circumstances (e.g., in a race, while playing football, etc.) should be chosen to evoke that exemplar. Better yet, to teach the generalized and sustained production of *-ing*, the clinician should present varied exemplars in which men, women, girls, boys, animals, and inanimate objects (e.g., cars, trains, airplanes) are involved in action and the present progressive is combined with varied verbs (e.g., *running, eating, reading, flying, jumping, racing*, etc.).

The target skill a child learns under varied stimulus conditions is likely to appear in natural settings, in which the circumstances that would naturally evoke the responses will be many and varied. Although it may be necessary to persist with a few, specific stimuli in the initial stages of training to establish the response, stimuli should be varied as soon as possible, so the responses come under the control of a wider range of stimulus conditions.

Giving sufficient treatment on all levels of response topography. Sometimes, student clinicians fail to give sufficient treatment to a child on all levels of response topography, especially at the all-important level of conversation. If treatment is terminated too early, for instance when the child was still learning specific targets only at the phrase or controlled sentence level, then the target behavior will not have received reinforcement at the conversational level, which is the naturally occurring response form. Some student clinicians fail to move swiftly through the treatment sequence to arrive at the conversational speech level. For example, a student clinician with a stricken look might approach a supervisor and announce that "This child has mastered the target

> Mastery of a target behavior at a lower level is good news! The clinician should move to the next level and advance to the level of conversational speech as soon as possible.

behavior I wrote for production of pronouns at the phrase level. It's only the middle of the semester! What do I do *now?*"

Perhaps this is excusable in a student clinician just beginning to practice, but, of course, this student is missing the entire point of treatment. The child should be treated at all levels of response topography, reaching the level of conversational speech as soon as possible, and then given adequate treatment at that level. This will then help an initial generalized production of the target skills so that parents and others may begin to reinforce those productions to promote their maintenance in natural settings.

Management of stimuli and responses, described so far, will help promote maintenance in the natural environment, but is it not sufficient. Further strategies that involve the final element of the S-R-C treatment chain, that of providing consequences for the child's response, also are required.

> Do you remember what S-R-C stands for?

Management of Consequences

Delivering a consequence that is contingent on the correctness of a response is the last step in the treatment chain. There are many strategies in managing consequences that will promote eventual maintenance of the target behavior in natural settings. These strategies include: (1) careful management of response consequences, (2) use of naturally occurring consequences as reinforcers, (3) teaching contingency management to significant others in the child's environment, (4) teaching the child self-monitoring skills, and (5) teaching the child to ask for reinforcement (contingency priming).

> "I do not reinforce children in language therapy because it is artificial." So claim some clinicians. They will admit to giving *feedback*, however. *Reinforcement* is a technical term that captures the essence of a social (verbal) interaction. If a speaker's verbal responses are not differentially responded to, there is no verbal interaction. *Differentially responding* to a child's verbal attempts is reinforcement or corrective feedback.

Management of response consequences. In Chapter 5, we discussed various ways in which the clinician responds to a child's correct and incorrect responses. Technically described as schedules of reinforcement or corrective feedback, such differential clinician reactions help establish and eventually help maintain the target skill in the natural environment. In the initial stages of treatment, the clinician should reinforce all correct responses and give corrective feedback for all incorrect responses (a continuous schedule of consequences). Differential and continuous feedback for correct and incorrect responses is efficient in establishing skills.

The eventual goal of treatment, however, is maintenance of skills in natural settings in the absence of the highly specialized reinforcement and corrective feedback the clinician provided in the clinic room. Therefore, as soon as possible, the clinician should move from a continuous schedule of consequences to an intermittent schedule in which the clinician refrains from responding to the correctness of some of the responses a child gives during treatment. A shift from continuous to intermittent mode should occur gradually so that the correct response rate is maintained and increased. If the correct response rate declines when shifted to an intermittent schedule, the clinician should reinstate a continuous schedule for a brief period of time. Eventually, the child's correct response rate should be maintained in the presence of reduced reinforcement; at the level of conversational speech, the need for reinforcement should be minimal.

In the initial stages of treatment, reinforcement or corrective feedback is delivered promptly when a response is made. Delayed reinforcement or corrective feedback tends to be ineffective or inefficient in establishing skills. Delayed delivery of consequences, however, is desirable in promoting maintenance of target skills in the natural environment where such delays are common (Baer et al., 1984; Dunlap et al., 1987; Stromer, McComas, & Rehfeldt, 2000). Any clinical procedure that resembles patterns of everyday interaction will help maintain clinically established skills. Therefore, in the final stages of treatment, the clinician should periodically delay the delivery of response consequences to see if the skills are still sustained. If they are, the clinician should delay response consequences more often. The duration of the delay should be increased in gradual steps, and the clinician should be prepared to decrease the duration of the delay at any point, if a decrease in the correct response rate is noted.

Use of naturally occurring consequences. In the clinic setting, the clinician may use specific verbal praise (e.g., "I heard that *s* at the end of the word! That is great!"), primary reinforcers (e.g., food items), or both. It may be necessary to use such reinforcers to get a response established during initial stages of treatment. Nonverbal children who have autism, developmental disability, or both may indeed need primary reinforcers in the initial stages of treatment. In the natural environment, though, the child is not likely to be reinforced in such a manner. Production of plural -*s*, for example, is not usually rewarded in the natural setting by specific verbal praise or a piece of popcorn being popped into a child's mouth.

As we noted earlier, the clinician fades all reinforcers to some extent. The fading is especially critical for primary reinforcers which are not normally used to reinforce verbal behaviors. Verbal approval is the most common verbal reinforcer for many kinds of language responses. When a child correctly names an object or produces a grammatically complex sentence, verbal approval is natural (e.g., "Yes, that is a giraffe!" or "That was a nice long sentence!"). Most specific kinds of verbal praise (e.g., "Yes, I heard that [plural] *s* this time!") may be faded into more general statements of approval ("Good!" "Correct!" or "I like that!").

Although primary reinforcers (food and other objects) are atypical, they are the reinforcers for one class of verbal behaviors called mands (requests, commands, questions, etc.; see Chapters 1 and 6). Mands specify their own reinforcers, and the best reinforcer is the one that a response specifies. Listener compliance is the most effective and natural reinforcer for all mands. For instance, if the target behaviors are requests (e.g., "Some juice, please" or "May I have that crayon please?"), the natural consequence would be to promptly provide what the request specifies. If the target behaviors are asking questions, the natural consequence would be to provide the children with answers to questions they ask (e.g., "What time is it?" or "What is your name?"). If the target behaviors are commands, the clinician should perform the action the child is being taught to command. During highly structured play activities, the child may receive natural reinforcement for production of adjectives by receiving the item the child correctly described. In all such cases, adding naturalistic verbal praise to the specified reinforcer might be beneficial. For instance, the clinician might say: "You requested nicely. Here is the crayon."; "You asked a right question! My name is Verbalena."; "You correctly told me to sit down. See, I am sitting down!"; and so forth.

> Technically, mands are a function of (caused by) a state of motivation (deprivation, need). To reinforce a mand, the causal need must be satisfied. They are unlike tacts, which describe or comment on events.

The use of conditioned generalized reinforcers (e.g., tokens, stickers, etc.) is a technique that mirrors what happens when people use money to buy "back-up reinforcers" (e.g., something the person may desire). As noted in Chapter 6, a back-up reinforcer may be an activity the child is allowed to engage in after earning a few tokens (e.g., 2 minutes of coloring). Offering the child an opportunity to "earn" enough "money" to "purchase" a backup reinforcer naturally lends itself to a concept commonly encountered in the child's environment. It is also a technique that can easily be taught to the child's parents or teachers.

There are many ways to structure therapy so that reinforcers more closely resemble those the child is likely to encounter in the natural setting. As noted before, the necessary use of reinforcement techniques that are more specialized to the clinic setting should be paired with reinforcement techniques that are more natural. The clinician should always give warm verbal praise along with other kinds of reinforcers. As the correct response rate becomes established, the clinician can then gradually withdraw specialized reinforcers, so that the response rate is maintained in the presence of warm verbal praise—a type of reinforcement people in the child's environment are more likely to use.

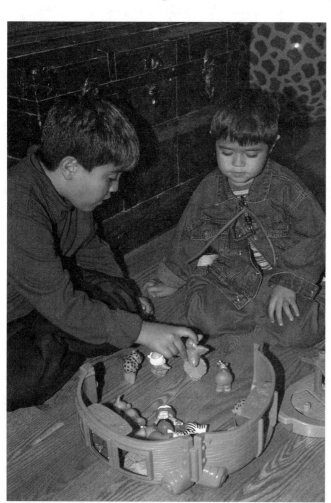

photo 9.3

A typically developing older brother helps his younger brother, who has a language disorder, play appropriately with a toy at home.

Teaching contingency management to others in the child's environment. This is the heart of extending treatment to naturalistic settings. If the people who regularly interact with the child begin to prompt the production of correct skills, reinforce such productions, give nonpunitive corrective feedback when the child makes mistakes, treatment then is extended to the natural setting. It may be noted that "extending the treatment and managing the treatment contingency in the child's environment" is a technical description of what should happen. For the family members and significant others, it is indeed an important change in their life: they need to become supportive and willing communicative partners with the child. This strategy underscores the view that extending treatment to naturalistic settings is the final treatment strategy.

In the beginning stages of treatment, family members and others in the child's environment should be encouraged to watch treatment sessions to familiarize themselves with methods used to evoke and reinforce target behaviors. As treatment progresses, all important individuals in the child's environment—parents, teachers, siblings, peers, caregivers, and others—should be taught to evoke, model, prompt, and reinforce target behaviors at home and in other nonclinical settings (see Photo 9.3 for an example of a sibling working with his brother). There is evidence that when multiple peers are recruited to offer treatment, skills tend to generalize better than when a single peer is involved (Pierce & Schreibman, 1995, 1997). Additionally, as discussed earlier, there is evidence that home-based treatment is efficient in promoting maintenance of target skills (Arndorfer et al., 1994; Derby et al., 1997; Krantz, MacDuff, & McClanahan, 1993).

> The clinician who asks parents to prompt and reinforce their children for target skill productions at home should prepare the child to receive such help from parents. A mother once reported that the first time she reinforced her son for producing a nice long sentence, the child said, "Why are you saying that? You are not Miss Jenny!" He was fine with the feedback when he learned that Miss Jenny wanted his Mom to help him.

The clinician should emphasize the importance of extending treatment to natural settings by teaching significant others to act in such a way that will support and maintain the child's newly learned language skills. Their support usually comes in the form of prompts, praise (plenty of it), gentle and subtle corrective feedback, an occasional model, periodic instructions, and, generally, attention to the child's communication. In this endeavor, the people in the child's environment should not only draw the child into social interactions, but strongly reinforce any attempt the child makes on his or her own to enter into such interactions. Above all, the significant others should interact with the child more often in ways that make such interactions highly reinforcing to that child.

In the school setting, the participation of the child's teacher in extending treatment to the classroom setting is important. The teacher should be given a written description of the child's target behaviors and should be shown how to evoke and reinforce those behaviors in subtle but effective ways. For example, if the child has been taught to ask for help, the teacher should respond positively when the child does so. If the target behavior is expansion of mean length of utterance, the teacher should prompt and reinforce lengthier expressions from the child. For a child who is learning to ask questions, the teacher should gently evoke that behavior (e.g., "Johnny, do you have a question?") and then promptly answer the question.

> Clinicians work with classroom teachers in a collaborative manner. Teachers should be involved at the very beginning of treatment, helping to guide the assessment of the child and suggesting possible treatment targets. If teachers' input has been carefully considered and acted on, the clinician's suggestions for classroom intervention will be warmly welcomed.

In essence, the clinician should work very closely with all significant others in the child's environment to maximize the potential for maintenance of language skills in natural settings. The clinician should also teach significant others how to recognize and reinforce all appropriate language behaviors the child may exhibit during daily routines, not just those behaviors that are targeted in clinic. It is important for everyone involved with the child to understand that the child's language skills will be maintained only when they come under the control of natural stimuli and consequences.

Teaching self-monitoring and contingency priming skills. While teaching significant others to extend treatment to natural settings is an effective maintenance strategy, it is even more effective to teach the child self-monitoring techniques that will maintain correct responses when no one else is around to help. Children can learn to self-monitor their communicative behaviors. They also can learn to seek out reinforcement when those in their environment fail to provide it.

Self-monitoring is a teachable skill that includes self-evaluation and self-correction. Several procedures have been researched (Rhode, Morgan, & Young, 1983; Sainato, Goldstein, & Strain, 1992; Shapiro, McGonigle, & Ollendick, 1980), but the most practical and simpler of them is to teach a child to judge the accuracy of his or her own productions. A child who is taught to chart his or her own production of morphologic, syntactic, and pragmatic behaviors will begin to self-monitor correct productions. This requires that the child understand the behavior that is expected and recognize the correct language form when it is produced. Therefore, the child is first taught to discriminate between correct and incorrect responses and then to contrast his or her own correct and incorrect responses. The clinician should give the child models of correct and incorrect productions (e.g., "The boy walking." "The boy *is* walking." or "two cup," "two cups"), using vocal emphasis to help the child discriminate between correct and incorrect responses.

> Once a 6-year-old boy who saw the clinician charting his production of the article *the*, asked the clinician, "What are you doing?" The clinician said, "I am counting how many times you say 'the' correctly. Do you want to count, too?" The boy eagerly agreed to count. He was delighted when the clinician handed him a sheet of paper and a pencil.

After the child has learned to discriminate between correct and incorrect responses, he or she is asked to evaluate responses along with the clinician, perhaps by charting correct responses with a plus sign and incorrect responses with a minus sign (or happy- and sad-face stamps, or whatever the system the clinician finds useful). To the extent possible, the clinician should give immediate feedback to the child on his or her self-monitoring skills. For example, a child who fails to make a plus or a minus sign can be prompted to do so. At the end of the session, the child's judgments may be compared to the clinician's.

The clinician can briefly discuss results with the child ("Oh, look! We agreed on three out of four responses that time!"), giving the child informative or corrective feedback, to ensure that charting skills will improve.

Charting responses can be intrinsically reinforcing to a child who is making good progress. The clinician might allow the child to keep track of progress session-by-session by plotting the correct response rate on a more comprehensive chart at the end of each treatment session, giving verbal praise when appropriate ("Look how many more you got right this time!").

Teaching children to self-correct is the next step. Children who can reliably chart their correct and incorrect responses may be asked to catch their own mistakes, stop, and rephrase or correct their mistakes. Whenever children thus stop and correct themselves, the clinician may verbally reinforce them. Whenever they fail to stop and correct themselves, the clinician may quickly stop them and prompt them to stop at the earliest sign of errors and correct those errors.

Teaching a child self-monitoring skills will ensure that even when no one else is around, the target behaviors will be monitored; the child is the only individual who can monitor the behavior all the time. When the child becomes his or her own therapist, maintenance of target behaviors in natural settings is considerably enhanced.

> Reinforcement priming is reinforcement begging! But it is desirable begging! It is the "Look at me!" request. The worst case of reinforcement priming is a show-off. People of all ages prime others for praise. A child who stopped his previously exhibited uncooperative behaviors (after differential reinforcement for not exhibiting them) came out of the session and announced to his Dad, "Dad, I didn't even act-up today!" and received a warm hug from his father. Listeners know what is expected when they hear: "Did you notice my new hair style?" "See, Miss Lyndee, I got new shoes!" or "Do you like my new tie?"

A potential problem children face is that the significant people in their lives may not reinforce desirable communicative behaviors that they have just learned to produce at home. Happy though they are that the child is communicating more effectively, some parents, in spite of a clinician's instruction, may fail to pay attention to their child's hard-earned communicative skills. Busy teachers, too, may fail to promptly turn their attention to desirable behaviors in children. Responses thus ignored are likely to be extinguished. In such cases, **contingency priming,** also known as **reinforcement recruitment,** might be useful (Craft, Alber, & Heward, 1998; Mank & Horner, 1987; Morgan, Young, &

Goldstein, 1983; Stokes, Fowler, & Baer, 1978). It is a technique of drawing out reinforcement (usually attention and positive comments) from ignoring persons. In using this technique, a child learns to prompt others in the environment to provide positive feedback for correct responses. In the present context, the child prompts others by drawing attention to his or her new language skills. Only those children who have learned to effectively self-evaluate (self-monitor) their skills can use this technique. The child who knows he or she has produced correct language responses may then draw the parents' attention to the behavior. Children can use contingency priming to remind parents, teachers, and others to reinforce correct productions. Contingency priming occurs every time a child says something such as, "Hey, Mom! I said, 'I ate the hot dog' instead of 'I eated' it! Pretty good, huh?" followed by warm verbal praise from the mother.

The maintenance strategies described in this section will help strengthen the language skills and extend treatment to naturalistic settings. The strategies also help teach self-monitoring skills and reinforcement priming in naturalistic settings. Taken together, the strategies help sustain the skills in natural settings. Even the most carefully designed maintenance program, however, will not guarantee that the child's language behaviors will be maintained forever, without additional clinical intervention. To guard against the possibility of language behaviors being extinguished post-dismissal, the clinician should plan on providing follow-up assessment and, if necessary, booster treatment (Hegde, 1998b; Hegde & Davis, 1999).

Follow-Up and Booster Treatment

At the time of dismissal, the child should be scheduled for follow-up assessment to monitor maintenance of language behaviors in natural settings. Although the schedule can be set up according to the clinician's judgment, a general rule is to provide follow-up assessment with decreasing frequency. For example, the clinician could schedule a child for follow-up assessment twice in the first 6 months post-dismissal, with one follow-up assessment scheduled after 1 year, and then perhaps another after 2 years. The follow-up schedule is always individualized and may be more or less frequent.

The follow-up assessment is a probe of conversational speech and consists of an analysis of language samples gathered in clinical as well as natural settings. The clinician can ask the parents or teachers to tape record the child's conversational speech at home, school, in the community, or any other setting. As an alternative, the clinician can visit the child at home or in the classroom, on the playground, or other settings to listen to the child's production of language. To establish reliability, at least two samples of the child's speech, each recorded in a different setting, should be obtained. The samples from the natural settings should be supplemented with a clinic sample.

If analysis of the language samples reveal that the language skills are maintained in the everyday conversational speech of the child, no further action is necessary until the next follow-up assessment is due. However, if the analysis reveals that the language skills the child learned in the clinic setting are not maintained in natural settings, or are produced at a rate that is judged to be unacceptably low, it will be necessary to provide booster treatment to the child to re-establish the behaviors previously taught.

Booster treatment consists of a brief round of therapy, which is offered after a period following dismissal from the original treatment. Booster treatment should not be as intense or as extensive as the original treatment. In many cases, it will be possible to reestablish the target behavior in as little as one or two sessions, although, if the deterioration of the response rate is severe, more sessions will be needed. Clinicians may use the same treatment that worked before, or some variation that has recently been proven to be effective.

Lack of maintenance following dismissal from treatment may suggest that the actions of significant others in supporting the child's communication skills have faded over time. If this is the case, the clinician should review the supportive behaviors (prompting, reinforcing) the parents and others were taught to strengthen the target skills in the child. Essentially, a brief refresher course in supporting the child's language skills, offered along booster treatment, may bring the skill levels back to where they were or should be.

Parents and teachers should be told at the very beginning of treatment that periodic follow-up assessments and possible rounds of future therapy may be necessary after the child has been formally dismissed from treatment. If the significant others in the child's life are informed of the need for follow-up assessment and booster treatment before treatment is even begun, they will be less likely to think treatment has failed if the language behaviors begin to deteriorate after the child is dismissed. They may also be more likely to bring the child back for follow-up assessment. Finally, the clinician should let the child's significant others know that they should report any noticeable change for the worse in the child's language production or comprehension. When people know that there are solutions, they are more likely to report the problem.

When language target behaviors are continuously maintained in natural settings, as revealed by periodic follow-up assessment of language samples, the clinician can consider the job done and the goals met. It is at that point that treatment is complete, and the child has realized his or her full communicative potential.

For some children, however, treatment is a continuous process. These are children who, because of some associated clinical condition, such as autism or developmental disability, will always need help with their language skills. For these children, certain modifications must be made both in assessment and treatment methods and procedures. The following chapters will examine several clinical conditions that are associated with language disorders and suggest ways in which assessment and intervention must be adapted to the needs of specific children.

Chapter Summary

Expanded social communication skills should be generalized to naturalistic settings and then maintained over time. Achieving this goal requires a partnership with the family and others involved in the life of the child. Generalization is a behavioral process in which learned responses are extended to new stimuli and new situations. The clinician should promote stimulus, setting, conversational partner, and response generalization. Discrimination is the opposite of generalization; it is a behavioral process of differentiating responses and concepts. Children learn generalization and discrimination through the behavioral principle of differential reinforcement, in which desirable responses to a specific stimulus are reinforced, and undesirable responses are not reinforced.

Maintenance, not generalization, is the ultimate clinical goal because generalized responses may or may not be maintained. To promote maintenance, the clinician uses a variety of strategies that include specific procedures to manage treatment stimuli, target responses, and response consequences. Among others discussed in the chapter, selecting naturalistic treatment stimuli; targeting functional and child-specific skills; teaching skills with multiple exemplars; giving sufficient treatment at the conversational level; switching to intermittent reinforcement schedules; delaying reinforcement; using naturally occurring consequences; teaching self-monitoring skills; and training parents to stimulate, prompt, and reinforce target skills will help promote maintenance of social communication skills in children. Periodic follow-up and scheduling booster treatment when the skills deteriorate will further the goal of maintenance.

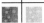 ## Study Guide

1. Discuss the two behavioral processes that are important in language learning and teaching: *generalization* and *discrimination*. Give examples from normal child language literature that illustrate the two processes at work. Show parallels in treatment of language disorders and point out the importance of working on the two processes in treatment of children with language disorders.

2. Critically evaluate the statement made in the chapter that "the final goal of treatment is maintenance, not generalization." Why was generalization defined the way it was in this chapter? How does it contrast with more common assumptions about generalization?

3. You have been working with a child in a school setting. You have made significant progress in teaching both the basic and more advanced language skills in your clinical room. However, the teachers have complained that the child in the classroom does not produce any of the skills you have targeted in your individual treatment sessions. You then decide to give a brief workshop on what the teacher can do to help the child produce the skills in the classroom and then promote their maintenance over time. Describe an outline of such a workshop and be specific about what the teacher needs to do. Use nontechnical language so the teacher can easily implement your suggestions.

4. Self-monitoring is a skill you can teach that will help promote maintenance of language targets taught in the clinic. Describe how you judge that a child is self-monitoring. Specify the measurement procedure. How would you teach self-monitoring to a 5-year-old child? Assume you are teaching pragmatic language skills.

5. Distinguish the various reinforcement schedules described in the chapter. Give examples of each type of schedule. Specify how you use them in a comprehensive treatment program that begins with the teaching of basic skills and moves on to more advanced skills taught in naturalistic contexts.

6. You have scheduled a meeting with the parents of a 7-year-old boy you have been treating for language disorders. Your agenda for the meeting is to teach the parents techniques that would help promote the maintenance of language skills you have taught the child. What suggestions would you offer the parents? Describe what the parents should do in nontechnical language. Describe also how you would monitor the parents' work, the child's progress, and how you would refine the parents' actions.

chapter 10

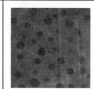

Supporting Academic Performance:
Language and Literacy

outline

Certain trends in the educational philosophy governing delivery of special education services have profoundly affected speech-language pathologists (SLPs) working in public schools. The distinction between special education and general education service delivery has been fading as advocates for disabled children have promoted full inclusion for all children in the general education classroom. The push toward full inclusion has been hastened by federal legislation mandating an appropriate and free education delivered in the least-restrictive environment to all public school children (see Box 10.1 for a summary of federal legislation affecting models of service delivery to children with disabilities). The pull-out model by which speech-language services have traditionally been delivered in the public schools is inconsistent with policies of full inclusion, and alternative models have been proposed to make delivery of those services more integrative. Delivery of services via alternative models has been necessitated by shifting educational dogma and large caseloads resulting from limited funding for special education services. Whether or not alternative models result in more effective intervention, however, is open to question (Kavale & Mostert, 2003).

Other trends in education have created another major change in the role of the school SLP. The scope of practice for SLPs now includes intervention for children who have problems with literacy. A position statement of the American Speech-Language-Hearing

box 10.1

Federal Legislation Affecting Models of Service Delivery to Children with Disabilities

The Education for All Handicapped Children Act (PL 94-142, 1975)

This act guaranteed to all children, regardless of the severity of their handicap, a free and appropriate public education (FAPE) delivered in the least restrictive environment (LRE). The act specified that children with disabilities should be provided with an individualized education plan (IEP) tailored for the needs of each student. The act further mandated that parents be given the right to participate in making decisions affecting their child's educational program.

Education of the Handicapped Act Amendments of 1986 (PL 99-457)

This act extended PL 94-142 to provide free and appropriate public education to preschool children, ages 3 to 5. The act also created a voluntary program to assist states in developing programs for infants from birth through age 2 with, and at risk for, disabilities. The act required eligible children and their families to be provided with an individualized family service plan (IFSP) detailing delivery of necessary services to the entire family, not just the individual child.

Individuals with Disabilities Education Act (IDEA) (PL 101-476, 1990)

PL 94-142 was reauthorized, amended, and renamed the Individuals with Disabilities Education Act (IDEA) in 1990. One of the provisions of PL 101-476 requires each student with a disability to have, at no later than age 16, an individual transition plan (ITP) included in the IEP to plan for the student's movement into adult living. The ITP therefore serves as a roadmap to vocational training, further education, and as independent an adult lifestyle as possible. IDEA was further amended in 1991, 1997, and 2004. Amendments included provisions for providing early intervention services in "natural environments" among typically developing peers and for transition procedures to facilitate movement of infants to preschool services and toddlers to public elementary schools. The most recent amendment, the Individuals with Disabilities Education Improvement Act of 2004 addresses many issues, among them a student's right to receive instruction delivered by highly qualified personnel trained in research-based methods (Council for Exceptional Children, 2004).

Association (ASHA, 2001) delineated this change by stating that SLPs have a "critical and direct role" in the assessment and remediation of children with communicative disorders who also have reading disabilities. ASHA also recognized a role for SLPs in promoting literacy for *all* public school children, stating that SLPs should support and make contributions to "the literacy efforts of a school district or community on behalf of other children and adolescents" (p. 69). Some SLPs have embraced such a role; others, pointing to burgeoning caseloads, have resisted it.

This chapter will begin with a more in-depth look at (1) trends in special education service delivery and (2) trends in literacy education. The chapter will conclude with a description of procedures to assess and treat literacy problems.

Trends in Special Education Service Delivery

Services for children with communicative disorders have traditionally been delivered via a **pull-out model** in which children receive either individual or, more commonly, small-group therapy in a clinic room. School SLPs who manage to give individual therapy at least two times a week for at least 40 minutes a session (admittedly a rarity in the school setting) enjoy the support of treatment efficacy research. Treatment procedures advocated in this book are based on one-on-one therapy in the clinic setting. It is this kind of treatment that has been supported by experimental research. It may be recalled that children with language disorders need special stimuli arranged in unique ways by professional SLPs who have the expertise to provide specialized intervention.

> Traditionally, services for children with communicative disorders have been provided using what kind of service delivery model?

In many ways, a public school is an ideal setting for carrying out this type of service delivery. The school SLP is frequently on campus (sometimes constantly), and is readily available to children and teachers. There are unlimited opportunities for school SLPs to observe children on their caseloads in natural settings—in the classroom, on the playground, in the cafeteria, and so forth. School SLPs who have nurtured respectful, mutually beneficial professional relationships with classroom teachers can collaborate effectively, advising teachers and demonstrating ways in which language target behaviors can be evoked and reinforced in the classroom setting. Also, public schools have unrealized potential as prospective laboratories to investigate efficacy of treatment procedures and models of service delivery.

Unfortunately, school SLPs are sometimes isolated from the daily routine of classroom and playground activities. Many school SLPs are itinerant—they travel from school site to school site. Consequently, it may be difficult for them to establish personal or professional connections with school personnel at any of the sites served. Sometimes the isolation has to do with physical placement of the "speech room"—perhaps a portable facility separated from wings of regular classrooms. Sometimes SLP's isolation is the result of an overwhelming and burgeoning caseload and piles of paperwork they have to complete. The result is that there is not enough time for involvement with general education activities. Some teachers may think remediating children's language difficulties is the SLP's job. Such teachers may resist the idea of receiving advice from SLPs and incorporating that advice into their classroom instruction and activities. In short, all too often, school SLPs delivering services exclusively on a pull-out model are buried in the clinic room, striving to deliver effective therapy to too many children and to keep up with paperwork. For many, establishing collaborative relationships with general education personnel has been a desirable but unattainable goal.

The quick answer to this dilemma is to reduce caseloads by increasing funding for special education services. Delivery of efficacious speech and language therapy is not difficult, if caseloads are reasonable. All too often, however, caseloads are not reasonable. In California, for example, state law requires that average SLP caseloads in a school district not exceed 55 children, and yet anecdotally, a single SLP may serve 100 children. Such horrendous caseloads are the result of a shortage of SLPs and increasingly limited funding available for special education services.

Increased caseloads have necessitated new methods of service delivery. ASHA (1996a) has approved the use of speech-language pathology assistants (SLPAs). These are paraprofessionals who are supervised by a credentialed school SLPs. Their scope of practice is limited; they cannot assess or prescribe a treatment plan, but they can deliver therapy a supervising SLP has prescribed. To date, evidence on the efficacy of SLPAs' services has not been gathered.

Besides increased caseloads, legislation and educational philosophy have dictated a shift to more integrated service delivery models. The goals of advocates for disabled people and the goals of legislators seeking to stretch federal and state dollars have meshed to produce a trend toward full inclusion of severely disabled students in regular education classrooms. The ultimate goal of many is to see the line between general education and special education erased, with the needs of all students being met within the general education framework. ASHA acknowledged this trend in a 1996 position statement, with some cautionary language, stating "ASHA believes that the shift toward inclusion will not be optimal when implemented in absolute terms. Rather, the unique and specific needs of each child and family must always be considered" (p. 35). Many special educators would agree that individual needs must not be overlooked in yet another "bandwagon effect"—the rush to fully include all disabled students in regular teaching arrangements.

The push for full inclusion has led to a rejection of the pull-out model by some school districts. It is thought that children are stigmatized by being singled out in such a manner, that valuable classroom instruction time is lost while children are in therapy, and that speech and language behaviors learned in a clinic setting are less likely to generalize to the classroom setting. School SLPs are encouraged instead to develop alternative methods of service delivery that are more in keeping with the educational philosophy and legal mandates of full inclusion. Two of the most commonly used alternative methods of service delivery include: (1) the consultative model, and (2) the collaborative model.

The Consultative Model

In the **consultative model,** speech-language services are delivered indirectly. Assessing, diagnosing, and planning for treatment are all functions that are carried out by the SLP. Intervention, however, is provided by others who are taught to evoke and reinforce language target behaviors in natural settings. SLPs may consult with parents, teachers, classroom aides, even with the child's peers who will then carry out a plan for intervention devised by the SLP. While the treatment plan is in place, the SLP should meet with all individuals

> True or False? In the consultative model, language services are directly provided.

involved with the child to monitor progress, to give feedback, and to make any necessary modifications to the treatment plan.

The consultative model may be beneficial for children who have a very mild language disorder. Too often, however, the consultative model is used as a way to manage unreasonably high case loads. Children with more severe language disorders will benefit by direct treatment and should receive it. In our experience, the consultative model is best used as a maintenance strategy—as a "bridge" between having met target behavior criteria in the classroom and eventual dismissal after having met the criteria in natural settings. In addition, there is no evidence that this model achieves its goal: remediating communicative disorders in school-age children.

The Collaborative Model

The **collaborative model** emphasizes the interrelatedness of the school SLP with other school personnel and is consistent with the mandated requirements that all special education services be directly tied to the curriculum and delivered in the least restrictive environment. While there have been numerous variations to the collaborative model proposed, some common elements include:

- Membership of the SLP in the educational team, including parents, teachers, administrators, providers of other instructional services, and the student (see Box 10.2 for types of professional teams)
- Shared responsibility for determining assessment procedures, writing treatment goals, devising treatment plans, and carrying out intervention
- Provision of special education services (e.g., language therapy) within the classroom and other natural settings

Working under a collaborative model requires a school SLP to become thoroughly familiar with the school curriculum, as legally mandated. It encourages inter-professional rela-

---

box 10.2 **Types of Professional Teams**

Three types of teams SLPs may work with are: (1) multidisciplinary, (2) transdisciplinary, and (3) interdisciplinary. Of the three, transdisciplinary is most suited for the collaborative model.

Multidisciplinary

In multidisciplinary teams, several disciplines are represented (e.g., the SLP, the psychologist, the school nurse, the adaptive physical education specialist, etc.). Each professional assesses and writes a separate evaluation, with little input from other members. Treatment is carried out by the professional most responsible for the type of treatment required, again with little input from other members.

Interdisciplinary

There is more interaction among interdisciplinary team members; a team member's suggestions may be adapted by another, assessment reports are collaboratively written, but treatment is again the responsibility of one team member.

Transdisciplinary

There is interaction among transdisciplinary team members in every aspect of assessment and treatment. Assessment is performed while all team members are present, assessment reports are written collaboratively, and treatment is the responsibility of several team members.

tionships focused on providing integrated, high-quality instructional services to students. For the collaborative model to be effective, school SLPs should function as welcome resources to classroom teachers.

Applied as it is conceptualized, the collaborative model involves providing intervention in the classroom setting. The SLP is in the classroom, either delivering whole class instruction while indirectly monitoring language behaviors of children on the caseload, or "floating" from child to child while the classroom teacher delivers a lesson. Another possibility is for the SLP to enter a classroom and pull children on the caseload aside for individual or small-group therapy.

While there are many aspects of the collaborative model that may sound ideal, there is a dearth of experimental research to support its efficacy. For the collaborative model to be fully embraced, it should be shown to be superior to the traditional pull-out model which allows direct treatment of communicative disorders. At the very least, it should be shown that language target behaviors can be established through the collaborative model with efficacy that is equal to that of the pull-out model. The problem, though, is that even the traditional pull-out model has not been experimentally evaluated for its efficacy.

It is possible to deliver language services using a combination of various methods of service delivery. It is best to establish language behaviors initially through direct one-on-one, or, at the very most, *small*-group therapy, in a clinic setting. That would require continued use of the traditional pull-out method. However, after language behaviors have been established, a combination of consultative and collaborative methods of service delivery may be useful in promoting generalization and maintenance of target behaviors in natural settings. There are obvious benefits to using more collaborative methods to establish the school SLP as a respected professional integrated into the daily routine of a public school campus.

> Consultative and collaborative models may help to promote generalization and maintenance of target behaviors.

What is urgently needed is the evidence that any of the service delivery models advocated or used in public schools are effective. New models are advocated for reasons other than their demonstrated effectiveness. Like most other trends in education and special education, new concepts are not based on experimental research. They are based on social, political, and economic exigencies.

Adapting to demands of changing service delivery models is not the only challenge facing today's school SLP. A number of trends in education have resulted in the identification of school SLPs as professionals likely to be of help in remediating children's difficulties in literacy. The remainder of the chapter will discuss those trends and provide methods for the assessment and treatment of reading and writing.

Trends in Literacy Instruction

Among the several reasons why SLPs are now involved with children's literacy, three new trends in education are important: (1) the adoption of an emergent literacy viewpoint over a reading readiness model, (2) a trend away from the use of the whole language instructional model in favor of instruction in explicit skills, and (3) a realization that reading and writing are language-based activities.

Emergent Literacy versus Reading Readiness

For many years, educators believed that a child should possess reading readiness skills before formalized instruction in reading and writing began. Various formal tests were used to determine whether a child had: (1) what were considered to be necessary visual, auditory, and linguistic skills, and (2) achieved a mental age of 6.5 years. It was believed that children without such skills could not benefit from instruction in reading and writing (Erickson, 2000; Polloway & Smith, 1992). Many children with cognitive deficits, even slight ones, were therefore excluded from direct instruction in literacy (Erickson, 2000). Unfortunately, the assumption that children without certain prerequisite skills or those with cognitive deficits do not benefit from instruction in **literacy skills** was not based on any experimental evidence. Therefore, it was an educational dogma that ensured low literacy skills in such children.

> The idea that children who do not show some presumed skills should not be taught certain other skills is the most detrimental psycho-educational myth. In most cases, teaching the target skills directly may be more beneficial than spending time on presumed prerequisites.

More recently, however, researchers have documented that children become aware of print and begin to develop rudimentary literacy skills long before they enter school (Gillam & Johnston, 1985; Snow, Burns, & Griffin, 1998; Sulzby, 1985; van Kleeck, 1990, 1998; Whitehurst & Lonigan, 1998). Such **emergent literacy skills** may be independent of any presumed "reading readiness" skills. For example, children notice environmental print in the home and in the community and may become aware of the meaning of labels, logos, and commonly encountered signs. This may be the very beginning of children's understanding of meaning from printed material.

Beyond a rudimentary understanding of print and its message, preschoolers differ widely in early literacy skills. Children who live in literacy-enriched households, with plenty of reading material and writing supplies available, tend to be more advanced in language and literacy skills than those whose home environments are literacy-impoverished. Children who are exposed to reading and writing materials at home learn to hold a book, turn the pages of the book, and begin to make the connection between the printed word and the meaning it conveys. Parents and caregivers who regularly read and write at home provide good role models for their children. Parents and caregivers who read to preschool children promote and reinforce early attempts at reading and writing in their children. As a result, they create positive and pleasant experiences with literacy activities for their children (Teale & Sulzby, 1986; Whitehurst & Lonigan, 1998).

Children who come from literacy-enriched households enter public schools well-equipped to benefit from formal literacy instruction. Unfortunately, many children come from households with few literacy materials, infrequent or nonexistent storybook reading, and adults who do not read or write. These children may enter public schools without having learned basic print concepts and with little in their learning history that would motivate them to learn to read and write (Hart & Risley, 1995; Whitehurst & Fischel, 2000).

While there is no definitive research available on the causal link between emergent literacy and future reading and writing skills, research on emergent literacy has fostered an even greater interest in early identification and treatment of children who are at risk for reading disabilities. School SLPs who serve on preschool assessment teams and have early elementary grade children on their caseloads are in a unique position to assess and help enrich a child's home literacy environment.

Whole Language versus Explicit Skill Instruction

The whole language approach was embraced for decades as an effective method of reading instruction, even though not a single, controlled experimental research study had shown it to be effective. The basic underlying presumption of the whole language approach was that reading and writing could be learned naturally, in much the same manner as listening and speaking is learned, without explicit instruction in basic skills such as word decoding (e.g., "sounding out" individual printed words), grammar, spelling, and punctuation.

Although the assumption that reading and writing skills are learned much like oral language without explicit instruction flew in the face of both empirical research and even common sense, the approach enjoyed acceptance for many years. The result, as many college professors will attest, was generations of young people who entered college without adequate reading and writing skills. Consequently, the unfounded belief in the merits of the whole language approach has been replaced by the realization that explicit instruction is necessary for children to become proficient readers and writers.

> Sweeping trends in education often take place without experimental evidence to support touted "new and improved" approaches.

Phonological awareness and phonemic awareness. Of particular relevance to school SLPs is a return to the use of systematic **phonics** instruction, a method in which children learn the names of letters of the alphabet and the sounds those letters represent. In much the same way as emergent literacy is thought to be a precursor to future literacy skills, the attribute of phonological awareness, including phonemic awareness, has been presumed to be a prerequisite to a child's ability to benefit fully from phonics instruction (see Box 10.3 for definitions). As a result, school SLPs are often expected to assess and treat phonological awareness in very young children. While instruction in letter-sound relationship and sound patterns may be helpful, it is not clear from research that phonological and phonemic awareness is necessary to further literacy skills in children. This issue will be critically evaluated in a later section.

Reading and Writing as Language-Based Activities

Perhaps no other factor justifies SLPs' involvement in literacy than the research-supported view that reading and writing are language-based activities, in contrast to past assumptions that reading disability was primarily due to visual deficits. It is now recognized that reading and writing are an extension of a child's oral language skills (Catts & Kamhi, 1999; Goldsworthy, 1996). The higher the proficiency in oral language, the easier it is to teach a child to read and write. Conversely, the lower the oral language skills, the greater the degree of effort involved in teaching a child to read and write. The prevalence of reading disability among children who have language disorders has been found to be as high as 60 percent.

> What is the prevalence of reading disability among children with language disorders?

Therefore, children with language disorders are at risk for the development of literacy problems (Lewis et al., 1998; Wiig, Zureich, & Chan, 2000). There is also evidence that children who are poor readers at the end of the first grade are likely to remain poor readers; maturation alone will not improve their reading (Catts et al., 2002; Flax et al., 2003; Justice et al., 2003; Whitehurst & Fischel, 2000).

Intervention is necessary to improve skills in both spoken and written language. While good oral language skills may be a foundation on which to build literacy skills, oral box 10.3   **Basic Definitions of Literacy Terms**

Literacy skills: Reading and writing.

Emergent literacy skills: Early skills that precede or are presumed to be prerequisites for later developing reading and writing skills.

Phonics: A method of reading instruction that emphasizes sound-letter correspondences and skills in "sounding out" (decoding) words.

Phoneme: The smallest part of spoken language that affects word meaning.

Grapheme: The smallest part of written language, represented by alphabetic letters. Graphemes represent phonemes; a grapheme may be just one letter or a combination of letters (e.g., *c* for /k/ or /s/; *ng* for /ŋ/; *ough* for /o/, /u/, or /au/).

Phonemic awareness: Skill in discriminately hearing, identifying, and manipulating individual phonemes, or sounds, in spoken words.

Phonological awareness: A term that includes phonemic awareness but also involves awareness and manipulation of rhyme, words, syllables, and onsets and rimes.

Syllable: Part of a word containing a vowel; the vowel can stand alone or be surrounded by one or more consonants (e.g., *ba-by*; *re-frig-er-a-tor*).

Onset and rime: Every word has an onset and a rime. The onset is the initial consonant(s) sound of the syllable. A rime is the part of the syllable that contains the vowel and all that follows it (e.g., the onset of the word *dog* is *d-*, the rime is *-og*; the onset of the word *bring* is *br-* and the rime is *-ing*).

language skills—even excellent skills—may not automatically result in acceptable literacy skills. In the evolution of human civilization, excellent oral skills existed for a long time without a trace of written skills. Even in the twenty-first century, many orally competent individuals do not read or write. Therefore, to establish or improve literacy skills, literacy skills must be explicitly taught. Because good oral language skills are a foundation for literacy skills, SLPs are well-equipped to provide intervention for the remediation of reading and writing disorders. Their technical training in assessing and treating language disorders will serve well in assessing and treating reading and writing disorders.

Many of the world's languages do not have a written form—a further indication that literacy is not a "natural" extension of oral language.

In recognition of the growing role of SLPs in assessing and treating literacy problems, the American Speech-Language-Hearing Association (ASHA) has published several papers describing the roles SLPs can play in supporting children's improved academic performance in schools. The papers also describe the training the SLPs need to have before they can help children and adolescents read and write better. According to the American Speech-Language-Hearing Association (2001), SLPs may design and implement programs to:

1. Prevent written language problems by fostering language acquisition and emergent literacy
2. Identify children at risk for reading and writing problems
3. Assess reading and writing
4. Provide intervention and document outcomes for reading and writing intervention programs
5. Provide assistance to general education teachers, parents, and students
6. Advocate effective literacy practices, and advance the knowledge base

Assessment of Reading and Writing

Before assessing reading and writing skills, SLPs should assess a child's receptive and expressive language skills. Therefore, the assessment procedures described in Chapter 4 are applicable to a child with reading and writing problems. Beyond oral language skills, the clinician may use certain standardized tests or child-specific measures to directly assess reading and writing skills.

There are many standardized tests available for the assessment of reading and writing. See Table 10.1 for a listing of reading and writing tests that are most commonly used in the educational setting. It is now within the scope of practice for SLPs to administer these tests, although additional training may be necessary.

Child-specific measures are many, varied, and will likely yield more useful information on a child's literacy skills than will the standardized tests. ASHA recommends the use

table 10.1

Tests for Assessment of Literacy Skills

Name of Test	Age Range	Skills Assessed
Comprehensive Test of Phonological Processing (CTOPP) Wagner, Torgesen, & Rashotte (1999)	5 yrs through adult	Phoneme manipulation, including sound deletion, sound and word blending, and segmentation of sounds, words, and syllables; includes assessment of "rapid naming"
Gray Diagnostic Reading Tests (GRDT-2) *Second Edition* Bryant, Widerholt, & Bryant (2004)	6 yrs through 13 yrs, 11 mos	Letter/word identification, reading vocabulary, subtests for reading comprehension, "rapid naming," and phonological awareness
Phonological Awareness Test (PAT) Robertson & Salter (1997)	5 yrs through 9 yrs	Rhyming, sound/letter association, word decoding, syllable segmentation, and phoneme manipulation, including isolation, deletion, and substitution; optional subtest on "invented spelling"
Test of Early Written Language-2 (TEWL-2) Hresko (1996)	3 yrs through 10 yrs, 11 mos	Emergent writing skills; also, spelling, capitalization, punctuation, sentence construction, writing stories about a picture prompt
Test of Reading Comprehension (TORC-3) Brown, Hammill, & Widerholt (1995)	7 yrs through 17 yrs, 11 mos	Comprehension of general vocabulary, syntactic similarities; answering questions regarding "story-like" paragraphs
Test of Written Expression (TOWE) Mcghee, Bryant, Larsen, & Rivera (1995)	6 yrs, 6 mos through 14 yrs, 11 mos	Writing skills, including essay writing in response to a "story starter" (e.g., student is required to continue a story to a conclusion)
Test of Written English (TWE) Anderson & Thompson (1988)	6 yrs through 17 yrs 11 mos	Screens for skills in written expression and paragraph writing; also assesses capitalization and punctuation
Woodcock Language Proficiency Battery— *Revised* Woodcock (1991)	2 yrs through adult	Measures of oral language, reading, and written language; includes English and Spanish forms

of child-specific methods to assess reading and writing skills at three developmental levels: (1) the emergent level (Preschool); (2) the early elementary level (Kindergarten through Grade 3); and (3) the later levels (Grade 4 and above; ASHA, 2001). While some of the procedures recommended still need research support, the ASHA statement offers useful suggestions on informal assessment of literacy at each of these three levels. First, the unique skills that need to be addressed at each level (the emergent, early elementary, and later grades) will be described. Subsequently, a few skills that may be assessed at multiple levels will be described and evaluated.

Assessment of Reading and Writing at the Emergent Level (Preschool)

The SLP should first conduct an assessment of the child's receptive and expressive language skills, including both formal and informal methods described in Chapter 4. If the child is found to have a language disorder, the SLP should also examine the home environment and the parental behaviors associated with literacy. Even if the child does not exhibit a language disorder, the SLP may suspect that the child's home environment and the parent behaviors could improve to promote literacy. This may warrant consultation with other professionals and parents.

For a child at the emergent (preschool) level, what should the clinician informally assess?

Informally, the clinician may assess: (1) the degree to which the home environment is literacy-enriched, (2) the child's beginning knowledge of print and its function, (3) assessment of parent behaviors that promote literacy, and (4) phonological awareness. Of these, phonological awareness is discussed in a later section

School SLPs often make home visits to assess a child's speech and language. They can also discreetly observe the amount of literacy materials present in the household.

Assessment of family literacy. The clinician should assess the child's home environment to judge whether or not it is sufficiently literacy-enriched. Home visits, parent or caregiver interviews, and questionnaires that parents and caregivers fill out will help make this assessment. Of these, direct observation through a home visit is the most reliable.

During the home visit, the SLP should observe whether literacy materials are evident in the household. Are there books, newspapers, and magazines present? Are writing materials, such as paper, pens, blackboards, dry-erase boards, easels, crayons, markers, chalk, and so forth, readily accessible to the child? Is there furniture suitable for reading and writing activities? Is there evidence that parents, caregivers, or both read regularly?

These observations should be made in a thorough, but sensitive manner. The SLPs should avoid stereotypes. They cannot automatically assume that a low socioeconomic household will be barren, although children living in poverty often do not have the benefits of a literacy-enriched home environment (Adams, 1990; Hart & Risley, 1995; Snow, Burns, & Griffin, 1998). Similarly, the clinician cannot assume that middle- or upper-class parents necessarily provide a literacy-enriched environment for their children. SLPs making home visits may need to carry books and writing materials with them, so the stimulus items, if not available at the child's home, may be used in assessment.

In our experience, some school SLPs, feeling sad over the lack of literacy materials in some households, have left books, crayons, markers, or some other literacy-related materials as small gifts for children they assessed at home.

Assessment of knowledge of print. The SLP should observe whether the child demonstrates an emerging knowledge of print and its purposes (a skill commonly referred to as print awareness). The SLP can show the child logos and signs commonly encountered in the environment. For example, the SLP might show the child a picture of a fast food restaurant's logo or a label from a can of soup and ask the child to name the associated products. Whether the child knows the meaning of common printed signs (*stop, exit, enter, men's room, women's room,* etc.) may also be a part of this assessment.

The SLP can also observe whether or not the child understands some basic concepts of print. If handed a book upside-down, does the child turn it right-side up (a task of correctly orienting the book)? Does the child turn the pages of a book when an adult reader pauses during reading? Assessment of more advanced preschool skills might include checking to see if the child can identify the boundaries between words, sentences, or paragraphs; if the child understands that print reads from top to bottom and from left to right; and if the child can identify letters or words in the context of an often-read book. These more advanced skills can be assessed by asking the child questions such as, "Where do I begin reading?" "Can you find the letter *m?*" "Can you find one word?" "How about a whole sentence?" "Can you count the words in this sentence?" "Can you count the sentences in this paragraph?" "Where is the end of the story?" and so forth.

> The need to teach basic concepts of print before providing direct instruction in reading and writing is yet another assumption; its validity has not been experimentally demonstrated.

> Parents permitting, SLPs can use stimulus items from the family's cupboards to assess a child's print awareness.

Clinicians should not presume, however, that these basic concepts of print are prerequisite skills to reading and writing. Research has not shown that reading and writing cannot be taught until the child demonstrates what are described as the knowledge of basic concepts of print. Therefore, the clinician should not necessarily consider those skills to be primary targets for intervention. Instead, the clinician should experiment with teaching reading and writing directly and then probe to see if knowledge of book orientation, word and sentence boundaries, and left-to-right directions emerges. If children who learn to read and write still do not have the knowledge of basic print concepts, then such knowledge is theoretical and empirically irrelevant.

> A print concept is that books have spines. Is this concept necessary to read books?

A child who has been exposed to a literacy-enriched environment is likely to exhibit pretend reading and writing. The SLP should observe these and related behaviors. For instance, does the child appear to enjoy looking at a book and turning the pages, as if reading? Can the child recite passages from a favorite book from memory while looking at the pages? Does the child pretend to write, by drawing or scribbling, and then ask the adult, "What does it say?" If the answer to these and similar questions is positive, it means that parents or others have reinforced such skills.

Children whose reading and writing have been positively reinforced show obvious pleasure in literacy-related activities. Therefore, the clinician may observe whether the child enjoys coloring, drawing, or scribbling. Does the child appear to be eager to be read to? Does shared book reading appear to be a pleasurable and desirable experience to the child? Can the child pay somewhat sustained attention to the printed word?

The answers to all of these questions depend, in part, on the actions of the adults in the child's environment. That is why it is also necessary to make observations regarding literacy-related behaviors of the adults having most frequent contact with the child.

Assessment of literacy-related behaviors of parents and caregivers. Because an intervention plan may include suggestions for modifying the child's environment, the SLP should interview and observe the parents and caregivers to assess their own literacy-related behaviors. While doing so, the SLP should consider cultural or socioeconomic factors, or both, that will affect the degree to which parents promote literacy in individual households. Some cultures, such as many Native American tribes, have oral traditions and do not necessarily place great value on the printed word (Kay-Raining Bird & Vetter, 1994). One recently immigrated group, the Hmong people from Laos, for many centuries had no written language until one was fashioned for them by French and American missionaries in the 1950s (Lindsay, 2004). Also, families in low socioeconomic status (SES) households have been found to place a low priority on literacy, because resources are necessarily directed toward basic needs for survival (Koppenhaver, Evans, & Yoder, 1991; Marvin & Mirenda, 1993).

Promoting literacy, however, should include advocating for effective literacy practices while taking into consideration such cultural and socioeconomic factors. Parents from diverse cultural backgrounds or low SES, or both, should be encouraged and supported to provide a more literacy-enriched environment for their children. Observing parental behaviors related to literacy will provide the clinician with necessary information on which to devise a home-based intervention program.

The clinician should therefore thoroughly assess the degree to which the child's parents and household environment support literacy. Are the parents or caregivers good role models of literacy? Do they read and write in view of the child on a daily basis? Do they display the child's written or drawn products on the refrigerator door or elsewhere in the home, indicating that they pay attention to the child's literacy efforts? Have they made any effort to teach the child to read simple words in storybooks and print the letters of the alphabet? Do they make positive comments regarding their child's beginning efforts to read and write?

The most important action the parents or caregivers can take is to read to the child on a daily basis. The SLP should assess how often the child is read to and what kind of material is read to the child. If shared book reading is a part of the household culture, the SLP should ask a parent or caregiver to demonstrate how he or she reads to the child and observe the interactions during reading. Is the child expected to sit and attend, without making comments or asking questions, while the parent or caregiver reads the book straight through? Or, is there an interactive style, with the parent or caregiver responding to the child's questions, or requiring the child to respond to questions? What is the seating arrangement? Do the child and the reading parent sit side-by-side so the child can see the printed material as the parent reads it? Does the parent draw the child's attention to pictures and expand on the information provided in the story? Does the parent point to words and sentences as they are being read? Does the parent ask the child to find a letter or a word on the storybook pages? To make valid observations, the clinician should request the parents to read in their usual manner and observe unobtrusively.

Assessment of Reading and Writing at the Early Elementary Level (Kindergarten through Grade 3)

Once again, assessment of speech and language skills should precede the direct assessment of literacy skills. At the early elementary level, the clinician should assess: (1) letter identification, (2) early reading skills, (3) elementary writing skills, and (4) other literacy-related tasks that are integrated into speech and language assessment. In addition, some researchers recommend measuring certain other skills in children because they are presumed to predict later reading performance. These skills include phonological awareness, rapid automatic naming, and phonological memory. The value of these skills will be briefly described and evaluated as to their value in literacy assessment and treatment.

> For a child at the early elementary level (Kindergarten to Grade 3), what should the clinician assess?

Assessing letter identification. Research seeking to establish a correlation between various factors and future literacy skills has shown that a child's knowledge of letter names is a robust predictor of later acquisition of literacy (Kaminski & Good, 1996; Scarborough, 1998a; Stevenson & Newman, 1986). This is not surprising as knowledge of letters is a part of literacy skills. It is important to assess whether a child can name letters of the alphabet with proficiency and ease. It also is necessary to assess whether a child can distinguish between the name of a letter and the sound the letter represents. The clinician should present various letters of the alphabet and request the child to name them. If the child names the letter, the clinician may say, for example, "Yes, it *is* a 'B'!" and then ask, "Do you know what sound it makes?" Assessment of this kind may be completed with the stimulus items the SLP carries or items such as books and toys the child has at home.

It is generally claimed that a child's demonstrated knowledge of letter names suggests a good prognosis for future literacy; conversely, a child's lack of knowledge of letter names in Kindergarten through Grade 3 suggests a poor prognosis. Children who lack such knowledge are predicted to be at risk for the development of reading disability. Such predictive claims are statements of the obvious. The child already has problems with literacy skills, especially the third grader who has no knowledge of letter names.

Assessing early reading skills. Gough and Tunmer's (1986) popular view of reading suggests that it consists of two processes: (1) decoding and (2) comprehension. According to the authors, *decoding* involves knowledge of sound–letter associations that transforms print to words. If a person has good decoding skills, the theory states, even words that have never been encountered can be "sounded out" as a preliminary step to making sense of it. Unfortunately, the unobservable decoding process is inferred from the observable sounding-out skill the children exhibit. Therefore, decoding means reading

> What observable skills can clinicians assess rather than unobservable "decoding" and comprehension processes?

aloud, sometimes by naming the sound of each letter in a printed word. Gough and Tunmer's (1986) theory simply states that reading *is reading* (and comprehension). Empirical clinicians, therefore, can be more productive in assessment and treatment if they target such observable skills in children as naming and printing the letters of the alphabet, reading words and sentences aloud, and answering questions about what they read (comprehension).

Reading (aloud or silently) and understanding what is read may be partly independent of each other. Some people with reading disabilities may read printed material without understanding it. People without reading disabilities also can read complex and unfamiliar material with little or no understanding. Therefore, in both assessment and treatment, the clinician needs to target comprehension as well as oral and silent reading.

Most school curricula require a child to be "sounding out" simple three-letter real or nonsense words by the time they leave Kindergarten. This skill can be assessed by presenting children with three-letter printed words and asking them to "sound it out" (e.g., /f/-/i/-/t/) and then "say it fast" ("feet"), if they have difficulty reading the word.

Fluency is another aspect of reading that SLPs should examine. This is done by having the child read material designed for that child's reading level, counting the number of words correctly read, and dividing that by the number of minutes the child read, resulting in the number of correctly read words per minute (e.g., 100 words read correctly in 5 minutes = 20 words correctly read per minute). SLPs can then judge whether the degree of observed fluency is acceptable.

To assess comprehension of reading, clinicians can have the child read a short paragraph and then ask questions regarding the material read. Comprehension also may be assessed by asking the child to paraphrase or retell what the child has just read.

Assessment of early writing skills. The clinician should obtain a sample of the child's drawing and writing skills. The clinician should have the child draw or write and observe how well the child attends to the writing task. The SLP should also notice if the child appears to have formulated a plan for the writing project and if the child seems to be able to carry that plan through, revising the composition as the project progresses. For example, as the child begins to write, does he or she hesitate, erase, or cross out what has been written, and start all over again and perhaps repeat this process? When asked, can the child explain the message the writing is meant to convey?

With the help of parents' formal or informal teaching, a very young child's drawings and scribbles begin to take on letter-like shapes by the time the child enters Kindergarten. SLPs should see if the child can independently print letters. If not, the clinician can ask the child to copy letters. If the child cannot copy the letters correctly, the SLP should observe whether or not the child can trace a letter outlined either with dashes or dots. The child who copies or traces letters shows the early signs of writing. The child who has difficulty copying letters will need instruction to do so.

For children with more advanced writing skills, the SLP should evaluate written mechanics and content of writing. Writing mechanics include sentence formulation, word usage, spelling, punctuation, and grammar. Content evaluation requires judgments regarding cohesiveness and logical sequence inherent in the child's writing. From the content of a child's written product, some researchers tend to infer the child's "story sense," which is presumably the recognition that a good story has a beginning, an end, and logical plot development in between. Whether young children have any such formal sense of "logical plot development" and whether such a sense is necessary to understand and enjoy a story are open to question, however.

Other literacy-related assessment tasks. The SLP may integrate the assessment of the following literacy-related skills into a comprehensive speech and language evaluation:

1. Naming common objects and concepts
2. Defining simple objects and concepts by describing attributes and functions (e.g., naming an object and talking about what it's used for and what parts it has; demonstrating knowledge of antonyms, synonyms, etc.)
3. Understanding and producing figurative language, such as idioms, similes, humor, puns, and irony
4. Retelling a story, paraphrasing it, and answering questions regarding paragraph-length material either read to the child or by the child

Assessment of Reading and Writing at the Later Level

Children who enter fourth grade encounter an increasingly difficult curriculum—a curriculum that shifts the emphasis from *learning to read* to *reading to learn* (Snow, Scarborough, & Burns, 1999). Children who are still struggling with the mechanics of reading will find it necessary to concentrate on reading itself, rather than on what is being read. These children will have difficulty in accessing the curriculum—a common criterion for qualification for special education services, including speech-language therapy. SLPs assessing literacy skills of children in the upper grades use methods that are specific to the level of the child being assessed. Those methods may include any of those described for the emergent and early levels. However, assessing reading and writing at higher levels may be necessary for students with milder reading disabilities.

> In Fourth grade, the curriculum shifts from *learning to read* to *reading to learn.*

Assessment of reading at the later level. SLPs should assess the student's more advanced knowledge of written language. Can the student distinguish between literary genres such as fiction and nonfiction, biography, poetry, and so forth? Can the student identify and describe the purposes of texts (e.g., to inform, to entertain, to persuade, etc.)? Can the student critically evaluate written material for mechanics and content?

The student should also be assessed for more advanced semantic, morphologic, and syntactic knowledge. Can the student identify affixes and describe how they change the meaning of root words? Can the student explain words with multiple meanings? Does the student demonstrate understanding of more advanced academic vocabulary of the classroom curriculum? Can the student explain the use of figurative language, such as similes, metaphors, and allegories in works of literature?

Assessment of writing at the later level. The SLP should obtain a sample of the student's writing and analyze it. Productivity should be assessed by counting the number of words in the writing sample. Syntactic aspects of the sample should be judged: does the student properly use complex sentence structures, including embedded clauses? The sample should also be analyzed for proper spelling and correct use of capitalization and punctuation. Besides mechanics, content should be evaluated. Is the writing sample cohesive, written in a logical sequence, with good paragraph construction?

> Clinicians should collect quantitative data on a student's writing. Percentages can be calculated for accuracy in spelling and punctuation (e.g., counting the number of times a student properly capitalized a word and dividing by the number of times proper capitalization was required).

Assessment of spoken language at the later level. A thorough assessment of the student's spoken language should be conducted, including literacy-related higher level spoken language skills. The SLP should analyze the student's language sample for evidence of increasing syntactic complexity. The student should use figurative language appropriately and should demonstrate knowledge of multiple word meanings, of synonyms, and of antonyms. In addition, the student should use, as well as understand, more complex academic vocabulary.

Additional Procedures for the Assessment of Reading and Writing

In addition to those listed, there are other procedures that are designed to assess supposed underlying processes or predictors of future difficulty with literacy, such as phonological awareness, phonological memory, and rapid automatized naming. Although there is no experimental evidence that suggests a need to assess these, SLPs commonly assess them because of expert advocacy. We mention them here for the purposes of critical evaluation. None of them should be used as the sole criterion by which a child is judged to be at risk for difficulties with literacy.

Assessment of phonological awareness. Because there is some evidence that there is a positive correlation between difficulties with phonological awareness and later reading disability, there may be some limited value in briefly assessing a child's **phonological awareness.** At the emergent level, children as young as 3 should detect and produce rhyme, recognize the syllable structure of words, and recognize alliteration (i.e., the similarity of beginning sounds in phrases such as *brown bear*). These skills can be assessed in the context of verbal play, using songs, books, and nursery rhymes as stimuli (Catts et al., 2002; Roth & Baden, 2001; Rvachew et al., 2003). Some researchers believe that a child's lack of phonological awareness in the early grades is a clear indication that the child is at risk for reading disability

By the end of the first grade, a child's phonological awareness should include phonemic awareness (manipulation of individual phonemes of a language). This can be demonstrated by asking the child to perform such tasks as:

1. Isolating a phoneme with a word (e.g., "What's the first sound in *bat?*")
2. Recognizing the same sounds in different words (e.g., "*Cat, catch, car*—What sound do all those words start with?")
3. Segmenting phonemes (e.g., "How many sounds are in *sit?*")
4. Deleting phonemes (e.g., "Say 'flag.' Now say it again without /f/.")
5. Substituting phonemes (e.g., "Say 'bar.' Now say it again, but change the /b/ to /f/.")

The evidence supporting assessment of phonological and phonemic awareness is mostly theoretical; anything empirical about it is correlational. Before spending much time asking a child to figure out the number of sounds in a word, to say a word by omitting or substituting a sound in it (which are done *too* well by children with articulation disorders), the clinician should seek evidence that shows that such an assessment has experimentally demonstrated treatment implications. Treatment research evidence should show that treatment of phonological awareness is necessary to establish literacy skills or to remediate articulation disorders. No such evidence exists. Therefore, it may be more fruitful to directly assess reading and writing skills rather than spending time assessing phonological and phonemic awareness. Tasks designed to have the child form letters, copy letters, read simple words, and understand the content of written material are more likely to provide an accurate assessment of a child's current literacy skills and past learning history. Clinicians who believe in the value of assessing phonological awareness should experimentally demonstrate its value in treating phonological, language, and literacy problems. For example, they should demonstrate that, with phonological awareness, training speech, language, or literacy treatment is more efficient than without phonological awareness training. Until such experimental evidence is produced, it is premature to recommend phonological awareness training to all children with speech, language, and literacy problems.

Assessment of phonological memory. Some researchers have attempted to establish a link between difficulties with reading and a child's performance on various tasks designed to measure supposed aspects of phonological memory. These tasks have included repetition of numbers, letters, words, and nonwords presented auditorily. A correlation between difficulty with these types of tasks and language impairment, poor phonological awareness, and reading disability has been reported in various studies (Montgomery, 1995; Torgesen & Wagner, 1998; Wagner et al., 1993). Whether such correlational evidence suggests that the clinician should then train such skills as repeating nonsense syllables is open to question. There is no experimental treatment evidence that demonstrates the necessity of assessing phonological memory.

Assessment of rapid automatized naming. Other researchers have reported a high correlation between difficulty with rapid naming tasks and future deficits in literacy. Rapid automatized naming (RAN) is measured by fast presentation of stimuli such as pictures of common objects, colors, shapes, or numbers (Bowers & Wolf, 1993; Scarborough, 1998b) that the child is required to name. Later researchers showed that it is much more useful to assess rapid naming of letters of the alphabet (Schatschneider et al., 2002). These later findings support the contention that it is more productive to teach literacy skills directly, rather than something that is presumably hiding behind those skills.

Again, research available on rapid automatized naming is correlational in nature; studies have only indicated that children who perform poorly in rapid naming tasks may also be at risk for failure to acquire literacy skills. But the question is, can a program of teaching rapid naming result in better literacy skills? Or, at the least, is it easier to teach literacy skills to children who have learned to name rapidly than to children who have not? Are there any clinical experiments that help answer these questions? Unfortunately, the answer is *no*, and hence, the best thing the SLP can do is to support only those activities that are supported by experimental data. If there are no experimental data, teaching the skills directly and documenting improvement will always make clinical sense.

Assessment of phonological awareness, phonological memory, and rapid automatized naming, if done at all, should be thought of as supplemental to other findings relative to the child's receptive and expressive oral language and demonstrated literacy skills. A diagnosis indicating the child is at risk for reading disability should not be made solely on the basis of these theoretical constructs.

Intervention for Reading and Writing

Effective treatment of literacy, similar to maintenance of language skills in natural settings, is the result of a strong partnership between the clinician, the classroom teacher, and the family members. Assessment of the three domains described so far—the child's oral language, home environment, and reading and writing—prepares the ground for building an effective literacy enrichment program that will help prevent or remediate reading and writing disability. To improve children's literacy skills, SLPs should: (1) collaborate with classroom teachers, (2) continue to provide intervention for oral language behaviors, (3) target parental behaviors that promote literacy in preschoolers, and (4) provide direct instruction in reading and writing.

Collaborate with Classroom Teachers

In various sections of this book we have emphasized that to design and implement effective language and literacy instruction for school-age children, SLPs should work closely with classroom teachers. For example, the clinician should consult with teachers (as well as parents) in selecting language treatment targets for the child. Teachers might suggest targets that are especially helpful in promoting literacy skills in the classroom. Academic words, quantitative terms, comparative terms, and so forth may be especially helpful. The techniques teachers use to teach reading and writing, if supported by evidence, may be borrowed so that both the clinician and the teacher use the same and similarly effective procedures. The clinician may invite the teacher to use a novel and effective procedure and demonstrate it for the teacher.

The teacher and the clinician may share instructional (treatment) stimuli. For instance, the clinician may show the teacher the stimuli she has prepared to teach various oral language skills. When the literacy skills are integrated into oral language training, as in target words or phrases printed below the pictorial stimuli, the teacher and the clinician may both promote both sets of skills simultaneously.

Continued Intervention for Oral Language Behaviors

Because literacy is directly linked to speech and language, intervention given to improve the phonologic, semantic, syntactic, and morphologic aspects of language may help improve literacy. Following assessment, the SLP should select client-specific target behaviors in consultation with the classroom teacher. Selected skills should be relevant to the child's curriculum. Words and syntactic structures taught in the classroom will be of special importance in language treatment.

In a later section we describe procedures for integrating literacy skills into the standard language treatment. In treating both receptive and expressive language skills, the clinician should include treatment targets and activities that help promote literacy skills. The treatment procedures, however, will not change because of added literacy skills to treatment targets. The procedures recommended in Chapters 5 through 9 will be useful in teaching both oral language and literacy skills.

Targeting Parental Behaviors That Promote Literacy

Because of the demonstrated link between parental behaviors and later literacy skills in children, SLPs should follow up on assessment of the home environment with suggestions to parents and caregivers as to how to better promote their children's literacy skills. Parents should be encouraged to: (1) provide a more literacy-enriched environment, (2) provide better role models of literacy to their children, (3) provide more practice in literacy skills, and (4) read more to their children, using techniques to make shared book reading interactive and focused on print.

The SLP should help parents gain access to low-cost means to provide a literacy-enriched home environment. The parents may be encouraged to borrow books from the local libraries.

Providing a literacy-enriched environment. The SLP should educate the parents about the importance of having reading and writing material available to the child at home. Parents should be encouraged to provide a variety of books, magazines, and newspapers that are regularly accessible to the child. Writing materials such as pencils, crayons, paper, blackboards, paint, and paintbrushes should also be available in the household.

If the family lacks resources, SLPs should give information on the locations of libraries, bookstores, and local public programs that may be available to support children's literacy. There may be sources of free or low-cost literacy materials in the community. Often, elementary schools will sponsor book drives in which books are donated and then distributed to any who request them. Some SLPs have actively solicited office supply companies or big variety stores to obtain donations of literacy materials to pass on to families they serve. At the very least, SLPs should be knowledgeable regarding the various literacy-related services available to families in their communities.

The parents should be asked to provide a setting within the home that is conducive to reading and writing activities. The household should contain furniture such as a child-sized table and chairs, an easel, and a bookcase or

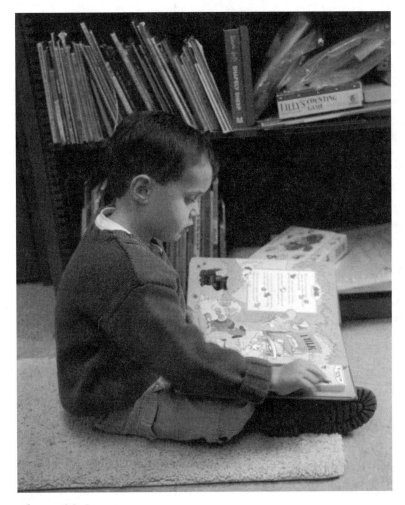

photo 10.1

Providing a cozy "book nook" for a child may reinforce literate behavior.

basket filled with reading material set beside a comfortable rocking chair or beanbag chair in a cozy corner of a room with good lighting. Colorful carpet samples children can sit on are low-cost alternatives to more substantial furniture and can usually be obtained free of cost through local flooring outlets. If children have a "book nook" all their own, they may be more likely to read and write.

Parents should also be encouraged to extend experiences in literacy beyond the home setting and into the community. Literacy-related community outings include visits to libraries or bookstores for story time. Parents may take their children to special occasions where children's book authors make presentations and sign books. If parents know a quality movie based on a children's book is about to be released, they can read the book to the child and then attend the movie. Parents might help children form a book club, similar to book clubs adults often have. Community activities that promote literacy as enjoyable and enriching will encourage children to become life-long, proficient readers.

Providing good role models of literacy. Children are likely to be motivated to learn reading and writing when the adults in their environment read and write on a regular basis. SLPs should encourage parents and caregivers to conduct literacy-related activities in view of their children. For example, suppose that the home literacy assessment has shown that a mother tends to wait until after she takes her son to preschool before she reads the newspaper. The SLP might suggest that she reorganize her morning routine, so that she reads at least a section of the newspaper while her son is close by. The mother may point out and read aloud any large print words, especially those that the child may be interested in (e.g., the pictures and the printed words in advertising supplements related to toys).

Other suggestions might be for parents to write out checks or grocery lists or write correspondence while their children are present. Adults can also describe or comment on their literacy activities. For example, a parent writing out a grocery list might make comments such as, "I need a list to help me remember what we need at the store! Let's see, we need milk . . . and cereal . . . and cat food," pausing after each item to write it down. Adults serve as good literacy role models when children can observe them engaged in functional daily activities connected to literacy.

Providing practice in literacy skills. Children should not be limited to merely observing the adults in the environment performing literacy-related activities. Adults should directly encourage children to participate in daily literacy-related activities. The adult writing out the grocery list, for example, may ask the child, "What else do you think we might need?" and then write in response to the child's dictation, drawing the child's attention to the word or words being written. If the child is beginning to write, the parent may manually guide the child's hand to write the words. Then, the child may be included in the trip to the grocery store, referring to the list, finding items, and checking them off the list. There are numerous ways in which adults can involve children in literacy-related activities throughout the day. Children can be encouraged to:

1. Help in the kitchen by following a written recipe
2. Read and follow instructions for a board game
3. Help assemble a household appliance or toy according to written instructions
4. Make a to-do list of the day's activities
5. Keep a colorful, personalized calendar, writing-in special events
6. Draw pictures or write various types of correspondence, such as thank-you notes, birthday invitations, letters to relatives, and so forth
7. Plan an outing or a vacation by looking at brochures, advertisements, and maps

This is not, of course, an all-inclusive list. Parents should be encouraged to be creative and consistent in providing their children with many opportunities to practice literacy skills in the context of daily activities. As always, children who participate in literacy activities should be praised and reinforced in other ways.

Shared storybook reading. Researchers have produced both correlational and experimental evidence suggesting early shared book reading can have positive effects on oral language development, the acquisition of literacy, and later academic achievement (Crain-Thoreson & Dale, 1992; Senechal & Cornell, 1993; Whitehurst & Lonigan, 1998). Often, parents will read a book to a child without engaging the child in conversation about the content of the book and without drawing the child's attention to print. This

> What two approaches have been shown to be effective in promoting language and literacy development during shared storybook reading?

is better than not reading to the child at all, but SLPs can teach parents techniques that will better promote a child's language and literacy development during shared storybook reading. Two approaches that have been shown to be effective are: (1) using dialogic reading and (2) using print-referencing techniques.

Whitehurst and his colleagues have investigated the efficacy of their program of shared book reading, called **dialogic reading,** conducting several studies involving children from diverse socioeconomic and cultural backgrounds (Arnold et al., 1994; Lonigan & Whitehurst, 1998; Valdez-Menchaca & Whitehurst, 1992; Whitehurst et al., 1988). The results of their experimental studies have shown that one-on-one dialogic reading has a positive effect on preschool children's language skills. Other researchers also have demonstrated the efficacy of dialogic reading techniques in preschool settings (Justice et al., 2003; Wasik & Bond, 2001).

Dialogic reading requires the adult to ask open-ended questions, add information to the text, and have the child retell the story. For example, the adult might ask the child questions such as, "What do you think is happening on this page?" or "What do you think might happen next?" The adult might add a comment to the narrative of the story or add information in response to the child's questions. Rather than require the child to sit quietly, the adult encourages the child to make comments, ask questions, elaborate on the story, and retell the story. The adult gradually requires the child to retell increasingly more of the story, until the child becomes the storyteller.

> Sometimes parents, or even teachers, believe that requiring a child to sit quietly when being read to is good preparation for success in a classroom setting. For younger children, however, an interactive storybook-reading style will reap far more benefits for early language and literacy development.

The use of **print-referencing** techniques was proposed by Justice and colleagues (Justice & Ezell, 2000, 2002a; Justice et al., 2002) as an explicit method of teaching early literacy skills to children through shared storybook reading. Compared to a control group, children who were read to by adults trained in the use of print-referencing techniques showed greater improvement in print awareness and alphabet knowledge.

Adults using print-referencing techniques use various prompts to draw children's attention to elements on a printed page. For example, the adult might ask the child:

- "Show me a word on this page."
- "Can you find the first word on this page? How about the last one?"
- "Count the words on this page with me."
- "Where's the letter *M* [or any other letter] on this page?"
- "Are there any letters on this page that are in your name, too?"
- "Where do you think the word *pop* is?"

The adult should give the child praise for correct answers ("Yes, that's the *M*—you found it!") and gentle corrective feedback for incorrect answers ("Oops! Not quite! Here's the *M*—see it?").

Shared storybook reading becomes more purposeful, interactive, and effective when adults learn to use techniques such as dialogic reading and print-referencing. SLPs should target such adult behaviors when intervening to improve children's literacy skills.

photo 10.2
Drawing a child's attention to print may help to promote early literacy.

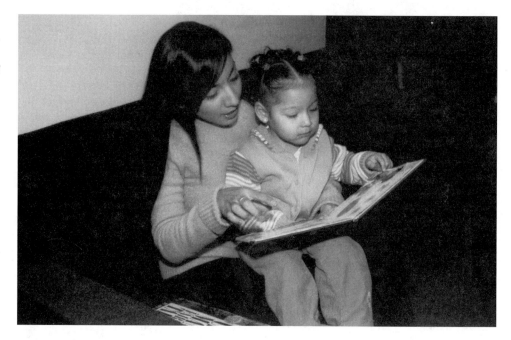

Providing Direct Instruction in Reading and Writing

Some have suggested that SLPs should take an indirect role in the remediation of reading and writing; that literacy instruction is best left to classroom teachers and reading and resource specialists. At most, it is said that SLPs should collaborate with other professionals in devising and carrying out a treatment plan for reading disability. This may be good suggestion if literacy training takes time away from oral communication training.

It is possible that the outpouring of interest in underlying processes such as phonological awareness, rapid automatized naming, and emergent literacy is partly the result of SLPs seeking a role they are comfortable with in literacy intervention. However, as has been discussed, there is no experimental evidence that causally links these presumed underlying skills to the acquisition of literacy skills. Furthermore, no evidence suggests that direct literacy skill teaching is inefficient compared to teaching presumed underlying skills. Therefore, SLPs who confine themselves to treating these underlying skills may not be making much of a difference in their clients' reading and writing.

It is not necessary to invent reasons for SLPs to be involved in literacy. A direct link between oral language and written language skills has been established, and the expanded scope of practice for SLPs clearly includes assessment and intervention for reading and writing. Many school districts, particularly those who do not have the resources to hire reading specialists, are providing additional training in literacy instruction for SLPs. Other SLPs who are drawn to literacy assessment and treatment are seeking out training on their own to enhance their knowledge and skills. While it is always beneficial to collaborate with other professionals, SLPs do not need to consider themselves to be secondary literacy professionals.

Therefore, rather than playing the role of a background professional or the one who targets underlying processes, SLPs should target directly reading and writing skills in children they serve for language intervention. This can be done within the context of traditional speech and language therapy. Treatment of all communication disorders provides an excellent context for literacy training. Treatment of articulation and language disorders is especially conducive to integrating literacy skill training. Furthermore, time and resources permitting and in conjunction with classroom teachers, SLPs may target basic reading and writing skills as independent intervention targets.

Treating Reading Skills in the Context of Speech and Language Therapy

There are many ways SLPs can integrate literacy instruction into speech and language therapy. To promote reading skills in children with communicative disorders, SLPs should always pair written material with pictured and modeled stimuli at every level of therapy. At the level of the isolated sound, the printed letter or letters (**graphemes**) should be presented; at the level of words, phrases, and sentences, the printed words should be presented. The clinician should draw the child's attention to the print, pointing or having the child point to it when responding. For example, instead of showing only a picture of common nouns selected for training, the clinician can have the word printed in large letters under each stimulus picture (e.g., printed words *sock, shirt, cup, hat,* etc.). Before asking the question, "What is this?" the clinician will point to both the picture and the printed word. Periodically, the clinician can probe to see if the child can sight-read the word presented without the picture. This general strategy can be effectively incorporated into articulation and language intervention in schools.

Often, storybooks can be used as stimuli when treating speech targets, language targets, or both. The storybooks should be selected carefully, assuring that they are relevant to the target behavior and will provide many discrete trial opportunities for the child to produce a response. For example, if the target behavior is the labeling of common nouns, there are many picture books that will provide numerous opportunities for the child to respond to the verbal stimulus, "What is this?" Similarly, any storybook depicting action sequences can be incorporated into discrete trial therapy for verb tenses, such as present progressive -*ing* ("What is he doing? Say, 'He's jumping!'"). While teaching a language target such as pronouns, the clinician might choose books such as *He Bear, She Bear* (Berenstain & Berenstain, 1974) or *Are You My Mother?* (Eastman, 1960). When reading, the clinician should first provide a model, by reading the entire sentence and then either asking a question or creating a sentence-completion task to evoke the response (e.g., "A mother bird sat on her egg. Whose egg is it?") There is no limit to creative ways in which books can be incorporated into therapy, but this must be done in a way that directly addresses the target behavior. SLPs should not spend valuable therapy time by merely reading to the child. See Table 10.2 for a brief listing of some favorite books with suggested verbal stimuli to use for various target behaviors.

> To integrate literacy training with speech and language therapy, pictured and modeled stimuli should always be paired with written material.

SLPs can also help older children read material during more advanced language training. According to the National Reading Panel (2000, 2001), repeated guided reading has positive effects on a child's word recognition, reading fluency, and comprehension of written material. **Guided reading** consists of having the child read aloud while giving the child direct feedback and guidance. The clinician may begin by reading a phrase, sentence, or

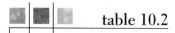

table 10.2

Storybooks as Stimuli for Commonly Targeted Language Behaviors

Here is a sample of storybooks that may be used during discrete trial therapy for selected target behaviors. They are simple, repetitive books that can be used to concentrate on one or several syntactic and morphologic skills or semantic concepts. They are suitable for toddlers through kindergarten-aged children.

Targeted Behavior	Suggested Books	Examples of Verbal Stimuli (Use Repeated Trials)
Present tense -s	*Watch William Walk* (Jonas, 1997) *Cleo on the Move* (Mockford, 2002) *The Little Sailboat* (Lenski, L., 1937)	Evoked: "What does William do?" Modeled: "What does William do? Say, 'He walks.'"
Adjectives	*Old Hat, New Hat* (Berenstain & Berenstain, 1998) *Big and Little* (Miller, 1998) *The Little Mouse, the Red Ripe Strawberry, and the Big Hungry Bear* (Wood & Wood, 1984)	Evoked: "What kind of hat is it?" Modeled: "What kind of hat is it? Say, 'Old hat.'"
Plural -s (/s/, /z/, /ez/)	*One Beautiful Baby* (Osborne, 2002) *Dogs, Dogs, Dogs* (Newman, 2002)	Evoked: "Baby has two _____." Modeled: "Baby has two _____. Say, 'eyes.'"
Prepositions	*Itsy-Bitsy Spider* (Trapani, 1993) *A Nap in a Lap* (Wilson, 2003)	Evoked: "Where did the spider go?" Modeled: "Where did the spider go? Say, 'up the tree.'"
Pronouns	*Who's Afraid of the Dark?* (Bonsall, 1980) *Our Granny* (Wild, 1994)	Evoked: "Who hears steps on the roof?" Modeled: "Who hears steps on the roof? Say, 'she does.'"
Comparative -ier	*Very Hairy Harry* (Koren, 2003)	Evoked: "Harry is hairy. What does he want to be?" Modeled: "Harry is hairy. What does he want to be? Say, 'hair*ier*.'"

What technique, known to increase children's reading fluency, can easily be incorporated into discrete trial therapy?

paragraph to provide the child with a model of fluent reading. The child can then read the material repeatedly, until an acceptable level of fluency is obtained. This is a method that lends itself very nicely to discrete trial therapy, giving the child repeated opportunities to produce whatever language structure is targeted, while at the same time providing intervention to improve reading skills.

When language treatment consists of phrases and sentences, the clinician can once again print those under the respective picture stimuli. For example, in teaching the regular plural morphemes at the phrase level, the clinician can print *two cups, many books,* and so forth under the respective picture stimuli. While teaching the present progressive *-ing* at the sentence level, the clinician can have such sentences as "The boy is running," "The Mom is reading," "The Dad is writing," and so forth. As suggested before, the training will continue with drawing the child's attention to both the picture and the printed stimulus. Probes may be conducted periodically to see if the child begins to read the phrases or sentences without the pictures. Similar strategies may be adopted in teaching phonemes to children with articulation disorders. The same reinforcers that the clinician uses to strengthen oral language skills will also be contingent on reading responses.

Treating Writing Skills in the Context of Speech and Language Therapy

Children may be required to write the letters of the alphabet, words, phrases, sentences, and paragraphs during speech and language therapy. The clinician may initially have to guide the child's hand to write the letter representing speech sounds under treatment or to produce written material representing language targets. Children who have good copying skills will not require this kind of manual guidance and can produce the written material independently. An intermediate step between manual guidance and independent writing would be to provide the child with outlines (consisting of dots or dashes) of letters to trace, gradually diminishing (or fading) the frame of the outline until the child is writing the material without it.

> Providing children with an outline to trace and then gradually diminishing the outline is an example of what treatment technique?

During advanced language training, such conversational skills as narration and story element sequencing lend themselves to writing exercises. The clinician should evaluate the child's written products for correct use of grammar and print conventions, such as capitalization, punctuation, and spelling. Direct feedback should be given for the quality of the writing, either praise for correct productions or corrective feedback for incorrect productions. The child should be given practice in rewriting erred productions, with much praise being given after getting it "just right."

Treating Reading and Writing Skills as Independent Targets

Justifiably, treatment of oral communication disorders is likely to remain a priority for most SLPs. Possibly, some clinicians may specialize in literacy assessment and treatment and provide both direct services to children and consultation to other clinicians and teachers. While not jeopardizing the treatment of oral speech and language skills, the clinicians may contribute to betterment of children's literacy skills. Therefore, time and resources permitting, SLPs should consider directly targeting reading and writing skills independently from other speech and language targets. This should be done in direct consultation and collaboration with any other professionals who may be involved in remediating the child's reading and writing difficulties in the school setting.

> By directly targeting literacy skills or integrating literacy training into speech or language therapy, SLPs ensure that intervention is solidly curriculum based.

SLPs should consult with parents and teachers to devise lists of functional words, phrases, and sentences taken from the child's home environment and school curriculum to be used as stimuli for teaching reading and writing. For a child with language disorders, the selected words, phrases, and sentences may very well be language treatment targets. For a child with articulation disorders, the selected targets may serve well in teaching phoneme productions. The clinician should begin by teaching the names of each letter of the alphabet, then moving to sound-letter associations and building to reading words, phrases, and sentences. Throughout this process, the child should be taught to write as well as read the material presented.

It is best to offer intervention to language, reading, and writing as integrated processes. It is not necessary, for example, to wait until children have achieved some level of competence with spoken language or with reading before teaching them to write. Research has shown that a balanced program, recognizing the integrated nature of language, reading, and writing, is most effective in improving children's literacy skills (Nelson, 1993).

The treatment of writing skills does not require any special techniques that are not used in oral communication training. The main difference is the stimuli presented to the child. While the traditional oral communication training did not emphasize printed material, literacy-oriented communication training will include printed language as stimulus material. The treatment procedures will include those that are known to be effective in teaching both verbal and nonverbal responses: instructions, demonstrations, modeling, prompting, manual guidance, fading, differential reinforcement, and corrective feedback.

Phonological Awareness and Rapid Automatized Naming (RAN) in Literacy Intervention

We have not suggested as intervention targets two popular skills: phonological awareness and rapid automatized naming (RAN) skills. Because of their popularity, we have suggested that these two skills may be assessed with a view to evaluate their usefulness. As noted earlier, the clinicians who treat children's speech and language disorders and offer direct intervention for literacy skills may then probe to see what changes take place in phonological awareness and rapid naming.

Research studies have not demonstrated a direct causal link between phonological awareness, including **phonemic awareness,** and a child's later reading performance. At most, a *correlation* between phonological awareness and reading difficulties has been demonstrated. Children who read and write poorly also tend to perform badly on phonological awareness tasks (Stackhouse et al., 2002; Stanovich & Siegel, 1994; Torgesen et al., 1997). Because the available evidence regarding phonological awareness is only correlational, it is not possible to determine what causes what. Do poor phonological awareness skills lead to poor literacy skills or vice versa? It is also possible that neither is the cause or the effect of the other: lack of phonological awareness may simply be a part of the larger problem of limited speech and language skills.

For treatment of phonological awareness to be warranted, research should show that unless phonological awareness is treated, literacy problems cannot be treated effectively.

Results of descriptive research have suggested that if children are deficient in phonological awareness skills, they tend to also be poor readers. This is what type of evidence?

Until such evidence is presented, SLPs should target skills that are more directly tied to literacy; valuable therapeutic time should not be used treating behaviors that are only presumed to be essential to the development of literacy. It is unclear why treating something (i.e., phonological awareness) correlated with a target skill (i.e., literacy) is more important than treating that target skill itself (literacy). Similarly, there is no controlled data that supports the teaching of rapid automatized naming.

It is best to target directly reading and writing skills, rather than presumed underlying processes or supposed precursors or predictors of future reading difficulty. Even the National Reading Panel (NRP, 2000, 2001), which recommended that a component of phonological awareness training be included in a balanced literacy program, suggested that such training: (1) should not take up more than 20 instructional hours in an academic year, (2) should not involve more than two types of phonological or phonemic awareness, and (3) should use the letters of the alphabet to teach children phonemic manipulations (see Box 10.4 for a summary of NRP findings). The last suggestion especially underscores the contention that direct instruction in reading and writing is more efficacious than treating skills which, at most, may have a correlational link to literacy.

box 10.4 | **Findings of the National Reading Panel**

The National Reading Panel (NRP)—composed of 14 individuals, including researchers, teachers, administrators, and parents—was called together by the U.S. Congress to "assess the status of research-based knowledge, including the effectiveness of various approaches to teaching children to read" (National Reading Panel, 2000, p. 1). The NRP analyzed more than 100,000 studies on selected literacy-related topics. Their findings are summarized in the following chart.

Topic Considered	Key Findings and Recommendations
Phonemic awareness	• Phonemic awareness is a teachable skill • Phonemic awareness helps children learn to read and spell • Children should be taught to manipulate phonemes by using the letters of the alphabet • Phonemic awareness instruction should be limited to only *one* or *two* types of phoneme manipulation, rather than several types • Phonemic awareness instruction should take *no more than* 20 hours of classroom time over a school year
Phonics instruction	• A systematic and explicit phonics instruction program significantly improves word recognition, spelling, and reading comprehension • Phonics instruction is particularly helpful for children who struggle learning to read or who are at risk for reading disability • Phonics instruction should begin early
Reading fluency	• Children's reading fluency improves with repeated reading of text and immediate feedback; guided reading is an efficacious technique in increasing reading fluency • Silent, independent reading with little guidance or feedback has not been empirically shown to be effective in increasing reading fluency
Vocabulary instruction	• Much of a child's vocabulary is learned indirectly, but some vocabulary should be taught directly
Reading comprehension	• Children benefit from instruction in comprehension strategies

Beyond Assessment and Intervention: Advancing the Literacy Knowledge Base and Advocating Effective Literacy Practices

In describing roles and responsibilities of SLPs in literacy, ASHA recommended that SLPs help advance the literacy knowledge base and advocate effective literacy practices. Throughout this chapter, controversial topics that have yet to be resolved through empirical research have been discussed. Far too often in education, a "bandwagon" effect takes place in which a popular idea becomes entrenched, without benefit of scientific scrutiny, and guides instruction of countless students for long, lost periods of time. It will be a fine day, indeed, when educational decisions are based on experimentally evaluated efficacy data, gathered *before* educational policies are put in place.

SLPs are in a unique position to advance the knowledge base regarding all of their areas of endeavor, including literacy. They should resist the urge to "jump on the bandwagon" and embrace every trendy idea that comes along. They should instead critically evaluate research regarding the efficacy of techniques for reading and writing instruction and, as in any other area, use only those methods that have been proven to be effective. When SLPs think that something they are doing to remediate reading and writing difficulties is working particularly well, they should devise their own studies, subjecting their methods to experimental evaluations and presenting or publishing the results. It is only through such efforts that ASHA's mandate to advance the knowledge base and advocate effective literacy practices can be realized.

Chapter Summary

Changing trends in education have resulted in changes in service delivery models and in the involvement of school SLPs in assessing and treating literacy difficulties. Clinicians may use the traditional pull-out model, the consultative model, or the collaborative model. Clinicians may use the pull-out model to establish language target behaviors and consultative and collaborative models to promote generalization and maintenance in natural settings. Another trend in pubic schools is that speech-language pathologists are increasingly involved in assessing and treating literacy problems in children with language disorders. Their involvement is appropriate because literacy skills are language based.

In the public schools, SLPs may assess literacy skills at the emergent, early elementary, and later levels. Such an assessment might be a part of the traditional speech-language assessment. Some research suggests that the clinicians should assess and treat such related skills as phonological awareness, phonological memory, and rapid automatized naming, although there is no strong evidence that such related skill assessment and treatment is superior to direct assessment and treatment of literacy skills.

Reading and writing can be assessed through formal methods that include standardized tests or through informal methods that the clinician designs to suit the individual child. In either case, an important task is to assess the child's home environment for literacy-related activities.

To help prevent and remediate reading disability, SLPs should: collaborate with classroom teachers, continue to provide intervention for oral language behaviors, and provide direct instruction in reading and writing. Furthermore, the SLPs should encourage families of children being served to provide a literacy-enriched environment, good role models of literacy, and systematic practice in literacy skills. The parents should be taught specific storybook reading that are known to promote literacy skills in children (e.g., dialogic reading and print-referencing).

Study Guide

1. Changes in services delivery models and views on the relation between oral language skills and literacy in children have prompted a greater involvement of SLPs in assessing and treating reading and writing problems. Describe these trends and summarize the position of the American Speech-Language-Hearing Association's position on the role speech-language pathologists should play in promoting literacy in school-age children.

2. Critically evaluate the research and theory on skills that educators and some speech-language pathologists consider prerequisites for reading and writing. Give a description of each of those presumed prerequisites. Based on the evidence presented, what conclusions would you draw? If you are working with a child with language and literacy problems, what approach would you take in helping the child in both realms (oral language and literacy). Justify your answer in light of research evidence.

3. Does the research support the assumption that literacy skills are acquired the same way as oral language skills? Why or why not?

4. Design an assessment plan for an 8-year-old boy with significant language and literacy problems. Assume that the child is at the early elementary level and is from a Spanish-speaking home. Specify the skills you would assess and the procedures of assessment. Justify the selection of your procedures.

5. You have been working with several children with language and literacy problems. Considering the importance of modifying parental behaviors in promoting literacy skills at home, you have invited them all for a mini-workshop. What specific suggestions would you offer them during this workshop? How would you monitor the progress of the child and the actions of the parents?

chapter

11

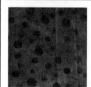

Children in a Multicultural Society: Implications for Assessment and Treatment

outline

- Cultural Competency: What Does It Mean and How Does It Help?
- Differences Are Not Disorders
- Understanding Each Other: Working with Interpreters
- Nonbiased Assessment of Multicultural Children
- Treatment for Multicultural Children: A Question of Generality
- Working with Children and Families of Varied Cultural Backgrounds
- Chapter Summary
- Study Guide

W alk any school corridor in many major urban areas of the United States, and you will likely find children of many different cultural and linguistic backgrounds coming together to receive an education. Children in the United States who come from culturally and linguistically diverse (CLD) backgrounds are increasing in number, due to continued immigration and to increased birthrates among some CLD groups (Roseberry-McKibbin & Hegde, 2005). In fact, all major ethnic groups in the United States are increasing, while the White population is decreasing. The 2000 U.S. Census revealed that one in every four people in the United States is nonwhite. Projected estimates are that by year 2020, a little more than one-third of the population will be nonwhite, and by 2050, half the population will be nonwhite (U.S. Census Bureau, 2000).

Of course, not all who describe themselves as "nonwhite" in census counts also identify themselves as culturally diverse. Cultural diversity is not determined by the origin of one's ancestors or skin color; many Americans who check "nonwhite" boxes in census counts consider themselves to be fully acculturated into what has been called "mainstream" American society. Therefore, cultural diversity as discussed in this chapter is not a matter of skin color; it is a matter of linguistic and cultural variations that affect social, academic, and occupational communication in the context of the larger U.S. society. Many people who have linguistic and cultural backgrounds other than those of mainstream Americans may exhibit communication patterns that do not negatively affect social, academic, and occupational life. Cultural diversity is determined by a number of factors, including, among others, linguistic background, religious beliefs, regional affiliations, educational levels, and socioeconomic status (Moxley, 2003) that create variations that demand scientific and clinical attention. Individuals who are likely to have a lesser degree of acculturation include those who have recently arrived in the United States, those who visit their country of origin frequently, and those who have limited contact with others outside their families or communities (Roseberry-McKibbin, 2002). These individuals

> People from specific cultural groups who have adapted American norms of behavior are said to have been acculturated into "mainstream" American society.

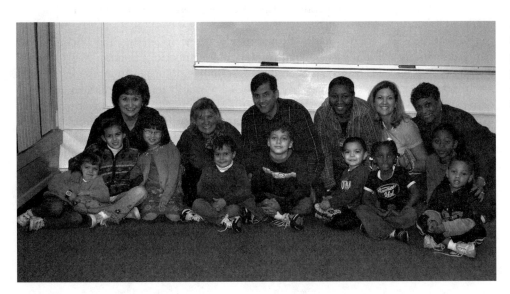

photo 11.1
The United States is becoming an increasingly multicultural, diverse society.

may have cultural beliefs and practices that bring them into conflict with prevailing American values and social mores. Because those conflicts may have an effect on the assessment and treatment of communicative disorders in CLD children and adults, there has been a call for SLPs to acquire what has been termed *cultural competence*.

Cultural Competency: What Does It Mean and How Does It Help?

As the population of CLD people has grown, authors and researchers in speech-language pathology have described a need for SLPs to become culturally competent. Cultural competency has been loosely defined as "a multi-dimensional concept that encompasses cultural awareness, cultural sensitivity, and cultural tolerance" (Wolf & Calderon, 1999, p. 5). It is felt that SLPs should understand how a client's cultural background might affect assessment and treatment of communicative disorders in culturally diverse individuals. SLPs may attain cultural competency by understanding their own value systems and then learning how value systems of other cultures might conflict with their own. SLPs working with varied students in the U.S. public schools may find that the values of children's families are not consistent with those of mainstream American values which permeate the educational system.

> Is the definition of cultural competency cited here an operational definition or a constituent definition?

Although respect for different cultures and tolerance for diversity are unarguably desirable characteristics, the quest for cultural competency should go beyond merely enhancing clinicians' intrapersonal qualities. We need evidence to show that cultural competence, once developed, will result in more efficacious therapy. In other words, it is not enough to ask clinicians to become culturally competent by learning about other cultures and linguistic differences; perhaps learning a few words of another language and understanding clashes between traditional American values and the values of other cultures. What is needed is to establish that such efforts will result in better treatment outcomes for children of all cultural and linguistic backgrounds.

Unfortunately, there is a dearth of experimental research investigating whether or not clinicians who are culturally competent conduct more efficacious therapy. Most of the research on multicultural issues has been both descriptive (nonexperimental) and directed toward assessment issues. Data have been collected primarily through interview, questionnaire, and survey methods. For the most part, published literature describes differences between mainstream American society and various multicultural groups in parent–child interactions, attitudes toward the disabled, value placed on education and oral communication, and unique linguistic characteristics. Discussion of treatment issues in most of the sources is limited (Battle, 2002; Coleman, 2000; Erickson, Devlieger, & Moon Sung, 1999; Goldstein, 2000; Johnston & Wong, 2002; Kamhi, Pollock, & Harris, 1996; Kayser, 1995; McNeilly & Coleman, 2000; Rodriguez & Olswang, 2003; Roseberry-McKibbin, 2002; Salas-Provance, Erickson, & Reed, 2002; Wilson & Wilson, 2000). Other studies have described levels of clinicians' cultural competency or sensitivity, pointed out areas of deficit, and recommended changes in university curriculum on multicultural issues or institutional in-servicing (Hammer et al., 2004; Roseberry-McKibbin & Eicholtz, 1994).

Research on multicultural issues has not translated into measurable clinical skills that are known to be effective in offering more appropriate assessment and treatment to children of diverse backgrounds. This is partly because the term *cultural competency* is far too broad and ill-defined and does not specify measurable clinical skills that result in cultural competency. Perhaps the next step that should be taken, then, is for researchers interested in multicultural issues to better define specific skills that clinicians should learn to gain cultural competency.

Ultimately, experimental research should demonstrate that specific clinical skills that presumably show cultural competence indeed result in effective services to children (and adults) with communication disorders. The greatest need is to find out whether existing treatment procedures are equally effective in treating children of various cultural backgrounds. On this question, there is little or no controlled evidence. We will return to the issue of treating language disorders in culturally diverse children in a later section.

In this chapter we will give an overview of major multicultural issues that affect clinical service delivery in speech-language pathology. Speech-language pathologists need to (1) distinguish language differences from language disorders, (2) work with interpreters to facilitate family counseling and clinical procedures, (3) conduct nonbiased assessment of CLD children, (4) evaluate the effects of treatment procedures and needed modifications, and (5) understand and work with children and families with varied cultural and linguistic histories.

Differences Are Not Disorders

We learned in Chapter 2 that a language disorder is impaired understanding and production of language; it refers to deficient verbal behaviors with negative social, personal, academic, and occupational consequences. **Language differences,** on the other hand, are variations mostly in language production (and to some extent in comprehension) that may be associated with a particular linguistic or cultural community.

African American English: A Case in Dialectic Differences

A popular mistake is to assume that a language spoken somewhat differently is a disorder. But no language is spoken in the same manner, even within a country or society. All languages have variations, which are called **dialects.** American English, for example, has its own dialects. There are such variations as Appalachian English, southern English, New York dialect, Boston dialect, and so forth. Consequently, the so-called Standard American English (SAE) is more of an abstract entity than a dialect spoken by individual speakers. Similarly, worldwide English dialects include, among its numerous variations, Canadian English, British English, Australian English, and New Zealand English. All of these and other variations may be called primary or native English dialects (Hegde, 2001a). Historically, no primary (native) English variations have been diagnosed as language disorders, although those that are due to the influence of another language (usually the first language of the speaker) have sometimes been mistaken for a disorder. For instance, English spoken as a second language by a Spanish speaker may be confused with a disorder.

Educators, SLPs, and the judicial courts faced the issue of American English dialects in the context of African American children who spoke a dialectical variation of English. In the 1970s, some African American parents in Michigan challenged their school district for lack of understanding of African American English dialect and the general insensitivity of educators toward the culture and communication patterns of African Americans. Agreeing with the African American parents, the U.S. Eastern District Court of Michigan ruled in 1979 that the school district should develop and implement a plan for increasing the educators' understanding and appreciation of African American dialect. The far-reaching consequences of this court ruling led to various changes in both general and special education, including language services offered to children who spoke dialectal variations of English.

The form of English spoken by most African Americans is known by many names: African American English (AAE), Black English, Black English Vernacular, and, most recently, Ebonics. Because a dialect is directly influenced by the community in which an individual lives, not all African Americans speak AAE, and AAE can be spoken by anyone of any ethnic or racial background, including White. From a behavioral point of view, children who speak AAE produce verbal behaviors that have been shaped through the principles of differential reinforcement by members of their community; what results is a manner of speaking that is different from SAE, but that is accepted and nurtured by the community in which the children are raised. From a linguistic point of view, children who speak AAE are using a rule-governed variation of the English language (Dillard, 1972). See Box 11.1 for more information on the Ebonics controversy and the linguistic viewpoint.

Clinicians working in public schools with large populations of children who speak AAE should understand that AAE is a systematic dialectical variation of American English. Clinicians need to know and appreciate the phonological, semantic, syntactic, and pragmatic rules of the dialect. Children who produce any social dialect according to the linguistic rules of the dialect do not exhibit a language disorder; their language is fully functional and acceptable within their communities. As stated in the ASHA (1983) position paper on social dialects, ". . . no dialectical variety of English is a disorder or a patho-

---

box 11.1   **African American English (AAE): Dialect or Language?**

There has been controversy in the past over whether AAE should be considered a dialect or a language that is altogether separate from English. In 1996, the Oakland School Board in California issued a resolution in which AAE, which was called Ebonics in the resolution, was declared to be a separate language—the primary language of the majority of students served by the Oakland Unified School District. The resolution declared that students should be taught in their primary language, with instruction in Standard American English (SAE) as a second language. This was seen by many as an attempt to "cash in" on federal money available at the time for bilingual students.

The Board later amended the resolution to delete any reference to Ebonics as a primary language, but not before a fierce battle had been fought in the media, calling widespread attention to the use of AAE. The Linguistic Society of America (1997) issued a resolution of its own in response to this controversy, calling attention to the validity of AAE as rule-governed, stating, "What is important from a linguistic and educational point of view is not whether AAVE [African American Vernacular English] is called a 'language' or a 'dialect' but rather that its systematicity be recognized."

logical form of speech or language. Each social dialect is adequate as a functional and effective variety of English" (p. 24). It is possible, of course, for a child to have a language disorder within AAE (or any other) dialect. Therefore, in diagnosing a language disorder in an African American child, the clinician has to judge the child's language skills against acceptable skills in AAE, not SAE skills. To this end, clinicians need to achieve the level of competency necessary to distinguish a normal dialect from a disorder *within* AAE. To properly diagnose a language disorder in an African American child, clinicians need to understand the rules of the AAE dialect. See Tables 11.1 and 11.2 for a listing of some phonologic, morphologic, and syntactic characteristics of AAE dialect.

Although a dialect is not a disorder or a deficiency, there are educational and vocational advantages to learning SAE. In the public schools, teachers who have a good understanding and appreciation of AAE would still be teaching SAE and various academic subjects in SAE. Much of the college curriculum is offered in SAE. Workplaces also mostly use SAE. Success and advancement in employment, especially in the technical fields, higher education, and professional settings, also is facilitated by standard English language skills.

     table 11.1

Some Phonological Productions Characteristic of African American English (AAE) Compared to Phonological Productions of Standard American English (SAE)

AAE Characteristic	SAE Production	AAE Production
Deletion of unstressed syllables	about	'bout
Prevocalic voicing of /p/	potato	botato
Devoicing of final consonants	mad	mat
Cluster reduction in final word position	cold	col'
	must	mus'
Metathesis in final /s/ + stop clusters	ask	aks
	clasp	claps
Deletion of final consonants	man	ma-
	five	fi-
Labialization of interdental fricatives	bath	baf
	thumb	fum
	together	togever
Stopping of interdental fricatives	that	dat
	with	wit
Stopping of voiced fricatives preceding syllabic nasals	heaven	heben
	wasn't	wadn't
/l/ phoneme deleted or de-emphasized	tool	too'
	always	a'ways
/r/ phoneme deleted or de-emphasized	more	moah
	professor	p'fessah
Substitution of /n/ for /ŋ/	thinking	thinkin'
	something	singin'
Substitution of /ɪ/ for /ɛ/ (before nasals)	hen	hin
	men	min

Note: Characteristics of the AAE dialect will vary according to region.
Source: Compiled from Craig et al. (2003), Pollock (2001), and Roseberry-McKibbin (2002).

table 11.2

Some Syntactic and Morphologic Characteristics of African American English (AAE) Compared to Standard American English (SAE)

AAE Characteristic	SAE Production	AAE Production
Use of *be* for auxiliary in present progressive tense	He *is* talking.	He *be* talkin'.
Auxiliary *is* used regardless of person	They *are* eating	They *is* eatin'.
Deletion of auxiliary in present perfect progressive tense	She *has been* writing.	She *been* writin'.
Past auxiliary *was* used regardless of number or person	They *were* talking.	They *was* talkin'.
Auxiliary omitted altogether	She *is* singing.	She singin'.
Deletion of past-tense markers	He *walked* to the store yesterday.	He *walk* to the store yesterday.
More frequent use of *had* + verb *-ed* in place of simple past tense	The car stopped. / She walked to the store.	The car *had* stopped. / She *had* walked to the store.
Multiple (or double) negatives	He has *nothing*.	He *don't got nothin'*.
Omission of present tense *-s*	He *eats* all the time.	He *eat* all the time.
Omission of plural *-s*	It costs two dollars.	It cos' two *dollar*.
Omission of contractive *-s*	*That's* not right.	*That* not right.
Omission of possessive *-s*	It's *Jack's* coat.	It *Jack* coat.
Done is combined with a past-tense verb—indicates an action that has been completed	She *cooked* the ham.	She *done* cooked the ham.
Copula *is* replaced with *be* when indicating actions and events over time.	She *is* often kind.	She *be* kind.
Them substituted for *those*	*Those* flowers are beautiful.	*Them* flowers *be* beautiful.
Pronoun used to restate the subject	My father takes me fishing	My father, *he take me fishin'*.

Note: Characteristics of both AAE and SAE will vary according to region.

Source: Compiled from *Encyclopedia: Black English Vernacular* (2004); Green (2004); Roseberry-McKibbin (2002); Ross, Oetting, and Stapleton (2004).

Therefore, it is likely that most parents who speak AAE and teach it to their children support the learning of SAE. They are likely to make attempts at preserving AAE while their children also acquire SAE in both spoken and written forms so their opportunities are not curtailed. What would be objectionable to African Americans and to everyone else in society is a mistaken notion that AAE is somehow pathological or degenerate.

> **Therapy given because a client or a client's family chooses to improve nonpathological speech or language is called what kind of therapy?**

It is acceptable for SLPs to offer treatment to children who speak AAE when parents ask for such services. It is acceptable to offer treatment to speakers of any dialect when the speakers themselves or their families request it, but such treatment should never be required because of a mistaken diagnosis of a language disorder. Treatment to modify a dialect is elective. SLPs may accommodate parents' wishes to have their children learn SAE, but may recommend therapy only for children who display a language disorder when judged against the standards of their own language. Treatment is never recommended based on a language difference (Hegde & Davis, 1999).

If direct service is precluded, the school SLP should serve as a consultant to the classroom teacher. The clinician may help the teacher understand some of the special characteristics of AAE. The clinician also may help the teacher distinguish a culturally rich dialect against a deficient disorder. The clinician may support the teacher's role of helping the child become bidialectal, proficient in both AAE and SAE. A **bidialectal** child is proficient in two variations of a language. In this case, the goal is not to eradicate or diminish the importance of the child's home dialects, but to create proficiency in an additional dialect needed for academic, social, and professional success. In this vein, Campbell (1993) spoke of teaching SAE as a second dialect—teaching "the language of education while simultaneously maintaining the integrity of the home linguistic variety" (p. 11). For example, a teacher may provide consistent models of SAE, requiring a student's imitated responses, while acknowledging that SAE is different from, but not superior to, the student's home language ("At home, you say 'I be goin' to recess.' At school, you say, "'I am going to recess.' Say it for me—'I am going to recess.' Good! You said it!"). See Box 11.2 for a common scenario involving a student who speaks AAE. We will return to the question of treatment for children of varied ethnocultural backgrounds in a later section

> What is the term used to describe children who learn to speak two dialects?

Dialects Due to Bilingualism

When a child has a **primary** (designated L1) and a **secondary** (designated L2) **language,** the secondary language may be spoken with a dialectal variation. This dialect may persist even as the child grows older and the second language becomes the dominant language. In this case, the secondary language is not secondary in importance or competence; it is secondary only in a chronological sense of learning. It was learned after another language was mastered. In some individuals, though, the secondary language may remain less proficient than the primary.

A child who has learned or is still learning two languages, may seem to exhibit a disorder in the second language simply because of the dialect in which the child speaks it. As in the case of a child with AAE, this seeming language disorder may not be a disorder. Again,

---

box 11.2   **Multicultural Scenario #1**

Deshawn's kindergarten teacher, Mrs. Smith, referred him to the school SLP for an assessment of his speech and language. Mrs. Smith reported on the referral form that she "doesn't understand a word he says!" The school SLP called Deshawn's mother who expressed surprise over the idea that anyone would think there was a problem with Deshawn's speech and language. The school SLP assessed Deshawn and found that all of his phonological, syntactical, and morphological errors were due to very heavy use of African American English (AAE). The SLP further observed Deshawn on the playground and saw that he seemed to be well-liked and had no difficulty communicating with his peers.

What Should This Clinician Do?

Because Deshawn is understood by his family and his peers, he is probably using African American English (AAE), which is a language difference, not a language disorder. However, if the kindergarten teacher cannot understand him, the clinician could decide to qualify Deshawn for services, because his dialect is interfering with his academic success. Treatment could be given *only* if Deshawn's family agreed it would be best for him to learn Standard American English. (See Box 11.7, which shows how to request parental permission for treatment targets.)

to diagnose a language disorder in the second language of bilingual children, the clinician needs to understand the linguistic rules and acceptable verbal behaviors of the primary language. In other words, the clinician should have a good knowledge of bilingualism—how children acquire and produce two languages and how to diagnose a language disorder in one or both of the languages.

Children who are raised in bilingual households, in which two languages are spoken and equally valued (reinforced), typically learn both languages as effortlessly as children do in monolingual households. Learning two languages at the same time is called **simultaneous bilingualism,** resulting in infant bilinguality (Genesee, 1988; Kessler, 1984; Schiff-Myers, 1992). Typically developing children will not be harmed by exposure to two languages; in fact, that is the ideal situation for learning two (or more) languages well. If a bilingual child has a language disorder, it is likely the result of factors unrelated to bilingualism.

> Some bilingual parents who have a child with a language disorder wonder if they have confused the child by introducing two languages at once. These parents need to be reassured that language disorders are not caused by exposure to two languages.

Some children will have learned their primary language at home and then get exposed to another language outside the home (school or larger social settings). Such children learn the second language (L2) sequentially, resulting in **sequential bilingualism.** Typically, such children learn their primary language at home and begin to learn English when they enter public school, often around the age of 5, if they did not attend a preschool program. Children who are sequentially bilingual show more variability in the development of L2 proficiency than those who are simultaneously bilingual (Kayser, 2002).

In the United States, children who do not have fluent English when they enter public school are described as English-as-a-second-language, or ESL, students. Technically, this is a wrong term because a *second* language should not always suggest a *weak* language. Unfortunately, it often is, and it means such in the U.S. public schools. Instruction offered to ESL children is highly variable across schools, ranging from bilingual classrooms in the primary grades to a "sink or swim" philosophy of total immersion in which children get no instruction in their primary language. Regardless of the amount of support received, ESL children are likely to exhibit patterns of language acquisition that are typical of second language learners.

Even well-trained SLPs may find it difficult to determine whether the communicative behavior observed in second language learners should be attributed to a language difference or a language disorder. It is especially critical, then, for SLPs to understand the distinction between characteristics of a language disorder versus those of bilingualism, especially the sequential variety. Some common processes include:

- Interference
- Silent period
- Fossilization
- Code-switching

Interference. Aspects of the first language generalize to the second language. This generalization is said to cause an **interference** with correct production of the second language. Aspects of the first language may interfere with phonologic, semantic, syntactic, and pragmatic aspects of second language production. Foreign accents are the result of the phonological system of the first language interfering with production of the second. Children are very likely to have difficulty in producing phonemes that do not exist in their first language. Russian children, for example, might struggle with producing the /θ/ phoneme, because it is not in the phonetic inventory of the Russian language. In the United States, clinicians most typically see children who speak Spanish or one of the Asian languages at home and are now learning English as their second language. Therefore, much descriptive research has accumulated on the speech and language characteristics of these two groups of children. See Tables 11.3 and 11.4 for some English articulation characteristics of speakers of Spanish and Asian languages.

Semantically, children may have difficulty with concepts that are not represented in the vocabulary of their primary language. A child from a tropical climate might not have words or phrases that are equivalent to *snow, snowmobile, coat, snowshoes, ice fishing, snowstorm,* and so forth. Also, figurative language does not directly translate between languages. A child's idioms of a primary language may interfere with the production or understanding of

table 11.3

Examples of Interference of Spanish as a Primary Language on Articulation of English Phonemes

Articulation Difference	How Spanish as L1 Contributes to Articulation Differences
Substitutions:	
b/v (*balentine* for *valentine*)	Spanish /v/ pronounced bilabially
ch/sh substitution (*chew* for *shoe*)	No "sh" phoneme in Spanish
/d/ or /z/ substituted for voiced "th" (*dem* for *them*)	No voiced or unvoiced "th" phoneme in Spanish
/t/ substituted for unvoiced "th" (*ting* for *thing*)	
Vowel substitutions (*beeg* for *big*, *bet* for *bat*)	Only five vowel sounds in Spanish (*ah*, short *e*, long *e*, *o*, *u*) and few dipthongs
y substituted for j (*yump* for *jump*, *yoke* for *joke*)	No single y phoneme in Spanish (*ñ* is a combination *n* + *y* sound as in *mañana*—"manyana")
/r/ phoneme produced with a flap or trill	Spanish /r/ produced either with a single flap (e.g., *pero*) or a trill (e.g., *perro*)
Deletion of /h/ in initial word position (*'ello* for *hello*)	In Spanish, initial /h/ is silent (e.g., *Hidalgo, helado*).
Insertion of a schwa before initial /s/ + consonant clusters (*esnake* for *snake*)	There are no words in Spanish beginning with consonant clusters containing /s/ as the first sound—a vowel sound precedes the cluster (as in *escuela* for school or *esposo* for husband).
Dentalization of alveolar consonants /t/, /d/, /n/, /s/, /z/	Spanish alveolars, especially /s/ and /z/, are produced with a more anterior tongue position.
Deaspiration of stops in final word position	Spanish words do not end with aspirated stops.
Final consonant deletion (e.g., *bo* for *boat*)	Spanish words most often end in vowel sounds; the only consonants produced in word-final position are /s/, /n/, /r/, /l/, /d/, compared to 24 consonant sounds that may occur in syllable-final position.
Differences in nonsegmental features (e.g., stress, pitch, intonation of questions and statements)	Spanish is less modulated than English; English production may sound monotonic.
	Spanish utterances begin with a lower pitch level with pitch change on first stressed syllable; English utterances begin with a higher pitch with pitch change on emphasized words.

Source: Compiled from Brice (2002); Goldstein (2001); Roseberry-McKibbin (2002).

table 11.4

Examples of Interference of an Asian Language as a Primary Language on Articulation of English Phonemes

Articulation Difference	How Asian Language as L1 Contributes to Articulation Differences
Final consonant deletion (*hi* for *hide, boo* for *book*)	Words more frequently end in vowels in many Asian languages
Syllabic differences:	
Deletion of syllables (*tephone* for *telephone, mato* for *tomato*)	Most words in many Asian languages are monosyllabic; some ESL speakers may therefore drop syllables.
Stress placed on the wrong syllable (*ef-fort'* for *ef'-fort, syl-la'-ble* for *syl'-la-ble*)	Syllable stress patterns in Asian languages are different from those in English; English stress patterns are especially difficult for speakers of tonal Asian languages, in which semantic information is conveyed by prosodic changes.
Substitutions:	
ch for *sh* and *sh* for *ch* (*chape* for *shape, shair* for *chair*)	These are all phonemes that do not exist in some Asian languages. Production of the phonemes is therefore difficult for ESL speakers with an Asian primary language.
Various phonemes for voiced and unvoiced *th* (*dese* for *these, sat* for *that, tink* for *think*) b/v (*base* for *vase*) a/æ (*hot* for *hat*)	
/l/ for /r/ and /r/ for /l/ (e.g., *light* for *right, rucky* for *lucky*)	In the case of confusion over /l/ and /r/, in many Asian languages those sounds occur in the same phonemic category.
Vowel length reduced in words; speech sounds "choppy" to American listeners	Vowels are properly short in many Asian languages; reduced vowel length is just one factor contributing to prosodic differences in English production by L1 speakers of Asian languages.
Consonant cluster reduction (e.g., *bake* for *break*)	Many Asian languages have few or no consonant clusters.

Note: Generalizations about Asian languages are *very* tentative because the continent is home to hundreds of languages that belong to widely different linguistic families.
Source: Compiled from Cheng (1987) and Roseberry-McKibbin (2002).

expression in a second language. For example, an ESL speaker for whom Spanish is the primary language might mistakenly say in response to a joke, "You're taking my hair!" English-speaking listeners would be perplexed by such an utterance, which is the literal English translation of the Spanish saying, "Me estas tomando el pelo!"—the equivalent of "You're pulling my leg!" (Burke, 1998). Another ESL speaker may literally interpret the English slang "Go fly a kite" as a command to fly a kite.

The syntactic and morphological structures of the first language can interfere with production of the second. Hispanic children speaking Spanish as a second language may produce such utterances as *dog big* or *I have hunger*, because those productions are consistent with rules of Spanish syntactic rules (e.g., *perro grande* and *Tengo hambre*). See Table 11.5 for more examples of how Spanish syntax and morphology interfere with English productions.

Conversational skills and routines vary widely in different cultures and may interfere with a child learning similar skills of a different language. For example, in the United States,

table 11.5

Syntactic and Morphological Interference of Spanish as L1 on English as L2

Spanish Syntax or Morphological Structure	Sample Spanish Production	Sample of Interference in English Syntax
Adjectives are most often placed after the noun.	la *casa grande* la *pluma azul*	the *house big* the *shirt blue*
Adverbs are placed between the verb and the direct object.	El maneja *muy rapido* el coche.	He drives *very fast* the car.
Superlatives are indicated by the word *mas*; no suffixes (such as *-er* or *-est*) to the root word.	El es *mas* viejo que su padre.	He is *more old* than your father.
Prepositional phrases indicate possession; no possessive *s* morpheme.	Este es la madre *de mi amigo.*	This is the mother *of my friend.**
Double negatives are properly produced in Spanish.	No tengo *nada.*	I don't have *nothing.*
Questions most often asked with rising intonation only; no alteration of declarative sentence.	Vas a ir a la oficina?	You're going to the office?*

*These are structures that occur less frequently in English, but are not technically incorrect.

direct eye contact is valued in conversation. It indicates that a person is listening intently. People who give direct eye contact are thought of as honest, straightforward people, in comparison to "shifty-eyed" people who do not maintain good eye contact. Children are expected to look at an adult when the adult is speaking; if they do not, adults assume they are not paying attention. It is not unusual to hear an American parent, when chastising a child, say, "*Look* at me when I'm talking to you!" In contrast, some cultures, especially Asian cultures, view direct eye contact as a sign of disrespect, in particular when a child is giving it to an adult. In those cultures, children being chastised should keep their eyes downcast, in a contrite manner. Children with such a cultural background are not likely to adapt quickly to American customs, and differences in their pragmatic language skills, such as eye contact, should not be viewed as symptomatic of a language disorder. For examples of pragmatic language differences in African American children, see Table 11.6.

> Conversely, clinicians should not always assume children's pragmatic behaviors are due to cultural influences. Children with language disorders may not give eye contact because they have learned to avoid situations that may require them to speak.

Silent period. Children learning a second language often go through a **silent period,** in which they listen much but produce little of the second language. This silent period may be a period of observational learning. The children may be covertly rehearsing what they hear. They are learning words and phrases but are hesitant to speak because they have not been reinforced yet for speaking a second language. Until the child has had some success and reinforcement, the new language will be produced infrequently and hesitantly.

> Anyone who has tried to learn a foreign language probably recalls being very reluctant to produce the language right away. When teachers of foreign languages in high school ask students to answer a question in Spanish or French, typically very few, if any, students eagerly raise their hands to volunteer.

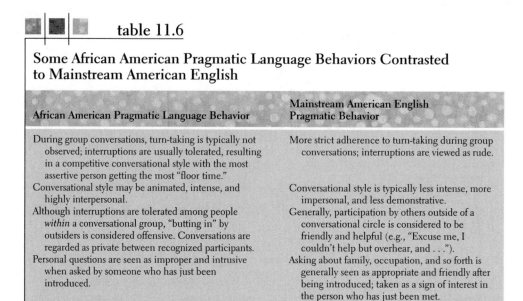

table 11.6

Some African American Pragmatic Language Behaviors Contrasted to Mainstream American English

African American Pragmatic Language Behavior	Mainstream American English Pragmatic Behavior
During group conversations, turn-taking is typically not observed; interruptions are usually tolerated, resulting in a competitive conversational style with the most assertive person getting the most "floor time."	More strict adherence to turn-taking during group conversations; interruptions are viewed as rude.
Conversational style may be animated, intense, and highly interpersonal.	Conversational style is typically less intense, more impersonal, and less demonstrative.
Although interruptions are tolerated among people *within* a conversational group, "butting in" by outsiders is considered offensive. Conversations are regarded as private between recognized participants.	Generally, participation by others outside of a conversational circle is considered to be friendly and helpful (e.g., "Excuse me, I couldn't help but overhear, and . . .").
Personal questions are seen as improper and intrusive when asked by someone who has just been introduced.	Asking about family, occupation, and so forth is generally seen as appropriate and friendly after being introduced; taken as a sign of interest in the person who has just been met.
Eye contact between children and adults is sometimes discouraged, particularly when children are being reprimanded; a child who makes eye contact may be seen as being disrespectful.	Children are encouraged to make eye contact with adults as a sign that they are listening respectfully.

Source: Compiled from Roseberry-McKibbin (2002); van Keulen, Weddington, and De Bose (1998); and Willis (1998).

Children who are going through a silent period may appear to be slow in their attempts at acquiring the second language. Professionals working with ESL children should warmly reinforce the children's attempts to produce the second language.

Fossilization. Even after acquiring a high level of proficiency in a language, there are some errors that may remain **fossilized,** meaning that they persist, although language production is otherwise excellent. The inconsistencies of the English language are often to blame for this. For example, every irregular plural word and every irregular verb is a separate response class unto itself; each must be individually learned. It is perhaps easy to understand why a child who otherwise speaks and writes English on grade level might persist in producing such errors as, "My foots hurt!" or "I blowed my birthday candles out!" even when the child produces most other irregular plurals and irregular verbs correctly.

Code-switching. Easily alternating between two languages is called **code-switching;** it is a behavior that is typical of fluently bilingual speakers. Code-switching can occur at the word, phrase, or sentence level. In multicultural communities in the United States, it is not unusual to overhear conversations in foreign languages that more or less frequently include English words or phrases.

Children who are bidialectic code-switch between two dialects, according to speaking situations.

Children in the early stages of bilingualism may substitute words or sentence structures from their first language (L1) for those in their

| box 11.3 | Multicultural Scenario #2 |

What Should This Clinician Do?

At an elementary school with a high percentage of children with English as a second language (ESL), an SLP ruefully looked at the pile of referrals she had received from primary grade teachers. Almost all of them were for the assessment of ESL students, and the SLP knew from experience that, after a full assessment in both English and their primary language (L1), the majority of them would be found to have no underlying language disorder. The high number of assessments necessitated by such referrals was a yearly frustration to the SLP.

An in-service designed to instruct teachers about normal processes of second language acquisition might help to keep inappropriate referrals down, especially if the clinician includes suggestions on how teachers might encourage and reinforce their students' emerging use of the English language.

second language (L2). In these beginning stages, code-switching may occur as a result of limited knowledge of L2. As children progress in learning L2, however, code-switching may become discriminative of the social situation or the conversational partners involved. While talking to a certain person, the speaker may use one language and immediately switch to another language while speaking to another person in the same situation. This is efficient and acceptable code-switching with good skills in both the languages. Many bilingual people code-switch; however, there is some research indicating that an over-reliance on code-switching might indicate a lack of proficiency in either language (Langdon & Cheng, 1992).

Often, professionals who have no knowledge of normal processes of second language acquisition may view ESL children as possibly exhibiting a language disorder. For example, school SLPs may receive a high number of unnecessary referrals for assessment of speech and language of ESL children who are simply in the process of learning the English language. In-servicing school staff on patterns of second language acquisition may help teachers recognize normal processes. School SLPs should expect to share information, to consult, and to collaborate with teachers to facilitate L2 development in ESL children. See Box 11.3 for a situation commonly encountered by school speech-language pathologists.

It is clear that in working with multicultural children, professionals should avoid the mistake of considering the influences of the first language on the second language as an indication of a language disorder. However, another mistake is for clinicians to attribute *all* difficulties multicultural children may have with language to differences resulting from cultural and economic background, social dialect use, or normal processes of second language acquisition. Language disability occurs in the same proportion among multicultural students as it does in the general population. Therefore, it is equally important to diagnose language disorders when they exist and provide appropriate intervention.

Understanding Each Other: Working with Interpreters

It is ethical and, in the public schools, legally required to assess a child fully in both English and the child's primary language. All forms and documentation, such as a listing of parents' rights under special education law, must be translated into the primary language, and oral communication with family members must be conducted in the primary language. To the extent it is practical, interpreters may help fulfill these ethical and legal requirements.

This is not always an easy task in the increasingly multicultural societies of the world. Many states in the United States pose significant challenges to SLPs to fulfill the legal and professional responsibilities of adequately serving children of diverse ethnocultural backgrounds. For example, Los Angeles Unified, the largest school district in the State of California, reported 56 primary languages spoken by students (California State Department of Education, 2004). Although the number of ESL children in the public schools is rapidly growing, the number of SLPs who are bilingual is not, at least not rapidly enough to keep up with the demand for assessment and treatment in a student's primary language. Of the total number of certified SLPs who were ASHA members in 2003, only 6.3 percent identified themselves as members of a racial minority, and only 2.7 percent were of Hispanic or Latino ethnicity (ASHA, 2003b). Of that very small percentage, there are even fewer who are bilingual.

Clinicians who do not speak the primary language of the child being assessed or treated may seek the help of an interpreter/translator (IT). An **interpreter** is one who converts an *oral* message from one language to another. A **translator** is one who converts a *written* message from one language to another. A person who is described as an interpreter/translator, then, can perform both functions; orally interpreting for children during assessment and treatment, and for families during meetings; and translating the various printed forms and reports related to the special education services into the primary language.

> What does an interpreter do? What does a translator do?

Selecting and Training an Interpreter/Translator (IT)

Interpreting and translating are technical and objective tasks that need training. Just fluency in two or more languages is not sufficient to do a competent job. Out of convenience, clinicians ask family members or support school personnel to serve as ITs, particularly during assessment procedures and meetings. Family members may be unsuitable ITs, because they are emotionally invested in the child and lack training in technical subjects. It might be tempting, for example, for a family member to give a child hints while interpreting instruction given during standardized testing.

In contrast, competent ITs are well-trained people with specific skills and knowledge. Desirable characteristics of ITs in speech-language pathology have been described by various authors (Langdon, 2000; Langdon & Cheng, 2002; Langdon & Quintanar-Sarellana, 2003; Roseberry-McKibbin, 2002). Effective ITs should:

- Have strong oral and written language skills in English and in the language of the child and family
- Adhere to professional ethics: maintain confidentiality, remain impartial, and respect other people's opinions and cultures
- Have good short-term memory skills so they can accurately convey messages and record information
- Help facilitate intercultural communication by explaining how cultural differences might be affecting an interaction

In addition, SLPs must provide training for ITs in specific skills and knowledge in speech-language pathology. Training for ITs should include:

- Familiarity with professional terms and with special education law
- Test administration procedures
- Information regarding normal processes of second language acquisition
- An understanding of the role of the IT on the special education team

Working with ITs: Three Phases in the Interpretive Process

Langdon and Quintanar-Sarellana (2003) have described three phases in the interpretive process: (1) the briefing, (2) the interaction, and (3) the debriefing. This three-step process has been abbreviated BID and includes specific tasks during each phase.

> What are the three phases of the interpretive process?

Briefing. During the **briefing,** the initial phase, the SLP consults with the IT and explains the goals of the upcoming interpretive task. If the IT is to help conduct an assessment, the SLP goes over the tests to be administered and describes the specific instructions for administering and scoring the tests. If the IT is expected to interpret at a meeting, the SLP describes the participants and the goals of the meeting. If the IT is expected to assist with the child's treatment, the SLP will describe the treatment plan, show the stimulus materials, and explain the data collection method to be used. The SLP should make sure the IT fully understands what the upcoming task entails and how to carry it out. If possible, the SLP should arrange for the IT to have a preliminary contact, either by telephone or in person, with the child, the family members, or both, to establish rapport and the beginning of a working relationship.

Interaction. The **interaction** is the actual event at which the IT will be providing services. The SLP *must* be present during the interaction. Letting the interpreter alone handle interactions with the child and with family members is an unethical and undesirable practice.

If the interaction involves a meeting with family members, the SLP should exhibit certain behaviors. First, when providing information, the SLP should look at the family, *not* at the interpreter. Cultural customs regarding eye contact should be respected, but under no circumstances should the SLP turn to the interpreter and say, "Tell them. . . ." Instead, the SLP should conduct the conversation *with* the family. Second, the SLP should speak in short sentences, pausing often to allow the IT to interpret the message to move on. An SLP who goes on and on, without a pause, will increase the likelihood of being misinterpreted by an IT who cannot remember exactly what was said. Third, the SLP should not use professional jargon which the IT may not adequately translate. The

> Conducting "sideline" conversations with other professionals while the interpreter is speaking to the family is rude and unprofessional.

SLP should instead use simple, direct language and should define a technical term that is unavoidable, just as the effective SLP would when talking to any family. Fourth, while the IT is interpreting what was said, the SLP and any other professional people present should sit silently and respectfully.

During the interaction, the IT should sit as close to family members as possible. The IT should carefully interpret everything that everyone says as accurately as possible. If

photo 11.2
What is wrong with this picture?

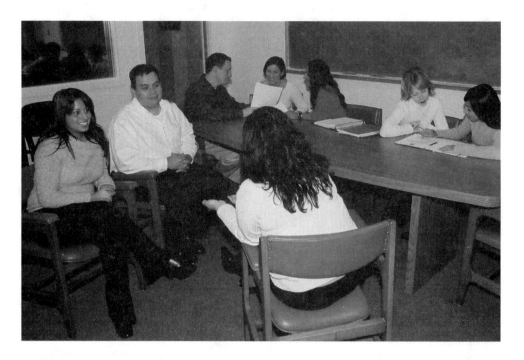

necessary, the IT should ask for clarification before interpreting a message that may have been misunderstood. Conducting a meeting using an interpreter naturally takes twice as long as conducting a meeting without one. Patience and respect are required of everyone involved. A successful interaction is one in which the goal of the interaction is achieved and the client-professional relationship is enhanced (See Box 11.4 for an example of what *not* to do during the interaction phase).

box 11.4 Multicultural Scenario #3

Jua, an 8-year-old special education student, was due for a 3-year full reassessment. The student's family, recent immigrants from Laos, spoke Hmong, and the school assessment team had found a Hmong interpreter in the community to help at the individualized education plan (IEP) meeting. The student's mother attended the IEP meeting and smiled at the professional people gathered to present their assessment findings to her. They smiled back, but then commenced to talk among themselves, furiously typing on their laptop computers, integrating their various reports into the one required multidisciplinary report. One by one, each professional person, including the school SLP, reported assessment results, talking directly to the interpreter.

While the interpreter spoke to the mother, the professionals continued their sideline conversations. At the end of the meeting, they asked the interpreter to ask the mother if she had any questions. She did not.

If You Were the School SLP, How Would You Have Interacted Differently with This Family?

When working with interpreters, professionals should talk directly to family members. While the interpreter is speaking, there should be no sideline conversations or report writing. Instead, the professionals should sit respectfully until the interpreter is done speaking.

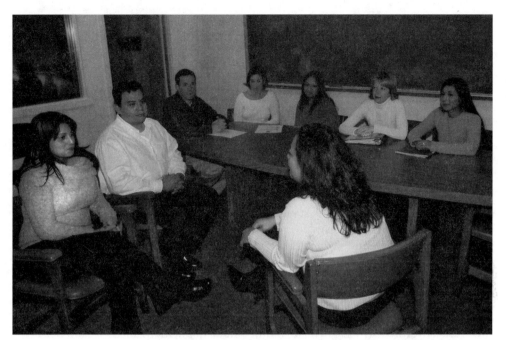

photo 11.3
Professionals should sit quietly and respectfully while their words are interpreted for the family members.

Debriefing. After the interaction, the SLP and the IT should sit down together for a **debriefing** session. During the debriefing, any problems that were encountered during the interaction should be discussed, along with suggestions for how future interactions can be improved. Conversely, the SLP and IT should also discuss what went well.

This is also the time when the IT might be invited to share his or her impressions of the family or child. While the SLP may consider the IT's observations when making an assessment or recommendations, the IT should never have full responsibility for diagnosis, school placement, or treatment decisions.

Working with interpreters is but one of several modifications that may need to be considered when assessing and treating CLD children. The following sections will discuss issues relevant to accurate assessment and effective treatment of CLD children, beginning with assessment.

Nonbiased Assessment of Multicultural Children

In Chapter 4 we described two types of procedures to assess language performance in children: (1) standardized tests and (2) child-specific procedures which include observation of the child and language sampling. Of the two, child-specific procedures are more likely to produce the type of in-depth information necessary to accurately diagnose a language disorder. Child-specific procedures, by definition, take into consideration the individual child, his or her linguistic and cultural background, and the family behavior patterns. Therefore, they are especially suited to assess CLD children. Most of the problems in assessing CLD children stem from the too common practice of administering standardized tests to children of varied cultural, linguistic, socioeconomic, and educational backgrounds. The following sections describe issues involved with the use of standardized tests in diagnosing language disorders in CLD children.

Bias in Standardized Assessment Tools

We pointed out in Chapter 4 that standardized testing raises questions about validity and reliability, the lack of adequate behavior sampling, and the applicability of normative data gathered from sampled groups of children to an individual child's language performance. Because of these problems, it was recommended that standardized testing be considered a supplement to child-specific measures of language performance. When assessing CLD children, the problems with standardized testing get compounded. In addition to all the problems discussed in Chapter 4, standardized tests tend to be culturally biased and yield results that may be totally or partially invalid for CLD children. The major problems with standardized tests administered to CLD children include the following:

- Test items do not reflect cultural and linguistic differences, particularly when the child tested is bilingual
- Samples of children on whom standardized tests are normed are often not representative of CLD children because they are excluded from the normative sample
- Tests advertised as designed for multicultural populations often lack validity and reliability
- Test modifications made by well-meaning clinicians weaken validity of results

Cultural and linguistic differences. Standardized tests are often devised without consideration of cultural differences and variations in structure and meaning across languages. Numerous studies have shown that CLD children do poorly on standardized tests that have been normed on samples drawn from populations of White, middle-class children. It has been suggested that differences in cultural tradition and socioeconomic background, rather than an underlying deficit in language, may be, in larger part, the cause of this poor performance (Campell et al., 1997; Fagundes et al., 1998; Long, 1994; Nelson, 1993; Wyatt, 1998).

Cultural bias can also occur because commonly held expectations regarding the testing situation may not be relevant to the child's cultural background. Test administrators typically expect a child to be cooperative, to attend to the testing tasks, and to strive to do their best to answer questions. In some cultures, however, children may be expected to be silent and respectful in the presence of adults (Matsuda, 1989; Roseberry-McKibbin, 2002). A CLD child may not be accustomed to being directly questioned by an adult or to being required to forthrightly answer questions. Furthermore, standardized testing is not as common in many countries as it is in the United States. Children from some countries may not be used to the *test culture* of mainstream United States and may find testing to be a novel and stressful experience. They will not have the experience of taking multiple tests in their educational setting as American children may be among the most tested. Even children who have mainstream American backgrounds are often shy with strangers—a CLD child may be even more likely to be uncomfortable with unfamiliar adults during testing. Cultural bias is likely to occur "if there is a mismatch between the interaction expected during testing and that which is familiar to the child" (Brice, 2002).

Standardized testing is also fraught with linguistic bias. Interference from the primary language may result in incorrect syntactical or morphological structures that are recorded as errors on standardized tests. Also, children who are learning English tend to make errors that are similar to developmental errors younger children commonly make (e.g., overgeneralized use of past tense *-ed*). Standardized test vocabulary may be confusing to CLD children, particularly those who speak English as a second language. Some children may know enough English to get along during everyday conversation, and may also know English vocabulary for school-oriented objects or concepts, but not much else. Some standardized tests may require the presentation of stimulus items that may be entirely absent in the child's cultural environment. Recently immigrated children, for example, may be confused by pictures of American sports, toys, fruits, vegetables, home appliances, and American holiday scenes. Some culturally diverse children may be puzzled by references to American nursery rhymes or fairy tales and storybook characters that are familiar to mainstream American children. Incorrect responses to such stimuli may not be symptomatic of a language disorder (Roseberry-McKibbin, 2002). Children who are still learning basic English skills should not be diagnosed with a language disorder because of their poor performance on standardized tests of vocabulary.

Lack of representation in samples drawn from the population. Samples of populations on which standardized tests are normed are often composed of predominantly White, middle-class, monolingual speakers of English. This is a practice that has been understandably criticized as being unfair to the many children in our society who come from CLD backgrounds (Washington, 1996; Wyatt, 1998). The *first* thing a clinician should do when selecting a standardized test to assess a CLD child is to look in the test manual to determine the ethnic and socioeconomic breakdown of the sample used for the generation of normative data. If there is insufficient representation of the group to which the child belongs, and there often is, then that test should not be used.

Authors of more recent editions of commonly used standardized tests have made some efforts to ensure that samples are more culturally diverse. However, geographic areas in the United States differ widely on the proportion of various ethnic groups in the local population. Therefore, it is difficult to imagine a sample that could be truly representative of children in all regions of the country.

Problems with tests designed for CLD children. Even if a standardized test is advertised as being specifically designed to assess a particular multicultural group, clinicians should critically examine the test before using it. Tests that are directly translated from English into another language have weak content validity because direct translations often do not reflect linguistic differences between the two languages. Some commercially available tests in Spanish, for example, are direct translations, slight modifications, or both, of existing English tests (Brice, 2002). One Spanish-language test, the *Spanish Preschool Language Scale-3* (Zimmerman, Steiner, & Evatt Pond, 2002b) was rigorously examined by independent researchers who concluded the test did not meet criteria for reliability and validity and that administration of the test resulted in overidentifying language disorders in Spanish-speaking children (Restrepo & Silverman, 2001).

Modifications of standardized tests. Some clinicians may attempt to make standardized tests culturally more "fair" by omitting items that they think may be particularly biased against the child being tested, by testing beyond the ceiling, giving extra time for the child to respond, giving subtle hints, and so forth. However, tests are *standardized* because the authors clearly specify the procedures for administering them and interpreting their results. Any time any alteration to a standardized test is made, the validity of that test is weakened.

When clinicians modify standardized tests, they turn the test into a criterion-referenced check of a child's language skills. This is acceptable if good information regarding a child's language skills is obtained, but there are better ways than modifying standardized tests to conduct a criterion-referenced assessment. Therefore, it is recommended that, rather than attempt to alter standardized tests to better fit the child, clinicians understand that standardized testing is *not* the best or the only way to diagnose a language disorder in any child, particularly a CLD child. There are alternative, child-specific methods of assessment that will yield results that are more representative of the child's language performance and will more reliably result in an accurate diagnosis.

Because of the many difficulties in applying results of standardized testing in a fair, valid way to CLD children, it is best to use child-specific methods of measurement when assessing children who are from diverse cultural backgrounds. If used at all, the results of standardized tests given to CLD children should always be reported with a disclaimer regarding the possible bias of the test. Many institutions provide SLPs with standard verbiage to that effect which is routinely included in diagnostic reports. We would ask, if data must be presented with such a disclaimer, why present it at all?

Alternatives to Standardized Testing: Child-Specific Procedures

The child-specific procedures described in Chapter 4 should be used in assessing CLD children. Observations of the child in naturalistic settings, language sample analysis, and interviewing parents, caregivers, teachers, and so forth will all contribute to a less biased and more accurate assessment of a child's language skills. In fact, there are very few modifications that need to be made in effective child-specific procedures when assessing CLD children. Craig and Washington (2000) found that a battery of commonly used measures of expressive and receptive language distinguished African American children with language disorders from those without. The assessment battery included language sample analysis, incorporating measures of mean length of communicative units (MLCU, similar to MLU discussed in Chapter 4) for words and for morphemes, analysis of vocabulary diversity, frequency of use of complex syntax, and, for receptive language, responses to *wh* questions and comprehension of passive and active voice sentence construction.

Some experts describe client-specific procedures as *informal*. But there is nothing informal about them.

Even without a particular assessment battery, a good language sample, taken with stimulus materials that are relevant to the child's language and home environment (see the next section), may be used to make an analysis of the child's vocabulary, syntactic constructions, morphologic features, and pragmatic behaviors. In addition, an analysis of the communicative demands made on the particular child will help design additional child-specific assessment procedures. For instance, the kinds of words the child is exposed to in the classroom, the literacy demands made on the child, and the grade level books the child is expected to read and understand, may all provide material for a child-specific assessment.

Some Special Considerations

In addition to child-specific procedures, CLD children need a few special considerations. In assessing such children, clinicians should: (1) conduct separate assessments in both languages, if the child is bilingual, (2) select culturally relevant stimulus items, and (3) apply knowledge of the values and traditions of the child's culture to the assessment process.

We have previously discussed the need to assess a bilingual child in both languages. This should be done separately, although it is a more difficult task to carry through during child-specific assessment than it is during standardized testing. Clinicians may be inclined to encourage a child to respond in either language, or clinicians, if they are bilingual themselves, may switch between languages to prompt responses during assessment. Intermixing languages during assessment will result in an unclear picture of the child's expressive and receptive language skills in either language. As much as possible, assessment should be conducted first in one language, and then in the other.

Another consideration is the selection of stimulus items that reflect the child's cultural background and home environment. Presentation of stimulus items that are not commonly found in the child's natural setting will result in a biased assessment that may lead to a misdiagnosis. A Hmong child who has recently immigrated from a Thai refugee camp will be unlikely to recognize pictures of objects such as a cactus, a penguin, or an aquarium (all pictures included in a commonly administered standardized test of expressive language). Most American toys, puzzles, dolls, and such play materials as play dough also will be inappropriate in evoking language from CLD children who have recently arrived in the United States. During assessment, it is desirable to avoid using biased stimulus items, because the goal is to make a differential diagnosis of a language disorder or normal language. During the initial interview, it may be helpful to show the selected stimulus materials (toys, pictures, objects, activities that involve materials) to the parents to ascertain whether the materials are familiar to the child. The ones that are not may be substituted with additional materials based on the parents' suggestions.

Child-specific assessment is more effectively carried out if the SLP has some knowledge of the values and traditions of the child's culture. A technique borrowed from the field of anthropology, **ethnographic interviewing** involves seeking out people from a particular culture and asking detailed questions regarding that culture (Roseberry-McKibbin, 2002). Clinicians who find themselves in a setting where a large proportion of the children are culturally diverse may choose to gather information regarding a child's home culture by engaging parents and other members of the community in this type of interview. Other ways in which clinicians may learn about a child's culture include direct observation, reading, consulting with other professionals, and attending conferences. When clinicians are knowledgeable about traditions and values of a child's culture, they become more able to accurately distinguish between a language disorder and a language difference. Also, with that knowledge, the clinician can select more suitable assessment materials for the child.

Treatment for Multicultural Children: A Question of Generality

Much of the writing on multicultural issues in speech-language pathology is on assessment issues. The importance of culturally appropriate assessment procedures cannot be overemphasized. Nonetheless, there is a need to move beyond the concept of culturally sensitive assessment procedures. The multicultural agenda needs to move on to treatment.

Unfortunately, most treatment efficacy research in communicative disorders has been done with White, middle- to upper-class samples. We do not know if treatment procedures that have been shown to be effective for the majority groups are also effective for members of minority groups. This is a problem of **ethnocultural generality,** a term that refers to the degree to which a treatment known to be effective with one ethnocultural group also is effective with other ethnocultural groups (Hegde, 2003a). Treatment procedures that are effective across diverse groups have ethnocultural generality.

> If a treatment method is experimentally shown to be effective with people from various ethnic groups, it is said to have what kind of generality?

There is little or no research on the efficacy of treatment procedures evaluated across clearly described ethnocultural groups. Treatment efficacy studies sometimes fail to give sufficiently detailed information on the ethnocultural background of participants. Furthermore, when diverse participants are recruited, the tendency is to give means (averages) for the groups. A failure to provide individual data on response to treatment makes it difficult to assess the effectiveness of procedures across culturally diverse participants. Ideally, we need experimental data to show that particular methods are indeed effective with particular ethnocultural groups. There is a great need to conduct such treatment efficacy research to demonstrate ethnocultural generality of widely used methods.

In the absence of negative evidence that certain treatment procedures will *not* work with particular ethnocultural groups, clinicians may select treatment procedures that have been experimentally evaluated and shown to be effective with at least some children with language disorders, even if the experiments did not sample diverse children. Treatment procedures whose effects have been replicated by different clinicians in different settings may be used with a greater degree of confidence; it is likely that widely replicated studies will have sampled some children of diverse background.

The treatment procedures described in this book are likely to be effective with a wide variety of children. The behavioral methods of modeling, instruction, prompting, positive reinforcement, differential reinforcement, shaping, extinction, and corrective feedback have been widely evaluated in both speech-language pathology and behavioral science (Hegde, 1998b; *Behavior Analysis in Developmental Disabilities, 1968–1985*). The generality of behavioral methods of treatment is now well established. Until studies produce contradictory evidence, there is no reason to suppose that some children are simply immune to the effects of these methods. It is also unlikely that children from different ethnocultural backgrounds need unique treatment procedures. It may be necessary to modify these procedures, but client-specific modifications are a part of treating any child or adult.

It is important to distinguish assessment and treatment issues in offering services to children of diverse backgrounds. Every important assessment issue is not necessarily important in treatment. For instance, it is inappropriate to select stimulus materials that are unfamiliar to the child and conclude that the child has a language disorder because of failed responses. Nonetheless, once a child is correctly diagnosed with a language disorder, the same unfamiliar stimulus materials may be excellent treatment stimuli. The recently arrived Hmong child in our earlier example may greatly benefit by learning words and concepts that are common in his or her new environment. To take another example, although it is inappropriate to diagnose a language disorder in an Asian child because of lack of eye contact, this and other pragmatic language skills may be appropriate treatment targets to enhance the child's academic and social success. When the selected treatment targets clash with the child's home communication patterns, the clinician should discuss the targets and obtain the parents' permission to teach them. The targets may be adopted, dropped, or modified as per the parents' wishes. In the next section, we suggest a method for obtaining parent approval for suggested treatment targets.

Working with Children and Families of Varied Cultural Backgrounds

Clinicians should enrich themselves and perhaps enhance their effectiveness as therapists by achieving a larger understanding of the culture, literature, and heritage of the families of the children they serve. Merely memorizing the linguistic differences across ethnocultural groups is not sufficient. Understanding the history of a people and reading literary works from different ethnic groups broaden the perspectives, increase the clinician's appreciation of cultural diversity, and culturally enrich the clinician.

While gaining richer understanding of children and families of different cultural backgrounds, clinicians should avoid the pitfall of stereotyping members of ethnic groups. Clinicians should not assume that families of different cultural backgrounds will reject mainstream values, for many have fully acculturated. Also, although there are many lists of cultural and communication features that typically characterize members of particular ethnicity, clinicians should not automatically assume that children of particular ethnic backgrounds they are about to evaluate will necessarily exhibit those features. Members of a particular ethnocultural group do not behave the same by the virtue of their group membership. This is true of African Americans, Hispanics, Asian Americans, or European Americans. Therefore, assessment and treatment that are client-specific will avoid many of the pitfalls of stereotyping a child or an adult of any cultural or ethnic background (Hegde, 2001a,b).

> Acculturation occurs when people who have immigrated to a different country adopt the values and behavioral patterns of that country. Many then become bicultural, staying involved with both the old and the new cultures.

In some cases, however, the values of a child's home culture and the values of mainstream America will collide in ways that affect delivery of effective intervention. For example, mainstream American values are highly individualistic; most Americans regard seeking self-fulfillment and the realization of individual potential as highly desirable goals in life. Many ethnic groups, however, have collective values. Individual needs are not as important as the needs of the group. There is much more emphasis on group loyalty and extended family. Children in some ethnic groups take on more responsibility for the well-being of the family than do mainstream American children. For the economic survival of the family, older children may be required to help support the family, working at various jobs, sometimes in labor-intensive jobs. In households with many children, older children may be expected to provide child care for younger siblings. These duties may result in high rates of absenteeism from treatment sessions and generally high drop-out rates as children set educational goals aside for the good of the family. There is little that an SLP can do when a student has either migrated with other family members to follow necessary work or dropped out of school entirely to support the family. To prevent a child from dropping out of school or to reduce absenteeism from treatment sessions, the school and the clinician may try to increase the parents' and the child's motivation to continue to receive educational and clinical services.

Clinicians who work in settings with large populations of families having divergent cultural values may find themselves in difficult positions. They are professionally obligated, and personally inclined, to advocate for the children on their caseload to receive quality intervention so that the children can succeed academically. On the other hand, clinicians are also obligated to respect and accommodate, when possible, cultural differences that may conflict with those goals. Clinicians who know and understand a child's cultural traditions are better able to work with families to reconcile conflicting values and provide more effective intervention.

Family hierarchy. Clinicians will be more likely to gain the cooperation of multicultural families if they pay close attention to the hierarchical structure of the family. In some cultures, mothers are not the primary decision-makers regarding their children. Fathers may have the most influence, or elderly family members might be the ones to have the "last say" in planning for a child's therapy. The observant clinician will determine who in the family is most likely to influence the course of a child's treatment and will direct recommendations and suggestions to that person or persons.

Diversity and disability. Views and behavioral dispositions toward disability may differ in some ethnic groups. Mainstream Americans, perhaps due to the emphasis on individual accomplishment, tend to admire disabled people who do everything they can to achieve as much as they can. The system of special education offered in the United States is designed to maximize the chances of disabled students living as independent a lifestyle as possible when they reach adulthood. Members of many other ethnic groups, however, may view a child with a disability as part of some divine plan that was not meant to be altered. Others may consider a disabled child to be a gift from God, sent to test the goodness of their character; how well they take care of the child will determine their personal worth. Such beliefs and dispositions may conflict with the goals of special education. It is not unusual for school personnel to gather to discuss a carefully devised individualized education plan (IEP) with family members only to find that the family has different, but equally well-formed, culturally influenced ideas on the child's future. Perhaps the plan is for one designated sibling to care for the child throughout life, or perhaps a future spouse will be responsible for the child's well-being. Because the child will be cared for within the family unit, it will seem irrelevant to family members to discuss goals designed to promote independence.

When clinicians are confronted with such values, it is best to acknowledge, validate, and accept a family's wishes. This does not mean, however, that clinicians should discontinue advocacy for further intervention for a child. If an adversarial relationship is diverted through acceptance and understanding of a family's wishes, the family may be more likely to accept a professional's recommendations for treatment objectives. See Box 11.5 for an example of how cultural values can affect the course of intervention.

Capitalizing on positive cultural influences consistent with SLP treatment. Different cultural values do not always conflict with mainstream American values. And, values that could conflict may be embraced in ways that actually enhance intervention. The emphasis on family that is present in many cultures can result in a desirable level of family participation during intervention. Many Asian groups place a very high value on education, practically revere teachers, and actively seek out intervention for children with academic difficulties or particular disabilities. In fact, clinicians may get better cooperation

box 11.5		Multicultural Scenario #4

In a middle school, special education personnel gathered for a yearly IEP meeting for a Pakistani female student with Down syndrome, Leisha. She had just had her 14th birthday, and, under state law, was due for a transition plan detailing goals for her adult life. The special education staff, including the school SLP, had worked hard to put together a transition plan which, they felt, offered her the opportunity to live as independently as possible, including a component of vocational training and suggestions for possible occupations. The family, who spoke English, listened patiently to the IEP team's recommendations. Then, they said that they had their own plans for Leisha. She would be married at the age of 18 to a Pakistani man who had already been selected. Her husband would take care of her and their future children in return for her dowry—the

monthly disability checks she will receive from the government when she turns 18.

How Would You Respond to the Family's Plan?

The family's plan for their child should be acknowledged, validated, and respected. The special education team should document the family's wishes. After letting the family know their plan is understood, efforts should be made to gain the family's acceptance for *additional* goals leading to vocational training. By accepting the family's ideas, the special education team will divert a possible adversarial relationship, making it more likely that the family will accept their recommendations for further education.

from some cultural groups than they do with some mainstream families. Clinicians who work with multicultural families should take advantage of cultural tendencies that can produce beneficial results in providing effective therapy. See Box 11.6 for an example of how a cultural tendency can be accommodated to enhance intervention.

When families know they are respected, they are more likely to accept a clinician's recommendations. They are even more likely to accept recommendations when they are given an opportunity to suggest treatment objectives for their children. The clinician who finds out that the social skills that are valuable to children in educational settings, such as eye

box 11.6		Multicultural Scenario #5

Miguel, a 10-year-old Hispanic male with a brain injury, was receiving his first speech and language therapy session at the outpatient clinic of a local children's hospital. Miguel's family, who spoke English as well as Spanish, accompanied him to the therapy session. There were, in all, eight of them—his mother, his father, his maternal grandmother, his paternal grandmother, his aunt, his uncle, and two cousins, ages 3 and 6. They all crowded into the SLP's therapy room. The SLP firmly told them, "I'm sorry, but I cannot give Miguel effective therapy if you are all here. You must wait in the lounge." The family reluctantly complied.

What Would You Have Done Differently?

Here is a cultural tendency that can positively affect treatment outcome. The clinician should welcome all family members initially and take some time for social talk—a custom called *simpatica*, which is practiced by many Hispanic families. Then, the clinician can gently suggest that one or two family members remain while the rest wait in the lounge. By accepting the family, understanding their need to be there, and establishing rapport, the clinician has set the stage for effective intervention. A little therapy time is lost, but future benefits will have been gained.

contact, asking for clarification, asking questions for further information, turn-taking, responding promptly to adults' questions, and so forth are not a part of a child's cultural upbringing, may get the family members involved in treatment planning. Families should be asked if they would like their child to learn targeted skills which will help the child function better within the educational setting. A trusting and respectful relationship built with the family will increase the probability that the family will approve the recommended treatment targets. See Box 11.7 for a suggested questionnaire seeking parental approval for common treatment targets that may represent cultural conflicts.

---

box 11.7 | **Please Tell Us What to Teach Your Child**

This form should be provided in the language spoken in the child's household.

Your child has been assessed and found to be in need of speech and/or language intervention. In preparation for the upcoming individualized education plan (IEP) meeting, please look at the following suggestions for skills that may be of help to your child in meeting educational goals. Please check the skills you would like your child to learn, sign where indicated, and return the form to your child's teacher.

I would like my child to learn:

_____ Unfamiliar English words

_____ About unfamiliar experiences (e.g., going to the zoo, going to the beach, attending sports events)

_____ How to ask questions about his lessons

_____ How to answer questions the teacher asks

_____ How to ask for help when the teacher's instructions are not understood

_____ How to take turns when speaking

_____ How to let the teacher know he or she is listening by looking at the teacher

_____ About customs and traditions of his home culture

_____ About customs and traditions of American culture

_____ About American rituals of politeness (e.g., how to greet someone, how to introduce people to each other)

_____ How to speak Standard American English (SAE)

_____ Other skills (please write them):

_____

_____

_____

Signed: _____   Dated: _____
        (Signature of Parent or Guardian)

Thank you! We are looking forward to working with you and your child!

SLPs are just beginning to understand issues involved with serving multicultural populations. As clinicians develop their practices, they will discover techniques that appear to facilitate relationships with CLD children and their families, perhaps contributing to the accuracy of assessment and the effectiveness of treatment. Clinicians who discover particularly promising treatment methods with a certain ethnocultural group should share those methods with their colleagues. More than that, they should conduct their own experimental studies on the efficacy of those methods and publish results. Only in this manner can we hope to discover the best ways in which to meet the needs of CLD children and their families.

Chapter Summary

Increased cultural and linguistic diversity of the U.S. population offers new challenges for the SLPs who are trying to serve the communication needs of diverse children. The clinicians now have to be competent not only in assessment and treatment procedures, but also in matters related to culture and communication. Clinicians need to know how to: (1) distinguish language differences from language disorders, (2) work with interpreters, (3) conduct nonbiased assessment of culturally and linguistically diverse children, (4) understand how the cultural background of a child may affect treatment, and (5) work with families of varied cultural backgrounds.

A language disorder is impaired understanding and production of language; language differences, on the other hand, are variations mostly in language production (and to some extent in comprehension) that may be associated with a particular linguistic or cultural community. No language is spoken in one fixed manner, hence there are social dialects (variations of a language and are not symptomatic of a language disorder). In the United States, African American English (AAE) is a special dialectal variation of English.

Some bilingual children speak an English dialect because of the influence of their first language. Children may acquire two language simultaneously or sequentially. The primary language may sometime interfere with the acquisition of the second language. Those who acquire two languages well may code-switch languages depending on their conversational partners.

Preferably, bilingual children should be assessed in both languages—English and their first language. SLPs may recruit the help of interpreters or translators in completing the assessment of bilingual children. Use of client- and family-specific procedures are important in assessing children of varied cultural backgrounds. Many standardized tests may be inappropriate because of their limited sampling of ethnoculturally different children during their standardization.

In selecting treatment procedures for culturally and linguistically diverse children, it is important to consider the degree of their ethnocultural generality. Much research is needed to show that many standard treatment procedures are applicable to children of varied backgrounds. Generally speaking, the behavioral treatment procedures described in this book have wide generality. While using these procedures with an ethnoculturally varied child, the clinician should carefully record the progress, so that the procedures may be modified at the earliest hint that they may not be working with a given child.

Study Guide

1. Distinguish between language disorders and language differences. Summarize the position of the American Speech-Language-Hearing Association on the question of dialects and disorders. Justify the statement, by examples of traditionally accepted variations of English as spoken in the United States, that dialectal differences are not a basis to diagnose a language or speech disorder.

2. How do children acquire two languages? What are the stages and potential problems of bilingual acquisition? Critically evaluate the statement that bilingualism does not negatively affect language competence in one or both languages.

3. You have been asked to assess the speech and language skills of a child who speaks limited English. The child and the family speak Spanish at home. How would you go about assessing this child? What kind of external help would you require? How do you make use of this external assistance? Why is it undesirable to use either family members or school support personnel to assist you in assessment?

4. Examine the statement that "many standardized tests of language skills are inappropriate for children with bilingual status or cultural differences." Offer suggestions to future test developers who are interested in standardizing tests that are culturally and linguistically appropriate for a wide variety of children.

5. A teacher has referred a 8-year-old African American boy for your speech and language assessment and potential treatment. What is your approach to assessing this child? What kinds of procedures would you use? Assuming that your assessment results are negative (i.e., the child does not have a speech or language disorder), how would you convey your assessment data and recommendations to the child's teacher? Be specific about the assessment procedures and the recommendations to the teacher.

6. Much of the research on culturally diverse children is about assessment procedures. Therefore, it is not clear whether the treatment procedures known to be generally effective are particularly effective with children of varied cultural backgrounds. In this context justify the statement that "certain issues that are relevant in assessment may not be relevant in treating children of diverse backgrounds." Give examples to sustain your justification.

chapter

12

Children with Developmental Disability

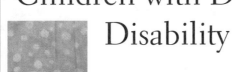

outline

In Chapter 3 we described children whose only diagnosis is a language disorder. They exhibit a disability that is specific to language, hence called specific language impairment. In this and the subsequent chapters, we describe children who have a language disorder and another disability. These are the children with dual diagnosis. For instance, the children we describe in this chapter have a language disorder *and* developmental disability (DD). These children need more than language intervention; but our primary concern is assessment and treatment of their language disorder. Speech-language pathologists (SLPs) will be the members of a team of specialists that will design and implement a comprehensive program that help children with DD.

Children with DD do not need entirely new assessment or treatment procedures. Nonetheless, they do need some special considerations. Their assessment and treatment procedures may need modifications or additions. Therefore, in this chapter, we will not repeat the treatment procedures that were described in the first part of this book; instead, we will point out what special considerations apply to children with DD.

Developmental Disability: Characteristics

Developmental disability (DD) is a complex phenomenon that may affect social, behavioral, intellectual, physical, and emotional development of a child. It has a significant effect on learning all kinds of skills, including language skills. Typically, this complex phenomenon includes such conditions as mental retardation, cerebral palsy, autism spectrum disorders, hearing loss, and so forth. However, in this chapter, we use the term in a more restricted way to refer to mental retardation in children.

> DD is prevalent in about 1 to 3 percent of the population. The prevalence of DD is slightly higher in boys than in girls.

SLPs need a basic understanding of DD, its causes and correlated conditions, general and language characteristics, and assessment and treatment modifications. We will start with definitions of DD.

Definition of Developmental Disability

There is no universally agreed on definition of DD or mental retardation. Parents and others, however, have no difficulty recognizing DD in their children, especially when the cognitive deficiency is significant. Most parents and teachers recognize DD by its behavioral deficiency, which includes limited intellectual performance. Some may also have congenital physical abnormalities or physical growth deficiencies. Almost all of them will be slower than the normal in learning skills—including language skills.

A frequently cited definition of DD is that of the American Association on Mental Retardation (AAMR, 2005). The association uses the term *mental retardation* in its definition and description of DD; in this chapter we treat the two terms as synonyms, although we recognize that DD may involve other clinical conditions (see Box 12.1 for a discussion of terms). According to AAMR:

> Mental retardation is a disability characterized by significant limitations both in intellectual functioning and in adaptive behavior as expressed in conceptual, social, and practical adaptive skills. The disability originates before the age of 18. (online)

| box 12.1 | | | | Developmental Disability versus Mental Retardation: A Choice of Terms |

We have chosen to refer to that group of children whose primary impairment is cognitive deficiency as *developmentally disabled* rather than *mentally retarded*. We recognize that this is technically at odds with definitions of developmental disability offered by many official organizations. The Administration on Developmental Disabilities, a branch of the U.S. Department of Health and Human Services, for example, defines *developmental disability* as:

a severe, chronic disability of an individual 5 years of age or older that—

(1) is attributable to a mental or physical impairment or combination of mental and physical impairments;
(2) is manifested before the individual attains age 22;
(3) is likely to continue indefinitely;
(4) Results in substantial functional limitations in three or more of the following areas of major life activity— [followed by a list of domains of life skills similar to that set forth by AAMR's definition of mental retardation] (Administration on Developmental Disabilities, U.S. Department of Health and Human Services, 2005, online).

The striking difference here is that, according to this definition a developmental disability manifests before the age of 22, while the narrower definition of mental retardation requires manifestation before the age of 18. Generally speaking, the term *developmental disability* is a broader term encompassing disabilities other than those necessarily marked by cognitive deficiency. There are individuals, for example, with autism, cerebral palsy,

and so forth who can be described as having a developmental disability but do not have any degree of cognitive impairment. Furthermore, many organizations advocating for the rights of people with mental retardation insist on using that term because there is a possibility services might be lost if that continued population was described as developmentally disabled. The nationally based organization Association for Retarded Citizens (ARC), for example, has defended its use of the term *mental retardation*, stating that any change in terminology "would have a direct impact on the availability of supports and services for people with mild mental retardation who do not fit the definition of developmental disabilities" (ARC, 2005, online).

We understand and acknowledge the political realities and heartfelt controversy surrounding terminology used to refer to people with cognitive deficiency. Our decision to use the term *developmental disability* was based on our consultation with many, many families we have served whose overwhelming preference was to refer to their children as having *developmental disability* rather than *mental retardation*. We believe our choice is in keeping with the style of writing recommended by the American Psychological Association (APA), which requires that we be "sensitive to labels" and "call people what they prefer to be called" (APA, 2001, p. 63). Therefore, in this chapter, and throughout the book, the term *developmental disability* is used in place of, but should be regarded as synonymous with, *mental retardation*.

The AAMR definition includes both intellectual limitations as measured by standardized tests of intelligence and behavioral deficits in terms of various skills. Generally, IQ test scores are 70 or below, combined with significant deficiencies in adaptive skills. Various conceptual, social, and practical skills are described as adaptive skills. Conceptual skills include language, reading, and writing skills. Social skills include interpersonal behavior, responsibility, rule following, avoiding victimization, and so forth. Practical skills refer to daily living activities, including eating, dressing, preparation of meals, taking medications, using the telephone, managing money, avoiding danger, and taking care of oneself (AAMR, 2005). This view of DD is clinically useful in that it includes all aspects of behavior and specific skills that need to be supported. The view emphasizes a need to understand various dimensions of a child's life to diagnose DD and to design support programs. The view

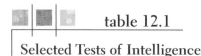

table 12.1

Selected Tests of Intelligence

Test Name	Age Range	Description
Comprehensive Test of Nonverbal Intelligence Hammill, Pearson, & Weiderholt (1997)	7 yrs through adult	Measures nonverbal reasoning skills; appropriate to assess individuals with limited language skills.
Kaufman Assessment Battery for Children, Second Edition Kaufman & Kaufman (2004a)	3 yrs through 18 yrs	Measures cognitive skills, including sequential and simultaneous information processing.
Leiter International Performance Scale— Revised Roid & Miller (2004)	2 yrs through 20 yrs, 11 mos	Appropriate for the deaf and children with cerebral palsy, non-English speaking, and those with low socioeconomic status (SES).
Merrill-Palmer Revised Scales of Development Roid & Sampers (2004)	2 mos through 6 yrs, 6 mos	May be used as a substitute for the Binet Scale.
Slosson Full-Range Intelligence Test Algozzine, Eaves, Mann, & Vance (1993)	5 yrs through 21 yrs	Measures both verbal and nonverbal skills.
Stanford-Binet Intelligence Scale—Fifth Edition Roid (2004)	2 yrs through adult	A verbal and nonverbal test of intelligence and cognitive skills.
Test of Nonverbal Intelligence—Third Edition Brown, Sherbenou, & Johnsen (1997)	6 yrs through adult	Useful in testing children with limited language skills.
Wechsler Preschool and Primary Scale of Intelligence—Third Edition Wechsler (2002)	3 yrs through 7 yrs, 3 mos	A verbal and nonverbal test of intelligence.
Wechsler Intelligence Scale for Children— Fourth Edition Wechsler (2003)	6 yrs through 16 yrs	Provides verbal, performance (nonverbal) and full scale scores.

discourages a diagnosis made solely on the basis of IQ test scores. See Table 12.1 for a brief description of selected tests of intelligence.

Limitations individuals exhibit should always be understood in terms of the social and cultural community to which the individual belongs (AAMR, 2005). The skill levels that are typical of the peers and the culture are important to consider, as a particular deficiency in one culture may not be in another. For instance, in cultures that value oral traditions, lack of reading and writing is not a sign of DD. The AAMR description also points out that children with DD do not exhibit only deficiencies; they also may exhibit particular strengths and that it is essential to understand those strengths as well as limitations.

Another well known definition of DD, or mental retardation, is that of the American Psychiatric Association (APA, 2000). According to APA:

> The essential feature of Mental Retardation is significantly subaverage general intellectual functioning (Criterion A) that is accompanied by significant limitations in adaptive functioning in at least two of the following skill areas: communication, self-care, home living, social/

interpersonal skills, use of community resources, self-direction, functional academic skills, work, leisure, health, and safety (Criterion B). The onset must occur before age 18 years (Criterion C). (p. 41)

The APA definition also stresses the need to evaluate adaptive living skills to make a diagnosis of DD. Consistent with other definitions or descriptions, APA suggests an IQ score of 70 or below, which is approximately 2 standard deviations below the mean. Persons who have IQs of 70 to 75 may still be developmentally disabled if they exhibit significant adaptive skill deficiencies. Conversely, individuals with IQs below 70 may not be developmentally disabled if their adaptive skills are adequate to meet the social and personal demands, suggesting appropriately that the scores on a test of intelligence are less important than how the individual can meet the demands of life. Intelligence testing should take into consideration the child's cultural and linguistic background. In addition, whether the child has sensory (e.g., blindness or deafness) or motor deficits (e.g., paralysis or paresis of hands) that will make it harder for the child to take the test should be considered in administering and interpreting tests of intelligence.

An IQ of 70 is how many standard deviations below the mean?

The criterion that the deficiencies must be evident before age 18, common to both the definitions, rules out the diagnosis of DD in individuals older than 18 whose adaptive skills are disrupted due to such causes as traumatic brain injury, neurological diseases, or psychiatric disorders.

Classification of Developmental Disability

Developmental disability may be classified in different ways. One classification is based on the severity of behavioral deficits, coupled with the different IQ scores. Another classification is based on etiologic factors.

DD is a matter of degree. It is not a disease that is present or absent. It is a behavioral deficiency that varies across children. Therefore, the APA (2000) classifies DD based on its severity, again using their preferred terminology of mental retardation:

- *Mild mental retardation.* About 85 percent of children diagnosed as DD belong to this category. The rough IQ range for this group is 50–55 to 70. Deficiencies of children with mild DD may not be evident until after age 5. They tend to appear nearly normal during their preschool years. They may acquire sixth-grade-level academic skills, may hold a job, and live somewhat independently. They may, however, need more or less consistent supervision and support.
- *Moderate mental retardation.* About 10 percent of children with DD fall into this category. The IQ range for this group is approximately 35–40 to 50–55. These children acquire communication skills during early childhood and benefit from vocational training. They need supervision to take care of themselves. They may be trained in most academic and social skills, although they may achieve no more than a second grade education. They most likely perform unskilled work or semiskilled work under supervision in sheltered workshops.
- *Severe mental retardation.* About 3 to 4 percent of children with DD have severe cognitive deficits. The IQ range for this group is 20–25 to 35–40. Language acquisition in this group is very limited. They may learn basic language skills during their

elementary school years. They may only sight read a few words. They can only perform simple tasks under strict and constant supervision.

- *Profound mental retardation.* About 1 to 2 percent of children with DD have profound cognitive deficits. The IQ range for this group is below 20 or 25. A genetic syndrome or a neurological condition is often associated with profound DD. Language and motor development is severely impaired. The children may have additional sensory deficits (e.g., hearing and vision problems). They usually also have neuromuscular deficits (e.g., paresis and paralysis).

The second classification, based on etiologic factors, recognizes two main categories of DD: (1) genetic/organic and (2) familial (Zigler & Hodapp, 1986). The two classifications are related to severity of behavioral and intellectual deficits, along with other characteristics:

- *DD with genetic/organic basis.* Compared to the familial variety, the more severe forms of behavioral deficits are associated with DD that has a genetic/organic basis. Many children with genetic syndromes and multiple sensory and physical impairments fall into this category. Therefore, these children are more easily identified as developmentally disabled. These children tend to have many health problems. Children whose DD is associated with genetic/organic factors tend to have IQs below 50. This type of DD is found in all segments of society. The siblings of affected children tend to have normal intelligence. Requiring more intensive and extensive assistance throughout their lives, the children in this category have a lower life expectancy than other children or children with familial retardation. People with this kind of DD are unlikely to marry and have children.
- *Familial DD.* As the term suggests, this is DD that is common to members of certain families. Heredity is thought to play an important role. IQs are generally higher than those found in children with genetic/organic DD, and are rarely below 50. Organic pathology, genetic syndromes, and multiple sensory and physical impairments are uncommon or nonexistent. More common in lower socioeconomic levels, parents and siblings of children with familial DD may also have below-normal intelligence. People with familial DD may enjoy relatively normal health, appearance, and mortality rate. They may hold certain simple jobs, and with some support, may lead relatively independent lives. They are likely to marry and have children, some or most of them with below-normal intelligence.

It should be noted that any classification of a disorder is somewhat arbitrary. The mild, moderate, severe, and profound categories are subjective, in spite of the suggested quantitative IQ scores. The distinction between the genetic/organic and familial may be unclear in many cases where mild physical or sensory impairments are associated with what appear to be familial DD. Speech-language pathologists will serve children with DD better if they make a client-specific analysis of the strengths and limitations of each child, instead of categorizing them.

Prevalence of Developmental Disability

It has been difficult to establish the exact prevalence of DD especially because it includes such varied conditions as mental retardation, autism spectrum disorders, and cerebral palsy.

Even if only mental retardation is considered, the prevalence figures vary from 1 to 3 percent of the population. The National Dissemination Center for Children with Disabilities (NICHCY at www.nichcy.org) states that 3 out of every 100 people in the country have mental retardation and that 1 out of every 10 children receiving special education services in public schools have developmental disability in the form of mental retardation. The U.S. Centers for Disease Control, which monitors the prevalence of developmental disabilities and birth defects in the greater Atlanta area, states that the prevalence of mental retardation is 9.7 per 1,000 children of 3–10 years of age (www.cdc.gov/ncbddd/dd/ddsurv.htm). This translates into roughly a 1 percent prevalence of mental retardation in the population.

Differences in prevalence rates reported in different sources may partly be due to the varying degrees of retardation studied, inclusion or exclusion of children who are institutionalized, and inclusion or exclusion of children with other developmental disabilities. For example, Larson et al. (2001) reported a prevalence rate of .78 percent of the population for noninstitutionalized mental retardation; a 1.13 percent for other forms of DD, and a combined prevalence rate of 1.49 percent for mental retardation and other forms of DD.

Developmental disabilities are more common among boys than among girls. DD, especially mental retardation, is more common in older children (ages 6–10 years) than younger (ages 3–5 years). Mild mental retardation is more common than severe retardation.

Causes, Correlations, and Explanations

DD has many causes. Most presumed causes of DD are based on correlation; that is, certain events precede the diagnosis or observation of DD in children. Whether those events are actually the causes or merely coincidental events is open to debate. In many cases, it is not possible to ascertain causes with any degree of certainty. The APA (2000) states that, in approximately 30–40 percent of individuals with DD, no clear etiology can be determined.

> Why is correlation not sufficient evidence of causation?

Nonetheless, it is important to understand potential causes and investigate their possible influence during assessment. Scientifically, it is more appropriate to discuss factors associated with DD rather than its causes.

There are a variety of potential causative (etiological) factors associated with DD. A factor may influence the degree of DD alone, but usually in combination with other factors. Therefore, in many cases, DD in a child is multiply caused. Even in the case of heredity as a factor, an interaction between genetic and environmental factors may determine the final outcome for the child.

Genetic Factors

The precise extent to which genetic factors, whether inherited or not, are responsible for DD is not clear. The estimates have a wide and imprecise range: 25 to 50 percent of cases may be due to genetic factors (Inlow & Restifo, 2004; Leonard & Wen, 2002; McLaren & Bryson, 1987). It should be noted that not all genetic conditions are inherited. The reason for this variability in estimating the influence of genetic factors is that DD is a characteristic of hundreds of genetic syndromes, some of them newly discovered. In their review of molecular genetic research, Inlow and Restifo (2004) concluded that by the year 2002, some

282 genes were recognized to be associated with an expression of DD, and hundreds more remain to be identified. The reviewers noted that 1–2 new DD genes are discovered every month (Inlow & Restifo, 2004). See Box 12.2 for a primer on chromosomal abnormalities that affect the function of genes, and consequently, cause DD and other genetic disorders.

Many genetic syndromes associated with DD also are associated with significant speech and language impairments. These syndromes, some more common than the others, include:

- *Down syndrome*. A common syndrome of DD, **Down syndrome** is due to a chromosomal defect. People with Down syndrome are born with an extra chromosome—47 instead of the typical 46. It is also called trisomy 21 because the extra chromosome is the third copy of chromosome 21. It is this small extra chromosome that is associated with the expression of the syndrome. The syndrome appears in 1 in every 800 live births.

 Down syndrome is associated with a higher risk of Alzheimer's disease later in life.

Maternal age is related to its incidence; older women, more than younger women, have a greater chance of giving birth to a child with Down syndrome. The characteristics of the syndrome include reduced muscle tone (hypotonia); flat facial profile; small ears, nose, and chin; short front-to-back head dimension (brachycephaly); shortened oral and pharyngeal structures; undergrowth of the mid face; narrow and high-arched palate; relatively large, fissured-tongue that tends to protrude; short neck with excess skin at the back; short

---

box 12.2 | **A Primer on Chromosomal Abnormalities That Lead to Genetic Syndromes**

- There are 23 pairs of chromosomes in each human body cell; they vary in size and are numbered 1 through 23. This includes two sex chromosomes: XX in females and XY in males.
- Chromosomes contain genes, which are made up of coded proteins that serve as the blue print of organisms.
- A small point of constriction on each chromosome (called a centromere) divides it into two sections, often called arms. One arm or section of the chromosome is smaller, and is called *p* for petite. The other, longer arm is called *q*.
- A chromosomal abnormality may be found in a particular numbered strand or section.
- Chromosomal abnormalities are various deformities including:

  - *Translocation*, in which a broken piece of one chromosome is attached to another.
  - *Ring construction*, in which the two ends of a chromosome join to form a ring.
  - *Deletion*, which is a general term for missing parts of a chromosome; in cri-du-chat syndrome,

a part of the short arm of chromosome 5 is deleted (5p-).
- *Duplication*, in which a portion of a chromosome or a whole chromosome is repeated; in Down syndrome, a whole extra chromosome 21 is found, resulting in 3 copies of it (hence the name, trisomy 21; *trisomy* means 3 bodies).
- *Inversion*, in which a broken section of an arm flips or inverts before it gets reattached.
- *Mosaicism*, in which cells within the whole body contain different number of chromosomes; normally, all cells in a human body will have the same chromosome number; in some individuals with Down syndrome, for example, trisomy may be found in 60 percent of the skin cells and only 5 percent of the blood cells.
- Partial loss of a chromosome results in survivable genetic syndromes, whereas a total loss of a chromosome is typically fatal. Similarly, 3 copies (instead of 2) of each chromosome is fatal.

fingers; and epicanthal folds. DD is typically mild to moderate, and speech, language, and hearing problems are common. A few individuals with Down syndrome may exhibit normal or even exceptional language skills (Rondal, 1998).

- *Fetal alcohol syndrome (FAS).* A congenital syndrome (noticed at birth, but not inherited), **fetal alcohol syndrome (FAS)** is caused by maternal alcohol abuse during pregnancy. The syndrome is completely preventable if women abstain from drinking alcoholic beverages during pregnancy. Prenatal and postnatal growth is affected because of the prenatal exposure to alcohol. According to the Centers for Disease Control and Prevention (CDC), FAS is found in 0.2 to 1.5 per 1,000 live births. The incidence of FAS is higher in American Indian/Alaskan Native populations (3 per 1,000 live births). Estimates of alcohol-related neurodevelopmental disorders and birth defects (not classified as FAS) are three times higher. More than 50 percent of women in their childbearing age drink; more than 50 percent of all pregnancies are unplanned; one in 30 pregnant women drink to an extent that exposes their fetus to the damaging effects of alcohol (CDC, 2004a). DD and physical growth deficiencies are common in children born with this syndrome. Physical symptoms include general physical growth deficiency, microcephaly (small head), small eye opening, maxillary hypoplasia (underdevelopment of the upper jaw), prominent forehead and mandible (lower jaw), short palpebral (eyelid) fissure, thin upper lip, epicanthal folds, cleft palate in some cases, heart anomalies, poor motor coordination, and kidney disorders. Such behavior disorders as hyperactivity, problems with daily living, delinquent or criminal behavior, inappropriate sexual behavior, problems with parenting, and poor judgment and reasoning skills are typical. Children born with FAS later tend to abuse drugs and alcohol. Speech and language disorders are common.

> Fetal exposure of 1 or 2 ounces of alcohol per day produces some negative effects of the fetal growth; more than 2 ounces a day will produce pronounced effects.

- *Fragile X syndrome (FXS).* A single-gene mutation on the X chromosome causes **fragile X syndrome (FXS).** The gene responsible for this condition is called the FMR1 (fragile X DD 1); abnormalities in this gene cause a failure to produce a protein thought to be necessary for brain function. The incidence of FXS is 1 in 2,000 male births; a smaller number of females are affected. More females (1 in 250) than males (1 in 700) carry the disorder. Generally, X-linked disorders do not affect females, but FXS is found in them. DD is more severe in affected males than in affected females (Shprintzen, 2000). Children with FXS, especially the males, have speech and language impairments, which include articulation disorders, sound repetitions, echolalia, jargon, telegraphic speech, missing morphologic features, unintelligible self-talk, and limited language production in social contexts. A notable language feature of the syndrome is perseveration on a word, phrase, or topic of conversation. Some children with FXS may show a marked weakness in their use of gestures (Roberts et al., 2002). Otitis media and conductive hearing loss may be found in some children (Abbeduto & Hagerman, 1998). Some children with FXS may talk like autistic children with tangential or irrelevant comments (Sudhalter & Belser, 2001). Physical characteristics may not be apparent in early childhood years. As the child grows, such characteristics as an elongated head, arched palate, large ears and hands, and flat feet tend to emerge.

> Deletion of the maternal chromosome 15 or receiving two copies of the same but both from the father causes a genetically different syndrome called Angelman syndrome. Different genetic syndromes that result from paternal or maternal gene abnormality are due to a genetic process called imprinting. PWS is the first known imprinting genetic disorder; children with Angelman syndrome develop no speech or language.

- *Prader-Willi syndrome (PWS).* Another genetic syndrome, **Prader-Willi syndrome (PWS)** is caused by a deletion of paternal chromosome 15 in the q11-q13 region or when the child receives two copies of chromosome 15 from the mother, and none from the father. Up to 70 percent of PWS cases have the deletion of paternal chromosome 15. One in 10,000 to 15,000 individuals have PWS; it affects males and females equally often (Cassidy, 1997; Lewis et al., 2002). Infants with PWS have feeding problems and hypotonia (reduced muscle tone). As children, they have voracious appetite and are obese. These children may exhibit temper tantrums, stubbornness, depression, compulsive behaviors, and inadequate social relationships. They may have a narrow palatal arch and a small lower jaw (micrognathia). Children with PWS have articulation disorders as well as hypo- or hypernasality. Their language disorders include below average mean length of utterances (MLU) with shorter phrases and sentences, limited vocabulary, and significant impairments in narrative and conversational skills. Language skills in children with PWS improve as they grow older, but may still remain impaired (Lewis et al., 2002).

- *Cri-du-chat syndrome.* Cri-du-chat means *cat cry* in French. Babies born with this **cri-du-chat syndrome** cry with a high-pitched voice that resembles the mewing of a cat. This is a rare syndrome with an estimated incidence of 1 in 20,000 to 1 in 50,000 births. The syndrome accounts for about 1 percent of all DD. The genetic basis of the syndrome is the deletion of a small portion of the short arm of chromosome 5. Therefore, the syndrome is also know as 5p– syndrome (5p minus). Besides the high-pitched cry, the syndrome is characterized by low birth weight, slow physical growth and motor development, small head (microcephaly), widely set eyes (hypertelerosim), cleft palate or cleft lip and palate, low-set ears that may also be malformed, partial webbing or fusing of fingers or toes, and low muscle tone. Behavioral disorders found in these children include self-injurious behaviors, repetitive movements, hypersensitivity to sound, and obsessive attachment to objects (Cornish & Pigram, 1996). Speech development is severely impaired in many children with cri-du-chat syndrome. Similarly, language skills are extremely limited although they may communicate their basic needs (Cornish & Munir, 1998; Cornish & Pigram, 1996). Conductive hearing loss associated with middle ear infections are common in these children.

- *Williams syndrome.* This is a rare syndrome of special interest to speech-language pathologists because some early research suggested that **Williams syndrome** is characterized by both DD and relatively intact language skills (Thal, Bates, & Bellugi, 1989). Based on this early observation, it was argued that language is an independent module that may be innately given in spite of severe intellectual deficits. Subsequent research has generally contradicted this characterization of the syndrome and the theory of language based on it, indicating that the language skills of children with Williams syndrome are comparable to their cognitive skills; that is, they do not have surprisingly better language skills than their intellectual levels (Karmiloff-Smith et al., 2003; Reilly et al., 2004; Stojanovik, Perkins, & Howard, 2001). In addition to DD, low birth weight, slow physical and behavioral development, learning disabilities, attention deficit, visuospatial deficits, irritability during infancy, various kinds of phobias, and speech-language disorders characterize the syndrome (Mervis, 2003; Vicari et al., 2002). Heart and blood vessel problems, dental and kidney abnormalities also are parts of the syndrome. A remarkable characteristic of the children with this syndrome is their hypersociability; they compulsively greet people, approach strangers, and strike conversations (Doyle et al., 2004). The disorder is traced to a deleted genetic material on chromosome 7 (specifically, 7q11.23).

Many other syndromes include DD and communication deficits. Speech-language pathologists need to consult other sources on DD and genetic syndromes (Baroff, 1999; Shprintzen, 2000).

Prenatal Factors

Prenatal factors associated with DD are adverse conditions a pregnant woman experiences. Such conditions may affect the growing of the fetus and cause brain deficiencies, leading to DD in the child. These factors include:

- *Rubella (German measles)*. Although this is no longer a frequent prenatal cause of DD, it is a potent factor. A single maternal infection, especially during the first 10 weeks of pregnancy, may cause fetal damage. Besides DD, the child may have hearing and visual impairments, and speech and language disorders commonly are present.
- *Maternal lead poisoning*. Inhalation of lead fumes by a pregnant woman can damage the fetus's brain. According to a report by the Centers for Disease Control and Prevention (CDC; 2004b), approximately 434,000 children aged 1–5 years have blood levels that exceed the recommended 10 micrograms of lead per deciliter of blood (CDC, 2004b). Because lead poisoning may not produce early symptoms, the problem often is unrecognized. Depending on its severity, lead poisoning can cause learning disabilities (including language disorders), behavioral problems, seizures, coma, and death. Lead-based paint and lead-contaminated dust within and surrounding old and deteriorating buildings are the two main sources of lead exposure. Although lead-based paint is no longer used, some 24 million housing units in the United States are known to be lead-contaminated (CDC, 2004b). Producing stained-glass windows, producing or recycling automobile batteries, and drinking water contaminated with lead are other sources of lead poisoning.
- *Maternal mercury poisoning*. When a pregnant woman inhales mercury fumes, the fetal brain may be damaged. Poor physical and mental development is typical of prenatal mercury poisoning. Many kinds of industries use mercury and expose their workers to potential mercury poisoning. For example, mercury is used in the production of alkaline batteries, electrical switches, lights, and medical equipment (e.g., thermometers, blood pressure measurement instruments). Various mining and chemical industries along with manufacturers of chlorine and caustic soda use mercury. Extraction of gold from ore needs mercury. People may be exposed to mercury when it is mishandled or spilled from devices used in the home or workplace. Other sources of mercury poisoning include eating food (e.g., fish) or water contaminated with it. Although reliable incidence of prenatal exposure of mercury poisoning is not available, a CDC report cites incidents in which hundreds of children were exposed to mercury fumes (Agency for Toxic Substances and Disease Registry, 2004).
- *Maternal anoxia*. Anoxia is lack of oxygen or significantly reduced supply of oxygen. Anemia and vascular diseases during pregnancy lead to fetal anoxia, which can cause fetal growth deficiencies, including potential fetal brain damage.

Prematurity is birth before the end of the 37th week of pregnancy. Low birth weight is less than 5 pounds and 8 ounces (2,500 grams). Very low birth weight is less than 3 pounds and 5 ounces (1,500 grams).

- *Prenatal trauma.* Various kinds of accidents a pregnant woman suffers may lead to fetal brain injury. Automobile accidents, especially during the later stages of pregnancy, are known to cause fetal brain injury.
- *X-ray and radiation.* Excessive exposure to radiation during pregnancy can adversely affect the fetal growth and damage the nervous system, including the brain.
- *Prematurity and low birth weight.* Children born prematurely and with low birth weight have a greater risk for DD and other physical impairments, including cerebral palsy. Prematurely born children generally tend to have low birth weights. More than 60 percent of low-birth weight babies are born prematurely. Some full-term babies may also have low birth weight; such babies are called small for gestational age or growth-restricted. In both the cases, prenatal factors restrict the growth of the fetus and have adverse effects on brain development. Annually, low birth weight affects about 1 in every 13 babies born in the United States and causes 65 percent of infant deaths.
- *Maternal drug abuse and alcoholism.* Maternal drug abuse may affect fetal growth. As noted earlier, maternal alcohol abuse may cause fetal alcohol syndrome (FAS).

Natal Factors

Factors that adversely affect the delivery of a child are called natal factors. These factors injure the child in the process of birth. Factors that affect the central nervous system are more likely to cause DD and include the following:

- *Fetal anoxia.* **Fetal anoxia** occurs when the brain of the newborn may be damaged because of reduced supply of oxygen when the labor is prolonged or the baby fails to cry (and breathe) soon after birth.
- *Other kinds of brain injury during delivery.* Several other factors may cause problems during delivery and lead to potential brain injury. For instance, an improper application of forceps, birth canal compression of the head, and malpositions of the baby may all cause brain injury.

Postnatal Factors

Factors that negatively affect the growth of the child, especially those that affect the growth of the brain, are **postnatal factors.** Technically, anything that affects the brain function after the child is born is a postnatal factor. However, postnatal factors are typically described as those that cause brain injury and growth deficiencies during the early childhood days. Some of the prenatal factors that affect fetal growth also may act as postnatal factors. Any kind of poisoning (e.g., mercury) or toxicity is an example. The postnatal factors include:

- *Post-immunization encephalitis.* Some children react negatively when they receive DPT (diphtheria, pertussis or whooping cough, and tetanus or lockjaw) immunization shots. The child may have high fever, convulsions, and coma. A slow recovery may be followed by sluggish responses and DD.
- *Rabies vaccine.* This vaccine may cause motor paralysis and brain damage, leading to DD.

- *Lead poisoning.* We noted earlier that lead poisoning in pregnant woman can damage the fetal brain. Similarly, a child may also come in contact with lead and experience central nervous system damage.
- *Mercury poisoning.* Another prenatal toxic factor may also be a postnatal factor when children come in contact with mercury fumes.

Traumatic Brain Injury

Traumatic brain injury (TBI) is an acquired injury to the brain, caused by external force or trauma. TBI is a fairly common cause of DD in children. Annually, some 200 to 250 per 100,000 children suffer TBI. Various factors, including automobile accidents, falls, domestic violence, child abuse, sport-related accidents, and pedestrian injuries may cause TBI. TBI does not include brain injury caused by prenatal and natal factors or diseases (e.g., tumors or strokes).

Chapter 14 includes a section on traumatic brain injury and its consequences. As noted in that chapter, cognitive impairments may be a permanent consequence in some children. In addition to speech and language disorders, children with traumatic brain injury are likely to exhibit a variety of behavior disorders (e.g., attention deficits, impulsive behavior, aggressive acts, and socially inappropriate behaviors).

Endocrine and Metabolic Disorders

Several endocrine and metabolic disorders are associated with DD. The most notable of the endocrine disorders associated with DD is **hypothyroidism** (thyroid deficiency). This hormone deficiency may begin prenatally or postnatally. If untreated in early childhood, hypothyroidism leads to DD. Hypothyroidism is often due to an autoimmune reaction that produces antibodies against the thyroid gland and thus limits the production of thyroxin (the hormone produced by the thyroid). The symptoms of hypothyroidism in children include jaundice (yellowing of the skin, eyes, and mucous membranes), hoarse cry, reduced appetite, umbilical hernia (a protruding navel), constipation, and slow bone growth.

> The *endocrine* is a system of glands and structures that secrete hormones and release them into the bloodstream. These hormones regulate growth and metabolism.

Major metabolic disorders associated with DD include phenylketonuria (PKU) and lipid metabolic errors. Occurring once in 10,000 births, **phenylketonuria** is a deficiency in metabolizing an amino acid called phenylalanine. A concentration of this acid is toxic to the body and causes nerve and brain damage. An absence of a liver enzyme is the cause of this metabolic disorder. Because the condition is effectively treated in early infancy, most states require a testing for PKU on all newborn babies. Consequently, PKU is not a common cause of DD in the United States, although it may be in some parts of the world.

Lipid metabolic disorders cause an accumulation of fat in neural tissue, leading to developmental disability and health problems. A well known lipid metabolic disorder is Tay-Sachs disease, a fatal and inherited genetic disorder in which excessive amounts of a fatty substance called ganglioside GM2 accumulates in the brain and the nervous system. Blindness, deafness, swallowing disorders, and severe DD follow. Speech and language acquisition is impaired. The disease is frequently found in descendants of Central and Eastern European Jews.

Cranial Abnormalities

Abnormalities in the formation of the skull and the brain are a well known cause of DD. Such abnormalities have several prenatal causes including maternal drug abuse, X-ray and radiation, vitamin deficiencies, and exposure to toxic agents. Genetic factors that may cause cranial abnormalities include chromosomal defects. Cranial abnormalities are a part of various genetic syndromes that are associated with DD and physical anomalies and disabilities. Some cranial abnormalities are incompatible with life while others are survivable:

- *Anencephaly.* A birth defect, **anencephaly** is the absence of the cranial bones and often the cranial skin. Due to various factors, the cranial structure fails to fuse during the embryonic period. With exposed brain and missing sense organs, this condition is incompatible with life. In the United States, some 1,000 to 2,000 babies are born with this cranial abnormality every year.
- *Macrocephaly.* Increased head circumference is called **macrocephaly.** A larger than the typical head size may run in certain families with no clinical implications. Clinically increased head circumference may be due to a variety of factors including hydrocephalus, but the prevalence of other causes distinguishes macrocephaly from hydrocephaly. For instance, certain rare brain diseases, including Alexander's disease and Canavan's disease, cause macrocephaly. These two diseases belong to a category called leukodystrophy which involves degeneration of the white matter of the brain, associated with the loss of fatty covering of the brain (demyelination) and formation of abnormal fibers in glia, the cells that support brain tissue. Mental and physical growth is retarded in children who have leukodystrophy. Speech and language acquisition is impaired.
- *Microcephaly.* A small head circumference in relation to the rest of the body is **microcephaly.** A child may be born with a small head or with a normal-size head that fails to grow in proportion to the rest of the physical growth. Syndromes associated with chromosomal abnormalities are often the cause of microcephaly. Delayed or impaired motor development, DD, hyperactivity, convulsions, and speech and language problems are common consequences of microcephaly.
- *Hydrocephaly.* As in macrocephaly, the head is enlarged in **hydrocephaly,** but this occurs for different causes. One of the most common cranial abnormalities (occurring in 1 out of 10,000 persons), hydrocephalus is an accumulation of cerebrospinal fluid (CSF) in the ventricles (channels or cavities) of the brain, leading to its enlargement and swelling. CSF is produced in various ventricles by a tissue mass called choroid plexus. The normally circulating fluid cushions the brain, provides some nutrients, and helps remove waste products. The fluid may accumulate because of lack of good circulation or excessive production. Congenital defects of the skull, brain tumors, and infections of the brain, among others, may block the fluid circulation. This fluid accumulation increases intracranial pressure; the brain is forced against the skull, causing tissue damage. The head expands if the condition develops before the different bones of the skull have fused; this fusion occurs around age 5. The child's growth is slowed and signs of DD appear. Lethargy, irritability, vision changes, loss of coordination, vomiting, headache, and other physical symptoms develop. Surgical intervention to improve CSF circulation is the main treatment, although drug treatment to control

the formation of the CSF is also available. Depending on the extent of brain tissue damage, the degree of DD will vary across children.

Speech and Language Skills

Speech and language skills of children with DD vary within a broad range; individual differences in language skills are significant. It is generally difficult to predict how language skills will develop in a given child (Brady et al., 2004), and making such predictions in the case of children with mild forms of DD is especially problematic. Communication skills of these children depend on the extent of DD, the presence of other deficits (e.g., hearing loss and motor deficits), effectiveness of rehabilitation services offered and the time at which they were initiated, and family support. Some children may only have a mild deficiency in their communication skills while others may have a profound deficiency, needing nonverbal means of communication.

In the past, experts debated whether children with DD are simply slow to learn their language but learn it in the normal sequence, or whether they follow an unusual, zigzag, abnormal sequence of language acquisition. Some experts had claimed that children with DD exhibit language patterns not seen in children developing normally, suggesting an abnormal pattern of language acquisition. Most investigators, believing that children with DD acquire language in the normal sequence but at a slower rate, disagree with this suggestion. Nonetheless, suggestion of an abnormal pattern in developmentally disabled children has not been completely discounted because children with Down syndrome may have better lexical skills than syntactic skills (Stoel-Gammon, 1990). Such uneven development of language skills is thought to suggest a pattern of language development that is qualitatively different from the typical pattern of language acquisition.

All aspects of speech and language may be affected in a child with DD. We will summarize the most common speech and language characteristics of children with DD, although our main concern is language disorders and their treatment.

Phonological Skills

Children with DD have difficulty learning to produce the speech sounds of their language. Consequently, disorders of articulation are common among these children. Up to 70 percent of children with DD may have speech disorders (Fristoe & Lloyd, 1979). The severity of articulation disorders depends on the degree of cognitive impairment and associated clinical conditions. The more severe the cognitive impairment is, the greater the problems of articulation. Children whose DD is a part of a genetic syndrome and orofacial anomalies (e.g., cleft palate) tend to have more significant articulation disorders than those whose DD is not associated with other complicating conditions. Hearing loss found in many children with DD also is a factor contributing to the severity of speech disorders.

Generally, children with DD exhibit speech disorders that are similar to those of other children with no cognitive impairment. Patterns of phonological processes found in persons with DD are similar to those found in others without cognitive impairment (Shriberg & Widder, 1990). Deletion of consonants, distortions of sounds, substitution of one sound for another are all found in children with and without DD; among these, deletion of consonants may be more prevalent than other kinds of articulation errors in children with DD. Generally, both phonological processes and individual sound errors tend to be more frequent and more severe in children with greater degrees of cognitive impairment (Bleile & Schwarz, 1984; Klink et al., 1986; Moran, Money, & Leonard, 1984; Shriberg & Widder, 1990).

Language Skills

In comparing the language skills of children with and without developmental disability, one can use either the children's chronological age (CA) or mental age (MA) based on IQ test scores. Significant differences between the groups emerge only when the two groups are matched on CA, but not when matched on MA. When matched on MA, the children with developmental disability will be older than those without.

As noted earlier, the rate at which children with DD learn language is slower, but they do not exhibit a markedly different pattern of acquisition. That children with DD are slow in the acquisition of language does not mean that they eventually catch up with their typical peers. The language skills of those with mild cognitive impairment who receive early and effective speech and language training along with consistent special education services in the school may develop language skills that approximate the typical. Those with severe DD, in spite of best speech, language, and special educational programs offered to them, may still retain certain language limitations. Nonetheless, speech and language services offered to children with DD are beneficial; language skills of children who receive effective treatment improve.

Like the speech disorders, the language disorders found in children with DD are similar to those found in children without cognitive impairment. Language skills of children with specific genetic syndromes, especially those with Down syndrome, have received much research attention (Eadie et al., 2002; Laws & Bishop, 2003; Miles & Chapman, 2002). Therefore, much of what we know about the language disorders of children with DD is specific to Down syndrome; research, however, is expanding into other genetic syndromes associated with DD (Abbeduto & Hagerman, 1998; Clahsen & Almazan, 1998; Cornish & Munir, 1998; Laws & Bishop, 2004; Lewis et al., 2002; Phillips et al., 2004; Uchino et al., 2001; Zapella, Gillberg, & Ehlers, 1998).

Comprehension of Spoken Language

Difficulty understanding spoken language (comprehension) is one of the characteristics of language impairment in general. However, the relationship between comprehension and production of language is complex. In some respects, there may not be a one-to-one relationship between the two. Generally speaking, especially with typically developing children, comprehension of certain language elements may be slightly ahead of production. That is, children may understand spoken sounds, words, phrases, or sentences that they have not mastered to produce yet. Simultaneously, though, children also may produce words and phrases whose meanings they do not understand (Hulit & Howard, 2002; McLaughlin, 1998).

In their comprehension of spoken language, children with DD are not drastically different from their typical peers. They also may comprehend some elements of speech and language before they gain full understanding of them and produce other elements without a full understanding. Generally, though, children who have DD can be expected to have difficulty comprehending complex and abstract words, complex and longer syntactic structures, and discussion of abstract concepts. Children with Down syndrome are known to have greater difficulty in understanding syntactic structures than individual words (Chapman, Schwartz,

& Kay-Raining Bird, 1991). Serious impairment in language production is likely to have negative effects on comprehension. Although better comprehension than production has been noted in children with Down syndrome (Stoel-Gammon, 1990), it is unlikely that children with DD will have comprehension skills that match the skills of their typical peers (Fowler, 1990; Laws & Bishop, 2003; Mahoney, Glover, & Finger, 1981; Miller, 1988, 1999).

Semantic Skills

Semantic skills refer to production and comprehension of words belonging to varied classes. Compared to their peers, children with DD generally have a limited vocabulary. Children with Down syndrome, for example, are known to have a vocabulary that lacks variety; although they continue to learn new words, they do so at a slower pace and learn fewer words than their typical peers (Miller, 1992). In essence, children with cognitive impairment produce and understand fewer words, shorter words, less complex words, and concrete words. They tend to talk about concrete events and objects. Children with cognitive impairment also have difficulty understanding or producing abstract statements, such as proverbs (Ezell & Goldstein, 1991).

Proverbs are an example of what kind of language?

As with other language skills and concepts, children with DD seem to learn semantic skills in the same sequence as do typical children (Kamhi & Johnston, 1982; Rosenberg, 1982). These and other semantic limitations found in children with DD are comparable to those found in children without DD (e.g., children with specific language impairment; see Chapter 3 for details). Similar to children with specific language impairment, children with DD (especially those with Down syndrome) also may show better vocabulary skills than morphological and syntactic skills (Laws & Bishop, 2003).

Morphological and Syntactic Skills

Morphological skills are generally poor in children with DD, although most studies have sampled only children with Down syndrome (Eadie et al., 2002; Chapman et al., 1998; Laws & Bishop, 2003; Rutter & Buckley, 1994). As noted, morphologic skills of children with DD may be poorer than their vocabulary. Morphologic skills of children with DD are roughly comparable to those of children with specific language impairment, described in Chapter 3. Generally, most children with DD, and especially those with Down syndrome may have difficulty producing various grammatic morphemes, including:

- Regular plural inflections
- Irregular plurals, although this may be less impaired than regular plural inflections
- Present progressive -*ing*
- Possessive morphemes
- Regular past tense inflections
- Irregular past tense words; although this may be less impaired than regular past tense inflections
- Third person singular
- Copula and auxiliary
- Prepositions
- Pronouns

The irregular forms of plural (e.g., *women, men*) and past tense (e.g., *went, spent*) are learned as whole words, as against the regular plurals (e.g., *cups, bags*) and regular past tense (e.g., *moved, painted*). This differential difficulty may be due to the children's greater difficulty in learning smaller morphologic components than whole words. Some difficulty in acquiring smaller inflectional morphologic features that are not stressed in adult speech may be due to a mild hearing loss found in a number of children with cognitive impairment, especially those with Down syndrome (Laws & Bishop, 2003).

Syntactic skills of children with DD also are below those of typical children. We noted earlier than children with cognitive impairment may have relatively better vocabulary than morphologic and syntactic skills. In essence, then, the greatest degree of difficulty is to be found in morphologic and syntactic skills. Children with DD tend to comprehend and produce relatively simpler sentences and have difficulty comprehending or producing more complex, compound, and less frequently used syntactic forms. Children with DD also have difficulty imitating longer or more complex sentences modeled for them (Eadie et al., 2002).

Children with DD may find it especially difficult to learn certain syntactic structures. For instance, they may learn to use the conjunction *and* relatively easily, but may find it difficult to correctly use *because* in conversational speech; they may overuse *and* (Kamhi & Johnston, 1982). Children with DD may ask fewer questions or may substitute *what* questions for all other kinds of questions (e.g., *where, when*).

Pragmatic Skills

Research on pragmatic language skills has included different types of cognitive impairment, but has been mostly concerned with children with Down syndrome. Whether children with different kinds of DD have differential pragmatic language skills or deficits is not clear. Nonetheless, it seems evident that children with moderate to severe DD have significant deficits in social communication and conversational speech skills. Once again, the pragmatic deficits of children with DD are roughly comparable to those found in children with no cognitive impairment.

The following kinds of social communication and conversational speech deficits have been documented:

- *Poor narrative skills.* Children with DD, especially those with moderate to severe cognitive impairment, may be relatively poor narrators of events, experiences, and stories. Children with Prader-Willi syndrome, for example, may be unable to retell a story or answer questions about the story; if they can retell a story, they may make significant errors (Lewis et al., 2002; Reilly et al., 2004). This deficiency is comparable to those found in children with specific language impairment. If story retelling requires immediate memory for what is told (short-term auditory memory), children with Down syndrome may have particular difficulty recalling what was told, even when such children are matched for MA with typical children (Kay-Raining Bird & Chapman, 1994). Miles and Chapman (2002) reported that children with Down syndrome who are matched on mental age, syntax comprehension, and mean length of utterance (MLU) may have narrative skills that are comparable to those found in typical children. This finding underscores the observation that whether differences emerge between the groups of children with and without DD depends on how they are matched. Obviously, if they are matched on language measures, there may not be any significant difference. But if they are matched on chronological age, differences in favor of the typical children usually emerge. In essence, children with Down syndrome may exhibit appropriate conversational skills but only at higher age levels (with greater life experiences) than those without cognitive impairment (Miles & Chapman, 2002).

- *Limited initiation of social exchanges.* Children with significant degrees of DD may be unwilling or unable to initiate conversation or any form of social exchange. These children may respond when spoken to, but often are reluctant to talk first. We noted earlier that children with Williams syndrome are an exception to this general observation; they almost compulsively greet strangers and start social exchanges (Doyle et al., 2004).

- *Inadequate topic maintenance.* Children with DD are less likely to abruptly introduce new topics. This may suggest good topic maintenance skills. However, their apparently good topic maintenance skill may partly be due to their difficulty in initiating new topics for conversation. In any case, their participation in conversation on the selected topic may be passive. They may continue to agree with their conversational partners by saying "Yeah" or "OK," while adding little of their own commentary (Abbeduto, 1991). In essence, children with DD help maintain a topic initiated (perhaps by someone else) but do not extend the topic by offering new information. In essence, these children do not play an active role in maintaining topics of conversation.

- *Potential difficulties in conversational turn-taking.* Conversational turn-taking is one of the better pragmatic language skills in children with DD, especially when the children talk with their mothers (Davis, Stroud, & Green, 1988; Tannock, 1988). However, whether children with DD also show appropriate turn-taking skills when interacting with strangers is not clear. Once again, the severity of DD may influence this skill; the more severe the level of cognitive impairment, the more children who interact with strangers may be expected to show difficulties in turn-taking.

- *Limited conversational repair skills.* These skills include appropriate responses when listeners fail to understand what is said and requesting clarification when one does not understand another speaker. Children with DD do exhibit a certain number of conversational repair skills. They are generally sensitive to listeners who do not understand them and do something to promote listener understanding. Even adults with severe to profound DD exhibit some conversational repair skills (Brady et al., 1995). Children with DD, too, try to modify their productions when listeners fail to understand them (Scudder & Tremain, 1992). Nonetheless, there is evidence to suggest that the repair skills are not independent of the degree of DD, and the quality and frequency of repair strategies may be less than what are found in individuals without DD. Children with greater degrees of cognitive impairment may repair less often than those with lesser degrees of cognitive impairment; most children may not repair often enough; some children may simply repeat what they said, instead of revising it or expanding it; children in community settings may attempt to repair their productions more often than those who live in institutions (see Brinton & Fujuki, 1991; Levy, Tennenbaum, & Onroy, 2003; and Brady et al., 1995 for a review of studies). Even children with Williams syndrome—who may have better language skills than children with other kinds of DD—also show pragmatic and social language problems (Laws & Bishop, 2004).

The research just summarized gives a broad picture of language skills of children with DD, although additional research is needed to obtain clarification on certain language skill levels found in such children. For instance, it is not clear whether children with DD do or do not have significant problems in topic maintenance or conversational repair strategies. Differences reported across studies are largely due to the differences in subject characteristics and the depth of the skills measured. The degree of cognitive impairment is an obvious factor. The claim that children with DD have acceptable conversational repair strategies could be potentially valid only with children whose cognitive impairment is not serious enough to severely limit expressive language. The claim that children with DD can exhibit conversational repair strategies may mean that they know when the listeners fail to understand them, may repeat what they just said, but may not always exhibit effective repair skills with sufficient frequency. Further research is therefore needed to examine the *quality* of the repair skills of children with DD.

Assessment and Treatment Modifications

Speech-language pathologists working with children who have DD are likely to be members of multidisciplinary teams. A team of professionals offer assessment and intervention services to children who have a congenital condition, such as Down syndrome. Children who are suspected of having DD later on are typically assessed by a multidisciplinary team who will recommend intervention if DD is diagnosed. In both cases, SLPs will be working collaboratively with special education specialists, psychologists, physical therapists, occupational therapists, adaptive physical education specialists, social workers, and others to provide a program of intensive early intervention designed to maximize the child's potential.

When assessing and treating children with DD, SLPs should keep in perspective the wide range of variability they are likely to encounter in the children's speech and language skills. Generally, speech and language skills will develop more typically and to a greater extent in children with mild degrees of DD. Children who have greater degrees of DD will exhibit greater difficulties with acquisition of speech and language, particularly if early intervention has not been offered. Even among people with severe DD, however, a "wide diversity of communication abilities" has been reported (McLean et al., 1999, p. 237). Such diversity is evident not only in language skills, but also in other social and motor skills of children with DD. As can be expected, the time at which intervention began, the quality and intensity of intervention, and the family involvement in the teaching program can make a significant difference in the skill level of a child with DD.

In any case, intensive treatment may make a profound difference in the lives of children with DD. Some modifications in assessment and treatment procedures may need to be made in consideration of the degree of cognitive impairment particular children have. The following sections will describe those necessary adjustments.

Modifications in Assessment Procedures

Although speech and language characteristics that are likely to be found in children with DD have been described in detail, clinicians should not assume that every child with DD will have all, or even most, of those characteristics. Also, clinicians should not rely overly much on lists of language characteristics commonly seen in children with DD to conduct their assessment of an individual child. Instead, as with any other child, clinicians should approach assessment of children with DD in a child- and family-specific manner. Clinicians who wish to administer standardized tests may do so, but it has been our experience that, even more so than other children, children with DD often perform less well on standardized testing than they do in conversational speech exhibited in natural settings.

> Sometimes children with DD are described as being "untestable" because administration of standardized testing to them is difficult. An SLP who uses child-specific measures of assessment, however, can describe the communicative skills of *any* child.

The assessment procedures outlined in Chapter 4 are generally applicable to children with DD. The following are some modifications that may be necessary to accommodate whatever the degree of cognitive impairment the particular child being assessed may have.

Observation and assessment of family communication. Initially, observing the child and the family may help select child-specific assessment procedures. A few minutes of informal talk with the child also will help gain an impression about the child's communication skill level. The clinician may take note of the patterns of verbal interactions between the family and the child: Is the child only minimally verbal? Does the child speak mostly in words, phrases, or sentences? Does the child exhibit relatively good language skills? Assessment of a child with minimal language skills will need more basic procedures than the assessment of a child with relative good language skills. The children in the latter group may be assessed for more complex language structures, including syntactic features.

The clinician should try to get as much information as possible about home interaction patterns because parent education is an important part of treatment of children with DD. Therefore, the clinician needs to thoroughly describe the manner in which people in the child's environment are currently interacting with the child. For example, do people in the environment respond to the child's attempts to communicate in an encouraging, responsive manner? Do they model good language production for the child? Do they require the child to produce verbalizations when attempting to express needs and wants? Are there siblings who speak for the child?

Assess the child in naturalistic settings. Children with DD are more likely to exhibit their communicative skills when given the opportunity to do so within the context of everyday routines; they find themselves at a disadvantage in formal testing situations. Therefore, more informal, less structured, more naturalistic settings may help evoke their communication skills better than the standard assessment setting. Once again, getting a sibling or parent involved in conversational exchanges may be helpful. Furthermore, getting recorded speech samples from home will help compare skills exhibited at home with those evoked in the clinic.

Identification of strengths and weaknesses. Children with DD exhibit both strengths as well as weakness in social and academic skills. Children with Down syndrome, for example, may be highly sociable and eager to learn. Other children may have good motor skills or free from distracting behaviors. Some children with DD have good rote memory skills. Other children may have relatively better nonverbal skills than verbal skills. Such strengths may be capitalized in language treatment. Therefore, the clinician should concentrate not just on the weakness of the child, but also on strengths.

Strengths and weaknesses of the family of a child with DD are also important to assess. For example, parents who are patient with the child, who read stories to the child to stimulate language skills, who are interested in learning new ways of helping their child, and who are willing to modify their work schedule to bring the child for treatment to strengths that another family may not exhibit. A child with a DD whose siblings are supportive and affectionate enjoys a strength that another child may not.

Assessment of associated deficits. Many children with DD have associated sensory and motor deficits. To design an effective treatment and rehabilitation for the child and the family, it is necessary to obtain accurate information on a variety of deficits that are associated with DD. The clinician should take note of the presence of behavior disorders, attention deficits, hearing loss, visual deficits, neuromotor problems, and a genetic syndrome. Such clinical conditions may require the clinician to make referral to other professionals. If the child has been seen by other professionals, the clinician should get their reports on the child.

Contacting the special education specialist. It is especially important to get information from the special education specialist who may be working with a school-age child with DD. The clinician should contact the child's special education teacher to learn about the educational plan for the child. Subsequently, in designing a communication treatment plan for the child, the clinician should consult with the educational specialists so that educationally relevant treatment targets are selected.

Considering the speech disorders of children with DD. For many children with DD, accompanying phonological and articulation disorders may make assessment of language production—especially the production of such grammatic morphemes as the plural *-s* and past tense *-ed*—difficult. It may be necessary to emphasize assessment of speech production, knowing that a treatment plan to increase intelligibility of speech may initially take precedence over increasing language skills.

Assessment of receptive language skills. The clinician may pay particular attention to how a child responds to verbal directions. The clinician should take note of the level at which the child experiences difficulty—at the level of one-step directions? Two- or three-step directions? Experiment with different prompts to see how the child responds. For example, can the child more readily respond to verbal directions if they are accompanied with a gesture, or perhaps manual guidance (such as gently guiding the child's hand to pick up a block when asked to "Put the block in the box.")? Observations such as these will help the clinician determine the initial level of treatment.

Assessment of present and emerging literacy skills. Some clinicians may think that, in view of the cognitive impairment, assessment of literacy skills in children with DD may not be a necessary step. However, many children with DD, especially those who are high functioning children with Down syndrome, can achieve certain levels of literacy. To ignore the area would ensure continued illiteracy.

Being alert to aggressive or self-injurious behaviors. Some children who have profound cognitive impairment or cognitive impairment and autism exhibit aggressive and self-injurious behaviors. A carefully taken case history will alert the clinician to this possibility (Lerman et al., 1997). A clinician who knows about such behaviors can take necessary precaution during assessment. For instance, the clinician may restrict the child's access to certain hard objects the child may throw at the clinician and arrange seating such that the child's movements are restricted.

Assessment of nonverbal or minimally verbal children. Children with profound disabilities may be nonverbal or minimally verbal. Potential for verbal communication training in such cases may be limited. Therefore, such children may be candidates for augmentative or alternative modes of communication. In such cases, the clinician may use specific assessment procedures described in Chapter 15 for the assessment of nonverbal or minimally verbal children.

Modifications in Treatment Procedures

Treatment procedures described in Chapters 5 through 9 are generally applicable to children with DD. Giving instructions coupled with demonstrations, providing modeling, corrective feedback, and positive reinforcement are principles that work well with all children, including children with DD. Intensity of treatment should be increased for children with DD; briefer but more frequent sessions during the week, instead of the typical twice-weekly sessions, may be offered. A total communication program, including a component of parent education and teacher collaboration should be put into place to support the child's emerging language skills.

Early intervention is important to any child, but, in the case of a child with DD, it is even more critical. Intervention must be started as early as possible to increase the child's potential communicative skill and the evidence for early intervention is favorable (Berglund, Eriksson, & Johansson, 2001). Collaboration with family members, teachers, and others in the child's environment may help develop a list of functional words, phrases, or sentences to serve as target behaviors. Selecting target behaviors that will have the most immediate, beneficial effect on the child's patterns of interaction in naturalistic settings, including the home and the school will be beneficial to both the child and the family. For example, teaching a child with DD to make requests or ask for clarification when instructions are not understood may most positively affect the child's social and academic function.

Several other suggestions may be useful in treating children with DD. Although many of the suggestions offered in the next sections are relevant to all children receiving language treatment, paying special attention to them will help achieve success in treating children with DD.

Selection and sequence of functional target skills. As with other children, the clinician should select target communication skills that are of immediate functional value to the child, the family, and for performance in academic settings. The clinician may select target skills in consultation with the family members and the regular and special education teachers. Depending on the academic demands made on the child, the clinician may select abstract language structures (e.g., idioms, metaphors, and proverbs) as clinical treatment targets (Ezell & Goldstein, 1992). The clinician should pay special attention to personal and story narratives and conversational repair skills (Haring et al., 1986; Scudder &

Tremain, 1992). Procedures described in Chapter 7 may be effective in teaching pragmatic language skills to children with DD.

The clinician may expect to use a relatively larger number of varied target behavior exemplars than normal. Target behaviors often need to be sequenced such that simple skills are taught first and the remaining skills are carefully sequenced to minimize errors. Small, incremental steps should lead to production of a language skill. The clinician may expect to use the shaping procedure more often than with children who are not developmentally disabled (see Box 12.3 for an example of a target behavior set up in this way). While using the shaping procedure, the clinician should initially reinforce better, rather than fully correct, responses. In graduated steps, the clinician should require progressively more accurate responses before offering reinforcement.

Careful selection of treatment stimuli. The clinician may prefer stimuli from the child's home environment, school, or both. The clinician should consult parents, siblings, other caregivers, and teachers about the child's preferences. Concrete objects as against line drawings may be more effective in evoking the target behaviors. Objects, when used, should be paired with pictures and words printed under the pictures (Welch & Pear, 1980) to make the eventual transition to less concrete stimuli easier. Realistic photographs or acted-out events as stimuli during clinic sessions may be especially effective with children who have DD. To be avoided are the ambiguous and nonrealistic line drawings. The use of stimuli taken from the child's school and classroom, when used with modifications, may be especially useful (Hart & Risley, 1974).

Children with DD enjoy a variety of stimuli although this variety should not be as excessive as to overwhelm them, resulting in distracting behaviors. An array of stimuli, not an isolated stimulus, may be more effective in teaching the same target exemplar. Varied stimuli also will help minimize the chances of stimulus overselectivity (tendency to respond

---

box 12.3 **Sequencing Target Behaviors**

Children with DD often need to have tasks broken down into small, incremental steps before they are able to learn the entire task. The following is an example of a series of target behaviors leading to the production of prepositional phrases.

Long-Term Objective

Production of prepositional phrases using *in, on, over,* and *under.*

Target Behavior #1

Production of one-word utterances (e.g., either *in, on, over,* or *under*) in response to the clinician's questions (e.g., "Where is the ball?") in the clinic setting with 80 percent accuracy.

Target Behavior #2

Production of two-word utterances, consisting of a preposition (e.g., either *in, on, over,* or *under*) and a noun (e.g., *in box, under table*) in response to the clinician's questions in the clinic setting with 80 percent accuracy.

Target Behavior #3

Production of three-word prepositional phrases, consisting of a preposition, an article, and a noun (e.g., *in the box, on the chair, under the table, over the bridge*) in response to the clinician's questions in the clinic setting with 80 percent accuracy.

only to one stimulus used in training; see Chapter 9) and promote generalization (Bailey, 1981; Dube & McIlvane, 1999). In teaching the production of the word *books*, for instance, the clinician may use books of different shape, size, and color.

The manner of stimulus presentation also may be varied. For instance, the clinician may place treatment stimuli on a desk, show them while sitting on the floor, or display them on a book shelf, and so forth. An array of stimuli, presented in a varied manner, helps promote generalized production at home, classroom, and so forth (Schussler & Spradlin, 1991).

Effective use of instructions, modeling, and prompting. Unlike children without SLI, those with DD may need simple instructions that are often repeated throughout the session. The clinician may ask the child to describe what he or she is supposed to do to check on the child's understanding of instructions. The clinician also may need to provide extensive demonstrations that accompany the instructions.

Target responses may have to be modeled and prompted more frequently than usual. Frequent and repeated models and prompts of target responses, especially in the early stages of treatment, will help reduce the error rate and insure a greater frequency of positive feedback given to the child. In addition to live modeling, the clinician may use the video modeling technique in which the children watch normal conversational patterns that they can emulate (Nikopoulos & Keenan, 2004). The frequently given verbal prompts should be paired with tactile prompts (e.g., touch) to which children with cognitive impairment may react favorably (Berg & Wacker, 1989). As with any children, the clinician should fade instructions, modeling, and prompts in gradual steps, and be prepared to reinstate any or all of them when any decrease in the correct response rate is noted.

Selection of functional and effective consequences. It is especially important to select child-preferred reinforcers by assessing the child's preferences. Consultation with parents about the child's preferred items and consequences that are effective will be essential. An experimentally evaluated method of letting the child choose reinforcers is to present two reinforcers at a time and selecting the one the child picks first. The method works best with such tangible reinforcers as an item of food versus a small toy or one toy versus another (Fisher et al., 1992).

Many children with DD, especially those with minimal verbal skills, respond well to primary reinforcers. Primary reinforcers (e.g., food) are especially useful in the initial stages of treatment. Whenever used, primary reinforces should be paired with secondary reinforcers as well. This will help fade primary reinforcers as soon as possible so that the child eventually responds to verbal praise given without primary reinforcement. As the child makes good progress, the frequency with which verbal reinforcers are given may also be reduced. This is especially important when the treatment moves to conversational speech. Such natural reinforcers that are inherent to conversation as a smile, a nod, agreement, general reinforcement for "talking well," telling a long or nice story, and so forth will help maintain the treated communication skills (Ducharme & Holborn, 1997).

Structure of the initial sessions. An intensive and well-structured treatment program is necessary for most children with DD. Intensive (more frequent) therapy is known to produce long-term positive effects in children with even severe cognitive impairment (Smith et al., 1997). Well-structured initial sessions will help establish the skill with minimal opportunities for distracting behaviors. The clinician should move as soon as possible to more naturalistic situations, however. For example, the clinician may teach past tense inflection on a phrase or sentence level through structured discrete trial therapy, but then move on to more naturalistic tasks such as talking about a past event in the child's life. Use of such naturalistic treatment procedures as milieu teaching and incidental reaching, which have been shown to be effective (Farmer-Dougan, 1994; Gobbi et al., 1986; Warren & Gazdag, 1990), will help establish the target skills in social communication.

Giving brief but frequent breaks from therapy may be beneficial to many children with DD. The clinician should make such free time contingent on acceptable task performance; when this is done, the target skills are known to increase (Zarcone, Fisher, & Piazza, 1996). For example, after a block of correct responses, the clinician may give a 2-minute period of free time.

Effectiveness of the time-delay procedure. The time-delay procedure has been found to be effective in increasing spontaneous speech in autistic and other children and is expected to be effective with other populations (Charlop, Schreibman, & Thibodeau, 1985a; Dyer, Christian, & Luce, 1982; Ingenmey & Van Houten, 1991; Matson et al., 1990). In the final stages of treatment, the clinician should delay modeling; after asking a question, the clinician should not model immediately as done in the initial stages. Instead, the clinician should wait for a few extra seconds as children with cognitive impairment tend to have a slower reaction time. Delaying the delivery of reinforcers also may help promote naturalistic speech because reinforcers in everyday situations are somewhat delayed compared to their delivery in clinical situations. The clinician may teach the child to delay his or her response by a few seconds after the stimulus presentation to reduce errors; a hand signal given to respond after the delay may be effective.

Reducing undesirable behaviors. The clinician should watch for the emergence of undesirable behaviors during language training. A potential reason for such behaviors might be task demands that are difficult for the child; the child who cannot perform the required tasks is likely to exhibit such undesirable behaviors as crawling under the table or refusing to pay attention to the clinical stimuli. If this happens, the clinician should reduce the demand and simplify the task. In Chapter 6 we described several types of undesirable behaviors and techniques to reduce them; these procedures mainly use reinforcement for alternative and desirable behaviors and are a variation of differential reinforcement. For instance, instead of repeatedly saying "No" to the child when he or she tries to leave the chair, the clinician may consistently and generously reinforce the child for sitting quietly.

Special concerns for maintenance. Teaching target behaviors in varied settings will help promote generalized production. The clinician should get siblings or peers, parents, and other caregivers involved in language treatment. To support the child's communicative attempts, the clinician should teach peers and siblings to be conversational partners with the child. The significant others should be trained to model and prompt target language skills, and to verbally praise the production of such skills (Goldstein & Wickstrom, 1986; Goldstein & Mousetis, 1989; Kaiser, 1993; Lancioni, 1982; Laski, Charlop, & Schreibman, 1988).

In the academic environment, the clinician needs to collaborate closely with the classroom teacher or special education teacher in developing and implementing a language treatment program for children with DD. That the teachers should have a say in selecting target skills has already been noted. Throughout the treatment period, the clinician should recruit teacher to help sustain and expand the clinically established language skills in academic sessions. The clinician may ask the teacher to reinforce the production of newly learned skills. To the extent possible, the clinician should teach the skills within the classroom setting, rather than in an isolated clinic room.

Teaching the child to recruit others to reinforce his or her target skill productions is another maintenance strategy. The clinician should teach the child to draw attention to his or her own newly acquired skills produced at home and in the classroom (Craft, Alber, & Heward, 1998; Morgan, Young, & Goldstein, 1983).

Evidence suggests that even mothers who are themselves developmentally disabled may be effectively trained by instructions, demonstrations, modeling, and positive feedback to increase meaningful social interactions with their children (Feldman et al., 1986). The clinician may use the pyramidal training program in which one family member trained to do treatment at home trains other family members. To monitor the progress the child makes under such programs, the clinician should collect systematic data on how others are doing and how the child is reacting (Kuhn, Lerman, & Vorndran, 2003; Neef, 1995).

Strategies for the nonverbal or the minimally verbal. If the child is nonverbal or minimally verbal, the clinician may consider strategies using augmentative and alternative communication described in Chapter 15. American Sign Language, alone or in combination with oral language, has been effectively taught to children with cognitive impairment (Gaines et al., 1988; Sisson & Barrett, 1984). Some evidence suggests that signs taught in the contexts of total communication (e.g., naming pictorial stimuli used in sign training) are acquired faster (Clarke, Remington, & Light, 1988). Also, in teaching nonoral communication to children with DD, an iconic system rather than a noniconic system may be preferred (Hurlbut, Iwata, & Green, 1982).

Even with the most intensive treatment program offered perhaps on a daily basis, outcome will depend to a great extent on the severity of the cognitive impairment. However, most people with DD live productive lives within mainstream society. Because of the efforts of advocates for the developmentally disabled, the risk of institutionalization, even for the most severely affected child, has been drastically reduced. Many children with DD go to school; they have friends; they learn an occupation. As adults, some may live almost entirely independently, with just minimal support from government agencies. Others live in group homes, with varying degrees of support. Intensive, effective intervention given by many professional people, including speech-language pathologists, increases the possibilities for children with DD. Working to help children with DD achieve their full potential is a rewarding endeavor.

▦|▦ Chapter Summary

In defining developmental disability (DD), the American Association on Mental Retardation (AAMR, 2005) emphasizes intellectual limitations and behavioral deficits; the American Psychiatric Association (APA, 2000) emphasizes subaverage general intellect accompanied by limitations in at least two adaptive skills. Two main etiologic factors—genetic/organic and familial—are typically associated with DD.

Among many others, Down syndrome, fetal alcohol syndrome, fragile X syndrome, Prader-Willi syndrome, cri-du-chat syndrome, and Williams syndrome illustrate the genetic basis of DD. Many negative prenatal, natal, and postnatal conditions are organic factors that affect the growth of the fetus and the subsequent development during infancy and childhood. In addition, traumatic brain injury, endocrine disorders, metabolic disorders, and cranial abnormalities contribute to DD in children.

Speech and language disorders are common among children with DD, although the actual skill levels vary within a broad range. Most of the research on speech and language skills in children with DD has been on children with Down syndrome. Impaired comprehension of spoken language, limited vocabulary, and deficient morphologic and syntactic skills characterize children with DD. These children are likely to have difficulty with complex and abstract words, complex and longer syntactic structures, and discussion of abstract concepts. Poor narrative skills, limited initiation of social exchanges, inadequate topic maintenance, potential difficulties in conversational turn-taking, and limited conversational repair skills also may characterize the language skills of children with DD.

In assessing children with DD, the clinician should modify procedures to concentrate on assessment in naturalistic settings, evaluating interactions of others with the child, describing accompanying phonological disorders, determining the extent of problems in receptive language, identifying weaknesses in literacy skills, and understanding their nonverbal communicative skills.

Modifications in treatment procedures for children with DD include increasing intensity of intervention, using structured treatment sessions, repeated use of modeling and instructions, simplifying the target skills, shaping more complex skills in gradual steps, devising a total communication program when needed, and including parent education and teacher collaboration.

Study Guide

1. Describe and compare definitions of developmental disability (DD) given by the American Association on Mental Retardation (AAMR, 2005) and the American Psychiatric Association (APA, 2000). What problems would a speech-language pathologist have in using the APA diagnostic criteria?

2. Describe some of the genetic syndromes associated with DD discussed in the text. Research the literature and describe some of the genetic syndromes that are associated with DD but are not discussed in the text.

3. A child with possible DD has been referred to you for assessment and potential language treatment. In taking an exhaustive case history, on what prenatal, natal, and postnatal factors would you seek information from the parents? Point out the importance of the factors on which you plan to question parents.

4. In assessing a child with DD, what kinds of modifications would you make in the standard assessment procedures? Justify and point out the importance of such modifications.

5. You are asked to treat a child with DD who has extremely limited language skills. The child speaks mostly in one-word or two-word utterances. In developing a treatment program for this child, what kinds of special procedures (target behaviors, stimuli, reinforcers) would you use? Justify the procedural modifications.

chapter
13

Children with Autism and Other Pervasive Developmental Disorders

outline

387

Few early childhood disorders attract such intense clinical interest as autism does. Also, few early childhood disorders cause such anguish among parents. Leo Kanner, who first described this clinical condition in 1943, thought that the children presented "fascinating peculiarities." Hans Asperger (1944), who, independent of Kanner, also described a few children with unusual behaviors, recognized the special educational needs these children would have and the special care they need for the rest of their lives. In his 1944 German paper (an English translation of which was published in 1991), Asperger noted that these "exceptional human beings must be given exceptional educational treatment . . ." (1991, p. 37). That children and adults with autism are special people with special educational and rehabilitative needs is still true today. Both Kanner and Asperger also recognized the essence of this disturbing condition: a profound difficulty in relating to people. Asperger wrote that the "social problems are so profound that they overshadow everything else" (1991, p. 37). Similarly, Kanner (1943) noted the children's profound lack of affective contact with people. See Box 13.1 for a glimpse at Kanner and Asperger and their work with children.

The diagnostic criteria for the clinical conditions Kanner and Asperger described have evolved over the years. As we will see shortly, debate continues whether the conditions the two experts first described are separate or the extreme ends of the same syndrome (Wing, 1991).

---

box 13.1   **Two Pediatricians and Their Children: The Story of Leo Kanner and Hans Asperger**

Two Austrian pediatricians described some unusual children who are now diagnosed with either autism or Asperger's syndrome. Both were immensely interested in the medical and educational aspects of children they worked with. Leo Kanner (1896–1981) published his first work on such children in 1943; Hans Asperger (1906–1980), unaware of Kanner's work, published his article on similar children in 1944. The two never met each other. Kanner used the term *autism* to describe the strange behaviors of his children, and Asperger used the German term *autistischen psychopathen* (*autistic psychopathy*) to describe similar behaviors of his children. Both Kanner and Asperger borrowed the term *autism* from the Swiss psychiatrist Eugene Bleuler (1857–1940), who is credited with the coining of another well-known term, *schizophrenia. Detachment from worldly reality* is the essence of both the terms.

Kanner, who migrated to the United States in 1924, wrote in English and quickly became well known. He is recognized as the first child psychiatrist in the country; he established the first child psychiatric clinic at Johns Hopkins Hospital in 1930. Asperger, who remained in Austria, wrote in German, and remained unknown outside his country until the British psychiatrist Lorna Wing (1981) published an article and named the symptom complex as Asperger's syndrome. Consequently, Asperger's work began to draw attention in the English speaking world. Controversy about the distinction between the two syndromes followed. Ironically, Wing (2000), who is responsible for the name *Asperger's syndrome*, does not now believe that it is different from autism. When Asperger (1979) eventually published a paper in English, he borrowed by-then-famous Kanner's term: *infantile autism.*

It is interesting to note that it is not necessary to observe large numbers of people to establish a valid clinical condition. Kanner's original report described 11 children; Asperger reported on just 4 boys, although both subsequently reported on other children. Their observations have been replicated by thousands of clinicians around the world. It is the keen and intense observations of individual children, not superficial observations of a large sample, that helped establish the syndrome of autism.

Children described by both Kanner (1943) and Asperger (1944) exhibited an extremely atypical pattern of language development. We now know that often the first indication a child may have autism or its variation is a failure to acquire language, or a pattern of language acquisition that is qualitatively different—language development may be oddly asynchronous, or children may acquire some language only to regress, losing whatever language they have until they become essentially mute. Language disorders associated with a diagnosis of autism are often tragically severe, making this group of children of particular concern to speech-language pathologists. Because children with autism often have serious behavioral problems, assessment and treatment procedures need to be significantly modified to effectively serve these children. Speech-language pathologists must become thoroughly acquainted with the early signs of autism, with its various diagnostic criteria, and with effective assessment and treatment procedures designed to help children with autism.

Pervasive Developmental Disorders or Autism Spectrum Disorders?

Childhood disorders that Kanner and Asperger described, along with a few other disorders, are called pervasive developmental disorders or autism spectrum disorders. **Pervasive developmental disorders (PDDs)** are serious and multiple impairments in child development and are typically diagnosed in young children, usually before the age of 3 (American Psychiatric Association, 2000). The concept of PDD is largely upheld by the American Psychiatric Association (2000). A group of independent researchers (Wing & Gould, 1979; Wing, 1988) have supported the concept of a spectrum of disorders that includes the classic autism and its variations. Both the concepts (pervasive developmental disorder and the spectrum of disorders) are controversial. Critics of the pervasive concept contend that autism does not negatively affect all aspects of development equally or with the same severity, as the term suggests; some individuals with autism have certain typical skills (Gillberg, 1991; Wing, 1991). Critics of the spectrum concept point out that the disabilities of autistic individuals indeed affect all aspects of life and that the spectrum concept suggests a continuity along variations of autism that may or may not be true (Volkmar & Cohen, 1991).

Characteristics common to all PDDs include impairments in social interaction and communication skills, and the presence of stereotypical behaviors, interests, or activities. There is often a degree of developmental disability associated with PDDs, although not all children with developmental disability are also diagnosed with PDD. In the past, children who exhibited symptoms of PDD were often labeled as *psychotic* and diagnosed with childhood schizophrenia. It is now believed that PDDs are distinct from childhood schizophrenia, although a child with PDD can also have schizophrenia as a co-occurring condition. Because there is no biologically based medical test (e.g., analysis of blood) for PDD, diagnosis of PDD is based on behavioral observations.

> What are four diagnoses contained within the category of pervasive developmental disorders?

PDD is not a diagnostic category, but it encompasses specific diagnostic categories as autism, Asperger's syndrome, Rett's syndrome, and childhood disintegrative disorder. Much of the basic and clinical research done on PDDs has been on autism. Although we will offer some basic and contrasting information on other forms of PDDs—especially Asperger's syndrome—this chapter is mostly concerned with children who have autism. Speech-language pathologists who have a caseload of children with PDD work mostly with children with autism. See Table 13.1 for an overview of PDDs.

Autism

Across children, the symptoms of autism (whether called PDD or a spectrum) vary in both severity and variety. As described later, some children are so minimally affected they may be mistaken for eccentric individuals. Conversely, some extremely eccentric but otherwise normal individuals may show characteristics that are autistic. Interestingly, social deficits that characterize autistic children may be more common in the general population than ever thought (Constantino & Todd, 2003), suggesting that the characteristics of autism are continuously distributed in the population. Other children are so profoundly affected that they need extensive and constant care. We will use the term *autism* to include the entire spectrum, although we will describe Asperger's syndrome separately, while recognizing the controversy about its classification. Although the notion of a spectrum suggests a continuum from mild to severe, there is controversy whether the different disorders included under the classification are on a continuum or are indeed distinct.

table 13.1

An Overview of Pervasive Developmental Disorders (PDD)

Specific Disorder	Prevalence	Main Characteristics
Autistic Disorder (also known as autism spectrum disorder, or ASD)	35 to 40 cases per 10,000 individuals	Impaired social interaction, disturbed communication, and stereotypical patterns of behavior, interests, and activities. May be associated with developmental disability.
Asperger's Disorder (Also known as Asperger's syndrome, or AS)	27 to 36 per 10,000 children	Impaired social interaction and repetitive and stereotyped patterns of behavior, interests, and activities (both as in autism), combined with relatively intact communication skills. Typically not associated with developmental disability; hence, some think those with Asperger's are high-functioning autistic persons.
Rett's Disorder	Between 1 to 3.8 per 10,000 live female births (Yale Child Study Center, 2004).	Apparently normal growth until 6 to 18 months; normal head circumference at birth but retarded growth of the head; severely impaired language skills; repetitive hand movements; shaking of the torso, and unsteady gait.
Childhood Disintegrative Disorder	None reported due to lack of definitive data; appears to be much less common than autism, and the condition is more common among males.	Loss of social skills, bowel and bladder control, language and motor skills, lack of play, lack of social development in a child during the third or fourth year who had been developing normally until then.
Pervasive Developmental Disorder—Not Otherwise Specified (PDD-NOS)	None reported.	Autistic symptoms that do not fully meet the criteria for a diagnosis of autism; a vague category with no specified criteria for diagnosis.

Definition. **Autism** is a pervasive developmental disorder that varies on a spectrum of mild to profound impairment marked by disinterest in typical social interaction; severely impaired communication skills; and repetitive, stereotypical movements, combined with narrowly circumscribed, obsessive interests. The condition affects virtually every domain of a child's development, although children with autism may demonstrate some age-appropriate skills in specific areas, such as fine motor or visual-spatial skills. A few may even exhibit some isolated but extraordinary skills. It is a lifelong disability. Children do not "grow out of" autism.

Diagnostic criteria. Because the physical cause of autism has not yet been identified, autism is diagnosed through observation of behavior, and the diagnosis is most appropriately made by physicians or psychologists. In the United States, criteria set forth by the *Diagnostic and Statistical Manual of Mental Disorders, Fourth Edition-Text Revision* (DSM IV-TR) (American Psychiatric Association, 2000) are most commonly used in diagnosing autism (see Box 13.2 for a sample of DSM IV-TR criteria).

---

box 13.2  **A Sample of Diagnostic Criteria for Autistic Disorder: DSM IV-TR (2000)**

To warrant a diagnosis of autistic disorder, the child should display characteristics in each of three areas: (1) social interaction, (2) communication, and (3) repetitive, stereotypical interests and activities. The DSM IV-TR sets forth criteria determining how many features in each area a child must exhibit before a diagnosis of autism is considered to be valid. Onset of these symptoms occurs before the age of 3. The following is a sampling of some of the characteristics the DSM IV-TR describes in each area.

Social Interaction

A child must exhibit at least two characteristics in this area, some of which include:

- Deficits in the production of nonverbal behaviors, such as eye gaze and other nonverbal pragmatic language skills
- No development of relationships with peers
- No establishment of joint reference (described by the DSM IV-TR as "a lack of seeking to share enjoyment, interests, or achievements," p. 75)

Communication

A child must exhibit at least one of several characteristics in this area, some of which include:

- No, or little, development of oral language
- For those who are verbal, production of language that is stereotypical, repetitive, or idiosyncratic (this would include the production of echolalia)
- No typical play (described by the DSM IV-TR as "varied, spontaneous make-believe play or social imitative play," p. 75)

Repetitive and Stereotypical Behaviors, Interests, and Activities

A child must exhibit at least one of several characteristics in this area, some of which include:

- Intense preoccupation with narrow, stereotyped interests
- Rigid adherence to nonfunctional routines
- Motor behaviors that are stereotypical, repetitive, or both (e.g., whole-body spinning, hand clapping, arm flapping, finger waving, rocking, etc.)

A diagnosis of autism is most appropriately made by a team of professionals that includes a pediatrician and a psychologist or psychiatrist.

Under these criteria, children who are diagnosed with autism exhibit deficits in three domains: (1) social interaction, (2) communication, and (3) stereotypical patterns of behavior, interests, and activities (American Psychiatric Association, 2000).

Of the three, social interaction and communication are inextricably entwined. Children with autism are frequently described as aloof and apparently disinterested in forming personal relationships with other people. There may be no eye gaze, and absent or inappropriate facial expressions and other "body language" associated with pragmatic language skills. Children with autism may not point to desired objects, may not appear to enjoy sharing objects or activities of interest with other people (e.g., no establishment of joint reference), and may not seek out approval from adults or peers. They may not appear to be aware of the social cues of others and may not respond typically to social praise or disapproval. They may not demonstrate emotional attachment to family members, family pets, or family friends. There is, in short, what the DSM-IV-TR describes as a "lack of social or emotional reciprocity" (p. 75).

> What are the three areas of impairment described by DSM-IV-TR criteria for diagnosing autism?

This lack of reciprocity is readily apparent in the severely impaired communicative skills of a child with autism. Speech and language are profoundly disordered, and approximately 50 percent of children with autism are nonverbal (Prizant, 1983). When children with autism do develop oral speech, the language they produce is often distinctively different from that produced by typical children, with the greatest deficits in pragmatic skills. They may fail to initiate and maintain topics of conversation, producing language that is stereotypical, repetitious, or idiosyncratic.

> Clinicians should not assume children with autism are totally disinterested in others or are incapable of communicating. They do attempt to relate and to communicate, but those attempts are so unusual as to be considered bizarre.

In addition to deficiencies in social interaction and communication, children with autism frequently exhibit stereotypical behaviors or activities and may have obsessive, narrowly conscribed interests or fixations with particular objects. A child may be observed flapping arms, clapping hands, twirling, or rocking incessantly—examples of typical stereotypical movements. There is an absence of spontaneous, make-believe play, either when playing alone or with peers.

There may be one or few very specific interests that preoccupy the child. For example, we have known an adolescent with autism who was fascinated with brand names of laundry detergents, eagerly running to the appropriate aisle during every outing to the grocery store to test his knowledge and to see if any new brands were being marketed. Still another listened to a classic 1950s rock-and-roll music station, and knew the lyrics, artist, record publishing company, and year released for virtually every Top 10 tune of the 1950s.

A child with autism might also be obsessively preoccupied with objects, such as toy trains or small cars. There is no observed typical play involved in such activities. Rather than digging "roads" and "bridges" in the backyard dirt for toy cars to roll over, the child with autism is much more likely to carefully line the cars up, perhaps sorting them by color, size, or shape, or repetitively spinning the wheels, consistent with the autistic child's tendency to fixate on parts of objects. Children with autism pursue such interests in the context of specific, nonfunctional routines or rituals of their own devising. Deviance from an established daily routine or ritual known only to the child who has fashioned them is unwelcome; the child with autism is typically inflexible, and may exhibit tantrum behavior when such routines are disrupted.

Children with autism do not always exhibit all of the characteristics described in the preceding paragraphs. Furthermore, many autistic children will occasionally produce behaviors that are inconsistent with diagnostic criteria for autism. For example, we have known children with autism who, without specific intervention, seem to seek out physical contact, occasionally exhibit typical play, or maintain eye contact (see Photo 13.1 for an example of eye contact in a child with autism). Criteria for the diagnosis of autism require only that a sufficient number of characteristics in each category be present, by the age of 3, to justify the diagnosis.

> Any change in routine is a possible trigger for a tantrum in a child with autism. One child, used to watching a popular TV game show at a certain time, became ragingly upset when the show was preempted to broadcast a football game. The parents quickly learned to keep a supply of videotapes of the game show handy for such occasions.

Associated clinical conditions. Various clinical conditions have been shown to be associated with autism. The National Institute of Mental Health (NIMH, 2004) has reported the following clinical conditions to be associated with autism: (1) sensory problems, (2) seizures, (3) Fragile X syndrome, (4) tuberous sclerosis, and (5) developmental disability.

Sensory problems in children with autism have been well documented and can take the form of either hyper- or hyposensitivity to sensory input, or a child may exhibit symptoms of both. Some children with autism may not be able to tolerate stiff, new clothing or rough-textured furniture upholstery. A child with autism may not react at all to the roaring sound of a jet plane, but may scream in terror at the musical ringing of a cell phone. Other children may appear to be seriously hyposensitive to pain or discomfort, not flinching while touching a hot stove burner, for example, or apparently not needing a jacket on a sub-zero winter day. The small percentage of children with autism who exhibit self-injurious

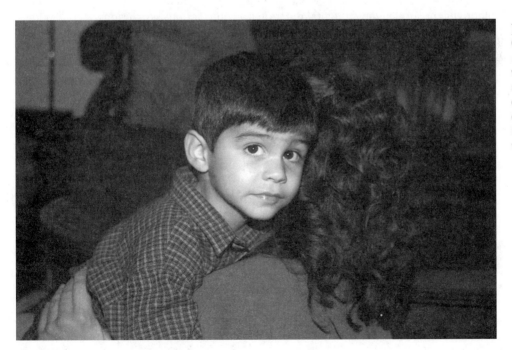

photo 13.1
Clinicians should *not* assume children with autism do not establish eye contact, or that they exhibit all characteristics associated with the diagnosis.

behaviors, such as banging their heads against the wall or biting their own hands, may be seeking out sensory stimulation they cannot experience otherwise (Kennedy Krieger Institute, 2004)

About 25 percent of children with autism develop **seizures,** the onset of which occurs most often either in early childhood or during adolescence (NIMH, 2004). A seizure results from abnormal electrical activity in the brain, and manifests itself in symptoms such as loss of consciousness, convulsions, or staring spells. Presence of seizures is confirmed through administration of an EEG (electroencephalogram), which measures electric currents produced in the brain. Anticonvulsant drugs may control seizures, but possible side effects dictate a conservative protocol in prescribing as little medication as is necessary.

> Self-injurious behaviors occur in approximately 5–17 percent of people with developmental disability, autism, or both (Kennedy Krieger Institute, 2004).

Fragile X syndrome is a genetic disorder that affects approximately 2 to 5 percent of children with ASD (NIMH, 2004). It is called Fragile X because, when examined under a microscope, a defective part of the X chromosome appears to be pinched or "fragile." Fragile X is a leading cause of developmental disability. Because males have only one X chromosome, they are more severely affected by the presence of Fragile X. Females have two X chromosomes, and, if only one is defective, the effects may be masked by the normal X chromosome. Parents who have a child diagnosed with autism should have the child checked for Fragile X, because if the disorder is present, any future male children will have a 50 percent chance of having it also (NIMH, 2004).

> See Chapter 12 for more on the Fragile X syndrome.

> What genetic disorder has been found to occur in approximately 2 to 5 percent of children with ASD?

Tuberous sclerosis is another genetic disorder that occurs in 1 to 4 percent of people with ASD. Effects of the disorder include the growth of benign tumors in the brain and other vital organs, epilepsy, mental deterioration, and various skin lesions. The condition has been found to co-occur with autism, although only a small percentage of cases of autism also have tuberous sclerosis (Bolton & Griffiths, 1997; Muhle, Trentacoste, & Rapin, 2004). Unfortunately, there is no effective treatment for this disorder (Anderson et al., 2002).

When autism was first clinically described, developmental disability was not believed to be part of the constellation of symptoms. It is now known, however, that many children who are diagnosed with autism also have some degree of accompanying cognitive deficiency: percentages of reported developmental disability in the autistic population have ranged from 25 to 70 percent (Klin, 2003).

An additional diagnosis of developmental disability is not always easy to make, because children with autism often have skills in specific areas of development that are age-appropriate or even highly advanced. Researchers have noted in the autistic population what appears to be a higher prevalence of the **savant syndrome**—the co-occurrence of high-level skills and generally low intelligence (Heaton & Wallace, 2004; see Box 13.3 for examples). Another condition, **hyperlexia**, is also observed with interesting frequency among children with autism, although it has also been noted in children with other diagnoses as well. Hyperlexia is the presence of precocious reading ability in children with severe language and learning disorders (Kupperman, Bligh, & Barouski, 2004). Children with hyperlexia read remarkably well, usually by the age of 5 with no formal instruction, although there may be little comprehension of what has been read (Klin &

> The co-occurrence of high-level skills and generally low intelligence is associated with what syndrome?

box 13.3   Autism and the Savant Syndrome: Some Examples

The prevalence of the savant syndrome is believed to be higher in the autistic population than it is in the general population, but exact figures are unknown. Estimates have been reported between .06 to 9.8 percent of children with autism have some kind of extraordinary skill that is inconsistent with other, generally low skills (Heaton & Wallace, 2004). There have been anecdotal reports of children who are remarkable musicians, artists, or poets. Others may have amazing skill in performing various mathematical calculations or in mechanical repair.

Anecdotal reports, while fascinating, do not constitute the type of systematic research that must be conducted before any cogent conclusions can be made regarding this interesting subgroup of children with autism. The authors, however, cannot resist describing some examples of savant syndrome in clients with whom one of us has been personally acquainted:

- One college-age young man with autism performed the "calendar trick," quickly calculating without fail what day of the week a date fell on—either in the past or in the future—in response to questions from a clinician referring to a 5-year calendar.

- While at the Special Olympics local winter games one year, a clinician noticed a nonverbal adolescent snowshoe athlete on his hands and knees, furiously digging in the snow. When she approached him, she found he had made, in perfect bas relief, a readily recognizable sculpture of two popular cartoon figures. His skills as a graphic artist, she later learned, were considerable.

- A 3-year-old boy was brought to a university clinic for evaluation. As he walked into the room, he spied the Peabody Picture Vocabulary Test (Dunn & Dunn, 1997) on the table. "Oh!" he said delightedly, pointing to each letter on the cover of the test, "/pʌ, pʌ, vʌ, tʌ/!" Evaluation of his speech and language warranted referral to a psychologist for further assessment of possible autism, with accompanying hyperlexia.

Volkmar, 1995; O'Connor & Hermelin, 1994; Tirosh & Canby, 1993). There is controversy over whether hyperlexia is symptomatic of disability or a promising skill suggesting a much better prognosis compared to children who are autistic but do not have hyperlexia (Grigorenko, Klin, & Volkmar, 2003; Kupperman, Bligh, & Barouski, 2004).

The presence of a remarkable skill is a strength that can be exploited in providing intervention for children with autism, but the severity of the overall impairments associated with autism should not be underemphasized. The argument over whether or not developmental disability is prevalent in children with autism is perhaps a moot one—most children with autism will function *as if* they have developmental disability, requiring intensive intervention and, most often, lifelong support.

Autism is a complex disorder with several identified associated clinical conditions and with several conditions under investigation (e.g., various genetic abnormalities, brain deformities, psychological conditions, etc.). The diagnostic picture is not at all complete, and further overlap of symptoms of autism with many other conditions is likely to be discovered.

Asperger's Syndrome

While autism is acknowledged as the most profoundly disabling of the PDDs, Asperger's syndrome (AS) is the mildest. There are many who would argue that it is incorrect to list AS as a separate diagnostic category—that it is only the other end of the autism spectrum (Asperger, 1991; Wing, 1991). These arguments are based on the difficulty of distinguishing between

AS and high-functioning autism (HFA), and, indeed, the diagnostic call is a difficult one to make.

Definition. **Asperger's syndrome (AS)** is a pervasive developmental disorder having as its most distinctive feature a severe impairment in social interaction. Unlike autism, acquisition of speech and language may not be delayed (although this is a controversial claim), and the child with AS rarely has accompanying developmental disability.

Diagnostic criteria. The DSM-IV-TR criteria for AS largely overlap with that set forth for diagnosing autism, and indeed are exactly the same for the first domain (social interaction) and the third domain (repetitive and stereotyped patterns of behavior, interests, and activities; see Box 13.2). However, the second domain, that of communication, is deleted in criteria for AS. Instead, DSM-IV-TR criteria state that, while "the disturbance causes clinically significant impairment in social, occupational, and other important aspects of functioning," there is *no* "clinically significant" delay in language or cognitive development (American Psychiatric Association, 2000, p. 84).

Clinically, children with AS display severe deficits in their pragmatic language skills. Children with AS are noticeably odd, seemingly unable to comprehend the feelings or points of view of others, or the give-and-take of normal human discourse. They develop intense interests in isolated topics (e.g., trains, snakes, public transit routes, etc.) and gather much factual information on those topics that they are eager to share. Conversations with a child with AS are one-sided, with the child engaging in a virtual monologue about his or her own narrow interests, without inviting a conversational turn from the listener. Children with AS have been described as not being able to "read" social cues and pay no heed to signals indicating the listener may be bored, in a hurry, or desirous of making a comment or changing the topic (Klin, 2003).

> Individuals with AS do best when engaged in an "interview format" type of conversation. They will respond eagerly to questions regarding their own interests, but will not ask questions to invite a conversational turn from their partner.

Researchers have noted that children with AS often express a wish to make friends, but they are pathologically awkward in approaching their peers, and their efforts at socialization are often rebuffed, sometimes cruelly (Klin & Volkmar, 1995; Volkmar et al., 2000).

The boundaries separating AS from other diagnoses are not distinct. As previously noted, there are many who would argue that AS represents the high end of the autism spectrum, and therefore, there is no need for a separate diagnosis (Klin, 2003; Wing, 1981, 1991). Bishop (1989) suggested that, rather than conceptualizing autism in terms of inflexible diagnostic categories, we should recognize that "the core syndrome of autism shades into other milder forms of disorder in which language or non-verbal behaviour may be disproportionately impaired" (p. 107). Reviewing the research on this issue, Howlin (2003) concluded that, although children with AS may be distinct from children with ASD, that distinction diminishes as the children age, and language becomes noticeably more impaired when adulthood is attained.

Those who would argue in favor of describing AS as a separate diagnosis clearly distinguishable from other PDD diagnoses point to case studies and analyses made by researchers who recommended its inclusion in the DSM-IV-TR (Ozonoff, Rogers, & Pennington, 1991; Volkmar et al., 1994). Language skills in children with AS were found by these investigators to be markedly superior to those found in children with autism. Prevalence of developmental disability is not as high in the AS population as it is in autism, although some AS children have been reported as having mild cognitive deficits (Klin & Volkmar, 1995). Furthermore, there is an apparent desire on the part of many children with AS to socialize with others. Children with AS are usually not withdrawn in the presence of adults and peers; they are eager to converse, albeit in the awkward, inappropriate manner previously described. Their social isolation is frequently the result of their own clumsy but overt attempts to interact. This is in sharp contrast to children with autism who typically appear to have no interest in interacting with either peers or adults in a social manner, and who are not at all bothered by rejection.

Another distinguishing feature of AS is a prognosis that appears to be quite a bit more positive than it is for children with autism. As children with AS mature, they become intellectually aware of their difficulties, and they can learn appropriate ways to socialize in the same way any of us learn a skill that is difficult. Follow-up studies have indicated some adults with AS have achieved impressive degrees of independence, with varying degrees of support. Although social difficulties persist throughout their lifespan, some adults with AS marry and have successful occupations (American Psychiatric Association, 2000; Bishop, 1989; Siegel, 1996; Volkmar et al., 2000).

Arguments over the validity of the diagnosis of AS are unlikely to abate any time soon. Clinically there is perhaps some danger in conceptualizing autism as a linear spectrum disorder, ranging from symptoms that are mild to profoundly severe. Such a conceptualization appears to imply that for those at the mild end of the autism spectrum, there is less need for intervention, or that less intense intervention is warranted. As pointed out by Klin (2003), children with AS are "mild" only in comparison to children with more severe symptoms of autism; they are still profoundly impaired compared to the general population. They are deserving of rigorous advocacy from professionals who understand their need for intensive intervention.

> Children with AS often need the same type of intense intervention as children with autism do. The focus for AS, however, will be on more advanced pragmatic language skills.

Rett's Syndrome

Rett's syndrome (RS) is included as a pervasive developmental disorder because, in the early stages, children with RS are frequently misdiagnosed with autism. Tsai (1992) argued that the disorder is sufficiently different from autism to warrant a separate diagnosis, citing various behavioral differences between children with RS and children with autism. Recently, the disorder has been found to be the result of a mutation of the MeCP2 gene on the long arm of the X chromosome (Xq28)—a discovery that established RS as a separate diagnostic category clearly delineated from autism (Amir et al., 1999).

Definition. **Rett's syndrome (RS)** is a genetically-based neurological disorder that is included under the category of PDD. It almost exclusively affects females, but there have been some recent reports of males who have mutations of MECP2 and who exhibit some of the symptoms of RS (Leonard et al., 2001; Schanen et al., 1998; Zeev et al., 2002).

Diagnostic criteria. Children with RS appear to develop normally during the first 6–18 months of life, meeting developmental milestones such as sitting, crawling, and, sometimes, walking at typical ages. Following this normal period of development, the child begins to lose purposeful movement of the hands; a characteristic wringing or "hand-washing" stereo-typical movement is one of the first signs of RS. Gait disturbances and decelerated head growth are also symptoms of RS. What little language may have developed begins to regress, resulting in a loss of expressive and receptive communicative skills. In the early stages of the disorder, children with RS appear similar to children with autism, exhibiting an autistic-like lack of social engagement. Some researchers have reported that this is a transient condition and that children with RS often become more social in later adolescence (Hagberg, 1989; Tsai, 1992). As they grow older, their autistic-like behaviors diminish while their physical deficits become more apparent.

Childhood Disintegrative Disorder

What percentage of parents report a period of normal development in the early months of their autistic child's life?

Approximately 20 percent of parents of autistic children report that their children appeared to be essentially normal during the first two years of development (American Psychiatric Association, 2000). The line separating those children from those with childhood disintegrative disorder (CDD) is a fine one, and some professionals have argued it is a line that should not have been drawn (Hendry, 2000; Rapin, 1997).

Definition. **Childhood Disintegrative Disorder (CDD)** is a pervasive developmental disorder marked by a prolonged (at least 2 years) period of normal development before the child begins to regress, losing social, language, self-help, and motor skills. CDD has a similarity to RS, due to the normal period of development that precedes onset and subsequent deterioration of skills. It is distinguished from RS because the period of normal development is longer and it affects primarily males. No genetic basis for CDD has been discovered, as is the case with RS (Amir et al., 1999).

Diagnostic criteria. The prolonged period of normal development is the major criterion for diagnosing CDD. This period must last at least 2 years, although onset is usually between 3 and 4 years of age. Regression can be abrupt or insidious. Some children with CDD lose skills suddenly; others, gradually—the particular course seems to have no effect on eventual outcome (Mouridsen, 2003). At some point, the loss of skills may plateau, and some improvement may even occur, but the impairments associated with the disorder are extreme and lifelong. Children with CDD are likely to be mute and have a severe to profound degree of developmental disability. After the condition has been established, they are indistinguishable from children with low-functioning autism (American Psychiatric Association, 2000; Mouridsen, 2003; Volkmar, 1992). So indistinguishable, in fact, that the validity of CDD as a separate diagnostic category has been sharply questioned (Hendry, 2000).

Pervasive Developmental Disorder—Not Otherwise Specified (PDD-NOS)

Symptoms delineating pervasive developmental disorders are difficult to definitively describe. As is evident by the preceding discussions of various PDDs, criteria for diagnosis frequently overlap, and children who have PDDs exhibit an infinite combination of various criteria; they are not at all a homogenous group. As a result, the validity of these diagnoses has been debated—children's symptoms often do not fall neatly into any one set of diagnostic criteria subsumed under the category of PDD.

Some children may have some symptoms of PDD, but not enough to warrant any of the specific diagnoses. Professionals may diagnose such a child as having **pervasive developmental disorder—not otherwise specified (PDD-NOS),** a diagnostic category loosely described in the DSM-IV-TR. This has been criticized as being a "catch-all" approach to diagnosing PDD (Filipek et al., 1999; Walker et al., 2004). PDD-NOS has been described as a "subthreshold" category which offers no specific guidelines for diagnosis (Yale Child Study Center, 2004a). Because PDD-NOS is an ill-defined diagnosis applied to a heterogeneous group of children, systematic research cannot be conducted on this condition. The category does, however, provide a way of recognizing children who appear to have atypical autism, presenting with a severe social impairment that does not fit the criteria of any existing diagnosis.

Prevalence of Pervasive Developmental Disorders

Because of shifting, often unclear, criteria for the diagnosis of PDD, accurate estimates of prevalence have been difficult to achieve. Different sources suggest different figures. Compared to other PDDs, prevalence of autism has received much attention from researchers. The American Psychiatric Association (2000) estimates the prevalence of autism at 2 to 20 cases per 10,000 individuals. The APA cites no prevalence figures for Rett's disorder, Asperger's Disorder (syndrome), or childhood disintegrative disorder.

The APA's extremely wide range (2 to 20 cases per 10,000) makes the estimate unreliable possibly because of differing criteria used in diagnosing the disorder and varied epidemiological methods used in collecting and analyzing the data. Generally, the lower estimates refer to the prevalence of autism defined in a narrow and classic sense (Wing & Potter, 2004); for many years, epidemiologists took the classic view in studying autism. The higher prevalence is more likely to be reported if the definition of autism is widened to include the entire spectrum. Also, the prevalence figures reported before 1985 are markedly different from those reported in the 1990s. Often reported pre-1985 prevalence of autism spectrum disorders (broader definition) is 4 to 5 per 10,000 children; for the classic autism, the pre-1985 prevalence is 2 per 10,000 children (Merrick, Kandel, & Morad, 2004). Worldwide prevalence estimates in the 1990s were already showing an increasing trend. A 1993 review of prevalence studies of autism in Europe, the United States, and Japan reported up to 16 per 10,000 (Wing, 1993). U.S. and European prevalence figures reported in the late 1990s to early 2000 suggested even higher numbers; about 17 to 40 per 10,000 children for the classic autism and up to 67 per 10,000 for the entire spectrum (Bertrand et al., 2001; Chakrabarti & Fombonne, 2001; Yeargin-Allsopp et al., 2003). Reported prevalence in Sweden is 71 per 10,000 children (Merrick, Kandel, & Morad, 2004). These figures suggest an alarming increase in the prevalence of autism.

> Only two characteristics define Kanner's classic autism: (1) a profound lack of emotional contact and (2) repetitive, elaborate ritualistic behaviors.

This dramatic increase has led many to question whether these reported prevalence rates are simply the result of broadening the criteria for diagnosing ASD, an increased awareness of the disorder, a combination of the two, or perhaps other factors (Coury & Nash, 2003). However, a systematic study in California (California Department of Developmental

Incidence is established by following healthy children for a period of several years and noting the number of children on whom a diagnosis is made.

Services, 2003) has found the increase in prevalence of autism to be a valid phenomenon (see Box 13.4 for information on prevalence of autism in California). What the California study showed is that there indeed is a dramatic increase in the number of children seeking services; this does not necessarily mean, however, that the *incidence* of autism has increased by the same proportion. Credible evidence that a disorder is on the rise comes only from an incidence study, not any kind of prevalence study. There have been no incidence studies on autism (Wing & Potter, 2004).

There may be an increase in the incidence itself, but the influence of other factors, cannot be ruled out. A careful examination of worldwide data on the prevalence of autism (Wing, 1993; Wing & Potter, 2004) raises some troubling questions. Is it likely that the incidence has increased worldwide, as the data seem to suggest? It is doubtful that the incidence of autism would simultaneously increase in many countries. Could it be that the autism spectrum concept has influenced the diagnosis of autism and such related conditions as Asperger's syndrome? There is some evidence that this may have occurred. It is not strictly correct to assume that a higher prevalence of autism spectrum disorders is noted only in the late 1980s and in the 1990s. A 1979 British study had reported that when only those children who had an IQ of 70 or below were studied, the prevalence of autism was 20 in 10,000, a number 4 to 5 times higher than what was typically reported for the classic autistic syndrome. Presumably, if the investigators had included children with IQs greater than 70, the prevalence would have been higher for children born during the years of 1956 to 1970. Until the early 1990s, there were no figures available for the prevalence of Asperger's syndrome. Then, in 1993 Ehlers and Gillberg conducted a study in Sweden on children who had IQs above 70 and were born during the years of 1975 to 1983 and reported preva-

box 13.4   Prevalence of Autism in California

The State of California is a particularly good laboratory for studying prevalence rates of developmental disabilities and possible causes of the reported increase. Passage of the state's Lanterman Act in 1969 guaranteed to developmentally disabled people a full range of services, to be administered by 21 independently operated organizations called regional centers. Data collected by regional centers have tracked the numbers of developmentally disabled people qualifying for services in California. In 1999, based on regional center data, the California State Department of Developmental Services reported a 269 percent increase from 1983 to 1995 in the number of autistic people receiving services from regional centers (California Department of Developmental Services, 2003).

Distressingly, the most recent reported prevalence figures for the State of California have documented an astonishing 634 percent increase in autism for the years from 1987 to 2002. Calculation of prevalence rates indicated an increase from 4 per 10,000 individuals in 1970 to 31 per 10,000 in 1997; a 774 percent increase. It is expected that, as children born between 1997 and 2002 are diagnosed, the number of children with PDDs receiving services in California will continue to sharply increase (California Department of Developmental Services, 2003).

These and similar data only show that there has been a phenomenal increase in the number of children and families seeking services for autism. The data do not show that the actual incidence of autism has increased worldwide. See the text for a critical review of prevalence data.

lence of 36 cases per 10,000 children. Thus, the total prevalence figures of the autistic spectrum including only the classic autism and Asperger's syndrome would be 56 per 10,000 (Wing & Potter, 2004). This high prevalence figure would still exclude the prevalence of such other spectrum disorders as Rett's disorder and childhood disintegrative disorders, even if they are relatively rare conditions. Furthermore, Ehlers and Gillberg (1993) also reported that an additional 35 per 10,000 children may also show social impairment of the autistic type even though they do not meet all the criteria for the autistic or Asperger's syndromes. Wing and Potter (2004) stated that if all children with social impairment of the autistic kind are counted, the prevalence may be as high as 91 per 10,000.

> Intensive studies in which a majority of children in a given area were directly evaluated have produced higher prevalence than studies in which either only a cross-section of children were studied or data were collected through case records and telephone contacts.

The prevalence of the entire spectrum of disorders may have been historically underestimated throughout the world, especially in children with IQs above 70. The California report (California Department of Developmental Services, 2003) recognized that autism in some children with developmental disability in the state may have been missed. The report also stated that the steepest increase in children with autism seeking services had IQs above 70—supporting the view that while the diagnostic criteria may not have changed, the criteria may have been applied to children who have higher IQs. Nonetheless, the prevalence figures estimated based on the number of children being served in California is 20.6 for children with IQs below 70 and 14.9 for children with IQs above 70, for a total prevalence in 1998 of 35.5 in 10,000. For children with IQs below 70, the estimated 20.6 is close to what Wing and Gould reported in 1979. For children with IQs greater than 70, California's 14.9 *is less than half* the Swedish figure of 36 per 10,000. The prevalence reported for the metropolitan Atlanta, Georgia, is 34.5, which is close to California's 35.5 (Yeargin-Allsopp et al., 2003). Among the recent U.S. regional studies, the Brick Township study in New Jersey reported one of the highest figures: 40 cases of autism per 10,000 and 67 for the entire spectrum (Bertrand et al., 2001; Centers for Disease Control and Prevention, 2000).

It is likely that in addition to any factual increase in the incidence of the disorder, the recent increases in the number of children and families seeking services may at least partly be a function of more accurate diagnosis of children who fall on the entire spectrum, higher social awareness of the disorder, increased funding for autism programs, more families seeking help for mildly impaired children, varied study methods, and such other factors.

Causes, Correlations, and Explanations

Behind the increasing number of those seeking services to children with autism are distraught families, struggling school districts that are trying to find the best way to educate those children, and cash-limited government entities that are trying to provide services—often lifelong services—to a growing population of people with autism. Interest in finding a cause, and ultimately a cure, for autism has never been greater. The desperation of parents and the pressure brought to bear on school districts and governments have fostered an interest in pseudoscientific discoveries of causes and promises of quick cures for autism, which we will briefly discuss. When a cause and a cure for autism are discovered, it will be the result of painstaking, intense research. Such research is currently being conducted, and this section will conclude with some promising, although inconclusive and tenuous, recent findings on the causes of autism.

Pseudoscientific Theories of the Etiology of Autism

Theories on the cause of autism have never been lacking. Unfortunately, many early and present-day theories are pseudoscientific, often rooted in coincidental events. Such theories may be advocated, sometimes by well-recognized experts, as having been scientifically verified even though they lack experimental support (Green, 1996; Herbert, Sharp, & Gaudiano, 2002). It is fine to speculate and propose reasonable hypotheses to answer scientific questions, but it is unethical to claim the validity of a theory without having first subjected it to rigorous scientific testing. Furthermore, treatment procedures that are based on unfounded theories are highly likely to be ineffective and, in some cases, actually harmful to people receiving such treatment. Examples of pseudoscientific theories on autism can be organized into two categories: (1) psychoanalytic theories and (2) theories regarding various physical causes.

Psychoanalytic theories. Early theories on autism posited that it is a psychological disturbance, caused most likely by a cold, detached mother who did not bond with her newborn baby. It was believed that children with autism chose to withdraw from such an unwelcoming environment, exhibiting a disorder similar to childhood schizophrenia.

In the 1960s, professionals described mothers of children with autism as "refrigerator mothers," with a cold, unfeeling affect toward their children. This baseless theory inflicted emotional trauma on many parents. Because there were often other, quite normal children in the same family, the theory was eventually discredited.

Bettelheim (1967) was an ardent advocate of this viewpoint, promoting a treatment regimen that entailed separation of children from their parents for extended periods. Such theories of the origins of autism have a complete lack of controlled evidence, although there are some modern-day psychoanalysts who continue to emphasize mother–child attachment dysfunction as a cause of autism (Rosner, 1996).

Theories on physical causes. Most scientists now believe that autism is biologically based. It is understandable, therefore, that there are a plethora of theories regarding the physical causes of autism. Some of those theories, to be discussed in a later section, may have merit, are being subjected to research, and are showing promise as possible explanations of autism. Many other theories have been proposed through the popular press or Internet and immediately taken by the public as valid. Families of autistic children may rush to procure, often at great expense, the latest popular "cure" for autism based on those theories (see Table 13.2 for a description of theories, resulting treatment methods, and efficacy evaluation).

One theory that met with immediate and intense attention was the idea that autism results from an adverse reaction to the measles, mumps, and rubella (MMR) vaccination that most children in developed countries receive by their 3rd birthday. As autism is typically diagnosed by the 3rd birthday, many saw a correlation between administration of the MMR vaccine and onset of symptoms associated with autism, ascribed to the presence of thimerosal, a mercury-based preservative, in the vaccine. In 1998, Wakefield and colleagues reported the presence of severe gastrointestinal symptoms in 12 children with autism. In their report, they noted that eight of the children's parents associated the onset of their chil-

Enterocolitis is an inflammation involving both the large and small intestine.

table 13.2

Some Pseudoscientific Theories of Causes of Autism and Resulting Ineffective Treatment Procedures

Presumed Cause	Proposed Treatment Methods	Evaluation of Evidence of Efficacy
The child has hypersensitive hearing	Auditory Integration Training (AIT); through headphones, the child listens to filtered, modulated music at various volumes and pitches (Berard, 1993; Stelhi, 1991)	Controlled research has found no benefit derived from AIT (Bettison, 1996; Gillberg, Johannsson, Steffenburg, & Berlin, 1997; Mudford et al., 2000; Zollweg, Palm, & Vance, 1997).
The child has sensory-motor dysfunctions	Sensory Integration Therapy (SIT); attempts to correct sensory-motor deficits through a variety of activities, such as swinging, applying brushes to the child's body, engaging in balance activities, and so forth (Ayres, 1979)	Although the children may enjoy the activities, controlled research has found no evidence of efficacy that is specific to SIT (Hoehn & Baumeister, 1994; Iwasaki & Holm, 1989; Mason & Iwata, 1991).
The child has a vitamin deficiency	Megadoses of various vitamins and minerals, most notably Vitamin B6 and magnesium (Rimland, 2003)	Anecdotal case studies; no controlled scientific evidence of the efficacy of megadoses of vitamins, which can have harmful side effects, such as nerve damage in the case of B6 and reduced heart rate and weakened reflexes in the case of magnesium (Deutsch & Morrill, 1993).
The child has a food allergy (Adams & Conn, 1997)	Various restricted diets, such as gluten- and casein-free diets, ketogenic diets, dairy-free diets, and so forth	There have been isolated reports of children who have seemingly recovered from autism following an adjustment in diet. However, there is no controlled scientific evidence showing that diet is a significant factor in autism.
The child has a yeast infection (*candida albicans*) causing a condition called candidiasis. Based on anecdotal reports that some children with candidiasis later develop symptoms of autism (Adams & Conn, 1997; Edelson, 2004)	Prescription of Nystatin, a medication for women's yeast infections	No controlled scientific evidence that candidiasis causes autism; Nystatin has no efficacy in treating autism.

Source: Compiled from Herbert, Sharp, and Gaudiano (2002); Rimland (2003); and other cited studies.

dren's behavioral problems and loss of skills with the MMR vaccine. The researchers concluded that they had identified a chronic enterocolitis in the children that could be related to their "neuropsychiatric dysfunction," and that onset of symptoms occurred after the MMR vaccination. They called for further research on this condition and its possible relation to the MMR vaccine (Wakefield et al., 1998).

Epidemiological studies have subsequently shown that there is no evidence, not even correlational evidence, supporting an association between autism and the MMR vaccine. Taylor et al. (1999) identified 498 cases of autism and found: (1) no difference in age of diagnosis in those vaccinated before the age of 18 months, after the age of 18 months, or who had never been vaccinated; (2) no temporal association between onset of autism and vaccination with MMR; (3) no clustering of developmental regression in the months after vaccination; and (4) no temporal clustering of first parental concerns with administration of the MMR vaccine. Madsen et al. (2002) conducted a retrospective cohort study involving all children born in Denmark from January 1991 to December 1998—537,303 children, of whom 82 percent had received the MMR vaccination. There was no significant difference in the prevalence of autism between the vaccinated and unvaccinated groups. Furthermore, there was no temporal clustering of cases of autism after immunization. Researchers have also found no evidence of a subgroup of autistic children with severe gastrointestinal problems caused by exposure to the MMR vaccine (DeFelice, 2003; Peltola et al., 1998; Taylor et al., 2002). In light of overwhelming scientific evidence showing no correlation between autism and the MMR vaccine, all but two of the original investigators in the Wakefield et al. (1998) study published a letter retracting their implication of a link between the MMR vaccine and autism. However, they also called for continued investigation into the gastrointestinal problems of children with autism, a subject that has received much attention from autism researchers (Murch et al., 2004).

It is perhaps unfair to describe this controversy under a heading of pseudoscientific theories of autism. Much that occurred during this process is consistent with acceptable scientific inquiry. An observation was made, much intense research was conducted, and valid conclusions were derived. But the idea that autism is caused by the MMR vaccine gained widespread popularity before it was properly investigated, causing some parents to postpone necessary vaccinations for their children, and sending parents of autistic children to unethical specialists who prescribed invasive treatments such as frequent enemas and chelation therapy to rid the body of supposed high levels of mercury caused by the MMR vaccine (See Box 13.5 for an explanation of chelation therapy). The harmful effects of this pseudoscientific theory are clear: children ran the risk of being denied

---

box 13.5 | **Chelation Therapy and Autism: An Example of the Harm Pseudoscience Can Do**

The presence of thimerosal, a mercury-based preservative, in the MMR vaccine led to the speculation that autism was the result of the introduction of heavy metals in the child's bloodstream. Similarities were pointed out between the symptoms of autism and the symptoms of lead poisoning (Bernard et al., 2001a,b). That line of reasoning led some parents to seek out chelation therapy for their autistic children.

Chelation therapy involves the administration, usually intravenously, of chelating agents—specific molecules that form complexes that inactivate heavy metals (such as mercury) which can then be eliminated through urination. It is a therapy that is used most appropriately for obvious cases of lead poisoning. Some parents have sought out chelation therapy for their autistic children, even though there is no indication

that autistic children have elevated levels of mercury in their bodies; one proponent of the treatment has even admitted hair analysis reveals that ASD children exhibit lower hair mercury than the non-ASD population (Kidd, 2002). Side effects of this treatment commonly include diarrhea and fatigue; more serious, but less common, side effects include liver enzyme elevation, abnormal blood counts, and mineral abnormalities (Holmes, 2002).

It has been our experience that chelation therapy did indeed produce strikingly noticeable fatigue and lethargy in a small client with autism being treated at our clinic. The parents were unconcerned, because they had been told by the specialist administering the treatment that children often get worse under the treatment before they get better.

necessary vaccines, and parents of autistic children were diverted from pursuing efficacious therapy.

Evidence-Based Theories of Autism

There is now much scientific evidence that a combination of genetic predisposition and early environmental (possibly in utero) insults may cause brain abnormalities leading to autistic behaviors (Herbert, Sharp, & Gaudiano, 2002). Although there have been no definitive conclusions drawn, genetic research and various investigations conducted on brain structures hold a great deal of promise for future scientific breakthroughs.

Genetic research. There is evidence that autism is genetically based. Reviewing the genetic research on autism, Muhle, Trentacoste, and Rapin (2004) have suggested that autism is "not a disease but a syndrome with multiple nongenetic and genetic causes" (p. 472). Evidence supporting a genetic basis for autism includes the disproportionate ratio of male to female children with autism (approximately 3:1), suggesting an X-linked disorder. The rate of autism in siblings of children with autism is 2 to 8 percent, significantly greater than the rate found in the general population (Chudley et al., 1998). Twin studies have shown that concordance rates for autism ranges from 60 to 91 percent in monozygotic (MZ) twins, and no concordance or no more than 10 percent concordance rates in dizygotic (DZ) twins (Bailey et al., 1995; Jamain et al., 2003; Steffenburg et al., 1989). Further evidence is seen in the high occurrence of conditions such as obsessive-compulsive disorder, communication disorders, and various phobias in family members of children with autism (Hollander et al., 2003; Smalley, McCracken, & Tanguay, 1995). Although discordance rates weaken a genetic hypothesis, evidence for a genetic basis for autism is compelling, and the identification of autism susceptibility genes responsible for the condition is the subject of much research.

> When a clinical condition exists in both members of an identical (monozygotic) twin pair, the condition is called concordant. If only one member is affected, then the condition is discordant.

To date, no specific gene or genes have been conclusively shown to be the cause of autism. In fact, the only pervasive developmental disorder for which a definite genetic basis has been identified is Rett's syndrome, recently discovered to be the result of the mutation of the MeCP2 gene (Amir et al., 1999). A mutation of the FOXP2 gene, recently identified as being responsible for speech and language disorders seen in the KE family, the subject of a longitudinal pedigree study (see Chapter 3), is not found in people with autism (Gauthier et al., 2003; Newbury et al., 2002; Wassink et al., 2002). Single gene mutation can be seen in children with autism who have a genetically based co-occurring condition, such as tuberous sclerosis, but the mutation cannot be said to be a cause of autism. Not all people with tuberous sclerosis are autistic, and the condition presents in only 2 percent of the autistic population (NIMH, 2004).

Researchers have discovered at least 10 genes that may be involved in autism. Potential genes on chromosomes 7, 15, and 17 are under investigation (Muhle, Trentacoste, & Rapin, 2004). It should be noted that in many cases, chromosomes initially identified as possible loci of gene abnormality may not be replicated across studies. Scientists also think that the genetic causes may be heterogeneous—implying that different genes cause autism in different families—and polygenic—implying that multiple genes are involved in any individual (Jamain et al., 2003).

Serotonin is a neurotransmitter affecting a person's mood. It is released and quickly reabsorbed via neural synapse. A selective serotonin reuptake inhibitor (SSRI) slows the reabsorption, thereby elevating levels of serotonin in the brain.

In addition to molecular genetic analysis, reaction to certain pharmacological treatments may provide clues to genetic susceptibility. If a particular drug appears to have a favorable effect on the symptoms of autism, genetic researchers view that as a clue as to where to look. For example, serotonin reuptake inhibitors (e.g., citolopram, fluvoxamine, sertraline) have favorable effects on behavioral symptoms of autism (Hollander, Phillips, & Yeh, 2003). Genetic researchers may, therefore, target the genes that code for receptors or neurotransmitters of serotonin.

Research on structural abnormalities of the brain. Autopsy and magnetic resonance imaging (MRI) studies on the brains of people with autism have yielded some promising and interesting results. Abnormalities have been found in the brainstem, in the frontal lobes, limbic system, and cerebella (Courchesne, 1997; Sokol & Edwards-Brown, 2004). There have been no consistent findings across autistic individuals, however, and no definitive marker of brain abnormalities for autism has been found, although some interesting observations have been made.

Courchesne and his colleagues have conducted retrospective studies, examining hospital records, clinical data, and MRI results in children diagnosed with ASD (Courchesne et al., 2001; Courchesne, Carper, & Akshoomoff, 2003). They have noted an abnormal pattern of head growth, or macrocephaly, during infancy. The pattern described indicated that children with ASD had, on average, a smaller head circumference than typical infants at birth. Head size then increased abnormally rapidly, beginning several months after birth, with a corresponding increase in volume of the cerebral cortex. By middle to late childhood, this accelerated head growth slowed, and by late adolescence, the head circumference of the children with autism was not significantly different from the typical average. This pattern of abnormal head growth has been verified through retrospective studies by several other researchers (Aylward et al., 2002; Bolton et al., 2001; Deutsch & Joseph, 2003; Gillberg & de Souza, 2002).

Macrocephaly is characterized by abnormal largeness of the head and brain in relation to the rest of the body.

Atypical head growth in infants with ASD may suggest several possibilities. First, the pattern of a small head circumference at birth followed by an unusually rapid increase in head size may be an early warning sign of risk for autism. Second, if accelerated head growth in infancy is a diagnostic sign of ASD, very early intervention can be offered and may be helped by the presumed plasticity of the developing brain. Third, if brain abnormality is present at birth, explanations for autism involving factors occurring later in life (e.g., adverse reactions to the MMR vaccination, exposure to environmental toxins, development of gastrointestinal difficulties, etc.) would seem to be unlikely causes.

These are tentative ideas based on unreplicated data. Not all children who have an unusually large head circumference during the early months receive a diagnosis of autism later in life. Conversely, not all children with autism have a history of accelerated brain growth in infancy (Wallace & Treffert, 2004). It has also been argued that a risk factor must precede the condition; macrocephaly may be simply another associated condition and not a cause of autism (Lainhart, 2003).

A better understanding of the causes of autism awaits further research. As we have discussed in other contexts, treatment is generally more effective when a cause is known rather than unknown, but it is still possible to treat communication disorders before their genetic or neurological causes are found.

Language and Communication in Children with ASD/PDD

Generally speaking, verbal children with PDD/ASD exhibit deficits in virtually all types of language skills, including phonologic, semantic, morphologic, syntactic, and, pragmatic skills. In addition, there is one characteristic, echolalia, that appears to be unique to children with PDD/ASD.

Echolalia. Echolalic speech is a hallmark of verbal children with PDD/ASD. **Echolalia** is a speaker's repetition of what has been said, either immediately or in the future, sometimes the far future. While this is a feature that parents and teachers may find irritating and disagreeable, there is some thought that echolalic speech may have a communicative effect on the listener (Prizant & Duchan, 1981). When an adult, for example, asks the child, "Do you want candy?" and the child replies, "Do you want candy?" it could be the child's only way of answering, "Yes!" Experimental research has shown, however, that echolalic responses can be inhibited either by teaching the child another general verbal response, such as "I don't know" (Schreibman & Carr, 1978), or by teaching the child correct responses, incorporating a pause before responding (Foxx et al., 1988; McMorrow & Foxx, 1986; McMorrow et al., 1987).

> Note that echolalia and imitation are similar, but different. Desirable imitative responses follow a model given to prompt that response. Undesirable echolalia is not contingent on a model given to prompt it.

Phonologic difficulties. Verbal children with PDD/ASD can exhibit the same types of articulation and phonological disorders that other children do. Suprasegmental phonologic aspects, however, are often noticeably impaired in atypical ways. Characteristics include:

- *Disordered prosody.* The child's speech might sound "sing-song," monotonous, or may have an inappropriate prosody that has no apparent pattern to it at all.
- *Inappropriate intensity.* The child may whisper or, conversely, shout loudly for no apparent reason.
- *Abnormal patterns of inflection.* The child's inflection may not correspond with the meaning of the sentence; for example, the child might produce a statement with rising inflection (abnormal), instead of a question (normal).

Semantic difficulties. Some children with PDD/ASD may appear to have an impressive vocabulary, particularly in connection with whatever interests they may have. There are, however, often some notable deficits in the semantic aspect of language, including:

- *Decreased receptive language.* The children may have difficulty in following even the simplest one-step direction (e.g., "Touch your nose," "Clap your hands," "Sit down")
- *Faster learning of* concrete *words as opposed to* abstract *words.* It is much easier for children with PDD/ASD to label objects than to label emotions or concepts.

- A *lack of generalization of words and concepts.* Children with PDD/ASD tend to use words in a restricted sense and context (e.g., they may learn that a familiar toy is a *ball* but fail to generalize the label to any other ball—also called underextension).
- A *lack of knowledge of the associations between words.* The children may know the meaning of the words *soap* and *water* but may not understand the relationship between those two words.

One mother decided to allow her high-functioning autistic son to order his own cake for his 11th birthday. He was able to tell the clerk taking his order what cartoon character he wanted on it, the flavor of the cake, and the color of the frosting. When she asked him what he wanted the cake to say, he lost patience. "Are you crazy?" he said. "Cakes can't talk! Just give me that one!" (Gilpin, 1993).

- *Production of idiosyncratic phrases and sentences.* Children with PDD/ASD may create their own ways of remembering to do things or telling others what they want (e.g., one girl was reported to say "Got a splinter!" whenever she was hurt or upset; another boy would let his parents know he needed to use the bathroom by saying, "Rusty zipper . . . yellow socks!") (Gilpin, 1993; Prizant & Wetherby, 1987)
- *No comprehension of figurative language.* Proverbs, idioms, and slang are likely to be taken literally.

Syntactic and morphologic difficulties. Verbal children with PDD/ASD may produce syntactic and morphologic structures that are commensurate with their mental age, with some peculiarities. Characteristics include:

- *Production of short, simple sentences.* Such productions contribute to a prosody that may sound "choppy."
- *Incorrect word order.* Children's word combinations may be unusual (e.g., "Green is her dress," "Now back home go we!").
- *Omission of grammatic morphemes.* Such omissions result in telegraphic, oddly inflected speech.
- *Pronoun reversal.* Substitution of *I* for *you,* and vice versa, is a common feature. Early psychoanalysts saw it as a sign of the autistic child's extreme egocentrism. Now, it is thought that the child's difficulty with abstract language and tendency to produce echolalic speech are more likely the cause of pronoun reversal.

Difficulties with pragmatic language skills. The essential deficit of PDD/ASD is found in the pragmatic aspects of language. It is the autistic child's difficulty with social interaction and pragmatic language skills that most clearly suggest the diagnosis. As previously discussed, there are some marked differences between children with Asperger's syndrome (AS) and children with other diagnoses within the PDD/ASD category, which will be noted. Difficulties include:

- *Absent or fleeting eye gaze.* This is one of the first signs of PDD/ASD
- *Lack of topic initiation.* Children with PDD/ASD are unlikely to seek out conversational partners. Children with AS, however, are likely to insist on initiating conversation with peers and adults when the topic is relevant to their own interests.
- *Lack of topic maintenance.* Children with PDD/ASD may make irrelevant comments during conversation or may abruptly terminate a conversation. Children with AS, on the other hand, maintain a topic of conversation for an inappropriately long period of time, conducting a one-sided virtual monologue regarding their favorite interest.

- *Impaired conversational repair skills.* Both children with PDD/ASD and children with AS seem to be unaware of the needs of their conversational partners for clarification. They do not amend their utterances to fulfill those needs and do not voluntarily seek clarification for themselves.
- *Generally inappropriate speech.* Both children with PDD/ASD and children with AS may produce utterances that are inappropriate to time, place, and person. For example, one Catholic family reported that their high-functioning autistic son shouted out, "Touchdown!" as their priest raised his hands to bless the host during Sunday Mass (Gilpin, 1993).
- *Limited turn-taking skills.* Children with PDD/ASD may interrupt with irrelevant comments and may have no sense of the give-and-take of human discourse. Children with AS in particular may talk incessantly on a particular topic, without inviting a turn from their conversational partners.

This listing is not meant to be used as a diagnostic checklist or even as the most comprehensive description of communicative behavior in children with PDD/ASD. The clinician should, as always, make child-specific observations and not be overly surprised if it is discovered that the child being investigated, while having a diagnosis of PDD/ASD, does not exhibit all of the characteristics described or does exhibit behaviors typically not noted in the literature.

Communication in Nonverbal Children with PDD/ASD

Recall that approximately 50 percent of children with PDD/ASD are nonverbal (Prizant, 1983). Without oral language, these children may attempt to express themselves in inappropriate ways, resulting in severe behavior problems and requiring intervention. In general, children with PDD/ASD who are nonverbal may:

- Tantrum for unexplained reasons, leaving caregivers to figure out what it is they want
- Take an adult's hand and guide it to a desired object or to perform a desired action, such as opening a door that is out of reach
- Scream or make unattractive growling, guttural noises, often suddenly and for no apparent reason
- Strike out physically, harming others and destroying property
- Display various other undesirable behaviors, such as spitting, kicking, biting, or pinching

Behavioral scientists have shown that, when given more socially acceptable ways to communicate, problem behaviors in children with PDD/ASD decrease. We will discuss reduction of undesirable behaviors in more detail in the following section.

Assessment and Treatment Modifications

In general, the child-specific assessment procedures and behavior-based intervention techniques discussed in previous chapters are applicable to children with PDD/ASD. There have been some controversial issues surrounding the administration of discrete trial therapy to children with autism. Arguments have swirled around the amount of time children should spend in discrete trial therapy, fueled by some exaggerated claims of "curing" autism through programs of applied behavioral analysis (ABA; Green, 1996; Lovaas, 1987; McEachin, Smith, & Lovaas, 1993). ABA has been described as "the use of behavior analytic methods and research findings to change socially important behaviors in meaningful ways" (Green, 2005, online). An ABA program includes a component of intense discrete trial training, but also incorporates incidental teaching methods to embed instructional, discrete trials in daily, ongoing activities. Although few children have been "cured" of autism through such treatment, replicated, well-controlled experiments have shown repeatedly that applied behavior analysis with discrete trials is of inestimable value in treating the symptoms of children with autism (Maurice, Green, & Luce, 1996).

Modifications in assessment and treatment procedures are mostly concerned with additional observations that should be made, with the degree of intensity required for early intervention, and with the need to include a plan for management of undesirable behaviors. We will discuss these modifications in the following sections.

Modifications in Assessment Procedures for Children with PDD/ASD

The lack of speech, language, or both is commonly one of the first indications many families have that there may be something wrong with their child's development. Therefore, SLPs are frequently the first professionals to see a child who may have a PDD/ASD, although the diagnosis is best made by pediatricians or psychologists. Clinicians can help by knowing the early signs of PDD/ASD, making a thorough assessment, giving an accurate description of the child's communicative behaviors, and making a referral to other professionals for further evaluation. See Box 13.6 for early warning signs of autism.

Assessment of unique language and communication pattern. The clinician should note the presence or absence of language impairments described earlier. The clinician

---

box 13.6 | **Early Warning Signs of Autism**

Clinicians should be alert to the following early warning signs of autism:

- No eye gaze (reciprocal gazing is typically seen in very young infants)
- No joint reference skills (e.g., looking in the direction a partner is looking; pointing with shifting gaze to direct a partner's attention toward an object) by 6 months
- No turn-taking as evidenced by participation in "baby games" (e.g., responding to parents' vocalizations with a "turn," playing peek-a-boo, etc.)

- Lack of babbling by 12 months
- No gesturing by 12 months (e.g., no waving bye-bye, pointing, etc.)
- No single words by 12 months
- No two-word spontaneous, noncholalic phrases by 24 months
- Loss of language or social skills at *any* age

Source: Compiled from Klin, Volkmar, and Sparrow (2000) and Woods and Wetherby (2003).

should take special note of communication patterns that are unique to PDD/ASD, including echolalic speech, pronoun reversal, incorrect word order, meaningless repetition of speech, inappropriate language, a general disinterest in communicating with others, a lack of reciprocity during social play, obsessive involvement with objects (e.g., spinning the wheels on toy cars, lining up puzzle pieces), and abnormal prosodic qualities (e.g., irregular pitch, pitch that is alternatively too high or too low, erratic rate of speech, wildly fluctuating intensity). In a client-specific assessment, the clinician should carefully note any idiosyncratic production of words, phrases, or sentences.

In some cases, the clinicians may have to observe the child and his or her family on multiple occasions. Observing the interaction between the family members and the child, especially with siblings, may more readily reveal the child's idiosyncratic behaviors.

Prudent use of norm-referenced standardized tests. Clinicians who rely on norm-referenced standardized testing to assess speech and language will find it difficult to assess children with PDD/ASD. Disruptive behaviors, lack of attention, irrelevant responses, and such other characteristics will make it difficult to administer standardized tests. In general, norm-referenced testing is an inefficient and perhaps invalid method of assessing the communicative behaviors of a child with PDD/ASD. If the child can attend to the tasks required by the test, any of the standardized instruments described in Chapter 4 may be used; many high-functioning children with autism may be good candidates for prudently selected tests that provide information in addition to such child-specific procedures as language samples. The clinician who administers traditional standardized speech and language assessment tools should interpret the results with caution as the test scores may or may not represent the child's communicative skills and deficits. There are also some standardized and criterion-referenced diagnostic instruments developed specifically to test children with PDD/ASD; see Table 13.3 for a description of selected tests.

Assessment of problem behaviors. Because some children with PDD/ASD have very severe behavior problems, the clinician should also note the presence of any self-injurious behavior (e.g., head banging, picking at skin, etc.), any aggressive behavior toward people or property, and stereotypical behaviors (e.g., twirling, flapping hands). To make an informal functional analysis of problem behaviors, the clinician should keep a keen eye on antecedent stimuli that appear to trigger the undesirable behaviors and their potential reinforcers. Documenting conditions under which a child behaves inappropriately (e.g., when the clinician asks the child to put a difficult puzzle together) will suggest potential antecedents. An inappropriate behavior that subsides when attention is withheld and increases when attention is paid is sustained by attention as a consequence. Such analyses help reduce the behaviors later during treatment sessions.

Many children with PDD/ASD are minimally verbal or nonverbal. Assessment of the communicative behaviors of children who are nonverbal, including those who have PDD/ASD, will be discussed in Chapter 15 on augmentative and alternative communication.

Sharing assessment findings with families. Diagnostic information suggesting or confirming that the child has PDD/ASD should be given to the family members with sensitivity, with knowledge of the devastation such a diagnosis brings, and empathy for the feelings of family members. Because the diagnosis is best made by other professionals, the SLP may

table 13.3

Assessment Instruments for PDD

Test	Age Level	Administration Time	Description
Asperger Syndrome Diagnostic Scale (ASDS) Myles, Jones-Bock, & Simpson (2000)	5 yrs through 18 yrs	10 to 15 minutes	50 *yes/no* questions designed to determine the likelihood of a child having AS; questionnaire format; standard scores and percentile ranks
Childhood Autism Rating Scale (CARS) Schopler, Reichler, & Renner (1998)	2 yrs and older	5 to 10 minutes	Distinguishes mild-to-moderate from severe autism; criterion referenced, questionnaire format
Differential Assessment of Autism and Other Developmental Disorders (DAADD) Richard & Calvert (2003)	2 yrs through 8 yrs	Will vary	Differentiates among developmental disorders in children; includes developmental disability and learning disabilities as well as PDD
Gilliam Asperger's Disorder Scale (GADS) Gilliam (2000)	3 yrs through 22 yrs	5 to 10 minutes	Distinguishes children with AS from children with autism or other PDDs; questionnaire format
Gilliam Autism Rating Scale (GARS) Gilliam (1995)	3 yrs through 22 yrs	5 to 10 minutes	Identifies autism and estimates severity; standard scores and percentile ranks
Pervasive Developmental Disorders Screening Test-II: Early Childhood Screener for Autistic Spectrum Disorders Siegel (2004)	18 mos and older	10 to 20 minutes	Identifies children at risk for development of PDD as early as 18 months; a parent-report screening measure

simply let the family know a recommendation will be made for further assessment by a psychologist or pediatrician. Any questions the family may have, however, should be directly, but gently, answered.

Most families want to know what the future will hold for their child with a confirmed diagnosis of PDD/ASD. In technical terms, they want to know what the prognosis for improvement will be, and what eventual outcome they can expect to see for their child. Prognosis for improved social and communicative behaviors in children with PDD/ASD is variable, depending on: (1) the presence of developmental disability, (2) the severity of developmental disability, if present, and (3) the level of oral speech and language skills. Children at the high end of the autism spectrum, who have good oral speech and language skills and no developmental disability have a better prognosis for improvement, perhaps even for normalization, than children who are nonverbal with a degree of developmental disability (Coplan, 2000; Szatmari et al., 2000). Obviously, the other, and perhaps the most important, factor affecting prognosis is the quality, intensity, and duration of intervention. As previously discussed, there is no easy answer to the question, "Will my child ever talk?" It has been our experience that if a child is not talking by the age of 5, it is necessary to explore other systems of communication, because oral language is not likely to develop.

It is best for families to know about the probable prognostic indicators and about the likelihood of the development of speech or improvement in existing skills. It is also important to let families know that an intensive program of early intervention is the best way to ensure that their child will develop to his or her fullest potential. Involvement of the family is vital to the success of intervention. Giving parents something tangible and helpful to do for their child will go a long way toward alleviating the shock, denial, and anger most experience on receiving the news that their child has PDD/ASD.

> What are three factors determining prognosis for improvement of social and communicative interaction in children with autism?

Modifications in Treatment Procedures for Children with PDD/ASD

Behavioral methods of teaching target behaviors, including verbal and nonverbal communicative behaviors, to children with autism have received extensive experimental support (Goldstein, 2002; Hegde, 2001b; Maurice et al., 1996; Reichle & Wacker, 1993). Discrete trial therapy has evolved since Lovaas (1987) introduced it as a way of "normalizing" autistic children. Although these children may not be normalized, their general and communicative behaviors improve significantly with discrete trial therapy.

Goldstein (2002) conducted a review of studies on treatment efficacy for procedures designed for children with autism. He found evidence of efficacy established by well-controlled, replicated studies for six broad categories of intervention programs: (1) interventions incorporating discrete trial training formats, (2) communication interventions incorporating sign language, (3) interventions implemented in natural environments, (4) interventions designed to replace challenging behavior, (5) interventions promoting social and scripted interactions, and (6) classroom and parent interventions applied to groups. Most if not all of these procedures are based on behavioral principles. The behavioral principles set forth in Chapters 5 through 9 on treatment can be used with confidence. Some additional considerations in treating children with PDD/ASD are summarized in the following section.

Careful selection of treatment procedures. As noted earlier, autism is a hotbed of new and revolutionary treatment techniques. Consequently, it is especially necessary to have a sophisticated knowledge of treatment efficacy research to accept or reject proposed methods. Clinicians need to employ hierarchical criteria when evaluating efficacy studies on treatment methods for children with autism (see Chapter 5 for a review of a hierarchy of treatment research evidence). The clinicians should consider the overwhelming amount of scientific evidence supporting behavioral principles of intervention; they should consider, also, the lack of evidence for such popular procedures as sensory integration therapy, auditory integration training, and facilitated communication.

Effective use of discrete trials. Discrete trial training is the cornerstone of behavioral intervention for children with autism. Discrete trials are those in which each stimulus presentation, response evocation, and consequence delivery is separated. In essence, attempts at producing target responses are separated by brief time intervals. Treatment is best initiated with discrete trial training to establish communication skills in children with PDD/ASD. Massed trials are especially useful in teaching skills to these children. Discrete trials include such treatment procedures as modeling, prompting, shaping, fading, and differential reinforcement and corrective feedback. Experimental research has indicated that discrete trial training is more

> What is the total communication approach?

effective when incorporated into natural settings (Delprato, 2001; Koegel, O'Dell, & Koegel, 1987). Brief periods of discrete trials, interspersed throughout the day, may be effective in strengthening communicative (and other) target skills at home and in the classroom.

Reducing challenging behavior. Research has shown that behavioral techniques that help increase alternative, competing, or incompatible desirable behaviors tend to have a beneficial side effect of reducing undesirable and challenging behaviors in children with PDD/ASD. Such desirable behaviors replace the desirable behaviors. For instance, strongly reinforcing a child for quiet sitting (instead of continuously admonishing the child for wandering around), will promote quiet sitting which will reduce the incompatible wandering. A boy who throws a temper tantrum because he cannot complete an assigned academic task may be taught to request help from the teacher; a child who requests (and gets reinforced by teacher's attention) is less likely to throw tantrums. In these and other techniques, the new skill taught helps obtain the same consequence (attention, help) that the old undesirable behavior helped attain. Such techniques that replace undesirable behaviors with desirable behaviors make the former unnecessary. These techniques are a part of positive behavior support—a behavioral approach to treating children with problem behaviors with an emphasis on improving their quality of life (Koegel, Koegel, & Dunlap, 1996).

Difficult task demands from the clinician also may increase undesirable behaviors. To control such behaviors, the clinician should gradually increase demands, task complexity, and session durations. Sitting directly in front of the child if necessary, with the child's legs between those of the clinician, may help physically restrain undesirable and distracting movements. In using this procedures, the clinician should gradually move the chairs closer to the table until it is possible to work off the table top. Such indirect methods of reducing undesirable behaviors by differentially reinforcing their counterpart desirable behaviors are described more fully in Chapter 6 and are reviewed in Box 13.7.

Techniques to promote social interactions. Interventions promoting social and scripted interactions, described in Chapter 8, have been shown to be effective in alleviating the social isolation of children with autism. Scripted social interactions help teach social routines to children with autism and peers. For instance, social scripts may describe a shopping trip, cooking, a birthday party, and such other social routines in which different children assume different roles. With the help of the clinician who models and reinforces correct role-playing, children learn social interactions. If the children can read, the use of written cues and prompts for specific actions (e.g., "Sing the birthday song.") will not only help evoke the right actions but also reinforce the children's literacy skills. Such scripts are typically faded as the target behaviors become established (Krantz & McClannahan, 1998; Sarokoff, Taylor, & Poulson, 2001; Thiemann & Goldstein, 2004; see Chapter 8 for a more detailed description of script therapy).

Classroom and parent interventions. Programs designed to help those who interact with children with autism the most in day-to-day routines were shown to increase numerous treatment targets (Goldstein, 2002). Although these programs were too multifaceted to be subjected to tightly controlled research, the benefits reported merited inclusion of these sorts of interventions in Goldstein's list of efficacious treatment methods. Such inter-

| box 13.7 | Review of Indirect Methods of Response Reduction |

Differential Reinforcement of Other Behavior (DRO)

In DRO, an undesirable behavior is targeted for extinction (ignoring), and the clinician reinforces *any other* desirable behavior, as long as the undesirable behavior is not occurring.

Example

A child with autism who screams may be reinforced for any other verbal behavior, as long as there is no screaming.

Differential Reinforcement of Incompatible Behavior (DRI)

In DRI, a behavior that is incompatible with the undesirable behavior is reinforced; most effective when the reinforced behavior is physically incompatible with the undesirable behavior.

Example

A boy with autism who pinches others may be taught to keep his hands in his pockets.

Differential Reinforcement of Low Rates of Responding (DRL)

In DRL, a child is reinforced for exhibiting a lesser rate of an undesirable response; the criterion for reinforcement is gradually reduced, requiring a progressively lesser rate of undesirable response before giving reinforcement. DRL will lessen, but not completely eliminate an undesirable behavior.

Example

A girl with autism who flaps her hands 10 times a minute may be reinforced for when she only flaps 8, 6, 4, and 2 times in that order; the child is reinforced during a period of no flapping, and by pointing out that she flapped only that many (fewer) times in the preceding one minute.

Differential Reinforcement of Alternative Behaviors (DRA)

In DRA, a child is taught a more socially acceptable way of expressing the communicative intent of an undesirable behavior.

Example

A boy with autism who tantrums when he needs to go to the bathroom may be taught the American Sign Language sign for toilet.

---

ventions help parents and teachers learn behavioral management techniques and methods to evoke and reinforce communication skills in naturalistic settings. See Table 13.4 for a listing of some recent efficacy studies on promising techniques for the treatment of autism.

Effective use of the time-delay procedure. In increasing spontaneous initiation of communicative interactions, the time-delay procedure has been shown to be effective (Charlop, Schreibman, & Thibodeau, 1985; Ingenmey & Van Houten, 1991; Matson et al., 1990; Taylor & Harris, 1995). In this procedure, the clinician presents a stimulus to evoke a response but delays the delivery of prompts to encourage the child to ask for something or comment on a situation relatively spontaneously. The duration of the delay may be lengthened gradually until the child produces the response without the prompt. (See Chapter 8 for a more detailed description of the time delay.)

table 13.4

Some Studies of Efficacy of Treatment Methods for Autism

Study	Participants	Method	Treatment Target(s)	Results
Buffington, Krantz, McClannahan, & Poulson (1998)	4 children, ages 4–6 yrs	Discrete trial training (DTT) incorporating modeling, prompting, token reinforcement, and praise	Gestural and verbal responses	Zero baseline; good increases across children and response categories
Charlop, Schreibman, & Thibodeau (1985a)	7 children, ages 5–11 yrs	Time-delay procedure	Requesting objects	Requesting quickly learned and generalized
Hwang & Hughes (2000)	3 preverbal children, ages 32–43 mos	Milieu teaching (MT); contingent imitation, expectant look, natural reinforcers	Eye contact, joint attention, motor imitations	Increases across behaviors and children; good generalization for eye contact, but minimal for joint attention
Koegel, Camarata, Valdez-Menchaca, & Koegel (1998)	3 children, ages 3–5 yrs	DTT; modeling, prompting imitation, reinforcing with desired items	Production of "what's that" questions; nouns	Questions learned and generalized; increased production of new nouns
Sarakoff, Taylor, & Poulson (2001)	2 children, ages 8 and 9 yrs	Scripted conversation	Comments about provided stimuli	Scripted comments were learned; some unscripted comments also produced
Thiemann & Goldstein (2004)	5 children, ages 6 yrs, 8 mos through 9 yrs, 1 mo	Peer training and written text cuing	Securing attention, initiating, and contingent response	Improved social communication; improved peer acceptance and friendship
Williams, Donley, & Keller (2000)	2 children, both 4 yrs	DTT; modeling, prompting, and reinforcement	Three question forms asking about hidden objects	Both children learned all three questions

Effective use of the video modeling technique. Research has documented that children with PDD/ASD who watch videotaped social interactions among their peers learn to exhibit appropriate social skills. The clinician may show videos of normal social interactive play for the children to imitate (Charlop & Milstein, 1989; Charlop, Schreibman, & Thibodeau, 1985b; LeBlanc et al., 2003; Nikopoulous & Kennan, 2004).

Potential use of augmentative and alternative communication strategies. Some children with PDD/ASD may be unable to acquire significant verbal communication skills in spite of best efforts. For such children, augmentative and alternative communication strategies may be appropriate. *Total communication*, in which the child learns to use both a sign language and his or her limited oral communication, may be helpful. Several studies have documented the benefits of sign language training in promoting social communication in children with PDD/ASD (Carr et al., 1978; Layton, 1988; Yoder & Layton, 1988), The clinician may consider other methods of augmentative and alternative communication discussed in Chapter 15.

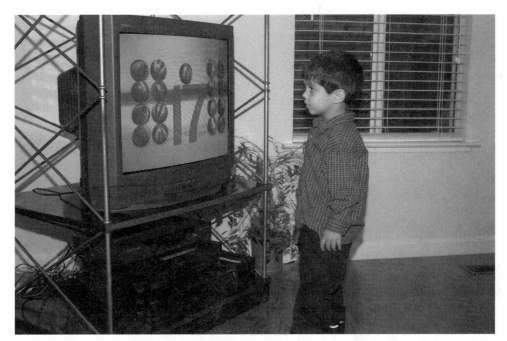

photo 13.2
Children with autism who are fascinated by videotapes may benefit from a technique called video modeling.

Techniques to promote maintenance of targeted behaviors. The variety of techniques described in Chapter 9 to promote maintenance of target language skills in naturalistic settings may be used in treating children with PDD/ASD. In essence, teaching behaviors that are likely to be rewarded in the natural environment, teaching family members intervention techniques, and treating in natural settings have been found to be effective strategies (Derby et al., 1997; Schepis et al., 1982; see Chapter 9 for details). Such naturalistic treatment procedures as milieu teaching (which includes the time-delay procedure described earlier) described in Chapter 8 also help promote maintenance. Programs of parent education that fit into the family's daily routine facilitate teaching throughout the day in natural settings. Such programs help decrease family stress and increase the child's communication (Koegel, 2000; Koegel, Bimbcla, & Schreibman, 1996; Schreibman, Kaneko, & Koegel, 1991).

Chapter Summary

A group of children have such serious and pervasive developmental disorders that they generally form a special diagnostic category. Pervasive developmental disorders (PDDs) are multiple impairments in child development that are typically diagnosed before the age of 3 and include autism, Asperger's syndrome, Rett's syndrome, and childhood disintegrative disorder. Autism is also called autism spectrum disorder (ASD) because, across children, the severity and variety of symptoms vary greatly.

Deficits in social interaction, communication, and stereotypical patterns of behavior, interests, and activities are diagnostic of autism. Children with autism may have sensory problems, seizures, Fragile X syndrome, tuberous sclerosis, and developmental disability. Some children with autism may have exceptionally good skills in specific areas.

Although children with classic autism have IQs below 70, those above 70 who otherwise exhibit certain symptoms of autism are diagnosed with Asperger's syndrome (AS). Children with autism may have much better language skills than those with classic autism, and their developmental disability tends to be less severe.

Rett's syndrome (RS) is a genetically based neurological disorder that predominantly affects females. It is the only PDD that has a known genetic cause. Childhood disintegrative disorder is distinguished from autism by a period of normal development during the first 2 years of life and subsequent deterioration in most skills.

Prevalence of PDD, particularly autism, has been reported to be increasing at an alarming rate; in the United States, what is more often documented is an ever-escalating number of children and families seeking services for autism, which does not necessarily mean that the incidence of autism is on the rise.

Children with autism tend to exhibit echolalia, phonological deficits, semantic difficulties, syntactic and morphologic problems, and severe pragmatic language impairments. Many children with autism have disordered prosodic features marked by inappropriate pitch, intensity, and inflection. Some autistic children, however, may have exceptional vocabularies and good syntactic skills. Unlike other children with language disorders, those with autism may exhibit unusual, idiosyncratic, or even bizarre expressions.

Generally, child-specific behavioral methods for assessment and intervention are applicable to children with PDD. The clinician should be proficient in recognizing early warning signs of PDD, making specific observations relative to symptoms of PDD, and note the presence of problem behaviors.

Behavioral treatment of language and related problems in children with autism has been found to be effective. Among others, discrete trial training, use of sign language, interventions implemented in natural environments, interventions designed to replace challenging behavior with more adaptive behaviors, interventions promoting social and scripted interactions, and classroom and parent interventions are especially effective.

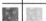 ## Study Guide

1. Discuss the issues related to pervasive developmental disorders (PDDs) versus autism spectrum disorders (ASD). Address the issue of Kanner's autism versus Asperger's syndrome. What conclusions do you draw from the controversy: do you see autism and Asperger's syndrome on a continuum or as separate diagnostic categories? Justify your answer by pointing out similarities or differences between the two diagnostic categories.

2. Summarize the current thinking on the potential causation of autism. Give a historical introduction by way of describing Kanner's views as well as the psychoanalytic views of causation. What evidence do you find in the literature about hypothesized increase in autism rate and the children's vaccines?

3. Critically evaluate the following two contradictory statements: (1) the incidence of autism has increased tremendously in all parts of the world; and (2) only the

demand for services has increased, not the incidence of autism. Examine the historical trends in the diagnosis of autism and Asperger's syndromes, increased public awareness, and increased funding for rehabilitation, along with any factor you might think that has increased the actual incidence of the disorder.

4. A 10-year-old boy with autism has been referred for speech-language treatment. You soon find out that the child exhibits a variety of undesirable, interfering, or destructive behaviors that make it difficult to treat. Drawing from the knowledge you have gained from earlier chapters on decreasing undesirable behaviors by increasing desirable behaviors through differential reinforcement, design a treatment program for this child to reduce such undesirable behaviors as pinching other children, grabbing objects from the clinician or another child, and throwing a temper tantrum when asked to perform a task. Use the technical terms to describe the procedures and point out why they are effective.

5. Describe the most effective treatment procedures that Goldstein (2002) reviewed and supported. What kinds of evidence did Goldstein cite in their favor?

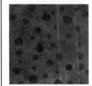
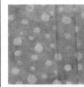

chapter
14

Language Disorders in Three Populations: Children with Traumatic Brain Injury, Cerebral Palsy, and Hearing Loss

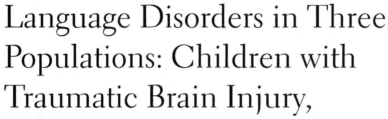

outline

- Children with Traumatic Brain Injury
- Children with Cerebral Palsy
- Children with Hearing Loss
- Chapter Summary
- Study Guide

In this chapter we describe three groups of children who exhibit language disorders associated with some additional problems. (1) children with traumatic brain injury, (2) children with cerebral palsy, and (3) children with hearing loss. We recognize that the three groups of children are distinctly different. We describe them in the same chapter for the sake of convenience and brevity.

For each group, the associated conditions and their causes will be discussed. Typical deficits in language associated with each condition will then be described. Each section will end with suggested modifications in assessment and treatment procedures that may have to be made to meet the unique and complex needs of children with these additional diagnoses

Children with Traumatic Brain Injury

Traumatic brain injury (TBI) is also known as craniocerebral trauma, head trauma, or head injury. TBI, especially when it is serious, causes an immediate medical emergency and results in longstanding disabilities. Children, adolescents, and young adults are especially prone to TBI. Currently, TBI is the most common cause of death and disability among younger populations in almost all societies. Physical and intellectual deficits that result from serious TBI have enormous personal, social, and economic effects on the person and the family. Severe TBI may permanently reduce the earning potential of many individuals. When medical and rehabilitation expenses are added to lost or reduced income throughout a life span, TBI may cost an individual and the family some $5 million or more (Hartley, 1995). The annual cost of caring for persons with TBI may be $25 billion or more (Adamovich, 1997; Bigler, 1990; Benson & Ardila, 1992). Professional care for children (and adults) with TBI includes medical treatment, rehabilitation, and speech-language services.

Traumatic brain injury is injury to the brain sustained by physical trauma or external force. This form of brain injury affects various intellectual and motor skills as well as general behavior. The term *traumatic brain injury* excludes all kinds of neurological diseases that cause brain injury (e.g., cerebral damage from strokes, tumors, infection, progressive neurological diseases, metabolic disturbances, toxic agents, and inherited or congenital conditions).

> What kinds of brain injury are not traumatic?

The terms *head trauma* and *traumatic brain injury* are often equated, but there is a difference. Brain injury almost always involves trauma to the head. A mild head trauma, however, may not damage the brain even though it may damage the facial structures. Cognitive and communicative deficits are more likely to follow significant *brain* injury than mild *head* injury.

Incidence and Prevalence of TBI

Estimates of TBI incidence in children vary mostly because of differences in studies. For example, some investigators include mild injury in their calculations, others do not. Some include TBI in children as well as adults; others include only children and adolescents; while still other investigators include only children. Furthermore, some investigators include only those who sustained

> What is the incidence of TBI in children?

brain injury while others include all who sustained any form of head injury with or without brain injury. Finally, some investigators may not count those who did not survive brain trauma while others may count them as well (Kraus & McArthur, 2000). In children, the incidence of TBI is estimated at 200 per 100,000 children with a mortality rate of 10 percent (Weiner & Weinberg, 2000). In the general population, suggested incidence figures are as high as 367 per 100,000 persons. Childhood leukemia is a major cause of death in children, but death due to TBI is 10 times higher. Annually, about 1 million children receive emergency treatment in hospitals and about 165,000 of them are hospitalized. More than 20,000 of them exhibit moderate to severe cognitive and physical symptoms needing extensive rehabilitation services, although many may not receive such services.

Several risk factors for TBI are well established. For instance:

> Another age group highly prone to TBI is the elderly. Among those who are 75 or older, the incidence of TBI is 3,000 per 100,000.

- *Age.* Adolescents and young adults in the age group of 15–24 have a very high prevalence rate of TBI. The prevalence is the highest for the age group 15–19 years (400 to 700 per 100,000, depending on the study).
- *Gender.* Boys are more likely to experience TBI and are more likely to die from it.
- *Living conditions.* TBI incidence is relatively high among people living in high-density urban areas and low socioeconomic status (Hartley, 1995).
- *Ethnocultural factors.* TBI is possibly more common in African Americans and Hispanics than in Whites. Head injury due to assault, gunshot wounds, and other forms of violence may be higher in ethnic minorities living in poor inner cities (Payne, 1997).
- *Time.* Most injuries are suffered between noon and midnight when children are likely to be out of school and engaged in various kinds of activities.
- *Setting.* TBIs occur most frequently on roads and in homes.

Causes of TBI in Children

There are a variety of causes of TBI in children. Some causes are longstanding, while others are relatively new. Some are specific to certain societies, others are universal. Some causes are found across all age groups, while others are more common in children. According to the National Pediatric Trauma Registry of Tufts-New England Medical Center (www.nemc.org/rehab/factshee.htm) and various other sources, the most common causes of TBI in children include:

- *Falls.* The most frequent cause, falls, account for more than a quarter of all TBIs (26 percent). Falls from stairs, high furniture (chairs, stools), balconies, and out of windows are the most common.
- *Automobile accidents.* Children as occupants of automobiles are exposed to the second most frequent cause of TBI. About 19 percent of TBI are due to automobile crashes. Up to 77 percent of children who suffer TBI due to auto accidents will not have worn seat belts or will not have been seated in protective car seats. Unrestrained children are tossed around in the vehicle or thrown out of the window.
- *Pedestrian injury.* This is the third leading cause of TBI in children. Children sustain TBI because vehicles crash into them while they are crossing the street, playing or walking on the sidewalk or street, or when they simply dart into a street.

- *Bicycle riding.* Falls from a bicycle due to various reasons (e.g., hitting stationary objects) or being hit by other vehicles while riding are significant causes of TBI in children.
- *Social and family violence.* Intentional and incidental violence cause severe TBI. TBI in 10 percent of children was due to gunshot wounds or stabbing. While a majority of these injuries are intentional, others are incidental in that the injured children are bystanders.
- *Child abuse.* Another form of intentional violence, child abuse, a class by itself, is often called inflicted brain trauma or injury. Hitting the child in the head is a frequent form of childhood abuse causing TBI. Another form of abuse, the shaken baby syndrome (also called inflicted childhood neurotrauma), is violent, intentional, repetitive, and unrestrained shaking of the child resulting in rapid acceleration-deceleration of the head, causing brain injury as well as other forms of injury (e.g., retinal hemorrhage), most typically in children younger than 3 (Forbes et al., 2004).
- *All-terrain vehicle accidents.* A relatively new cause of TBI and more common in some western societies is the use of all-terrain vehicles and consequent accidents. In the United States, the frequency of TBI due to all-terrain accidents is on the increase. More males than females are injured, and one third of all-terrain vehicle accidents involve children (Carr et al., 2004).
- *Sports-related injuries.* In one study, 87 percent of all sport-related pediatric injuries were to the head and neck (Schalomon et al., 2004). In addition to such sports as football, basketball, and baseball, downhill skiing, ice skating, skateboarding, and other sports all contribute to TBI. One study reported that TBI was the leading cause of child deaths in downhill skiing accidents (Xiang, Stallones, & Smith, 2004).
- *Farm-related injuries.* Accidents involving agricultural machinery is yet another cause of TBI in children (Smith et al., 2004). Accidents causing TBI may be related to animals (often involving horses) or farm machinery (e.g., riding on tractors that roll over).
- *Domestic accidents.* Various kinds of accidents that occur in homes can cause TBI in children. Accidental discharge of guns, dangerous toys that cause facial and head injuries, fireworks-related accidents, and misuse of power tools and machinery (including riding on lawn mowers) are among the more common domestic accidents that can cause pediatric TBI.

As children increase their use of motorized toys, more head injuries may be expected. Although no specific data exist, motorized scooters (two wheelers) have recently been reported to cause many injuries to children. Although falls are a leading cause of TBI and death among children, the combined incidence of TBI due to vehicular accidents (including auto accidents, pedestrian accidents, bicycle accidents, and all-terrain crashes) exceeds that due to all other single causes. A majority of TBIs that are due to vehicular accidents are preventable as only a small number of children involved in them will have used protective devices (e.g., seat belts, helmets).

Neurological Effects of TBI

The neurological effects of head trauma vary depending on the severity of the trauma, the type of trauma, the rate at which the force is applied, and several other factors. Two types of injuries are often evident: penetrating and nonpenetrating.

Penetrating injuries are those in which the skull is fractured, meninges (brain coverings) are torn, and the brain tissue is damaged. There is an open wound in the head, thus these injuries are also known as open head injury. Bullets, knives, nail guns, and so forth that penetrate the head cause this type of injury. Fragments of penetrating objects (e.g., bullets, glass pieces) may be lodged in the brain. Some penetrating brain injuries are fatal. Neurological effects of penetrating brain injuries in surviving individuals include an immediate increase in the intracranial pressure, fluctuating blood pressure, reduced cerebral blood flow, destruction of brain tissue, subsequent infection, swelling of the brain, physical disabilities (e.g., paralysis or weakens of limbs), sensory deficiencies (e.g., defective vision), intellectual (cognitive) deficits, and communication problems.

Nonpenetrating injuries are those in which no foreign bodies or particles enter the brain; the meninges remain intact; and the brain is damaged with or without skull fracture. Accidents, falls, blunt blows to the head, and various forms of child abuse (including the shaken baby syndrome) tend to create nonpenetrating injuries. Because there is no open wound in the head, nonpenetrating injuries are also known as closed head injury.

> Is it possible to have brain damage with an intact skull?

Acceleration-deceleration injuries and nonaccelerating injuries are the primary consequences of nonpenetrating head injuries. **Acceleration-deceleration injuries** are those that are caused by initial violent movement of the head and the subsequent slowing down; these are caused by forces applied to a movable head. The head that receives the impact of a moving object will first receive an impact trauma (trauma at the point of contact with the external force or object). Injury to the brain tissue at the point of impact is called the **coup injury.** But more critically, as the head begins to move violently, the brain inside the skull also will move forward or backward (depending on the direction of impact). When the head movement slows or stops, the brain inside still moves and crashes against the inner and opposite side of the skull, causing **contrecoup injury** (pronounced *contra-coo*). Thus, the coup injury occurs at the point of impact and the contrecoup injury at the opposite side of the brain. **Nonacceleration injuries** are those that are caused by forces applied to a fixed (immovable) head. A blow delivered to the head of a child who is lying on a hard surface, for instance, will cause a nonacceleration injury. There is little or no movement (acceleration or deceleration) of the head and the brain in such cases.

> Where do coup injuries occur? Where do contrecoup injuries occur?

A serious neurological consequence of acceleration/deceleration forces of nonpenetrating brain injury is **diffuse axonal injury** (DAI), which consists of torn nerve fibers in widespread areas of the brain. Patients who survive severe TBI and remain in vegetative states have extensive DAI of the long neural tracts throughout the hemisphere or hemispheres. Other effects of head trauma include **diffuse vascular injury** (ruptures in the brain's blood vessels) causing bleeding in the brain, **brain stem injury,** often resulting in coma, and primary focal lesions, which cause localized and restricted brain tissue damage.

There are many secondary consequences of TBI, which occur sometime after the trauma was sustained. These include pooling of blood in the brain or in the skull (intracranial or intracerebral hematoma), accumulation of blood in the space between the brain and the skull (epidural hematoma), death of brain tissue for lack of blood (ischemic brain damage), seizures, and infection.

Neurobehavioral Effects of TBI

Traumatic brain injury changes a child's general behavior. Some treatment modifications that SLPs need to make in working with children who have sustained TBI are related to their behavior disorders. Initially, TBI causes altered levels of consciousness. With mild injury, a child may simply be **dazed** (reduced awareness of the surrounding) and recover soon. More severe injuries may cause **stupor** (the child is unresponsive except for pain and strong stimuli) or **coma** (unconscious and unresponsive). Following TBI or following the regaining of consciousness, most children will be confused and disoriented to time and place. They may experience headache, blurred vision, dizziness, lethargy, and mood changes and mood swings. Impulsive behavior and some aggressive behaviors also may characterize children with TBI. The children also may exhibit socially inappropriate behavior.

> Of daze, stupor, and coma, which is the most serious condition?

Cognitive impairment is a common feature of children with TBI. A particularly disabling problem is loss of memory, especially for events just preceding and following the trauma. Children with TBI experience memory problems mainly associated with either reduced level of consciousness or a state of excessive arousal, called **delirium.** More or less subtle memory problems may persist, however. Other aspects of cognition affected in children with TBI include reasoning and problem solving skills. These children do not think of steps to be taken in solving a problem, fail to recognize missing or inconsistent information, do not anticipate difficulties in solving a problem, and generally fail to approach problems in ways that are useful. It is thought that when the frontal lobe is injured, planning, reasoning, and task execution functions are negatively affected.

Other neurobehavioral symptoms children are likely to exhibit include swallowing problems (dysphagia), seizures, vomiting or nausea, weakness or numbness of the extremities, loss of balance or coordination, restlessness, and agitation. Some children may cry persistently and refuse to eat. Difficulty concentrating on external events and stimuli is a common consequence of TBI. Such attention deficits affect the child's communication. A few children, as they come out of coma or a state of confusion, may experience hallucinations (false sensory experiences as seeing things that do not exist) and delusions (thoughts not based on reality as the false belief that someone is going to hurt them).

> Families often find behavioral changes to be the most difficult factor in learning to cope with residual effects of a child's TBI.

Recovery from TBI

TBI in a child is an insult to a developing brain. There has been some debate whether children with TBI recover more easily and more fully than adults. Many investigators have argued that they do because of their brain plasticity. Presumably, a growing brain can better handle injury than a fully developed brain. Uninjured portions of the brain can take over the functions of injured brain.

More recent investigators have questioned this traditional line of reasoning. Although longstanding effects of mild TBI is less well understood, moderate to severe brain injury in children, even when the skills seem to recover, may leave permanent and subtle effects on complex and abstract skills. Their academic performance may suffer in subtle ways. Therefore, it is prudent to continuously evaluate a child for possible deficiencies and offer professional help as needed. Contrary to earlier beliefs, some studies suggest that in mortality rates associated with automobile accidents, children do not fare better than adults (Johnson & Krishnamurthy, 1998).

Speech and Language Disorders Associated with TBI

The SLP, while taking into consideration the neurological and behavioral symptoms of the child, is especially concerned with the speech and language problems that follow TBI. The general effects of brain injury complicate language disorders. Depending on the severity of the injury, the clinical picture of children with TBI changes over time. Their communication skills, too, change as they either recover from their TBI or experience neurological deterioration.

An initial communication problem associated with TBI is a speech disorder known as **dysarthria,** a complex set of communication problems due to impaired neural control of muscles involved in speech production. Dysarthria affects all aspects of speech production: respiration, articulation, rate of speech, prosody or rhythm of speech, voice quality, and resonance. Another form of motor speech disorder, apraxia of speech, also may be associated with TBI. **Apraxia of speech** is a motor planning disorder in the absence of muscle weakness. Apraxia is evident when the child cannot position articulators correctly for speech production even though there is no muscular problem. Scientific and clinical literature on motor speech disorders is extensive and will not be reviewed here as we are more concerned with the treatment of language disorders associated with TBI. See Box 14.1 for a primer on dysarthria and apraxia.

> Is there muscle weakness or paralysis in apraxia of speech?

---

box 14.1   **A Primer on Dysarthria and Apraxia of Speech**

Dysarthria and apraxia of speech are motor speech disorders. In dysarthria, there is impaired neural control of the speech muscles. The speech muscles may be paralyzed or weakened. In apraxia, there is no muscle paralysis or weakness, but there is impaired planning of motor movements involved in speech production—more a central than a peripheral problem.

Roughly 30 to 35 percent of patients with TBI exhibit dysarthria. As a result of TBI, the child may have limited breath support for speech. Production of consonants may be imprecise, resulting in partly or mostly unintelligible speech. The stress patterns in speech may be abnormal. The rate of speech may be slow. The child may speak with monotonous pitch. Speech loudness may be limited. The child may exhibit hypernasality. The voice may be hoarse or harsh in quality.

Because the speech muscles are weak or paralyzed, nonspeech movements (smiling, chewing, swallowing) may also be affected.

As a result of TBI, children may exhibit apraxia of speech, which is characterized by inconsistent and variable errors in articulation of speech sounds, especially on consonant clusters; presumably due to a failure to plan the movements needed to produce speech, not a difficulty in actually moving the articulators. The speech attempts are typically described as groping; transposition or reversal of phonemes (e.g., saying "maks" for *masks* or "soun" for *snow*); addition of phonemes (e.g., saying "clat" for *cat*); and prolongation or repetition of speech sounds. Pure apraxia is rare. A child with TBI may show a combination of symptoms characteristic of both dysarthria and apraxia of speech.

Brain injury in adults is a significant cause of **aphasia,** a loss or impairment of language skills. The incidence of aphasia in children with TBI is very low. Many aphasic symptoms may be seen in the acute stage of TBI. However, as the child's general status improves, most aphasic symptoms tend to disappear. A few aphasic symptoms (e.g., word finding problems) may persist, however.

> Aphasia is diagnosed in older individuals who have had a history of normal language but lose it to varying extents because of a recent brain injury. The term is not used in cases of children who sustain TBI.

Language disorders associated with TBI are less remarkable than the neurobehavioral symptom complex. However, if the child sustains moderate to severe TBI before language acquisition is complete, then that acquisition may be slowed. Unfortunately, systematic studies of language acquisition in children with TBI are lacking. Therefore, statements about language acquisition in such children are extrapolated from other sources. Possibly, the child is likely to learn new words and new sentence forms more slowly than other children. The child's vocabulary may consist of simpler and more concrete words. The child may have marked difficulty in learning complex and abstract words, expressions, idioms, and proverbs. The child's acquisition of grammatic elements may be slowed. Understanding of spoken language may be limited or impaired. This difficulty in speech comprehension may be due partly to the child's attentional deficits, however. The child may have difficulty concentrating on what is said.

Soon after the trauma, a few children may exhibit a transitory muteness (total lack of speech). The most significant language problems of children with TBI are likely to be pragmatic, however. Their language difficulties tend to be more global than what are seen in children with specific language impairment (SLI), described in Chapter 3. Because TBI produces significant neurobehavioral problems, the child's overall interaction with people and

> What notable language problems are associated with TBI?

events is affected to an extent that is not found in children with SLI. Therefore, the language problems of children with TBI are more appropriately described as an overall communication problem.

Pragmatic language problems are typically evident in social dialogue. Children with TBI may be somewhat impulsive (disinhibited), inattentive, and may fail to use gestures that normally accompany communication. In the early stages of the trauma, the disoriented child may make irrelevant, bizarre, inappropriate, incoherent, and confused comments. As the child improves, these problems may subside. Word finding problems may persist for longer durations, however. Because the child cannot produce the specific words, the language productions may be imprecise, marked by circumlocutions (e.g., "beating around the bush"), filled with interjections (*uhs* and *ums*), word and phrase repetitions, and long pauses. The child may fail to initiate conversation; may speak only when spoken to. When somehow conversation is initiated, the child may fail to take turns during conversation and interrupt speakers. A failure to maintain topics of conversation may be a notable deficiency in children with TBI. Narrative skills may be severely affected as well. The child may tell a story with no regard for temporal sequence, and the narration itself may be sparse and impoverished. Once again, most of the pragmatic language impairment may be due to the child's inattention.

> Review Chapter 2 for details on pragmatic language problems.

> What might account for most of the pragmatic language problems a child with TBI may have?

A child who has mastered grammar before the TBI will generally retain it. Purely linguistic deficits (e.g., ungrammatical sentence productions) are not as frequent as pragmatic language problems described. In spite of retained syntactic structures, the child does not communicate effectively because of the neurobehavioral effects of the TBI (e.g., memory loss, impulsive behavior, and inattention).

Modifications in Assessment Procedures for Children with TBI

In assessing language disorders in children with TBI, the clinician can use most of the procedures described in Chapter 4 (on assessment). All procedures previously described, however, may need modifications to a lesser or greater extent to fully understand and treat children with TBI. Generally, in assessing children with TBI, the following special considerations or procedural modifications are needed (Bigler, Clark, & Farmer, 1997; Blosser & DePompei, 1994; Gillis, 1996; Hartley, 1995; Hegde, 2001a; Mira, Tucker, & Tyler, 1992).

See Chapter 4 for general procedures of assessment.

Assessment as a team effort. Assessment of children with TBI is a team effort. Unlike those who exhibit SLI, children with TBI experience a complicated set of neurological, behavioral, and communicative problems. This requires the services of medical specialists, psychologists, physical therapists, speech-language pathologists, and other specialists, depending on the symptom complex of the child. The SLP should develop his or her assessment plans in consultation with other specialists.

Obtaining information on the premorbid status of the child. The case history and the interview, in addition to the standard format, will especially be structured to obtain information on the status of the child before the trauma. The child's premorbid health, general development, social and communication skills, cognitive skills, and academic performance (when relevant) will be of great concern. This information is essential to help evaluate the degree of change in the child's skills subsequent to the trauma.

Review of reports from other specialists. Before developing an assessment plan, the clinician should review the most current reports of other professionals. The medical condition will have a significant effect on assessment procedures. For example, if the medical reports suggest that the child is still confused and disoriented, the communication assessment will have to be limited and brief. Medical records help clinicians understand the severity of the child's injury that may affect the current behavior and the extent of expected recovery. Among others, the results of traditional radiological tests, computed scanning of brain structures, and neurological examinations will help determine the extent of injury and the immediate consequences the child will have suffered. Reports from psychologists, physical therapists, nursing staff, and other specialists on the team will give additional and relevant information on assessment and treatment planning.

Bedside examination and interview. A brief observation of the child at his or her bedside will help establish the extent to which the child is oriented and the degree to which he or she can be expected to participate in assessment procedures. Simple questions like "What is your name?" "How old are you?" "What time is it?" "What day is it?" "Where are you?" and so forth help establish orientation and attention. This bedside examination will also note whether the child has motor deficits that may limit participation in assessment procedures. The clinician can then select assessment procedures that suit the child and his or her present behavioral dispositions.

Standardized testing. Very few tests have been standardized for children with TBI. Some tests help assess the general state of the patient, such as awareness and consciousness, regardless of age. Clinicians may modify test items to suit the needs of children and clinically evaluate the results of such testing without reference to test norms. In every case, the clinician should critically evaluate the test standardization sample, and its reliability and validity. Generally, careful and systematic observation may often result in more reliable results than the administration of standardized tests. Because of confusion and attention deficits, children may not perform to the extent they can on some of the standardized tests. As always, client-specific procedures are preferable. Tables 14.1 through 14.3 list a sample of selected standardized tests designed to evaluate a variety of speech, language, and cognitive skills.

Integration of information. As the final step in assessment, the clinician should integrate information from different specialists to get a comprehensive view of the strengths and the limitations of not only the child, but also of the family. This integrative report will clearly describe the communicative performance of the child, physical and cognitive limitations that are still present, prognosis as suggested by other professionals, and prognosis for communication training. The assessment report will suggest potential language treatment targets and strategies.

Modifications in Treatment Procedures for Children with TBI

In treating children with TBI, such procedures as selection of client-specific targets, modeling, shaping, differential reinforcement, corrective feedback, and so forth described in the chapters in Part II will be essential. A description of some special treatment considerations

table 14.1

Assessment Tools for Attention and Memory

Test	Age Range	Description
Children's Auditory Verbal Learning Test—2 Talley (1995)	6 yrs, 6 mos through 17 yrs, 11 mos	Assesses presence and level of severity of memory impairment in children
Detroit Tests of Learning Aptitude—Fourth Edition Hammill (1998)	6 yrs through 17 yrs	Offers 10 subtests on skills such as sentence imitation, word sequences, and story sequences
Goldman-Fristoe-Woodcock Test of Auditory Discrimination Goldman, Fristoe, & Woodcock (1978)	3 yrs, 8 mos through adult	Assesses skills in speech sound discrimination
Mental Status Checklist—Children Dougherty & Schinka (1992)	5 yrs through 12 yrs	Assesses psychological difficulties and helps plan for treatment
Wide Range Assessment of Memory and Learning, Second Edition Sheslow & Adams (2002)	5 yrs through adult	Assesses memory including immediate and delayed recall

table 14.2

Assessment Tools for Academic Achievement

Test	Age Range	Description
Differential Ability Scales Elliott (1990)	Preschool: 2 yrs, 6 mos through 5 yrs, 11 mos School age: 6 yrs through 17 yrs, 11 mos	Measures cognitive abilities and academic achievement
Kaufman Assessment Battery for *Children, 2nd ed.* Kaufman & Kaufman (2004)	3 yrs through 18 yrs	Measures cognitive skills including sequential and simultaneous information processing
Kaufman Test of Educational *Achievement—II* Kaufman & Kaufman (2004)	4 yrs, 6 mos through 25 yrs (comprehensive) 4 yrs, 6 mos through adult (brief)	Assesses strengths and weaknesses in reading, spelling, and mathematics
Peabody Individual Achievement Test— *Revised—Normative Update* Markwardt (1998)	5 yrs through 22 yrs, 11 mos	Measures academic achievement
Woodcock Language Proficiency *Battery—Revised* Woodcock (1991)	2 yrs through adult	Measures of oral language, reading, and written language; includes English and Spanish forms

and procedural modifications follows (Bigler, Clark, & Farmer, 1997; Blosser & DePompei, 1994; Gillis, 1996; Hartley, 1995; Hegde, 2001b; Mira, Tucker, & Tyler, 1992).

Treatment is a team effort. Treatment plans for children with TBI should be developed in consultation with other specialists, including medical and medical rehabilitation specialists, psychologists, occupational therapists, and physical therapists. How other specialists manage their tasks will affect the work of speech-language pathologists. For instance, how the medical team manages the physical symptoms and how the neuropsychologists manage the behavior problems may affect communication treatment. A child whose confusion and disorientation is better controlled, or whose impulsive and aggressive behaviors are reduced, will be more productive in all kinds of rehabilitation programs, including speech and language treatment.

Inclusion of family members and teachers. Treatment of children with TBI is not only a specialist-team effort, it also is a family effort as the behavior of these children affect the lives of all in the family. Family members should be involved in selecting treatment targets and should take part in treatment sessions. They may offer suggestions on selective familiar and effective stimulus materials for treatment. The family members may also know about potential reinforcers that may be used in treatment. By observing and taking part in treatment sessions, the family members may learn to control the undesirable behavioral effects of TBI and to promote productive behaviors, including communication skills.

In an educational setting, including the child's teachers in the treatment plan is essential. The clinician should seek suggestions from the teachers on target skills that may be especially useful in attaining academic success. Ways of integrating language and academic

table 14.3

Assessment Tools for Speech and Language Skills

Test	Age Range	Description
Frenchay Dysarthria Assessment Enderby (1983)	12 yrs through adult	Designed to provide a differential description and diagnosis of dysarthria
Peabody Picture Vocabulary Test (3rd ed.) Dunn & Dunn (1997)	2 yrs, 6 mos through adult	Receptive language: point-to-picture task
Pragmatic Communication Skills Protocol Academic Communication Associates (2004)	3 yrs through 11 yrs	Assesses various pragmatic language skills, including expressing feelings, requesting information, maintaining conversational topics; nonstandardized
Test for Auditory Comprehension of Language—Third Edition Carrow (1973)	3 yrs through 9 yrs, 11 mos	Assesses receptive skills in understanding word classes, grammatical morphemes, and sentence structures
Test of Language Development—Primary	4 yrs through 8 yrs, 11 mos	Subtests include oral vocabulary and grammatic understanding
Test of Language Development—Intermediate Newcomer & Hammill (1997)	8 yrs, 6 mos through 12 yrs, 11 mos	Subtests include sentence combining and correcting "silly" sentences (malapropisms)
Test of Word Finding—2 German (2000)	4 yrs, 4 mos through 12 yrs, 11 mos	Both tests assess picture naming (nouns and verbs), sentence completion naming, and other word finding skills
Test of Adolescent/Adult Word Finding German (1990)	12 yrs through adult	
The Token Test for Children DiSimoni (1978)	3 yrs through 12 yrs	A screening measure of receptive language dysfunction
The WORD Test—R Huisingh, Barrett, Bowers, LaGiudice, & Orman (1990)	7 yrs through 11 yrs, 11 mos	Six subtests assessing expressive and receptive knowledge of associations, synonyms, and other skills
The WORD Test—Adolescent Bowers, Huisingh, Barrett, Orman, & LaGiudice (1989)	12 yrs through 17 yrs, 11 mos	Four subtests assessing expressive and receptive knowledge of synonyms, definitions, and other skills

goals may be discussed with the teachers. Teachers may further enhance generalized production of language skills by prompting and reinforcing the skills the clinician teaches.

Management of problem behaviors. Various problems behaviors that interfere with language treatment is a special consideration. Children with TBI are likely to be distracted, easily fatigued, impulsive, and uncooperative during the early stages of treatment. To make the treatment sessions productive, the SLP should have a clear grasp of procedures to reduce undesirable and interfering behaviors. Generally, extinction (ignoring) and differential reinforcement of desirable behaviors instead of only corrective feedback for undesirable behaviors will be effective. Teaching alternative, desirable behaviors that replace the undesirable behaviors are known to be effective (Carr et al., 1994; Koegel, Koegel, & Dunlap, 1996). Several brief treatment sessions spread across a day may be more effective than one or two long sessions. Relatively longer sessions should have frequent breaks. Also, holding the treatment sessions in a quiet and distraction-free room will help reduce undesirable behaviors.

> Review Chapter 6 for procedures to reduce undesirable behaviors.

Working with other members of the TBI management team. To make communication treatment more effective for the child, the SLP should work closely with other members of the TBI management team. For example, if the child is drowsy during treatment because of a prescription drug, perhaps the physician will be willing to reduce the dosage administered before communication treatment. Similarly, the SLP may request the psychologist to design a program to reduce the uncooperative behaviors, increase the child's attention span, and so forth. Conversely, the clinician may give suggestions to other specialists on effectively prompting and reinforcing communicative behaviors. In the initial stages of rehabilitation, the clinician may design a simple communication board the child can use while interacting with all specialists on the team.

Dynamic treatment targets that change over time. A necessary treatment modification for children with TBI is the changing nature of treatment targets. A few grammatical errors that may be initially noted are not immediate treatment targets, although they may be if they persist. Linguistic accuracy is not important in treating children with TBI, especially in the early stages. Effective communication with whatever the means is the most meaningful initial treatment target. The clinician may encourage expression through gestures, signs, pointing, nodding, blinking, words, phrases, sentences, or any other creative means to get the messages across. As the child's medical condition improves, progressively more complex oral language skills may be targeted for treatment. In the later stages of treatment, including literacy skills in language intervention might be especially helpful in the school setting.

The special relevance of treating pragmatic language skills. Teaching conversational skills is the most important aspect of language treatment. Coherent and relevant expressions, initiation of conversation, maintenance of conversational topics, turn-taking during discourse, and narrative skills should be the treatment targets. Ignoring irrelevant comments, prompting correct responses as soon as a question is asked (e.g., "What is today? *Today is Thurs. . . .*") may help reduce irrelevant or impulsive responses.

Shaping of skills. Starting with what the child can do and moving on to progressively more difficult tasks is especially important in treating children with TBI. The child can easily get frustrated and start exhibiting undesirable or uncooperative behaviors if the treatment task demands are too difficult. Therefore, shaping is the technique of choice in the initial stages of treatment. Chapter 6 describes the shaping procedure.

Minimizing corrective feedback and maximizing positive reinforcement. If the brain injury is severe to profound, the clinician may need to use primary reinforcers (food and drink) to motivate the child. Such reinforcers are used in the initial stages of treatment and faded as the child's correct response increase and stabilize. As noted in Chapters 5 and 6, primary reinforcers should always be paired with secondary reinforcers (e.g., verbal praise) so that the clinician can eventually fade the former and keep the response rates high with only the latter.

Integrating cognitive skill training with communication training. Instead of spending time exclusively on cognitive skills, the clinician can more efficiently integrate them into communication training. For instance, instead of trying to improve attention by such tasks as cancellation of letters or geometric shapes that do not fit a pattern printed on a sheet (a nonfunctional attention task), the clinician may reinforce good attending behavior during communication training. The clinician may reinforce the child for quiet sitting, looking at the stimulus pictures used in communication training, and for progressively longer durations of sustained work.

Training others to accept all means of communication. Teaching parents, other care givers, siblings, peers, and teachers to accept any means with which the child can communicate will result in immediate improvement for the child. Parents and teachers may not immediately recognize the importance of gestures and signs in a child who communicated with complex verbal expressions. However, for a child recovering from TBI, any means of communication is an improvement and in some cases, an achievement. Family members, peers, and teachers should be taught to accept and applaud such efforts from children with TBI. Such training of significant others also will help promote maintenance of target behaviors in natural settings.

Alternative and augmentative communication skills. Assessing whether a child with TBI needs an augmentative and alternative system of communication is an ongoing concern. If the child has sustained severe brain injury, and has made little progress on regaining oral communication under a systematic training program, then the possibility of teaching augmentative or alternative forms of communication should seriously be considered. Chapter 15 describes various options and strategies for minimally verbal or nonverbal children who need augmentative and alternative forms of communication.

> See Chapter 15 for details on alternative and augmentative communication.

Community reentry programs. A program designed to have the child reenter his or her former environment with as much of normal skills as possible reinstated is a special feature of treating a child with TBI. The child may have been in a hospital-based rehabilitation program for a long duration; the child may have been in and out of a hospital frequently and for too long. Such a child's reentry to the community (e.g., the home and the school) may be fraught with anxieties and uncertainties for both the child and the family. In spite of the best rehabilitation efforts, the child may have sustained moderate to severe TBI and may be left with significant residual deficits in intellectual, adaptive, and communicative skills. Therefore, how, when, and with what special assistance the child can go home and reenter school need to be planned with the help of family members and educators. Depending on the residual disabilities, the home and the child's classroom environment may have to be restructured to support the child. See Box 14.2 for suggestions on helping the child succeed at home and school.

Children with Cerebral Palsy

Children with cerebral palsy are another group in whom language disorders are part of a larger clinical picture involving neurological impairment. The term is a misnomer as its literal meaning is *paralysis of the brain*. **Cerebral palsy** refers to a complex set of

> True or False? Cerebral palsy is a progressive neurological disease.

box 14.2 **Suggestions on Helping the Child with TBI Succeed at Home and School**

To design a program to return the child with significant residual disabilities, the SLP (and the team of specialists treating the child) should:

- Make a thorough assessment of the child's residual deficits and needed environmental modifications along with support systems before discharging the child from clinical services.
- Counsel both the family members and teachers to support effective communication through whatever the means, but especially with the means of clinically established skills. Depending on the child's need, for instance they may be asked to (1) talk slowly and in simpler and shorter sentences while addressing the child; (2) emphasize or repeat key words; (3) repeat instructions, give them in writing as well, ask the child to repeat the instructions; (4) model or prompt correct responses, provide manual guidance, offer visual cues; (5) define all new terms, give examples, illustrate them concretely by showing pictures or drawings; (6) give extra time to respond; (7) give background informa-

tion on topics of discussion; (8) make special efforts to include the child in interactions; and (9) reinforce such conversational skills as topic initiation, turn-taking, and topic maintenance.

- Counsel both the family members and teachers to redesign the living and learning environment to support the child. The clinician may ask them to: (1) reduce visual and auditory distractions for the child; (2) eliminate physical barriers for the child with limited mobility; (3) teach and reinforce the use of such special learning devices such as calculators and computers that help learning; (4) encourage the child to keep his or her belongings in a specific place; (5) teach the child to consult notes, directions, instructions, and so forth before implementing a task; (6) read slowly to the child and ask frequent questions to test understanding; (7) offer manual guidance in writing; and (8) provide for any special seating arrangements in the class to help child stay focused on the teacher.

neuromotor and developmental disorders caused by an injury to a still developing nervous system. Cerebral palsy is not a disease, but only a name for a group of symptoms. The condition is not progressive; in fact, children improve as they grow older (Koman, Smith, & Shilt, 2004; Mecham, 1996; Yorkston et al., 1999). Sometimes, cerebral palsy is considered a part of the developmental disability, described in relation to mental retardation in Chapter 12.

In the United States, the incidence of cerebral palsy is variously reported to be 1.5 to 3 per 1,000 children, with a more commonly suggested figure of 2.5 per 1,000 children (Cans et al., 2004; Dabney, Lyston, & Miller, 1997; Koman et al., 2004; Yorkston et al., 1999). As such, it is a relatively common childhood disability, requiring extensive, and in some cases lifelong, special care. Medical treatment and various kinds of rehabilitation of individuals with cerebral palsy is expensive; the estimates range from 8 to 11.5 billion dollars annually (Centers for Disease Control and Prevention, 2004; Koman et al., 2004). The lifetime medical and rehabilitation expense of one individual with cerebral palsy approaches $1 million.

Causes of Cerebral Palsy

Although often described as a congenital disorder, cerebral palsy is not always evident at the time of birth or soon after birth. Neurological deficits may become evident only after many months after birth; it may be diagnosed anytime during the first two years of life. Some studies have included children up to age 10 in calculating the prevalence of CP (Yeargin-Allsop et al., 1992). Strictly congenital conditions are caused by prenatal factors (causes that affect a fetus) or perinatal factors (causes that affect the delivery of a baby). Multiple factors cause cerebral palsy; they include prenatal, perinatal, and postnatal factors, along with a few other risk factors not easily classified. Postneonatal cerebral palsy is found in 1.26 per 10,000 live births (Cans et al., 2004). Although many potential causes are known, causes may not be clear in some 40 percent of children with cerebral palsy.

A congenital disorder is diagnosed at, or soon after, birth.

Prenatal factors are negative variables a pregnant woman experiences which cause brain injury in the unborn child and lead to cerebral palsy. These include:

- Maternal rubella
- Maternal infections (e.g., mumps, influenza)
- Maternal anemia
- X-ray and radiation
- Maternal anesthesia
- Maternal involvement in automobile and other accidents

Perinatal factors are negative variables a baby is exposed to, which in turn cause brain injury to the child during the process of birth and lead to cerebral palsy. These include:

- Prolonged labor
- Breach delivery

Postnatal factors are negative variables that cause brain injury in a child during his or her first two (or more) years and lead to cerebral palsy. These include:

- Anoxia (lack of oxygen to the brain)
- Traumatic brain injury, mostly automobile accidents resulting in brain injury in the child; about 18 percent of cases are due to traumatic brain injury
- Infections and diseases including mumps, scarlet fever, measles, whooping cough, meningitis, and encephalitis; these diseases cause 50 percent of cases with postnatal causes
- Lead and mercury poisoning (the latter being controversial)
- Vascular diseases, including strokes; these are uncommon in children, but they do occur; about 20 percent of children with postnatal cases may have vascular causes

Other risk factors that are associated with cerebral palsy include:

- Premature birth; there has been an increase in the incidence of cerebral palsy among prematurely born children, presumably because of improved care that has reduced mortality (but not disability)
- Low birth weight
- Multiple births

Neuromotor Effects of Cerebral Palsy

Impaired posture and movement are the two main neurological effects of cerebral palsy. In different children, cerebral palsy results in different patterns of neuromotor problems. These patterns of symptoms give rise to four major types of cerebral palsy.

- *Spastic cerebral palsy.* Increased muscle tone is spasticity. Rigidity or stiffness of the muscles is the dominant symptom of **spastic cerebral palsy**. This is also the most common type; about 70 percent of children with cerebral palsy have spasticity. Because the opposing muscles are simultaneously active, the movement is awkward, rigid, jerky, and stiff. Damage to upper motor neurons, which are motor fibers that lie within the central nervous system, causes spastic cerebral palsy.
- *Athetoid cerebral palsy.* Slow, involuntary, and writhing (worm-like) movements are called athetosis. Hands, arms, and feet are affected the most; face and tongue may be affected in some, causing speech problems. Posture is often affected. Damage to the basal ganglia and its connections is the typical cause of **athetoid cerebral palsy**.
- *Ataxic cerebral palsy.* Balance disorders are called ataxia. The main symptoms of **ataxic cerebral palsy** include impaired balance, stumbling and awkward gait, and clumsy and uncoordinated movements. The muscles may lack tone (flaccidity). Damage to the cerebellum, which controls balance and coordination, causes ataxic cerebral palsy.
- *Mixed type of cerebral palsy.* About 25 percent of cases have **mixed type of cerebral palsy**. Both spasticity and athetosis may be present in the same child, although typically one or the other will be the dominant symptom. Extensive brain damage produces the mixed type.

Paralysis and paresis are two characteristics of abnormal muscles. **Paralysis** implies muscles that cannot be moved. **Paresis** is muscle weakness, and paretic muscles can move, although inefficiently and with reduced strength. In cerebral palsy, paralysis or paresis may affect various parts of the body. See Box 14.3 for common types of paralysis and paresis.

A neurologically significant and diagnostic feature of children with cerebral palsy is the persistence of some primitive reflexes that are mediated by the brainstem. Primitive reflexes are all present at birth in full-term babies but they disappear after the first 6 months or become increasingly difficult to elicit. For instance, sucking is a primitive reflex elicited by touching the lips of an infant; this reflex may persist in children with cerebral palsy. Another persistent primitive reflex is flexion of the fingers when the palm is scratched.

> At what age do primitive reflexes tend to disappear?

---

box 14.3   Types of Paralysis or Paresis

Paralysis or paresis may be found in one or both sides of the body and only in like parts (e.g., legs only or arms only). The common types of paralysis and paresis include:

- *Diplegia.* Paralysis or paresis (muscle weakness) that affects like parts on both the sides of the body (e.g., either two legs or two arms). About 33 percent of children with cerebral palsy may have diplegia.
- *Hemiplegia.* Only one side of the body (either the right or the left) is affected. Some 13 percent of children may have right hemiplegia and 10 percent may have left hemiplegia.
- *Paraplegia.* Only the lower extremities (lower trunk, including legs) are affected.
- *Monoplegia.* Only one limb is affected.
- *Quadriplegia.* All four limbs are affected. Diffuse brain injury causes quadriplegia. Forty percent or more of children with cerebral palsy may have quadriplegia.

Persistence of these and other reflexes help make an early diagnosis of cerebral palsy (Zafeiriou, 2004). Another neurological feature that helps make an early diagnosis in an infant is muscle hypotonia, which is lack of muscle tone.

Additional Problems Associated with Cerebral Palsy

As noted before, cerebral palsy presents a complex and varied set of symptoms. In addition to neuromotor symptoms, children with CP exhibit:

- *Developmental disability.* Up to 30 percent may be developmentally disabled.
- *Hearing loss.* Some 13 percent may have hearing loss; middle ear infection is common in children with cerebral palsy.
- *Visual impairments.* Between 20 and 40 percent may have visual-perceptual problems.
- *Learning disabilities.* Most children may exhibit some limitation in academic performance. Most severely involved children may have significant learning disabilities.
- *Seizures.* About 35 percent experience seizures.
- *Distractibility.* Children with cerebral palsy may have a short attention span and difficulty in controlling their response to varied stimuli. This feature is likely to contribute to the children's learning disabilities in school.
- *Emotional problems.* Emotional instability or overreactivity is common, as also are frequent episodes of emotional upsets.
- *Breathing abnormalities.* Because of weakness in the muscles of respiration, the child's breathing may be effortful, noisy, or tensed; as can be expected, these abnormalities affect speech production.

Speech and Language Disorders Associated with Cerebral Palsy

Depending on the extent of brain injury, communication disorders in children with cerebral palsy are variable across children. While some may only have a mild communication disorder, others may have a significant disorder involving both speech production and language skills. Technically, cerebral palsy, being a motor disorder, should affect only speech production. The clinical literature on speech disorders in children with cerebral palsy is more extensive than that on language disorders. Children with cerebral palsy also may have language disorders, however. This is mainly because of such associated clinical conditions as developmental disability and hearing loss that cause difficulties in language learning. We will only give a brief description of speech disorders associated with cerebral palsy as our emphasis in this book is language disorders.

Speech disorders are dominant communication problems in children with cerebral palsy. As noted before, dysarthria is a characteristic of speech in children and adults who have sustained brain injury and as a consequence have motor deficits. Children with cerebral palsy, therefore, are likely to exhibit dysarthria (see Box 14.1). Estimates of the prevalence of dysarthria in associated with cerebral palsy vary from a low of 31 percent of children to a high of 88 percent (Yorkston et al., 1999). Obviously, the greater the severity of the neuromotor deficits is, the higher the likelihood of dysarthria. Children with cerebral palsy are likely to exhibit articulation disorders

Is dysarthria a functional disorder?

characterized by jerky, effortful, and irregular speech with reduced intelligibility. These children may have a pronounced difficulty in producing tongue-tip sounds. In addition, the speech characteristics of children with cerebral palsy include weak voice, reduced loudness and unpredictable variations in loudness, monotone, and breathiness in some cases. Children with cerebral palsy are also more likely to stutter than are those without it.

As noted, there is little systematic research on the language characteristics of children with cerebral palsy. However, because of developmental disability and hearing loss in many such children, their language acquisition is likely to be delayed. There is no strong evidence that the language disorders associated with cerebral palsy are unique, requiring special treatment procedures. Language disorders, when present, are likely to involve the same features that were described in Chapter 2. Limited vocabulary, slow learning of new words, omission of grammatical morphemes, production of simpler sentences, difficulty understanding or producing complex sentence forms are likely features. In addition, children who do show language problems are likely to exhibit deficiencies in conversational speech. Such pragmatic skills as topic initiation, topic maintenance, narration of personal and objective events, request for clarification, and appropriate response to requests for clarification from listeners are all likely to be impaired to varying extents. The same difficulties may be found in children with developmental disability without cerebral palsy.

> Does cerebral palsy produce a unique type of language disorders?

Modifications in Assessment Procedures for Children with Cerebral Palsy

Assessment of children with cerebral palsy requires a team of specialists. The team may consist of speech-language pathologists, neurologists, pediatricians, orthopedic surgeons, physical therapists, occupational therapists, audiologists, otorhynolaryngologists (ear, nose, and throat specialists), psychologists, ophthalmologists and optometrists (vision specialists), medical social workers, and so forth. The child's medical problems have to be constantly monitored and managed.

The overall goal of assessment is to make a functional analysis of child's communication skills, self-help and other daily living skills, social behavior, and academic demands and performance. As a member of the team of specialists, a speech-language pathologist makes a communication assessment to develop and implement a treatment program. In a school setting, the clinician will work closely with the classroom teachers and special education specialists working with the child.

There are no special language tests designed to exclusively assess children who have cerebral palsy and a suspected language disorder. Therefore, the clinician will use the procedures described in Chapter 4. Standardized tests and client-specific procedures, including language samples, will be useful.

A description of some of the needed special considerations or procedural modifications needed in assessing children with cerebral palsy follows (Hegde, 2001a; Mecham, 1996; Yorkston et al., 1999).

Investigation of potential factors associated with cerebral palsy. In addition to obtaining standard information about the child, the case history and the interview will be especially concerned with the maternal health during pregnancy, child delivery and reported difficulties associated with it, prematurity, birth weight, child's early motor development, difficulties in swallowing, parental concerns about the child's hearing, and speech and language development. It is a common practice to establish prenatal, natal, and postnatal risk factors that the child may have been exposed to.

Review of assessment reports from other professionals. Prior assessment and treatment reports from other professionals will help assess the extent of new assessment needed and will help guide the selection of procedures. Medical records, especially from the child's pediatrician, neurologists, and orthopedic specialists will be particularly helpful. Prior diagnoses of developmental disability, hearing loss, or both will help alert the clinician to the presence of speech and language disorders. Frequent and prolonged hospitalization also may suggest a possible language disorder, even if it is temporary.

Integration of information from different specialists. To get a comprehensive view of the neuromotor, general medical, and speech-language status of the child along with associated deficits (e.g., hearing loss or developmental disability), the clinician should integrate information from different specialists. The clinician should gain a good understanding of the strengths and the limitations of not only the child, but also of the family.

Modifications in Treatment Procedures for Children with Cerebral Palsy

Children with cerebral palsy are candidates for various kinds of orthopedic surgery to correct postural and movement disorders. Improvement of muscle strength and range of motion through physiotherapy, braces, electrical stimulation of muscles, and a combination of these and other methods will be a priority (see Photo 14.1 for an example of adaptive equipment).

Children with cerebral palsy need a comprehensive communication training program. They need treatment for both speech and language disorders. In treating these disorders, the clinician should incorporate such evidence-based treatment procedures as modeling, shaping, differential reinforcement, corrective feedback, and so forth described in the chapters in Part II. A summary of some of the special considerations in treating children with cerebral palsy follows (Hegde, 2001b; Mecham, 1996; Yorkston et al., 1999).

Integrating communication training with educational programs. The SLP needs to work closely with the regular teachers and special education specialists in devising and implementing a communication training program. Similarly, including parents and other family members in treatment is necessary for the success of a child with cerebral palsy. As with all other children, the clinician should consult with the family members and educators before finalizing a list of target skills to be taught. The language targets selected for the child should help enhance academic success of the child.

Consultation with other specialists. Frequent consultation with other specialists, including orthopedic surgeons, physical therapists, psychologists, and special educators will help improve the child's performance in communication training. For example, physical therapists may have suggestions on postural adjustments for the child. A child with significant

photo 14.1

Professionals, such as physical therapists and occupational therapists, part of the professional team, can provide special adaptive equipment, such as this stander, for children with cerebral palsy.

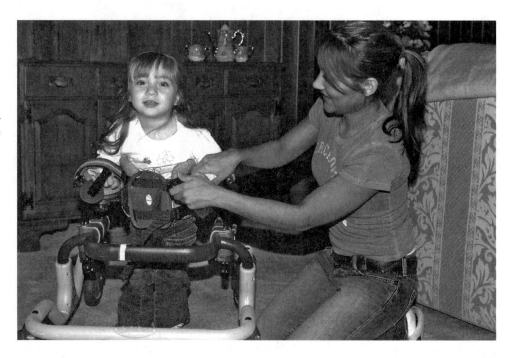

Review Chapter 6 for procedures to reduce undesirable behaviors.

neuromotor problems may have difficulty in sitting quietly during treatment sessions. Physical therapists may have designed procedures or mechanical aids (e.g., braces) to stabilize the child's posture and may suggest strategies for muscle relaxation to improve functioning. Adopting such techniques during communication training might be necessary for conducting the treatment sessions effectively and efficiently.

Use of techniques to reduce unwanted and interfering movements.   Uncontrolled movements elsewhere in the body of a child with cerebral palsy may affect speech muscles and speech production. The clinician should use techniques or devices that have been recommended to control such unwanted movements during communication training. For example, a chin strap may reduce uncontrolled movements of the jaw. Just holding the hand may control its slow, writhing movements. Such measures may have a noticeable effect on speech production (Mecham, 1996).

Attention to significant swallowing, chewing, and drooling problems.   To achieve success in communication training, it is necessary to devise programs to reduce swallowing, chewing, and drooling problems some children with cerebral palsy exhibit. It is within the scope of practice of SLPs to address these types of feeding and oral issues, although specialized training is required. Unless trained in swallowing therapy, the speech-language pathologist should refer the child to an SLP who is competent in it.

Effective communication, not necessarily grammatic accuracy.   With children who have multiple handicaps including severe to profound developmental disability, effective and functional communication, rather than grammatical accuracy, is the most functional treatment target. As with children who have TBI, the clinician may encourage expression through gestures, signs, pointing, nodding, just blinking, words, phrases, sentences, or any other means to achieve functional communication. Parents and teachers also may be asked to accept and reinforce such functional communication attempts from the child.

Integrating literacy skills with language training. Working closely with the classroom and special education teacher, the speech-language pathologist may integrate reading and writing skills into speech and language training. Including written stimuli along with pictorial stimuli to be used in language training will be a good start. See Chapter 10 for various ways in which communication training and literacy training may be combined.

Candidacy for augmentative and alternative communication training. Some children with severe cerebral palsy and multiple associated disabilities may make only minimal progress in oral communication training sessions. Such children may be considered for augmentative and alternative communication training. These children may be trained to use simple communication boards or more complex electronic devices as described in Chapter 15. The child must be thoroughly evaluated for such candidacy to maximize the use of an augmentative or alternative communication (AAC) device within the context of the child's neuromuscular limitations. See Chapter 15 for a more thorough discussion of evaluating a child's physical capabilities when selecting an appropriate AAC device.

Children with Hearing Loss

Children with hearing loss form another special group for whom language assessment and treatment procedures need to be modified. This is also a varied group with different degrees of hearing loss and different types of loss. A hearing level of 25 dB HL or higher in adults and 15 dB HL or higher in children who are still learning their language suggests hearing loss (Alpiner & McCarthy, 1999; Hull, 2001; Martin & Clark, 2003).

> Hearing loss is measured in terms of decibels. A decibel is $1/10$ of a Bell, a basic unit of sound energy, named after Alexander Graham Bell. Hearing level (HL) is the lowest intensity of a sound that the human ear can detect.

Congenital hearing loss (i.e., hearing loss present at birth) has the most significant effect on oral language acquisition. Hearing loss acquired after the acquisition of language or during adulthood has relatively little effect on communication, although individuals in this category may need amplification (e.g., hearing aids) to functional effectively in social situations. The incidence of congenital hearing loss is not known precisely; studies suggest hearing loss in 1 to 6 in 1,000 newborns (Cunningham & Cox, 2003; Kemper & Downs, 2000). About 1.2 percent of children with disabilities who receive special services in schools have hearing loss (U.S. Department of Education, 2002).

The term *hearing loss* includes all individuals with reduced hearing acuity. People with hearing loss may be further classified into two categories based on the severity of their loss: the hard of hearing and the deaf. Individuals who are **hard of hearing** have reduced hearing

> The degrees of hearing loss are classified as: *Mild:* 16–40 dB HL; *Moderate:* 41–70 dB HL; *Severe:* 71–90 dB HL; and *Profound:* 90+ dB HL.

acuity but nonetheless acquire oral language primarily by hearing the language spoken around them. As children, they learn language mostly like hearing children do. Depending on the severity of the loss, the hard of hearing may use a hearing aid and speechread (lip read) to understand some of the spoken language. The **deaf** are individuals whose hearing loss is severe to profound and who cannot use their residual hearing to acquire oral language. Deaf children more naturally acquire sign language than oral language, and most deaf individuals cannot benefit from amplification (e.g., hearing aids).

Typical oral language acquisition requires adequate hearing sensitivity. Regardless of the varied theories of language acquisition, a universal observation is that children learn to speak the language they hear. If they cannot hear well or hear at all, oral language learning may be delayed or severely disturbed. In this context, an issue of importance is that language may be nonoral, as in the case of American Sign Language (ASL), which is a fully developed language with its own syntactic rules. As mentioned earlier, deaf children acquire sign language with relative ease. Therefore, we do not mean to say that deafness prevents language acquisition per se; we only mean that it may prevent or impair the acquisition of oral (spoken) language. In fact, many people who are deaf point out that, in communities where ASL is produced, their disability is minimized to the extent that it becomes insignificant. They therefore consider themselves to be a part of a separate culture—the Deaf culture, with a capital *D*—by virtue of their nonoral language.

> The Deaf consider themselves a cultural group and deafness a natural state, not a problem.

An issue of importance is that the Deaf, who consider ASL their natural and complete form of communication, may reject oral forms of communication. A sound position for SLPs is to consider it the parents' right to seek whatever intervention they wish for their child with hearing loss.

If the parents seek oral forms of communication with or without other means (e.g., amplification, cochlear implants) for their child, speech-language pathologists should offer their services. The rest of this section should be understood in this context.

Hearing Loss: Types and Causes

Types of hearing loss have differential effects on language learning and social communication. Hearing loss is classified according to the location of pathology (cause) within the auditory system. See Box 14.4 for a brief description of the auditory system.

The common classification includes three types of hearing loss, each with a different set of causes:

- *Conductive hearing loss.* Sound is normally conducted through the outer and middle ear into the inner ear (cochlea). In **conductive hearing loss,** efficiency of this sound conduction is reduced. In essence, the cochlea does not receive all of the sound energy that enters the outer ear. It may be congenital or acquired after birth. Causes include deformities of the ear canal including atresia (partially or fully closed ear canal), swelling, and bony growth that obstruct sound conduction; impacted cerumen (ear wax); foreign objects in the ear canal; perforations (ruptures) or thickening of the tympanic membrane (ear drum); fixation of the small, normally vibrating bones of the middle ear; and middle ear infections.

- *Sensorineural hearing loss.* Hearing loss due to damage to the cochlea is called **sensorineural hearing loss.** The cochlea contains both sensory hair cells and the nerve cells that pick up the sound and carry it to the brain. Cochlear damage, therefore, produces

| box 14.4 | | **A Brief Description of the Human Auditory System** |

The human hearing mechanism consists of the ear, the auditory nerve, and parts of the brain that receive and interpret auditory stimuli. It starts with the outer ear, with two parts: the pinna and the external auditory meatus, which is a 2 to 3 cm canal that secretes wax and ends at the eardrum (tympanic membrane). The middle ear begins at the tympanic membrane, which is thin, elastic, and cone shaped; it vibrates when sound waves strike it. Past the tympanic membrane lies a chain of three small bones (ossicular chain): the malleus, one end of which is attached to the tympanic membrane; the incus, which is attached to malleus; and the stapes, which is attached to incus at one end. The other end, or foot, of the stapes is inserted into the oval window, a small opening in the bone that houses the inner ear. The sound vibrations of the ear drum are transferred to the ossicular chain. The middle ear is connected to the nasopharynx (part of the back throat that opens into the nasal passage) by way of the auditory tube.

The inner ear is a system of interconnected tunnels called labyrinths in the temporal bone. The tunnels are filled with a fluid called perilymph. The inner ear contains two functionally separate systems. One, the vestibular system, consists of semicircular canals and is responsible for balance. The other, the cochlea, is a coiled structure filled with a fluid called endolymph and is responsible for hearing. The cochlea contains several thousand hair cells that respond to sound waves. The inner ear receives the sound waves though the stapes, the foot of which is attached to the inner ear. The cochlea is also the place where the auditory branch of the acoustic nerve (cranial nerve VIII) terminates and carries the sound to stimulate the primary auditory area of the brain, housed in the temporal lobe.

The Human Ear

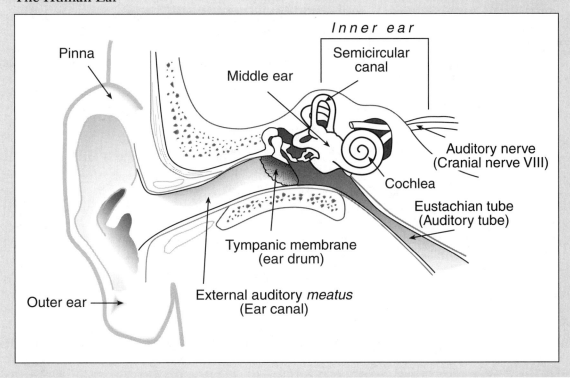

hearing loss that is both sensory and neural. This type of hearing loss also can be congenital or later-acquired. In some cases, sensorineural loss may have a genetic basis as it runs in certain families. A symptom of many genetic syndromes is sensorineural hearing loss. Among others, maternal rubella, alcohol abuse (resulting in fetal alcohol syndrome), drug addictions, acquired immune deficiency syndrome (AIDS), herpes infection (cytomegalovirus) are prenatal causes of sensorineural hearing loss in infants. Anoxia (oxygen deprivation during birth) and any kind of head trauma during birth may be a natal cause in some children. Postnatal causes (all causes that operate after the child is born), include head injury that affects the cochlea, certain antibiotic drugs prescribed to children (e.g., streptomycin and others of the "mycin" family of drugs), certain cancer drugs, meningitis (inflammation of the layers that cover the brain), acoustic trauma (sudden exposure to damagingly loud sound or prolonged exposure to harmful noise), degeneration of the cochlea due to excessive X-ray, childhood mumps, and Mènière's disease.

> Mènière's disease is characterized by dizziness, vomiting, and sensorineural hearing loss.

- *Mixed hearing loss.* When both the middle ear and the inner ear do not function normally, the result is called **mixed hearing loss.** Causes of mixed hearing loss include a combination of those that are associated with conductive *and* sensorineural hearing loss.

Air is the medium of sound conduction through the outer and middle ear. However, the sound also sets the bones of the skull into vibration. This vibration may be felt by the cochlea; therefore, sound is also conducted by bone. Thus, air and bone conduction are the two ways of sound conduction. They are differentially affected in conductive and sensory neural hearing loss. In conductive hearing loss, only the air conduction of the sound is affected; the bone conduction is normal. Conductive hearing loss, therefore, is never as profound as sensorineural loss. A damaged cochlea, which causes sensorineural loss, cannot respond to bone vibrations.

> Which type results in the more profound hearing loss—conductive or sensorineural?

Factors That Affect Language Learning

Roughly 28 to 30 percent of children with oral language disorders also may have a moderate to severe hearing loss (Douniadakis et al., 2001). Although normal hearing is critical to oral language acquisition, the severity of language disorders found in children with hearing loss depends on several factors. In other words, the same degree of hearing loss does not produce the same effects in all children. Among others, the major factors that affect the level of oral language skills are:

- *The degree of hearing loss.* Although two children with the same level of hearing loss may have different language skills, generally, the higher the loss, the greater the severity of language disorders. Generally, profound sensorineural loss produces the most damaging effects on oral language acquisition.
- *The time of onset of hearing loss.* A congenital hearing loss has a greater effect on language learning than the one that is acquired sometime during, or after, language

acquisition. The later the onset of hearing loss, the less severe the effects on communication skills.

- *The time at which the hearing loss was detected.* The earlier the detection of hearing loss, which is followed by prompt and effective services, the better the language skill compared to late detection. Of course, early detection that is not followed by effective intervention may produce no desirable effects (Yoshinaga-Itano, 2003; Yoshinaga-Itano et al., 1998).

- *The time at which the intervention was initiated.* As implied in the previous bullet, the earlier the intervention, the better the language skills. Infants who receive language stimulation acquire better language skills than those who receive it much later Yoshinaga-Itano, 2003; Yoshinaga-Itano et al., 1998).

- *The quality of intervention programs.* Intervention may be more or less effective; therefore, just early intervention may not make a significant difference. A sustained and effective intervention program may produce better language skills than weak, ineffective, or intermittent intervention.

- *Family involvement in intervention.* Parents who are more actively involved in intervention and who work regularly with the child at home according to the recommendations of specialists will see better language skills in their child with hearing loss than those who are not similarly involved.

- *Educational programs in schools.* Educational programs that emphasize oral communication and continue to offer oral language treatment to children in the schools may promote better oral language skills in children with hearing loss than those in which such skills are deemphasized.

Otitis Media and Language Learning

Often mild and sometimes fluctuating conductive hearing loss due to middle ear infection (otitis media) is common in children. By their third birthday, some 75 percent of children will have had at least one episode of otitis media (National Institute on Deafness and Other Communication Disorders, 2002). Average hearing loss due to otitis media across children is about 20–25 dB, although it can be as high as 50 dB in some cases. Hearing loss of any severity may be found in 50 percent of children who have otitis media with ear discharge (Balbani & Montovani, 2003).

What is a common cause of fluctuating hearing loss in children?

Whether conductive hearing loss during the first 3 years of life has a significant negative effect on speech and language learning has been debated. Although research is extensive, the evidence is contradictory. While some early studies suggested negative effects of otitis media on later language learning, more recent studies suggest only a weak effect (See Casby, 2001; Roberts, Wallace, & Henderson, 1997; Shriberg et al., 2000 for review of studies).

Clinicians evaluating a child with a history of otitis media should take into consideration the degree of loss and the duration of the disease. A more severe hearing loss associated with a persistent and prolonged otitis media may be considered a risk factor for potential speech-language delay. Children with such a history may be evaluated more thoroughly for potential effects on communication skills.

Hearing Loss and Communication Disorders

Hearing loss affects all aspects of communication, not just language skills. It affects speech production, voice quality, and overall fluency of oral expression. Therefore, the SLP working with children with hearing loss should understand their speech, language, voice, and fluency disorders.

Speech and language disorders associated with hearing loss are mostly due to two problems. First, the children cannot fully hear the speech sounds and language structures produced around them. Therefore, they are trying to learn something they have heard only partly or not at all. Second, children with hearing loss cannot monitor the speech they themselves produce because of lack of the immediate feedback hearing provides. Hearing speakers constantly monitor their speech production, their syntactic structures, voice quality, and fluency. The voice of speakers with hearing loss is usually high-pitched, and lacking typical intonation; it tends to be hypernasal, although hyponasality also may be a problem. Because of lack of self-monitoring, children with hearing loss make errors in all aspects of speech and language production.

Speech and Language Disorders Associated with Hearing Loss

Children with hearing loss have difficulty learning to produce the speech sounds of their language. Consequently, intelligibility of their speech may be limited. Speech disorders commonly associated with hearing loss include the following:

- Omission of initial and final consonants in words; omission of /s/ in most word positions
- Omission of consonants in blends
- Substitution of speech sounds (e.g., substitution of voiced sounds for unvoiced; nasal for oral; some vowel substitutions)
- Distortions of most speech sounds, especially of stops (/t/ and /d/) and fricatives /s/, /z/, /θ/, /tʃ/, and /ʃ/
- Imprecise production of vowels with increased durations with breathiness before their productions
- Addition of sounds
- Atypical flow and rhythm of speech
- Limited fluency of speech

Some children with unilateral hearing loss (loss only in one ear) may also experience some difficulty learning speech and language skills. Up to a third of them may repeat grades and need special education assistance (Lieu, 2004).

Hearing loss in children does not produce a unique type of oral language disorder. With minor variations, these children tend to make the same errors as those without hearing loss. Language disorders associated with hearing loss include the following:

- A *slow rate of language learning*. The overall rate is slow, even though the sequence is roughly the same.
- *Smaller than the normal vocabulary*. Children with hearing loss do not learn new words as fast as those with normal hearing.
- *Limited comprehension of language*. Children with hearing loss tend to have difficulty understanding the meaning of unusual words, abstract words, and multiple meanings

of words; they have difficulty understanding proverbs, simile, irony, slang, and other forms of language usage; they may interpret proverbs and slang expressions literally.

- *Slower acquisition and improper use of grammatic morphemes.* Children with hearing loss tend to omit grammatic morphemes including the plural and possessive inflections, the present progressive *-ing,* tense markers, auxiliaries and copulas, conjunctions, and prepositions; many of these are perhaps not predominant (e.g., the plural -s may be produced softly) in speech, and therefore, the children with reduced hearing acuity do not hear them. Present progressive *-ing* may be somewhat easier for them to learn than other grammatic morphemes. Consequently, their speech consists mostly of nouns, giving it a telegraphic quality.
- *Difficulty learning verb forms.* Verbs are also difficult for children with hearing loss. Missing present progressive *-ing,* regular past tense inflections, and so forth make their verb usage inappropriate. The children may have a pronounced difficulty with tense inflections and the third person singular present tense inflection as in *walks* or *reads.*
- *Limited syntactic skills.* Syntactic structures that are difficult to learn for hearing children also are difficult—only to a greater extent—for children with hearing loss. Children with hearing loss tend to produce relatively simple sentences. Production of complex, compound, and embedded sentences may be limited. Passive sentences (e.g., "The ball was hit by the boy.") and negative passives (e.g., "The ball was not hit by the boy.") are especially difficult as are clauses that are embedded (e.g., "The girl *who could not see* still scored very high."). The present perfect tense (e.g., *have written*) also is especially difficult for children with reduced hearing acuity.
- *Somewhat limited pragmatic language skills.* Children with hearing loss generally do well on certain pragmatic language skills while showing deficiencies in others. Verbal expressions of these children may include gesture, facial expressions, vocalizations, and formal or informal signs as those of hearing children. Children with hearing loss take conversational turns well and maintain conversation. Nonetheless, these children may have difficulty initiating conversation (especially in educational settings) and responding appropriately to requests for clarification when listeners fail to understand them. In response to such requests, children tend to repeat what they just said, instead of modifying their expressions (Most, 2002).
- *Reading and writing problems.* The deficiencies the children with hearing loss show in oral language are reflected in their reading and writing skills. Their reading comprehension of complex and abstract material may be limited. Deaf students who graduate from high school have only, on average, a fourth-grade reading competence (Paul, 2001). In writing, they tend to omit many grammatic morphemes. Simple sentences, a limited variety of sentences, concrete vocabulary, and grammatical errors characterize their writing.

Amplification and Implants: Electronic Aids to Language Learning

Historically the standard method of helping children acquire oral language is to amplify sound so the hearing mechanism with reduced acuity can hear the sounds, including speech. **Hearing aids** that amplify sound are still the main rehabilitation device for most children with hearing loss. A variety of powerful and progressively smaller (hence inconspicuous) hearing aids are now available. See Box 14.5 for a primer on hearing aids. Most children the SLPs work with to increase their oral language skills may wear a hearing aid.

box 14.5 | A Primer on Hearing Aids

Hearing aids are electronic instruments that amplify sound and deliver it to the ear. There are two major types of hearing aids. The traditional analog aids were big enough to be worn on the body, but now they are small enough to be hidden inside the ear canal. All analog aids contain a microphone that picks up the sound, an amplifier that makes the sound louder, a receiver, a power source (batteries), and volume control. Analog aids convert sound to voltage patterns in a manner similar to sound wave patterns. Newer digital aids rapidly sample the sound waves and convert each sample into a binary system of zeros and ones. A computer then processes the numbers and is capable of amplifying selected sounds, suppressing unwanted noise, and thus creating sound patterns that are especially suited to the individual's hearing loss.

There are several models of hearing aids. The biggest is the body-worn type; though small enough to be inserted into a shirt pocket, it is now less popular. The behind-the-ear (BTE) type fits behind the pinna and many children and adults use them. In-the-ear (ITE) models are smaller than the BTE and sit at the opening of the ear canal. In-the-canal (ITC) types are smaller than the ITE; therefore, they may be fitted deeper into the auditory canal. The smallest is the completely-in-the-canal (CIC) type, which is fitted closer to the tympanic membrane and may be invisible. The smaller aids are esthetically attractive to people, but they are harder to take care of. Adjusting the volume on them can be difficult for some children and many older individuals.

Four Types of Hearing Aids

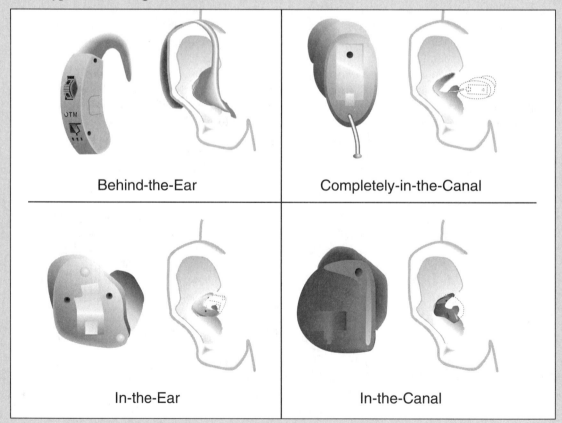

Behind-the-Ear

Completely-in-the-Canal

In-the-Ear

In-the-Canal

A relatively recent innovation in the rehabilitation of children with hearing loss is cochlear implants. **Cochlear implants** are electronic devices surgically placed in the cochlea and other parts of the ear to directly deliver the sound signal to the auditory nerve endings in the cochlea. Thus, the device helps bypass a defective ear that cannot transmit sound to the nerve endings. It consists of a microphone that is either worn on the body or mounted on an earmold and placed in the ear canal. The microphone picks up the sound, converts it into electrical energy, and sends it to a speech processor worn on the body. The processor suppresses noise and sends only useful sounds to an external transmitter—a magnetic coil worn on the skull, somewhat like a behind-the-ear hearing aid. Another magnetic coil (a receiver), implanted under the skin and just behind the external transmitter receives the sounds from the external transmitter. A ground electrode is implanted somewhere outside the cochlea, and up to 22 active electrodes are implanted inside of it. The sound signals pass from the microphone to the speech processor, external transmitter, internal receiver, and the implanted electrodes. The electrodes stimulate the nerve endings in the cochlea. The auditory nerve carries the signals to the auditory center of the brain. See Figure 14.1 for an illustration of a cochlear implant.

Children who receive cochlear implants are profoundly and prelingually deaf. They do not benefit from hearing aids and typically have hearing parents. Many deaf parents or those who consider deafness a natural state are unlikely to consider implants and often

figure 14.1   A 22-Electrode Cochlear Implant

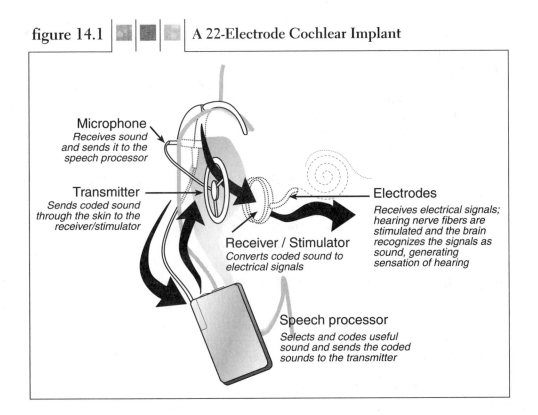

Microphone
*Receives sound
and sends it to the
speech processor*

Transmitter
*Sends coded sound
through the skin to the
receiver/stimulator*

Electrodes
*Receives electrical signals;
hearing nerve fibers are
stimulated and the brain
recognizes the signals as
sound, generating
sensation of hearing*

Receiver / Stimulator
*Converts coded sound to
electrical signals*

Speech processor
*Selects and codes useful
sound and sends the coded
sounds to the transmitter*

Prelingually deaf children are those in whom deafness is present before language acquisition.

offer arguments against it. Selection of children for implantation requires a thorough assessment of the child and the entire family by a team of specialists that includes otologists, audiologists, and speech-language pathologists.

The number of children receiving cochlear implants is on the rise. Implants help individuals to recognize sounds, hear and monitor their own voices, and learn speech sounds and language structures better than without implants or with hearing aids. Reading skills are also known to improve after implantation (Svirsky et al., 2000; Tomblin, Spencer, & Gantz, 2000). Long-term follow-up studies of implantation confirm its continued and beneficial effects on communication and academic performance (Waltzman et al., 2002). Speech intelligibility and language skills may improve to an extent that the children may be enrolled in oral educational programs, although their speech may be less intelligible than the speech of hearing children (Chin, Tsai, & Gao, 2003). Nonetheless, without intensive speech training, implanted children may continue to experience difficulty learning consonants and language structures correctly. The best outcomes are expected when implants are performed before the age of 2 and are followed up by effective, intensive, and prolonged speech-language services (British Medical Journal, 1999). Therefore, SLPs play an important role in the rehabilitation of children who have received cochlear implants.

Rehabilitation of Children with Hearing Loss

Assessment and treatment of children with hearing loss requires a team effort. Most likely, the clinician will be working with the regular and special educators, especially the educator of the deaf, educational audiologists, and the team of medical specialists (pediatricians and otologists) that may be involved in managing the child's hearing health (e.g., ear infections). If the child has received a cochlear implant, the speech-language pathologist needs to be in constant touch with the medical team (which will include an audiologist) in charge of the post-implant management of the child. The medical team may want to know the effects of cochlear implant, combined with communication training, on the child's speech perception and production. In all cases, the child's communication treatment must be integrated with the academic demands and tasks.

Although our main concern is language assessment and treatment in this chapter, it should be noted that treatment of communication disorders in children with hearing loss takes a total approach to remediating speech, voice, fluency, and language disorders. Such a remediation program is conducted in the context of a larger special educational program designed for the child and his or her family.

Modifications in Assessment Procedures for Children with Hearing Loss

In assessing children with hearing loss, it is necessary to follow the procedures described in Chapter 4. In addition, the following special considerations or procedural modifications are needed (Alpiner & McCarthy, 1999; Hegdé, 2001a; Hull, 1997).

Assessment of the risk factors. In obtaining a detailed case history, the clinician should concentrate on the potential prenatal, natal, and postnatal causes of hearing loss in children. The mother's health during pregnancy, the delivery process, and the child's health (especially middle ear infections) and development (especially of speech) during infancy and childhood are of special interest. The child's response to sound (e.g., looking in the direction of sound), speech (e.g., response when the name is called), and the mother's voice are important early indicators of normal or impaired hearing acuity. Information on cooing and babbling at expected ages and the appearance of the first words and other language skills will help assess the child's communication deficits and potential hearing loss. The child with a hearing loss may begin to babble at a normal age, but may soon stop because of lack of auditory feedback. The child's high-pitched voice and hypo- or hypernasality may give a clue to potential hearing problem.

Review of audiological assessment reports. It is important to know the results of an audiologist's examination and his or her recommendations for the child. If an audiologist has not seen the child, the child should be referred for an audiological examination. The communication disorders of a child with hearing loss can be fully understood only in the context of that child's audiogram. The audiologist may prescribe a hearing aid and an aural rehabilitation program for the child.

> An aural rehabilitation program may include training in the use of hearing aids or other systems of amplification, along with communication and educational intervention.

Assessment of speech, voice, and fluency. In addition to assessing language skills, the clinician also should assess speech, voice, and fluency in children with hearing loss (Haynes & Pindzola, 2004; Hegde, 2001b). Speech samples and selected standardized tests may be used to assess these skills. Standard procedures with suitable modifications will help assess these skills.

Assessment of varied oral language skills. Different children with the same level of hearing loss may have vastly different oral language skills. Therefore, selecting procedures that are appropriate for the level of skill a child exhibits is an important consideration in assessment. Assessment procedures that are tailored to each individual child will help obtain more valid information on the speech and language skills of the child. Many standardized speech and language tests and language samples may be practical in the case of children with substantial oral language skills. Such procedures may be impractical with children with extremely limited oral language skills. Child-specific procedures, then, are the most useful means of valid assessment.

Assessment of oral reading skills and reading comprehension. In most educational settings, SLP's work with children is done in the context of academic skills, especially the literacy skills. Therefore, assessment of reading and writing skills is a part of the child's overall educational plan. The SLP needs to collaborate with the child's classroom teacher, educator of the deaf, or both, to help make a complete assessment of the educational needs of the child.

Assessment of the amplification needs of the child. Most children with hearing loss may be candidates for hearing aids. A child an SLP begins to serve may already be using a hearing aid. If not, an audiological consultation should be recommended. If the child is using a hearing aid, the SLP needs to make sure that during the assessment session, the child is wearing it and that the aid is working properly.

Modifications in Treatment Procedures for Children with Hearing Loss

In treating speech and language disorders in children with hearing loss, such evidence-based treatment procedures as modeling, shaping, differential reinforcement, corrective feedback, and so forth described in the chapters in Part II will be effective. As with most other children, the significant others should be included in treatment. Parents, other family members, deaf educators, regular and special education teachers should help suggest treatment targets and assist in promoting the targeted skills. A summary of additional special treatment considerations and procedural modifications that may be needed follows (Alpiner & Jerome, 1999; Hegde, 2001b; Hull, 1992).

Starting an early language stimulation program. An early language stimulation program conducted at home will help minimize later negative consequences for oral communication. Parents may be taught to talk to the child as frequently as possible to counter the tendency to stop talking to the child because "he or she does not hear anyway." The parents should be taught to imitate the baby's babbling, and to reinforce the baby's attempts at vocalization by a gentle tickling, picking up, cuddling, and so forth. They should talk slowly and clearly to the child. They should read stories aloud while showing the words and pictures as they would while reading to a hearing child.

Preparation of a priority list of treatment targets. Teachers and parents should be invited to offer suggestions on what they think are more immediate treatment targets. Because the child has multiple needs (speech, voice, language, and reading and writing skill training), it is necessary to design a sequence in which they will be taught. Perhaps the child's articulation disorders need to be addressed first; language next. Perhaps language and literacy skill training can be integrated as described in Chapter 10.

Need for an auditory training program. If the family has just purchased a hearing aid for the child, the clinician should implement an **auditory training program** in which the child is taught to understand and appreciate the differences in amplified sounds that he or she is perhaps hearing for the first time. Presenting different kinds of taped sounds along with matching visual stimulus is a starting point (e.g., a dog's bark paired with the picture of a dog). If the clinician is not trained in auditory rehabilitation, an audiologist or an educator of the deaf who is may be contacted.

Facilitating speech reading. This is an important aspect of working with children with hearing loss. Even with powerful hearing aids, children with hearing loss may still speechread (lipread) to some extent. Therefore, the clinician should make speech reading easier for the child during speech and language treatment by arranging seating such that the clinician's face is well lighted. A slightly slower speech rate and sufficient mouth opening during speech production also will help.

Integrating technical devices into communication training. While working with children who have hearing loss, it is essential to integrate such technical devices as hearing aids, desktop auditory trainers, and FM amplifiers. Before starting therapy, the clinician must check to see if the child's hearing aid is working properly and that the child is wearing it, that it is turned on, and that the volume setting is correct. Treatment offered to children in a small group may use a desktop auditory trainer, which consists of a desktop unit which receives the clinician's speech, amplifies it, and feeds it to the children's ears through headphones they wear. This is more effective than individual hearing aids children wear. A wireless system that can be used to train individuals or small groups is known as the frequency modulated (FM) auditory trainer, which consists of a transmitting unit and a receiving unit. The clinician and each student wear both the units, so they can transmit and receive speech from each other wirelessly. With wireless FM trainers, the participants are free to move around.

Emphasis on visual stimuli. In teaching the meaning of various sounds, the clinician should use visual stimuli. For example, pairing pictures or objects with their associated sounds will facilitate a child's learning of language concepts. To the extent possible, and especially during the early stages of treatment, the clinician should use objects, colorful pictures, or enacted events to teach language skills. In teaching a set of basic nouns, for example, the clinician might use objects and pictures. In teaching verbs, video representations (e.g., people involved in various actions) or computerized programs may be especially useful.

Abstract language training. Teaching abstract language concepts is a priority for children with hearing loss. Language training needs to include multiple meanings of words, proverbs, common sayings, slang, and all kinds of abstract words the children are known to have problems with. Abstract language training is usually done during the latter stages of language treatment when the basic grammatic and syntactic skills are mastered. A selection of academically useful words, common proverbs, typical expressions, and so forth may be selected for teaching their multiple and abstract meanings.

Conversational skill training. Conversational skills are somewhat variable across children with hearing loss, only those that are needed to be taught may be targeted based on the results of assessment. Conversational repair (revising one's own expressions when someone fails to understand what was just said) is most likely target for children with hearing loss. Such other targets as narration and speech initiation in group or classroom settings also may be useful targets.

Speech, voice, and rhythm training. Most children with hearing loss need training in speech production, normal voice qualities, and a natural speech rhythm. While traditional methods of treatment are effective, some modifications may be necessary. In speech sound training, the child needs maximum visual feedback on the position of the articulators. Computerized programs or a simple mirror help demonstrate the movements of the articulators. Instruments such as VisiPitch help give feedback on speech and voice productions on a computer screen. Such feedback acts as instant reinforcement for correct behaviors (e.g., a lower pitch, reduced nasality) and corrective feedback for undesirable behaviors.

Nonverbal communication training. If oral language training is not successful, or was ruled out from the beginning, nonverbal means of communication, such as American Sign

Language, may be the next choice. If the child has physical disabilities coupled with developmental disability, augmentative and alternative modes of communication may be considered. See Chapter 15 for details.

Integrated or independent treatment of literacy skills. This is especially important in view of low reading and writing skills of children with hearing loss. Visual stimuli to be used in teaching basic words may also include printed words the child constantly looks at. Words, phrases, or sentences may be printed below pictures that are used in language treatment. Independent literacy skill training may be typically handled by the educator of the deaf or hard of hearing. In such cases, SLPs can serve as collaborators or consultants on literacy skill training.

Parent training in maintenance. As with all children who receive language treatment, implementation of procedures to promote maintenance of oral language skills is necessary to have the skills last over time and expanded in complexity. Parents should be taught to recognize target skills in their children, model and prompt them, and positively reinforce their production at home and other natural settings. See Chapter 9 for details on maintenance techniques.

With early intervention, good support for learning oral or sign language, and advanced education, many people with hearing loss, including those with profound deafness, have achieved a level of verbal competence that is even uncommon. Highly accomplished hard of hearing or deaf people, among whom are poets, scientists, writers, professionals, and performing artists, testify to this. Therefore, whether the target is sign language or oral language, a systematic, intensive, and sustained program of intervention, started early in the child's life, will help avoid difficulties in communication and remove barriers to success in life.

▓ ▐ ▓   Chapter Summary

In this chapter we described three groups of children, who in addition to language disorders, have significant associated problems. Two of the three groups have neurological impairment (traumatic brain injury or cerebral palsy) associated with their language disorders. The third group has hearing loss and the associated language problems.

Traumatic brain injury (TBI) is injury to the brain caused by physical trauma and/or external force; it excludes brain damage due to neurological diseases (e.g., strokes or tumors). A major medical problem, TBI may be caused by falls, automobile accidents, pedestrian accidents, bicycle riding, social and family violence, child abuse, all-terrain vehicle accidents, sports-related injuries, farm-related injuries, and domestic accidents. TBI can produce a variety of neurological injuries that are classified as penetrating, nonpenetrating, acceleration-deceleration, coup, contrecoup, diffuse axonal, diffuse vascular, and brain stem.

Neurological symptoms of TBI include confusion; stupor; disorientation to time, place, and persons; reduced attention span, mood changes, impulsive and aggressive behaviors; cognitive deficits including memory problems, and deficits in planning and reasoning skills. Communication disorders associated with TBI include dysarthria (a motor speech disorder), apraxia (a motor planning disorder in the absence of muscle weakness), confused language, word finding problems, narrative problems, and difficulty with complex and abstract words and phrases. Assessment and treatment modifications of children with TBI is a dynamic process as their physical condition improves and communication and cognition change over time.

Cerebral palsy, a complex set of neuromotor developmental disorder caused by an injury to an immature brain, is another neurological disorder that affects speech and language skills. Adverse prenatal, natal, and postnatal factors are associated with cerebral palsy. Classified into spastic, athetoid, ataxic, and mixed types, cerebral palsy is associated with dysarthria. Children with CP may have significant language problems if they also have developmental disability and hearing loss, as many do. Assessment and treatment modifications for these children need to take into account their neurological deficits.

Hearing loss in children also produces significant communicative problems. Hearing loss is 25 dB HL or higher for adults and 15 dB HL or higher for children who are still learning language. Hearing loss may be conductive (diminished air conduction of sound to the inner ear due to problems in the ear canal and the middle ear), sensorineural (impairment due to a damaged cochlea), or mixed (both kinds of problems). Children with hearing loss may be classified as *hard of hearing* or *the deaf*.

The severity of communicative disorders associated with hearing loss depends on the degree of g loss; the time of onset and diagnosis; and the time, intensity, and quality of intervention. Speech disorders associated with hearing loss include errors of articulation, especially of stops and fricatives, addition of sounds, atypical rhythm, and limited fluency. Language disorders of children with hearing loss are characterized by semantic, syntactic, and pragmatic difficulties and difficulties with abstract language.

Amplification through hearing aids and cochlear implants are the two main technical means used in the rehabilitation of children with hearing loss. SLPs may offer speech-language services to those who wish to acquire and maintain oral language skills. Assessment and treatment modifications include the use of amplification and helping the child use visual as well as auditory modalities during training.

 ## Study Guide

1. The nature of brain injury depends on the way the physical forces acted upon a skull that was either stationary or moving. Within this context, describe the various kinds of brain injuries. Include in your description how the varied physical forces acting upon the head can cause different sets of injuries and neurological consequences.

2. You are doing your clinical externship in a hospital that specializes in head trauma. There, you have been asked to make a bedside evaluation of an 18-year-old man who has sustained severe head injury in an automobile accident. How would you prepare for this bedside evaluation? What kinds of behavioral, neurological, and communicative deficits do you expect in this young man? What standardized or nonstandardized tools would you use?

3. Discuss the classification of cerebral palsy. Relate the classification to both the etiologic factors and neurological consequences. Define all the technical terms you use in your description.

4. A teacher, who has referred a child with cerebral palsy for your assessment and treatment, has asked a specific question: "What is the prognosis for significantly improved communication skills in this child?" To give a reasonable answer to the teacher, what kinds of observations and assessment procedures would you use? What kinds of reports would you seek from other professionals to better understand the strengths and limitations of the child that may have an effect on prognosis? What kinds of treatment would you recommend to offer a more positive prognosis?

5. Drawing from the knowledge you have gained in courses on audiology, describe in detail the different types of hearing loss and their auditory pathology. What are the consequences the different types of hearing loss have on the acquisition of oral language skills? Address the issue of early fluctuating hearing loss and its effects on language learning.

6. You are working on a team of specialists on cochlear implants for children with severe hearing loss. On occasion, you are asked to make presentations to parents of children with hearing loss on the beneficial effects of cochlear implants on oral communication skills. Considering the views of some members of the Deaf community, how would you present the information in a sensitive as well as professional manner?

chapter

15

Augmentative and Alternative Communication

outline

There is a wide range of oral language skills among children who have additional clinical conditions described in the preceding chapters. Some children with developmental disability, pervasive developmental disorder (PDD) or autism spectrum disorder (ASD) are quite verbal, although their language will often be marked by profound deficits. Others will remain nonverbal or only minimally verbal throughout their life span. Children who are hard of hearing will develop intelligible oral language to the extent the degree of hearing loss and the intensity of oral language training will allow. Children with neurological deficits, such as cerebral palsy or brain injury, will also show great variation in their production of oral language. In each of these populations, there will be a percentage of children for whom oral speech and language will not be a practical method of communication.

Children who are nonverbal or remain minimally verbal even after extensive oral language intervention need nonoral means of communication. Such nonoral means may augment (supplement) the minimal oral language skills or may provide an alternative means of communication when oral skills are not functional. Speech-language pathologists will assess these children to help determine which of many systems of augmentative and alternative communication (AAC) may be the key to unlocking a world of social interaction previously inaccessible to such children. Before selecting an AAC system that is likely to be functional, the clinician should make an assessment that includes observations of the child's physical, sensory, communication, and cognitive skills; an analysis of the child's various environments; and an evaluation of the amount of support available to the child. Treatment procedures will be modified to teach the child and the people in the child's environment to access the AAC system, and then to provide ongoing support and consultation once the system is in place.

What does *AAC* stand for?

This chapter will begin with a definition of AAC and a description of various AAC systems. Then, we will discuss modifications to assessment procedures to emphasize evaluation of nonverbal communicative skills, motor skills, sensory limitations, and cognitive function. We will then discuss considerations for selecting an appropriate AAC system, based on results of the assessment. Modifications to treatment will include procedures for instructing the child in the use of the AAC system, consultation with people in the child's environment, and follow-up support. The chapter will conclude with a look at what the future may hold in technological advances and what those advances may mean to nonverbal individuals.

Augmentative and Alternative Communication: Definition and Types

Technological advances, changing educational philosophies, and legislation pertaining to the rights of disabled individuals have resulted in expanding communicative options for children who are nonverbal or minimally verbal. In 2003, 51 percent of school SLPs reported working with children who use AAC (ASHA, 2004a). Children with disabilities in inclusive classrooms and in the community employ a variety of AAC systems, with the support of their parents, caregivers, teachers, peers, and professional specialists. This section will describe the expanding definition and various types of AAC.

Definition of AAC

Augmentative and alternative methods of communication are nonoral means of either supplementing limited oral skills with nonoral methods or providing nonoral methods as the primary means of communication for individuals who are functionally nonverbal. Supplementing limited oral skills with nonoral means is augmentative. **Augmentative means** of communication enhance and enlarge available, though deficient, oral language skills. Providing nonoral methods as the primary means of communication is *alternative*. **Alternative means** of communication replace oral communication skills. The definition of AAC, then, is multifaceted—augmentative, because systems of AAC expand and enhance an individual's limited oral communication; alternative, because systems of AAC can serve as substitutes for oral communication, when the individual has very little, if any, functional oral speech. Individuals do not have to be nonverbal to benefit from using AAC; people with highly unintelligible speech also may be likely users of AAC.

Types of AAC

We will describe types of AAC in this section very briefly, and then offer more details when we discuss selecting a specific system of AAC for a child, based on child-specific assessment results. Broadly speaking, systems of AAC can be **unaided** or **aided.** The system selected depends on a detailed

 What are two broad categories of AAC?

evaluation of the child's communicative needs, and an assessment of the child's motor, sensory, and cognitive capabilities.

Unaided systems of AAC. Systems of AAC that do not rely on instruments or other external aids are called unaided. These methods of communication systematically use gestures, signs, and facial expressions to supplement, or substitute for, oral communication. See Box 15.1 for examples of unaided systems of AAC.

Aided systems of AAC. These are systems of AAC that use various external aids, such as picture books, alphabet boards, or computerized devices. A wide range of aided systems

---

box 15.1 | Examples of Unaided Systems of AAC

Gestural systems to indicate *yes* and *no*

- Head movements (e.g., up and down for *yes*; side-to-side for *no*)
- Eye movements (e.g., up for *yes*, down for *no*; blinking once for *yes*, twice for *no*)
- Hand movements (e.g., thumbs up for *yes*, thumbs down for *no*)
- Foot movements (e.g., right foot moves for *yes*; left foot moves for *no*)

Pointing, or purposefully moving any body part toward, desired objects

Pantomiming concepts that communicate various communicative needs

Established manual systems of communication

- American Sign Language (ASL)
- American Indian Hand Talk (AMER-IND)

of AAC are available, from low-technology to high-technology systems. Low-technology systems of AAC use no or very little electronic technology. There are no computerized software programs, voice output activators, message storage systems, or printed output. Examples of low-technology systems of AAC include direct selection of objects, various picture systems, and alphabet boards. High-technology systems of AAC employ sophisticated electronic devices, including computers, to generate synthetic speech or printed messages.

Because of the many options available, selecting a system of AAC for a child involves thorough evaluation of a child's nonverbal communicative skills, and motor, sensory, and cognitive capabilities. Assessment methods must be modified to accommodate the need for these additional observations. The next sections will describe those modifications and considerations.

> Give two examples of low-technology, aided AAC systems.

Assessing Communicative Skills in Children Who Are Nonverbal or Minimally Verbal

The road to devising an effective system of communication for a child who is nonverbal or minimally verbal begins with a thorough assessment of the child's nonverbal communicative skills, as well as any verbalizations or limited speech the child might produce. Observations will have to be made even more carefully and intently than usual, because the communicative attempts of children with severe disabilities can be very subtle. The SLP will have help in making these observations—assessment of children who are nonverbal is typically carried out by an interdisciplinary team of specialists, each playing a special role in designing a plan of services for a nonverbal child. Also, in good models of interdisciplinary team assessment, family members are included as team participants.

> People unfamiliar with the broad scope of practice described for SLPs might ask how a child who has no speech can benefit from speech and language services. Trained SLPs know that there are many ways to communicate that do not involve oral speech.

The Assessment Team

While SLPs often work as part of interdisciplinary teams, in the case of nonverbal children, the need to do so is intensified. Physical, sensory, and cognitive deficits of the child must be observed and described. While the SLP will make valuable contributions, professionals such as physical therapists, occupational therapists, and psychologists provide valuable information on the child's various skills and capabilities. The following is a description of the roles some other professionals take, the types of assessments they make, and their contributions toward devising an AAC system for the child (Anderson et al., 2002; American Speech-Language-Hearing Association, 2004b).

Physical therapist. A **physical therapist (PT)** is a licensed professional qualified to assess physical limitations and provide treatment to maximize the independence of people who have physical disabilities or limitations. As part of the interdisciplinary team, the PT will assess various parameters of the child's motor abilities, including balance, coordination, muscle strength, and range of motion. The PT can also recommend various types of adaptive equipment for children who need that type of physical support.

Occupational therapist. An **occupational therapist (OT)** is a licensed professional qualified to assess daily living skills, vocational skills, and degrees of sensory or motor impairment in individuals who are limited by physical injury, cognitive deficits, social impairment, or developmental disability. The OT will assist in the assessment of the child's mobility and muscle control. The OT will also assess the adequacy and function of any adaptive equipment the children use, particularly noting the sitting position of children who use wheelchairs. Based on such assessment, the OT may make recommendations for altering equipment to provide better support.

Psychologist. The **psychologist** specializes in the study and assessment of behavior and is especially qualified to assess the intellectual skills and cognitive deficits of individuals. Children being assessed for AAC often already have diagnoses of various types of cognitive impairment, and determination of a degree of developmental disability does *not* imply the child is not a candidate for AAC (see Box 15.2 for a discussion of the old candidacy model in AAC assessment). Complexity of the system chosen, however, will depend, to some extent, on the child's cognitive levels.

Depending on the needs of the child, other specialists will be included in the interdisciplinary team. Those specialists might include the child's pediatrician, other physicians who specialize in rehabilitation, social workers, educators, and professionals involved with developing, designing, and marketing AAC devices and switches.

| box 15.2 | | "Candidacy" and AAC: Should *Any* Child Be Denied a Chance to Communicate? |

In the past, the goal of assessing nonverbal individuals was to determine whether or not a person was a "candidate" for receiving a system of AAC. It was believed that a child should have certain prerequisite skills and demonstrate an adequate cognitive level before being introduced to a system of AAC. Such a line of thinking excluded children with developmental disability, autism, and severe physical and sensory impairments from AAC intervention. Treatment instead focused on teaching isolated, meaningless "readiness" skills, endlessly preparing children for the day they would be allowed access to a system of communication. The result was increased isolation and segregation of nonverbal, multiply disabled children from the experiences and instruction that might have provided them with the means to express their needs and preferences, and to interact socially with others (Beukelman & Mirenda, 1998).

In response to the efforts of advocates for people who are disabled, and to changing federal and educational

law, the emphasis on determining candidacy for AAC has been replaced by assessment procedures that determine the communication needs of an individual, through a functional assessment of the environment (Beukelman & Mirenda, 1998). Using the communication needs model, clinicians can assess children with any degree of cognitive impairment, describe their current communicative skills, and prescribe possible systems of AAC that may result in increasing those skills. Beukelman, Yorkston, and Dowden (1985) described the following steps in implementing an assessment based on the communication needs model:

- Document an individual's communication needs
- Observe how the individual is currently meeting those needs
- Introduce systematic AAC intervention to reduce the number of unmet communication needs

The functions of the members of a professional team overlap to some extent. Professionals on teams that function well will welcome those overlapping efforts, collaborating with each other, and teaching each other about their special-

What professional is primarily responsible for determining: (1) level of cognitive functioning? (2) degree of motor and sensory impairment? and (3) degree of physical limitation?

ties. Many of the observations SLPs make will often complement assessments other professionals make. As we shall see in a future section, SLPs can also assess a child's seating position and make recommendations for changes. SLPs can determine whether or not a child has the muscle control to point to a picture, access a computer keyboard, purposefully move any part of the body to access any type of control switch, or give direct eye gaze to specified pictures or objects. In other words, SLPs make many of the same observations other professionals might make, but the emphasis is on communication and the suitability of a particular AAC system.

Observing Nonverbal Communicative Skills

The assessment procedures described in Chapter 4 are generally applicable to children who are nonverbal. There are some standardized and criterion-referenced instruments available, but the most important data, as always, will result from child-specific measurement of communicative skills.

Standardized and criterion-referenced instruments. It is rarely best to rely on results of standardized testing to produce an adequate, detailed description of a child's communicative skills. That some children who are nonverbal need speech and language services will be obvious. Nevertheless, clinicians might find themselves in settings where quantifiable data are necessary to qualify a child for services.

Many nonverbal children can respond to test items on standardized tests of receptive language that are used for verbal children. Typical tests of expressive language are obviously unsuitable. There are, however, some standardized and criterion-referenced tests that are designed to assess the communicative skills of nonverbal individuals. Some also provide a systematic means of making the observations necessary to determine possible AAC systems (see Table 15.1 for a listing of assessment instruments).

Child-specific assessment tasks. There are many child-specific ways to measure communicative behavior in children who are nonverbal. Recall that these are not "informal" measures—they are systematic, quantitative, and qualitative observations of a child's communicative behaviors. The communicative behaviors observed might be production of

Describe some communicative functions that should be assessed in children who are nonverbal.

verbalizations—some minimally verbal children may produce words or two-word combinations—but will more likely be gestures, atypical vocalizations, facial expressions, displays of emotion, and, possibly, aggressive or otherwise undesirable behavior. The clinician should observe if and how the child: (1) requests desired objects or actions,

Although we use the term *nonverbal children,* few, if any, are totally nonverbal. Vocalizations, including grunts that communicate something, are verbal responses.

(2) protests to others, (3) interacts socially, (4) initiates a communicative interaction, (5) establishes joint attention, and so forth. The clinician should arrange the environment so that the child is encouraged to interact in whatever way he or she can.

table 15.1

Tests for the Assessment of Nonverbal Communication Skills or Possible AAC Use, or Both

Test	Description
Achieving Communication Independence (ACI) Gillette (2003)	Assesses communicative skills in individuals across the life span, from infants to adults. Also assesses potential communication partners and opportunities in various environments.
Communication and Symbolic Behavior Scales Developmental Profile—First Normed Edition (CSBS DP) Wetherby & Prizant (2003)	Assesses communicative behavior and symbolic development of children with a chronological age of 9 months to 6 years, who have functional communicative ages of 6–24 months. Incorporates checklists, caregiver questionnaires, and systematic use of "communication temptations" to judge the presence or absence of communicative behaviors.
Sequenced Inventory of Communication Development—Revised (SICD-R) Hedrick, Prather, & Tobin (1995)	Assesses early communication skills of children with and without developmental disability who have functional skill levels between 4 and 48 months of age. Uses parent report and direct observation of receptive and expressive language behavior.
The Nonspeech Test Huer (1988)	Criterion-referenced (skill is present or absent) checklist of expressive and receptive oral language and nonverbal communicative behavior. Measures skills typically seen in children from 0 to 48 months; yields an age equivalency score.

To assess the manner in which a child requests objects or actions, the clinician can involve the child in a variety of activities, interrupt the activity, and see how the child responds. Some suggested activities:

- Engage the child in a familiar game (e.g., "Row, row, row your boat!"), stop, and wait for the child's response
- Blow bubbles, close the bubble jar, put it on a shelf, and wait for the child's response
- Activate an appealing wind-up toy, let it run down, and wait for the child's response
- Place a desired food item (with the parent's prior approval) in a clear plastic tub; wait for the child's response
- Blow up a balloon, let it go and let it fly around the room until completely deflated; wait for the child's response

Children who have good requesting skills will indicate what they want in a variety of ways. Good, positive responses include:

- Moving body parts to indicate more (e.g., rocking back and forth on the clinician's lap to request more "Row, row, row your boat!")
- Either pointing to an object, picking up an object and handing it to the clinician, or shoving the object toward the clinician
- Manipulating the clinician's hand toward a desired object or to perform a desired action
- Directing eye gaze toward object or the clinician, changing facial expression, or moving any body part in any way toward a desired object
- Vocalizing, either atypically or with a verbal approximation of a discernible word

The clinician must be sharply observant of any manner in which the child requests desired objects or actions. Sometimes, parents, caregivers, teachers, or others may miss the child's unconventional, often subtle, attempts to communicate. Clinicians can help by pointing out the many ways in which a child may be attempting to interact.

There is frequently no need to set up special opportunities for children to protest during assessment sessions. If necessary, the clinician can ask parents beforehand about a child's less preferred toys or activities, and offer them to a child to see if the child rejects them in some way. It is the clinician's job to describe the ways in which a child expresses displeasure and rejection of objects and activities:

> Such routine procedures as hearing screenings and orofacial examinations often provide adequate stimuli to evoke protesting behaviors.

- Pushing undesired objects away, or interrupting an action by pushing the clinician's hand away
- Running from the clinician
- Hitting, pinching, kicking, spitting
- Crying; perhaps exhibiting full-blown tantrum behavior
- Verbalizing; either appropriately, by saying or verbally approximating *No!*, or inappropriately, by screaming, growling, or producing some other idiosyncratic noise

Many of these are undesirable behaviors, but they communicate. Children who are nonverbal often express themselves through aggressive, destructive, and sometimes self-injurious behaviors. Such undesirable behaviors have been experimentally shown to reduce when children are provided with a more appropriate means of communication, such as a system of AAC (Carr & Durand, 1985; Charlop-Christy et al., 2002; Frea, Arnold, & Vittimberga, 2001).

Besides requesting and protesting, clinicians should also assess the child's skill at interacting socially. Does the child initiate communicative interaction? Does the child respond to interaction initiated by others? Does the child attempt to establish joint reference with a communicative partner? Does the child "show off" for the benefit of observers? Does the child maintain good eye contact? Take turns? Show affection toward others? Many of these behaviors can be observed during tasks designed to assess requesting and protesting, but some further suggested activities for evoking social interaction include:

- To evoke initiation of social interaction, clear the room of all appealing objects, except for one toy or book. Sit with your back to the child and play with the toy or read the book aloud. Observe if the child initiates communicative behavior indicating a desire to join you.
- To assess joint reference, use a shared storybook reading activity. Observe if the child directs his or her gaze toward a picture you point to; also observe any time the child might point to a picture and look at you, perhaps shifting eye gaze between you and the picture several times.
- To assess a gestural social response, observe any instances of the child returning your smile or expressions of delight or pleasure.

The clinician should collect both quantitative and qualitative data on the child's communicative behavior. Separate frequencies of different types of communicative behaviors exhibited during the session should be noted. By totaling the number of instances of com-

| box 15.3 | Example of Data Analysis for an Assessment of a Child Who Is Nonverbal |

Tommy is a nonverbal, 4-year-old boy who was assessed for speech and language. During one 30-minute assessment session, the clinician observed Tommy exhibiting communicative behavior 20 times. He verbally approximated the word *no* 3 times, moved the clinician's hand toward an object 10 times, screamed in protest 2 times, and screamed in protest in combination with pushing an object away 5 times. The clinician analyzed the data as follows:

Total number of communicative behaviors observed: 20

Communicative Behavior	Probable Intent	Number	Percentage of Total
Verbal approximation of *no*	Protesting	3	15%
Moved clinician's hand toward object	Requesting	10	50%
Screamed	Protesting	2	10%
Screamed plus pushed object away	Protesting	5	25%

municative behavior, the clinician should calculate percentages for every type of behavior observed. Each type of behavior should be qualitatively described. See Box 15.3 for an example of data collection and analysis for a child who is nonverbal.

> What types of data should be collected during a child-specific assessment?

Assessing receptive language. Children who are nonverbal may have receptive language skills that are better than their expressive language skills, particularly if their physical disabilities are not associated with substantial cognitive impairment. The clinician should use child-specific assessment tasks that are typical of those used for verbal children, with some modifications to allow for whatever physical limitations the child may have. For example, a child with cerebral palsy may be asked to "Look at . . . " a particular picture in a field of two, to check for identification of pictures of common objects. It is also possible to devise tasks to check for understanding of more complex grammatical and morphologic structures. To check for understanding of pronouns; for example, the clinician might hold up pictures of a boy eating, a girl eating, and a group of people eating, and ask the child to point to, or look at, or otherwise indicate, "They are eating" and alternatively, "He is eating" or "She is eating."

The clinician should also give the child simple directions to follow to check for language comprehension and understanding of basic concepts. The clinician can ask the child to point to, or otherwise indicate, body parts, shapes, colors, numbers, or letters. Depending on the child's motor abilities, the clinician can ask the child to perform certain actions (e.g., stand up, sit down, clap your hands).

A child may indicate *yes* and *no* in some way; either through head nods and shakes, pointing or looking at a red card for *yes* and a green card for *no*, or, if there is some literacy skill present, pointing to cards saying *yes* and *no*. The clinician can check for language comprehension in such cases by asking obvious *yes* or *no* questions (e.g.,

"Are you a boy?" "Is this your classroom?" "Are we in the library?" etc.). If the child does not have a means of indicating *yes* and *no*, the clinician should teach one as a primary target behavior.

Assessing literacy. It is particularly important to check for emerging or existing literacy skills in children who are nonverbal. If the child is literate, or has the potential to become literate, it will make a vast difference in the child's ability to access an AAC device. The child will not, of course, read aloud to demonstrate literacy skills, but there are tasks the clinician can present that will help assess them. Assessment of present or emergent writing skills will depend on the adequacy of fine motor skills. The clinician can assess the child's skill in:

- Matching logos to the products they represent (e.g., matching a commercial soup label to a picture of a bowl of soup)
- Matching letters to letters
- Matching uppercase letters to lowercase letters
- Matching words to words
- Matching words to the objects they represent (e.g., matching a stimulus card with the word *ball* on it to a picture of a ball in a field of four)
- Drawing, coloring, scribbling, or otherwise producing marks on paper; if no skills are apparent, the clinician should attempt to evoke them by providing models, hand-over-hand guidance, or both
- Writing letters, words, sentences, or paragraphs; either independently or by copying a model

Assessing possible higher-level speech and language skills. Even though the indications are that the child is essentially nonverbal, the clinician should not give up on evoking speech and language. Assessment should probe slightly higher levels to make sure the description of the child as nonverbal is a valid one. Sometimes, people in the child's environment may resign themselves to the idea that the child does not talk, and will therefore not attempt to directly evoke speech. The clinician should do everything possible to evoke spontaneous production of speech and language, just as in any assessment of any child. The clinician should also check the child's skill in imitating a modeled production. If the child has any imitative skill at all, it is a good sign for the possibility of achieving some oral speech and language.

Prognostic Indicators for the Development of Oral Speech

Perhaps the most difficult question a parent could ask of a clinician is, "Will my child ever talk?" When parents ask, clinicians must answer—if the news is not good, it should still be delivered, gently, but directly.

With very young children who have no clearly identifiable primary diagnosis, the direct answer could very well be, "It is difficult to predict. Mary needs intervention, and we will all work hard to give her the best chance of developing speech. We will have to see how she does." But, sometimes assessment findings may indicate that there is little chance of a child becoming an oral communicator. Poor prognostic signs for the development of oral speech include:

What is a *prognosis?*

- The presence of a primary diagnosis which characteristically indicates a high likelihood of a lack of speech and language development (e.g., severe autism, profound developmental disability, serious neuromuscular disorders)
- A history of regression; the child had a few words early on in development, but those words have disappeared and no new language skills have developed
- Lack of demonstrated skill in imitating verbalizations; no stimulability for oral speech (Carr et al., 1978; Carr & Dores, 1981; Yoder & Layton, 1988)
- Age; the older the child is, the less likely it is that oral speech will develop

Even when it is the clinician's best professional judgment that oral speech is not likely to develop, parents should be reassured that professionals treating their child will not "give up" on evoking speech and language from the child. This is so because professional judgments are only judgments; only serious attempts at teaching a skill will either confirm or refute that judgment. Sometimes families are hesitant to embrace the idea of a system of augmentative and alternative communication for their child, thinking that introducing such a system will have an inhibiting effect on oral speech production. Controlled experimental research, case studies, and descriptive longitudinal research, however, have indicated that a system of AAC is more likely to facilitate, rather than inhibit, oral speech (Clibbens, 2001; Goldstein, 2002; Kravits et al., 2002; Powell & Clibbens, 1994). Pointing out such research evidence will reassure many parents. AAC is rarely used as a total replacement for oral speech; the *augmentative* function is much more often applicable than the *alternative* function.

Assessing Physical, Sensory, and Cognitive Skills

In addition to assessing communicative skill—a goal of any language assessment—there are additional observations an SLP must make to assist in determining an appropriate system of AAC for the child. The SLP must assess: (1) physical skills—the degree to which a child has voluntary control over movement of any part of the body; (2) sensory capabilities—the presence or absence of functioning hearing or sight, or both; and (3) cognitive levels, which will affect the complexity of the system of AAC selected.

> What additional observations should an SLP make when assessing a child who is nonverbal?

Assessing Physical Skills

An important question in assessing a child for possible use of an AAC system is: How can the child access an AAC device? Ancillary questions are: Can the child point? Purposefully direct eye gaze? Purposefully move any part of the body? Clinicians ask these questions to understand how a child might access an AAC device. If the child has voluntary control over any part of the body, there will be some kind of AAC system available to that child. There are children who, if they do not have purposeful movement of their hands, can activate AAC systems by pressing switches with their feet, or thighs, or heads, or elbows or *any* part of the body over which they have volitional control. There are even systems of AAC that can be accessed by eye

> One child seen on a consultative basis was reported to have no means of accessing a switch. After a more thorough assessment, it was found that the child could purposefully hit a switch, if it was located so that she could hit it with her right upper thigh.

movement. Physical skills can be assessed in a hierarchical fashion; if the child has good control over fingers, hands, and arms, there is no need to assess other body parts. However, clinicians should assess any movement the child is capable of to activate an electronic AAC device.

The clinician should assess:

- Mobility and dexterity of the hands first. The most efficient way to access an AAC device is through pointing, typing, and so forth. Therefore, the hand movements are the primary targets of initial observations.
- Functional integrity of the muscles of the neck and face next. If the child has volitional control over movement of the neck and face, various facial expressions, head nods, head shakes, eyeblinks, or eye gaze can be used for AAC. Also, the client may activate a switch with a head movement, if the hands and arms are immobile.
- Functional integrity of the legs and feet last, and only if there is very limited mobility and dexterity of hands, neck, and face.
- Motor skills necessary to directly access an AAC device or method. Can the child point? Can the child use a mouse to move a computer curser? Can the child access a keyboard? Purposefully hit a switch with any part of the body?
- Hand and finger mobility and fine motor skills, if a sign language system is being considered.

In the case of a child using a wheelchair, the clinician should also assess the adequacy of the wheelchair in supporting the child's upright seating position. If a child with cerebral palsy, for example, is left slumped over in a chair that does not offer the proper support, recommendations can be made for alterations to the chair. Consultation with physical or occupational therapists will likely result in joint recommendations for alterations to a child's seating arrangements to: (1) provide a symmetrical seating position for the child, (2) provide a stable base of support, (3) decrease the influence of atypical muscle tone, and (4) accommodate fixed deformities and correct flexible deformities (Beukelman & Mirenda, 1998). When a child achieves an optimal seating position, opportunities to access an AAC system are also optimized (See Photo 15.1).

Assessing Sensory Skills

The clinician should assess the presence or absence of functional vision and hearing. Any AAC system requiring symbol selection depends on the child's functional vision. Some systems present a series of audio-recorded messages the child can select by hitting a switch—those systems depend on functional hearing. The clinician should therefore assess:

- *Functional hearing.* Does the child respond to and try to localize sound? If not, the child should be referred to an audiologist with expertise in the assessment of the hearing of severely disabled individuals.
- *Functional vision.* Does the child maintain eye contact with a communicative partner? Does the child look at objects of interest? Can the child track an object with eye gaze? Up and down? Side to side? Can the child scan an array of objects, before making a selection?

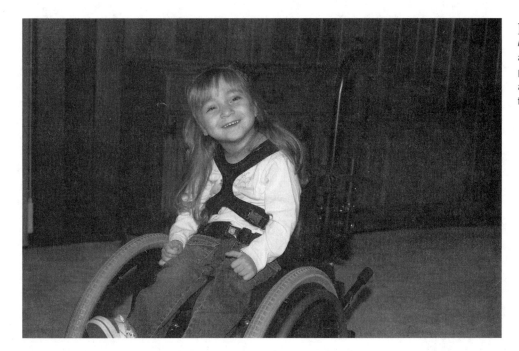

photo 15.1
A child who achieves an upright sitting position while using a wheelchair is ready to communicate!

Assessing Cognitive Skills

The clinician's observations can help assess the cognitive level of the child, although that determination is usually made by a psychologist on a multidisciplinary team. The clinician can supplement the psychologist's assessment of intellectual skills by reporting:

- How well the child attended to task
- How well the child followed directions
- The presence of any literacy skills noted
- Demonstrated knowledge of basic concepts (e.g., identifying shapes, colors, etc.)
- Any evidence of problem-solving skills (e.g., perhaps the child moved a stepping stool closer to a shelf to gain access to a desired object)

At the conclusion of the assessment, the clinician should have enough quantitative data and qualitative observations to judge whether or not a system of AAC is likely to be helpful to the child. In the case of nonverbal children, the answer to that question is often *yes*. The next task is to make a recommendation for a system of AAC that will be functional for the child and logistically feasible for those in the child's environment to support.

Looking for the Best Fit: Selecting an AAC System

The line between where assessment ends and intervention begins is even more blurred than usual when clinicians intervene by suggesting a system of AAC. Before a system is recommended for a child, the clinician should consider whether the child's environment offers opportunities or limitations for developing communicative skills. Based on an assessment of the child's skill level, the communicative demands the child faces, the family strengths and weakness, and logistical considerations, the clinician will make recommendations for a system of AAC. Recommendations may be for a particular system, a combination of systems, or for trial periods for a variety of systems that may be suitable for the child's social and educational needs, environmental factors, and the parents' preferences. The clinician will then teach the child and the child's potential communicative partners to use the AAC system. Once the system has been learned to at least a minimally functional extent, the clinician will continue to teach and give ongoing support to the AAC-using child, the family members of the child, teachers, and others in the child's environment. Assessment will be ongoing throughout treatment; constant re-evaluation of the functionality of a child's AAC system must be accomplished, with any necessary adjustments.

Evaluating the Child's Environment

An assessment should be made of the child's environment. The clinician should address the following questions:

- What is the level of support among significant others in the child's environment for the adoption of a system of AAC?
- What opportunities exist within the environment for the child to communicate?
- How is the child currently communicating?
- How are the family members communicating with the child? What are their preferences, strengths, and limitations (e.g., could they use a complicated high technology system?)?
- How could the child's communicative attempts be improved?
- What logistical barriers might there be to the introduction of a high-technology system of AAC (e.g., some high-technology systems of AAC are bulky and difficult to transport)?

To answer such questions, the clinician must consult with significant persons in the child's life, observe the child in naturalistic environments, and experiment with several possible communicative modes before recommending a system of AAC.

Consulting with others. A clinician may think that a particular system of AAC would be perfect for a child, or maybe the clinician has a bias favoring one system of AAC over the other, but it would be a mistake to make a recommendation based only on the clinician's professional judgment. The most well-considered treatment plans will go awry if the clinician has not included suggestions from significant people in the child's environment. Considerations must be made according to the level of support potential communicative partners will give to the AAC-using child. Do they have a commitment to the basic idea that AAC will be advantageous for the child's developing communicative skills? If so, do the people in the child's environment agree with the adoption of the particular recommended system? Are they resistant to the idea of learning whatever gestural system may be proposed? Are they comfortable with the logistics of operating and transporting a more high-technology system, such as an electronic device?

Clinicians involve family members, caregivers, and teachers from the very beginning of the assessment process. If people in the environment are regarded as equal members of the assessment team, and if their input is sincerely listened to and acted on, the chances of having a recommended system of AAC accepted will be greatly enhanced. There is little chance of a child succeeding with a system of AAC if that system is not accepted and supported by those in the child's environment. Conversely, if the child's attempts to communicate with AAC are greeted with consistent responsiveness, enthusiasm, and encouragement, the number and quality of a child's interactions should increase because of such social reinforcement.

Evaluating communicative opportunities. Observations should be made in naturalistic environments of the communicative opportunities the child encounters during daily activities and how the child reacts to those opportunities. For example, in a preschool setting, is the child given opportunities to participate in various activities, such as responding during circle time, interacting during storybook reading, conducting art activities, playing during recess, and so forth? If not, suggestions should be made to preschool teachers and aides to increase those types of communicative opportunities. If so, the clinician should observe how the child is currently responding. For instance, does the child:

- Actively engage during circle time, either through vocalization or appropriate movement (e.g., swaying in time to songs, clapping hands, etc.)?
- Have any means of commenting, responding to questions, or establishing joint attention during storybook reading time?
- Have any means of requesting necessary items or assistance during art projects?
- Interact with peers during recess? Greet peers? Take turns? Engage in cooperative play?

The clinician who is watching how the child is currently reacting to environmental opportunities afforded to communicate should consider how those reactions can be improved, augmented, and increased. Also to be considered are the ways in which others react to the child and how those reactions may be modified to improve the effectiveness of the AAC system being used.

Similar observations should be made of the child at home. In particular, the clinician should evaluate the extent to which family members evoke communicative interaction from the child. In some families, there may be a tendency to anticipate the child's needs without requiring the child to expressively indicate those needs. Or, maybe the family members consistently respond to such inappropriate behaviors as crying, kicking, or hitting by quickly supplying the child with whatever they think the child wants, thereby reinforcing those behaviors and ensuring that those behaviors will persist and increase (see Box 15.4 for a discussion of procedures to decrease such undesirable behavior).

Experimenting with various AAC systems. Often, it is not possible to pinpoint a specific type of AAC that is most likely to succeed with a particular child in a particular environment. Therefore, target behaviors for AAC users should be flexible, for example: *A variety of unaided and aided systems of augmentative and alternative communication will be explored to determine an appropriate method of AAC for Johnny to use in classroom, home, and community settings.* While not defined in strictly operational terms, this target behavior reflects the experimental nature of initially introducing an AAC system to a child and to those in the child's

box 15.4 | Decreasing Undesirable, but Communicative, Behavior Using AAC

Differential Reinforcement of Alternative Behavior

Recall from previous chapters that one method of decreasing behaviors is differential reinforcement of alternative behavior (DRA). Because the alternative behavior taught is a more socially acceptable way of expressing the same communicative effect, DRA has also been called *functional equivalence training*; other authors have referred to DRA as functional communication training (FCT). This is a method that is particularly applicable to children who are nonverbal and behaviorally difficult. Mirenda (1997) conducted a review of studies showing the efficacy of DRA in reducing undesirable behaviors when individuals are trained in various systems of AAC as functionally equivalent behaviors and identified the components of effective programs, some of which included:

- A thorough functional analysis of the communicative function of the problem behavior. This can be accomplished through observation and through experimentally exposing the child to stimuli simulating naturally occurring environmental events that may be antecedent to the challenging behavior. For example, if it is suspected that the behavior occurs

so that the child can escape an undesired activity, the clinician can repeatedly expose the child to known undesired activities, note if the behavior occurs, and, if it does, terminate the activity. If the behavior is reinforced by termination of undesired activities, an increase in the behavior will be noted, and the clinician can reasonably conclude that the function of the undesirable behavior is to request, or demand, that an activity be discontinued.

- A "response match" between the assessed function of the challenging behavior and the messages conveyed by the selected system of AAC. The new communicative behavior must be the functional equivalent of the undesirable behavior. A child who exhibits a temper tantrum to obtain a desired object, for example, might be taught to sign *I want* followed by pointing to the object.

- The new communicative behavior should obtain the desired response. Parents, teachers, and caregivers should be prepared to give the AAC-using child access to desired objects or activities requested, or to respond to a child's comments. If they do not, the challenging behavior will not decrease, and the new communicative behavior will eventually be extinguished.

environment. Most vendors of electronic devices will allow a trial period free of charge or for a nominal rental fee. In many large urban areas, there are AAC "libraries" where potential consumers can check out AAC devices for a trial period before making a final selection. Similarly, many large school districts keep a sampling of AAC devices on hand to lend to children and their families to select a system before incurring the expense of purchasing the device.

Selecting the AAC System

Although there may be a need to experiment with various systems of AAC before finding one that is functional for the child and the family, the selection of a system of AAC is not a haphazard process. Any experimentation is limited, not totally open; a few systems selected based on the child and the family assessment will be evaluated for their usefulness. The clinician should consider the following questions: (1) Would the child and the family do best with an unaided or an aided system of AAC? (2) Should a low-technology or a high-technology system be tried? (3) If an aided system is recommended, what type of symbols should be used? and (4) How will the child access the system?

Unaided or aided? As noted, unaided systems of AAC do not rely on external devices; they are gestural systems that employ only the child's purposeful movements. For example, American Sign Language (ASL) is a gestural language system that serves as an alternative to oral speech (review Box 15.1 for more examples of unaided systems of AAC).

Advantages of unaided systems of AAC include:

- *Spontaneity of output.* Children using unaided systems of AAC produce gestures within naturalistic settings, without needing to locate, for example, a picture book or AAC device. They are limited only by the extent of their sign (gestural) vocabulary. Children who have been taught unaided systems of AAC can communicate independently, so there is never any question as to the authorship of their message. As we shall see later, this is not the case with some other systems of AAC.
- *No financial cost.* Unaided systems of AAC are expense-free and therefore accessible to any child in any situation. Funding is not a concern.
- *Ease with which people in the child's environment can support the child's communicative attempts.* It is usually no problem for busy parents, teachers, and others familiar to the child to learn to recognize and properly reinforce a child's repertoire of gestures. There is no need to remember to program a computer or to locate pictures, symbols, or objects needed for aided systems of AAC.

> If possible, children should be taught gestures that are commonly recognized (e.g., nodding the head for *yes*).

Disadvantages of unaided AAC include:

- A *limited applicability beyond the child's immediate environment.* The child may not be understood by people in the community unfamiliar with the gestural system employed.
- *Lack of immediate feedback.* There is some thought, but little empirical evidence, that children initiate and respond to communicative interaction more often and more proficiently if they are provided with a **voice output communication aid** (**VOCA**). These are systems that provide a synthetic voice for the child, thereby providing immediate auditory feedback—a feature that is lacking in unaided AAC systems.

Despite these disadvantages, we will confess to having a bias toward trying unaided systems of AAC with a child first, if the child has sufficient gross and fine motor skills to be taught a gestural system. Goldstein (2002) conducted an exhaustive review of research efficacy studies investigating treatment methods for children with autism and found good empirical support for using a total communication approach, incorporating both signing and oral speech. Also, it has been our experience that even children with severe cognitive impairment can learn signs for basic needs and wants, if consistently taught and demanded by those in the environment before reinforcement is given. The authenticity of the child's messages, the spontaneity with which those messages are produced, and the ease with which they are reinforced are advantages that, in our opinion, outweigh any limitations of unaided systems of AAC.

> What is total communication?

There will be other clinicians who will favor aided systems of AAC, systems that employ various external devices or materials to help the child communicate. Recall that aided systems of AAC range from low-technology to high-technology.

Low-technology or high-technology? In selecting an aided system of AAC that may prove to be functional for a child, clinicians should consider the many options available, from low-technology systems to high-technology systems. Decisions should be based on results of the assessment, an analysis of the child's environment, and a realistic appraisal of sources of funding that may be available.

Low-technology systems of AAC can consist of something as simple and low-cost as pasting pictures or symbols to various manila folders, with each folder containing symbols that are relevant to particular activities (e.g., in a classroom setting, one folder for circle time, another for art projects, still another for requesting playground equipment, etc.). The SLP can collaborate with teachers, parents, aides, and others to devise child-specific systems designed to meet the needs of the child and the demands of the environment.

Two types of low-technology systems of aided AAC have some experimental validation of efficacy: (1) the **Picture Exchange Communication System** (PECS; Bondy & Frost, 1994), for spontaneous expressive language, and (2) **visual schedules,** for receptive language (Bryan & Gast, 2000). In the PECS, children learn to exchange picture cards for desired items, so that manding (requesting) is the first unit of verbal behavior taught (see Figure 15.1

figure 15.1   **A Picture Exchange Communication System (PECS)**

A Picture Exchange Communication System (PECS) binder turned to a page showing preferences for food.

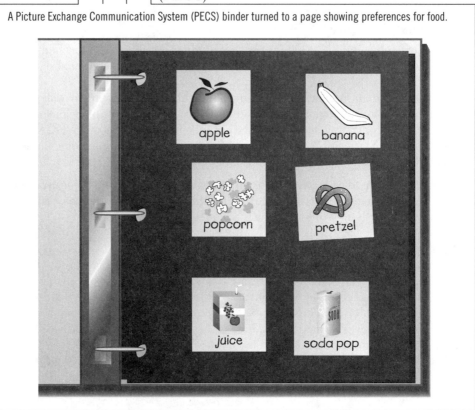

for an example of a PECS binder turned to a page indicating preferences for food). Reinforcement is immediate, with the communicative partner supplying the child with whatever has been requested. No verbal prompts are given during training for PECS, so the child does not become over-reliant on prompting and learns to independently initiate communicative interaction.

Besides manding, children can also learn to make comments (tacting) and respond to questions using PECS. Using a multiple baseline across subjects experimental design (Hegde, 2003), Charlop-Christy and her colleagues demonstrated increases in spontaneous speech and social-communicative behaviors and decreases in problem behaviors in three children with autism who were trained to use PECS (Charlop-Christy et al., 2002). Another experimental study has demonstrated that PECS is more effective than manual signs in teaching mands to children with severe to profound developmental disability (Chambers & Rehfeldt, 2003). Several clinical reports also have documented significant improvement in communication of children with autism and other disorders with PECS (e.g., Kravits et al., 2002; Magiati & Howlin, 2003; see Bondy & Frost, 2001, for a review of studies). See Photo 15.2 for an example of a child using PECS to communicate with an adult.

Visual schedules can be used for several purposes, most frequently to keep children with PDD on task and engaged during classroom activities. The exact form of a visual schedule can vary according to the needs of particular settings and children, but the basic principle is to devise a pictorial representation of daily activities to which nonverbal children can refer (see Figure 15.2 for an example of a visual schedule for a bedtime routine). Bryan and Gast (2000) used an A-B-A-B withdrawal research design (Hegde, 2003) to investigate the effects of a picture activity schedule on four children with high-

> Children can also learn to do various tasks by referring to a series of pictures sequencing a task broken down into small steps, another function of a visual schedule.

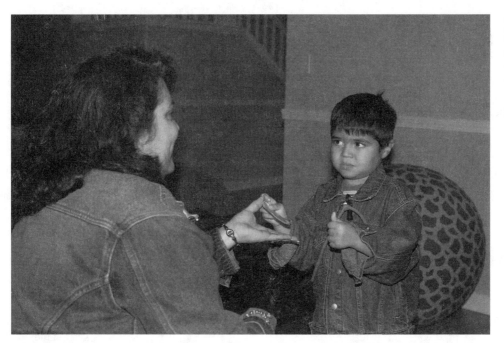

photo 15.2
Children first learn to mand with PECS; here a child asks for a favorite toy by handing over a PECS symbol.

figure 15.2 | A Visual Schedule for a Bedtime Routine

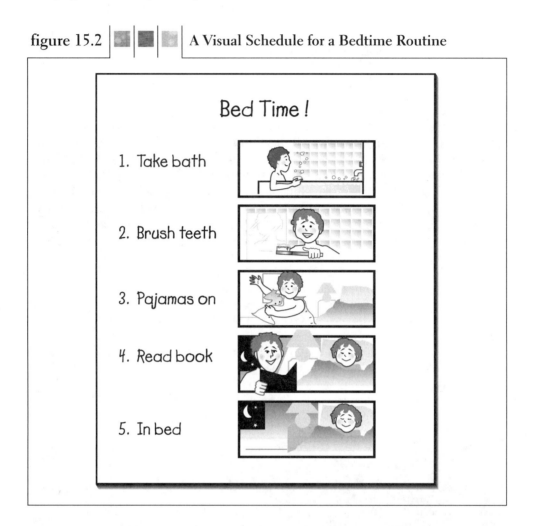

functioning autism in a special education classroom setting. These children were verbal, but receptive language was not sufficient for classroom functions. The children showed increases in on-task and on-schedule behavior when the picture schedule was introduced, with those behaviors decreasing when the picture schedule was withdrawn, followed by an increase when the picture schedule was reintroduced. Further research is needed to validate this and other visual schedules in teaching children to perform various tasks.

There are advantages and disadvantages to low-technology systems of AAC. Advantages to low-technology systems of aided AAC include low-cost, portability of materials (as opposed to more cumbersome electronic devices), and the ease with which such systems can be customized to meet the needs of a particular child in a specific environment. Disadvantages include a more limited repertoire of communicative functions (compared to more sophisticated high-technology systems), the need for individuals in the environment to update and revise symbols used, a lack of spontaneity, and a question as to the authorship of the messages.

Authorship of messages is a particularly troubling issue. For both low-technology and high-technology aided systems of AAC, the child must rely on others in the environment to set the system up, maintain it, and make carefully considered guesses about what the child might like to communicate. There may be messages the child might prefer to convey, but cannot, if the system is not set up to provide the means to convey those messages. Also, perhaps the messages the child is provided with do not represent what the child might like to communicate, but the child accesses them anyway, because they are available, and the child has been trained to do so. These are the types of limitations that will be more thoroughly discussed in a further section on ethical issues in the field of AAC.

High-technology systems of AAC are generally thought to be more versatile than low-technology systems. There is a wide variety of communicative functions that the AAC user can produce, such as engaging in social conversation, making comments or "small talk." Some are voice output communication aids (VOCAs), supplying a child with a digitized or synthetic voice to relay a message. Mirenda (2003) described some limited retrospective and case study research supporting the efficacy of VOCAs in increasing communicative skills and providing a means of more naturalistic interactions with peers and teachers in both special education and inclusive classroom settings (Light et al., 1998; Mirenda, Wilk, & Carson, 2000; Schepis et al., 1998). Certainly, VOCAs provide a means of communication that can be understood by anyone the child may communicate with, in any setting. However, it has not been experimentally demonstrated that VOCAs, which can be quite expensive, are superior to other systems of AAC in increasing communicative interactions of the VOCA-user (see Figure 15.3 for an example of a VOCA).

> What does *VOCA* stand for?

There are some disadvantages to high-technology systems of AAC. The most obvious is the high cost of some systems, often thousands of dollars. If there were clear empirical evidence supporting the superiority of these systems over unaided or low-technology systems, this additional cost would be justified, but no such evidence exists. High-technology AAC devices can also be quite complex, challenging the technological know-how of SLPs, teachers, and parents who must initially program and continuously update computerized devices. Lack of portability is another drawback—busy parents and teachers may find it difficult to transport an electronic device during a community outing or transitions to the playground or cafeteria. As a result, spontaneity of communication is hampered, because the device must be available, properly programmed, and ready to go when the child is ready to communicate. Finally, the same reservations regarding authorship of messages conveyed apply to high-technology systems as they do to low-technology systems, perhaps to an even greater extent. If an individual cannot directly access a device, alternative methods require people in the environment to program messages they *think* the individual might want to express. As we shall see, there are some troublesome ethical issues regarding the authorship of an AAC user's message when others are involved in generating those messages.

If the clinician recommends an aided system of AAC, there are other decisions that must be made. Those include: (1) the type of symbol system to be used and (2) how the child will access the system.

What type of symbol system? In unaided systems of AAC, the symbols used include various gestures, facial expressions, and other body movements produced by the child. Aided systems of AAC incorporate symbols such as objects, line drawings, photographs, various

figure 15.3 | 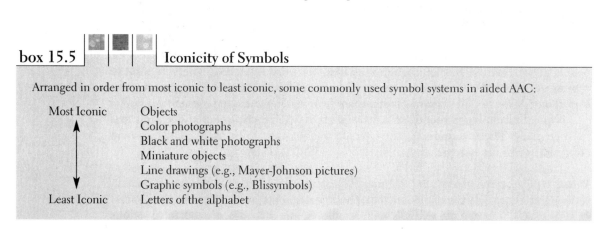 | **A Voice Output Communication Aid (VOCA) with Scanning Option**

graphic systems, or letters of the alphabet. Both unaided symbols and aided symbols vary in their degree of **iconicity,** the degree to which they directly resemble their referent—that which they are meant to represent. The more a symbol resembles its referent, the more iconic it is. The most iconic is the object itself (e.g., a cup to hand to a partner to indicate "I want a drink."). Letters of the alphabet are examples of symbols that are much less iconic (see Box 15.5 for a spectrum of iconicity in symbol systems used for aided AAC).

True or False? The more iconic a symbol is, the less it resembles its referent.

In general, less iconic symbol systems are more versatile than iconic symbol systems. Children who are literate and can produce alphabetic writing (or typing, or pointing) generate an unlimited number of messages compared to the limited communicative functions

box 15.5 | | **Iconicity of Symbols**

Arranged in order from most iconic to least iconic, some commonly used symbol systems in aided AAC:

Most Iconic   Objects
  ↑   Color photographs
                       Black and white photographs
                       Miniature objects
                       Line drawings (e.g., Mayer-Johnson pictures)
  ↓   Graphic symbols (e.g., Blissymbols)
Least Iconic   Letters of the alphabet

available to children who rely on an object symbol system. However, children learn symbols that are more iconic more easily than they learn less iconic symbols (Fuller, 1997; Luftig & Bersani, 1985). Children with cognitive impairments should initially be taught a more iconic symbol system, moving to less iconic symbols as the children's communicative skills improve (See Figure 15.4 for an example of objects used in an AAC device.

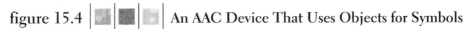 True or false? Symbols that are more iconic are easier for children to learn than symbols that are less iconic.

How will the child access the system? Especially for children with severe physical disability, the clinician must consider how the child will access the AAC system, or what the interface between the child and the AAC system will look like. There are two major types of interface between the child and the AAC system: (1) direct access and (2) scanning.

In **direct access,** the child selects symbols from an array either by keyboarding, pointing, touching, with eye gaze, or with the help of an adaptive pointing device. On a PECS activity board, for example, a child can select a picture card indicating a desire to go outside, and hand it to the classroom teacher. On various VOCA electronic devices, a child can push a picture to produce a synthetic voice saying, "I want to go outside." A child with good control over head movement, but little use of hands, arms, or legs, may access a symbol through fixed eye gaze. A less physically impaired, literate child can point to letters on an alphabet board to convey messages. Others might have functional keyboarding skills and will generate messages in that way; typing on a keyboard is the most versatile type of direct access.

What are two major types of interface?

A child who cannot gain direct access to an AAC system can use an alternative method called **scanning,** an indirect method of symbol selection. With scanning, an array of options is presented to the child through visual, auditory, or both modalities. The child

figure 15.4   **An AAC Device That Uses Objects for Symbols**

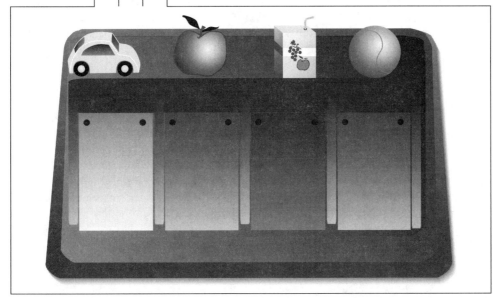

listens, watches, and, when the desired symbol presents itself, activates a switch to "freeze" the device on that symbol. Many AAC electronic devices have both direct access and scanning capabilities. Switches can be set up so that the child can activate them with any part of the body that has been determined to be under the child's volitional control. Physically involved children can push switches with their heads, their feet, knees, chins, and so forth. While direct selection of symbols is always the preferred method, scanning may be the only option available to children with severe physical disabilities.

Guidelines for AAC selection. Taking into consideration the advantages and disadvantages of the various types of AAC systems available, the following guidelines are offered for recommending an AAC system:

- Consider the child's potential for the development of speech; some systems have good research supporting their efficacy in facilitating development of oral speech (e.g., see sections on ASL and PECS)
- Consider the child's cognitive level; prefer unaided systems or less complex aided systems using iconic symbols to establish a basic communicative repertoire for children who have cognitive impairment
- Consider the child's motor and sensory capabilities to assess how the child will access the AAC system
- Consider cost; know the sources of funding that may be available (e.g., health insurance, grants, charitable organizations), if an expensive device is selected
- Consider complexity—do the people in the child's environment have the technological knowledge necessary to program and maintain complicated devices?
- Select AAC systems that people in the child's environment have indicated a willingness to support

Even the most carefully selected method of AAC may prove to be nonfunctional for a child. That is why, in the initial stages of treatment, it may be necessary to experiment with various types of AAC, perhaps exploring the child's skill in learning manual signing while also providing a picture system of communication. Regardless of the system selected, there will be necessary modifications made to basic treatment procedures to teach and support a child using AAC.

Supporting Children Using AAC in Naturalistic Settings: Modifications to Treatment Procedures

With many systems of AAC, it may be necessary to establish basic skills and an initial repertoire of communicative functions, by teaching a child in a clinic setting, using procedures described in previous chapters. The recommended treatment procedures for teaching a child to use the PECS, for example, begins with intense discrete trial therapy to establish the behavior of handing a card to the clinician to gain access to a desired item. Other behaviors that may be established in the clinic setting include those that the child will need to access an AAC system—pointing or using a body part to activate a switch, for example.

As quickly as possible, however, treatment for a child learning to use an AAC system should move to naturalistic settings, with discrete trials embedded in the day-to-day routine in the child's home or classroom. To learn to effectively use a system of AAC, the child must have many opportunities to communicate throughout the daily routines. Even more than usual, then, the clinician must evaluate a child's environment and assess the adequacy of opportunities given to the child to communicate. The clinician should teach the significant persons in the child's environment to increase communicative opportunities for the child and to use various techniques to encourage (e.g., prompt) and reinforce communication. Treatment, then, is extended not only to the child, but to those who will be supporting the child's communicative attempts in the natural environment.

Identifying Communication Opportunities in Naturalistic Settings

During assessment, the clinician should observe and evaluate communication opportunities that are available for the child in naturalistic settings. The same kind of observations should be made to monitor and support the child's progress in using the AAC system in various environments. Reichle, York, and Sigafoos (1991) proposed taking an ecological inventory of communication opportunities given to AAC users. There is no one way to format an ecological inventory, and it can be taken for a variety of reasons. Before treatment begins, the clinician can devise a child-specific assessment tool which will provide a description of opportunities given to the child to communicate and make observations as to what might be done to increase those opportunities. During treatment, the clinician can take another ecological inventory to see if communication opportunities have increased and how well the child is responding to those opportunities. If adjustments must be made, or one AAC system abandoned in favor of another one, the clinician can take an ecological inventory to examine the effects of those adjustments.

To illustrate this technique, let us suppose that a clinician has been teaching a nonverbal 5-year-old boy, Johnny, with cerebral palsy to use a VOCA mounted on his wheelchair to request items and actions and engage in greeting and leave-taking social rituals (see Figure 15.5 for a drawing of a wheelchair-mounted VOCA). Johnny can directly access his VOCA, with some difficulty, by using his left index finger to push the desired symbol. The clinician observes Johnny in the classroom to see how many communication opportunities he is given to use his VOCA. When he arrives in the classroom, he is greeted warmly by the classroom teacher and the aide, who encourage him to respond by activating the *Hi! How are you doin'?* symbol on his VOCA. During circle time, he smiles and makes body movements, but is not asked to participate in activities such as answering simple questions, singing along with the rest of the class, or choosing activities. During an art project, he is given an ample amount of art supplies, and an aide gives him hand-over-hand guidance to complete the project. For recess, he is parked by the supervising teacher under the shade of a tree, watching, but not participating in, playground activities. In the cafeteria, an aide prompts him to select a drink, and he hits the *juice* symbol on his VOCA. The aide then gives him hand-over-hand assistance to eat the very adequate amount of food he has been given. Box 15.6 shows an ecological inventory the clinician devised as a result of these observations.

figure 15.5 | A Wheelchair-Mounted Voice Output Communication Aid (VOCA)

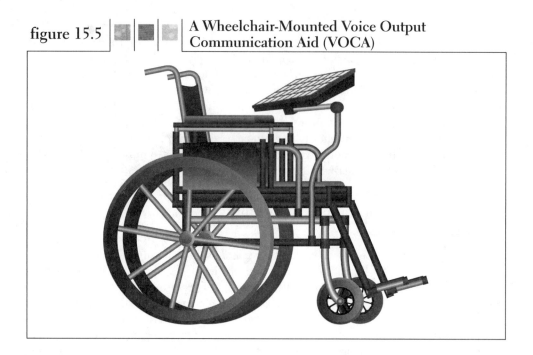

Creating Communication Opportunities in Naturalistic Settings

An ecological inventory such as the one described in the preceding section can be taken in each of the child's natural environments. The inventory should describe the communication opportunities created for the child, and the manner in which those in the child's environment prompt a response. It is usually necessary to teach parents, teachers, caregivers, aides, and others to create more opportunities for communication and prompt for response initiation. Sigafoos (1999) discussed the following ways to "engineer" the environment to create a need for the communicative functions of requesting or rejecting: (1) missing-item format, (2) interrupted-behavior chain, (3) incomplete presentation, (4) delayed assistance, and (5) wrong-item format. It may be noted that some of these techniques overlap with our discussion on milieu teaching in Chapter 8.

The missing-item format requires adults to withhold one or more items needed to engage in or complete a desired activity (Cipani, 1988; Sigafoos et al., 1995). For example, during an art project, necessary supplies such as glue or scissors might be left off the table to prompt a request from the child. In the interrupted-behavior chain technique, a child is interrupted from completing a just-initiated action to prompt a comment or a request. A child who is heading out the door for recess, for example, may be blocked by a teacher standing in the doorway to create an opportunity for the child to request, "Out, please!" (Goetz, Gee, & Sailor, 1985; Hunt et al., 1986). For incomplete presentation, the child might be given a puzzle, for example, without all of the pieces. If the child asks for the pieces, the adult might provide one or two additional pieces, and then wait again for the child to ask for more

A child who is nonverbal and has autism has learned to set the table for snack time in his preschool class. The teacher hides the plates and waits for the child to ask for them by giving her a PECS symbol for *plates*. This is an example of what language-evoking technique?

Child's Name: Johnny Doe   Grade: Kindergarten
Age: 5   Teacher: Mrs. Smith

Activity	Communication Opportunities Observed	Given	Not Given
Arrival in the classroom	Greeting the teacher	X	
Circle time:			
Calendar activity	Answering simple questions (e.g., "What day is it today?")		X
Singing songs	"Singing" along		X
Storybook reading	Choosing a favorite book		X
Art project:			
Making a snowman	Asking for necessary supplies		X
	Asking for help		X
Recess	Greeting peers and interacting with peers (e.g., "Hi! Can I play?")		X
	Asking for an activity (e.g., "I want to play ball!")		X
	Asking for a break (e.g., "I'm tired! Can I take a rest?")		X
Cafeteria	Choosing a drink	X	
	Asking for assistance		X
	Asking for more food or drink		X

Notes for the Classroom Teacher and Aide:

Great job on prompting the greeting ritual! Also, I was happy to see the VOCA programmed for choosing either *milk* or *juice* for lunch; he seemed to enjoy having that choice. I do have a few suggestions.

1. Record choices on the VOCA for circle time activities:

   - Let Johnny be the "calendar kid" occasionally by giving him a "day of the week" symbol programmed with the day and date
   - Record the song you are planning to sing; let Johnny activate the recorder so he can sing along
   - Occasionally allow Johnny to select the book to be read during circle time by offering him a choice of two or three books

2. During art projects:

   - Be a little "sneaky" and don't give Johnny everything he needs for his art project. Program the VOCA with choices such as *More glue, please,* or *I need the scissors, please*
   - Rather than have the aide automatically help him, have Johnny hit his *I need help* symbol

3. During recess:

   - Appoint two or three peers to be Johnny's special "playground pals" for the day. Teach the children to prompt Johnny to interact (e.g., "Hi, Johnny! Do you want to play?")
   - Have an aide present to assist with Johnny's participation (remember to allow Johnny to ask for help!) in playground games, such as playing catch
   - Be alert for signs of fatigue, and encourage Johnny to ask for a break, if he needs one

4. During lunch:

   - Have the aide sit and look expectantly at Johnny to prompt, "Help me, please!"
   - Try giving him a little less food than usual; prompt him to ask, "More, please!"

(Duker, Kraaykamp, & Visser, 1994). Delayed assistance is a technique that can be used when an adult in the environment notices the child requires assistance in completing a difficult activity (Reichle, Anderson, & Schermer, 1986). A child might be struggling to open a package of cookies during preschool snack time, for example, and an aide might move closer to the child, to invite a request for assistance. The wrong-item format can be utilized to teach rejecting or protesting. The adult may place an array of appealing items in front of a child, and when the child reaches for a preferred item, the clinician quickly hands the child the wrong item by "mistake" to create the opportunity for the child to say, "No!," thus rejecting the item (Sigafoos & Roberts-Pennell, 1999).

For all of these techniques, if the child does not initiate the proper response, a verbal prompt should be given (e.g., "What do you need?"), but the prompt should be systematically faded until the child spontaneously produces the correct response. The clinician should promptly reinforce the child's correct responses or appropriate communicative attempts. The techniques lend themselves to the daily routine at school, home, or in the community. They are appropriate for children using a variety of AAC systems, such as signing, picture systems of communication, and electronic devices. Adults in the child's environment can easily be taught to use these techniques, creating many discrete trial opportunities for communicative interaction embedded in naturalistic settings.

To summarize, modifications in treatment procedures necessary to support the AAC-using child in natural environments are:

- Teach basic skills necessary to learn and access an AAC system using discrete trial therapy in the clinic setting, but move treatment into naturalistic settings as quickly as possible
- Identify the communication opportunities given to the child in naturalistic settings
- Suggest ways in which communication opportunities can be increased
- Teach adults in the child's environment to "engineer" the environment to increase communication opportunities, to prompt responses, to fade prompts, and to provide immediate reinforcement for correct responses
- Provide ongoing support to the AAC-using child and to the child's communicative partners

Some Ethical Considerations

In our discussion of advantages and disadvantages of various systems of AAC, we discussed spontaneity and authorship of the messages generated as important factors to consider. We made an argument that, before all else, unaided systems in which the child uses body movement to convey messages, be tried. There can be no doubt when the child is using unaided AAC that the messages generated are coming from the *child*—that those messages are truly what the child communicates. Similarly, in aided AAC, the messages of a child who is literate and can access a keyboard or alphabet board can also be assumed to be authentic, although production will be less spontaneous.

When children do not have the motor or cognitive skills necessary to learn an unaided system of AAC or to access directly an aided system, interventionists must settle for a system that depends on others in the environment to decide on what it is the child *might* want to communicate. Even systems children can directly access have some problems with authenticity, because they provide the child with only a limited number of options, selected by others. To take an innocuous example, let us say a child's teacher programmed a VOCA to order chicken nuggets, a hamburger, or a cheeseburger at a popular fast-food restaurant during a class outing. The child directly selected "I want cheeseburger, please," and a cheeseburger was then purchased for the child. Later, when talking to the child's family, the teacher discovered that the child's favorite meal from that particular restaurant is a fish sandwich—an option that was not given to the child, who was given no other means of communicating that preference.

This is a simple example of an ethical dilemma. A more extreme example is the phenomenon of **facilitated communication (FC)**, a controversial practice that is still common in some parts of the country, even in the face of overwhelming controlled experimental

---

box 15.7 **The Phenomenon of Facilitated Communication: Beacon of Hope or Pseudoscience at Its Worst?**

Facilitated communication (FC) is a technique by which a "facilitator" sits beside a person who is nonverbal, and usually autistic, to give hand-over-hand manual guidance while the person accesses a keyboard, pecking away laboriously with one finger to produce messages, but, curiously, often not looking at the keyboard (Shane, 1994). The technique was developed in Australia initially as a method to teach pointing skills (Crossley & McDonald, 1980). However, it quickly developed into what has been called the "facilitated communication craze" (Wolfensberger, 1994), when introduced and promoted by Biklen (1990) as a method to give people with autism a method of communication.

Miraculously, by virtue of simple "physical, communication, and emotional supports" (Duchan, et al., 2001, p. 140), many children and adults with autism, previously nonverbal and presumed to be illiterate, began typing messages of incredible complexity and astonishing insight. Professionals hailed FC to be a major breakthrough in our understanding of what autism is, and what it is not. All this, without the benefit of any controlled scientific research providing evidence of the efficacy of FC.

When individuals using FC began generating messages alleging they had been sexually abused, determining the authorship of the messages became a pressing legal issue (Shane, 1994). Scientific research subjected the facilitator (the person giving hand-over-hand assistance) and the facilitated (the nonverbal person) to a variety of controlled experimental conditions. For example, a picture of a common object would be shown to the facilitated person, but not to the facilitator, or the facilitator would be shown a picture of an

object and the facilitated person a picture of a different object. Facilitated people, many of whom had previously been reported to be capable of generating sophisticated messages, could not type the name of the common object presented. When a different picture was shown to the facilitator, the typed message identified the object as being that which the facilitator saw—not the one the facilitated person saw. Other similar types of tasks produced the same results (see Green, 1994, for a review of these studies).

In the light of such overwhelmingly negative scientific evidence, it should seem obvious that FC should have been discredited. However, this has been a controversy that refuses to die. Proponents of FC have proven to be quite resistant to abandoning the method, pointing to a few case studies as proof of efficacy, and criticizing the controlled scientific experimentation that has been conducted as imposing artificial, invalid tasks on people who communicate much better in naturalistic environments when supported by people who respect them as competent communicators (Cardinal & Biklen, 1997; Janzen-Wilde, Duchan, & Higginbotham, 1995). One group of authors has proposed "guidelines" for SLPs who wish to use FC or other controversial methods in their practice. The seven guidelines include using "specially designed informed consent procedures" and preparing for "eventual challenges" (Duchan et al., 2001).

We would propose but one guideline: when a method has been subjected to controlled, replicated scientific experimentation that has produced negative evidence of efficacy, DO NOT USE IT.

evidence that the messages generated by many FC-users are not theirs but the messages of their "facilitators" (see Box 15.7 for a discussion of facilitated communication).

To guard against the possibility of "putting words into the mouths" of children with disabilities, clinicians should adhere to the following guidelines:

- If it is necessary to use an AAC system with preprogrammed symbols and a limited number of communicative options, consult thoroughly with those in the child's background to determine the child's preferences; make sure those preferences are available to the child when programming the AAC device.
- When analyzing a child's communicative skill, take into account only those behaviors that are clearly observable and measurable. Probe behaviors that are at a higher level than what might be expected for the child, and rejoice if they are found; but do not assume extraordinary hidden talents in every child assessed.
- Treat children respectfully as potential communicative partners, but make a realistic appraisal of the limitations exhibited by many children with severe disabilities and set reasonable goals for treatment.

A Look into the Future: Technology, Communication, and Children

AAC is still in its infancy, expanding over the last two decades as technology has improved, and consumers have been included in the development process, identifying their needs and driving innovations in design and quality (Blackstone, Williams, & Joyce, 2002). Perhaps in the future technological advances will result in the creation of AAC high-technology devices that overcome the disadvantages of high expense, complexity, and lack of spontaneity and authenticity of messages generated (See Box 15.8 for an example of NASA-developed new technology that could have applicability to AAC).

Unfortunately, because the emphasis on developing AAC technology has been on the needs of adult users, much of the technology available today is not suitable for young chil-

---

box 15.8   **Speaking through the Muscles: An Innovation from NASA**

When a person "talks to himself" or reads silently, the tongue and vocal cords receive speech signals from the brain. Scientists at the National Aeronautics and Space Administration (NASA) have found that small, button-sized sensors placed under the chin and on both sides of the "Adam's apple" (the bulge in the throat made by the thyroid cartilage of the larynx) can pick up those nerve signals, send them to a processor, and then to a computer program that translates them into words. The result is a system that translates silent muscle movements associated with speech into communicative messages.

Further experimentation will include controlling a simulated Mars rover with silently spoken words. There are other applications pertinent to astronauts and space travel, but, as one scientist stated, "A logical spin-off would be that handicapped persons could use this system for a lot of things" (NASA, 2004, online).

Could this be the beginning of AAC devices that produce effects on listeners by translating silent muscle movements into communicative messages? If so, future possibilities for cognitively intact, nonverbal people are virtually open-ended.

dren. Some research has been conducted to determine how AAC technology might be modified to better meet children's needs. Drager, Light, Speltz, Fallon, and Jeffries (2003) investigated the efficiency with which 30 typically developing 3-year-old children could gain access to symbols arranged in different ways on three VOCAs. The authors found that all of the systems were difficult for the children to learn—the children demonstrated low levels of accuracy across all four training sessions. How much more difficult, the authors pointed out, it must be for very young children with multiple disabilities to learn to access such a device.

A further study by Drager and her colleagues investigated the variable of menu display (e.g., the manner in which symbols are presented) and its effect on the ease with which 30 typically developing 3-year-old children learned to identify vocabulary items using those displays. Two groups of 10 children used displays exhibiting symbols representing both concrete and abstract vocabulary items in a traditional "grid" design—lined up in rows on an AAC device. The third group used a display that embedded symbols into a contextual scene depicting a cutaway house revealing rooms and common household scenes within those rooms. Results indicated that each group of children initially had difficulty learning to identify symbols representing specific vocabulary words. However, by the second learning session, children in the group using the contextual scene menu display performed significantly better, a trend that continued throughout the remainder of the sessions. Although typically developing children were used in the study, and results may not be generalizable to children with disabilities, the authors concluded that embedding symbols into contextual scenes may be a more appropriate, effective way to present AAC symbols to young children (Drager et al., 2004). More research of this kind is needed to examine the effects of different variables on teaching children to access AAC devices.

Light and Drager (2002) called for a renewed effort to "ensure that young children with communication disabilities attain the power of communication, language, and literacy in their lives" (p. 17) through improving the design of AAC technologies for young children. They suggested that, ideally, new technological designs should:

- Be appealing to young children. Designs should be colorful, incorporating much decoration; one study has shown that children like systems that look "cool"—not just functional, but fun (Light & Pitkin, 2003).
- Be integrated into children's daily activities. Children often must leave an activity to access an AAC device; it is difficult to play *and* use a device. Light, Binger, and Kelford Smith (1994) investigated storybook reading interactions between AAC-using children and their parents. They found that children did not have ease of access to their AAC device; it was simply too difficult to balance the child, the book, *and* the device on the parent's lap. Future designs should emphasize improvement of portability and accessibility, so that AAC can be easily incorporated into play and language learning activities.
- Be easy for children to learn and use; also, be easy for families, professionals and others to learn and maintain.
- Be reflective of the cultural and linguistic diversity of American society. Many times, the only language available through an AAC device is English. Children from families who are monolingual and speak a language different from English cannot use the device to communicate with, and are therefore isolated from, their family members.

Future designs should "better support the needs of children from different cultural and linguistic backgrounds and their families" (Light & Drager, 2002, p. 21).

Future innovations in AAC devices may provide means of communication previously inaccessible to children who are nonverbal. Speech-language pathology will be greatly affected by such innovations. If it is progressively more possible to effectively treat people who are speechless, the clinicians will be even more effective in teaching those with some oral skills. Speech-language pathologists have the training and the expertise to make a difference in the lives of children who have language disorders, even those whose disabilities are severe. It is hard to imagine a more satisfying, rewarding experience than to help a child become a competent communicator.

■ ■ Chapter Summary

In this chapter we described children who, because of their severe mental and physical disabilities, have only extremely limited oral language skills that do not meet their social and academic needs. Such children need augmentative and alternative communication (AAC), which can either enhance (augment) the limited oral language skills or provide an alternative form of communication. AAC involves both aided and unaided systems. Unaided systems are gestural systems that do not require external aids. Aided systems use various external aids; they range from the low-technology communication boards to high-technology computerized systems.

Candidacy for an AAC system must be carefully determined by a thorough assessment. Both standardized and criterion-referenced assessment instruments are available for children who are nonverbal or minimally verbal. In addition, child-specific assessment that concentrates on such functional targets as requesting, protesting, commenting, and initiation of social interactions will be useful. Clinicians should not neglect receptive language, literacy skills, and possible higher-level speech and language skills in nonverbal children. Physical, sensory, and cognitive skills as well as the child's environment and family support should be assessed to determine what type of AAC device might be useful for the child, and how the child will access the device.

Devices and AAC programs vary in iconicity, which is the degree to which a symbol resembles its referent; generally, it is easier to learn to use symbols with a high degree of iconicity, although less iconic symbols are more versatile. Some devices allow direct access to the messages while others allow scanning of various options to select a desired message. Future advances in technology should result in improvement in the design of AAC devices, especially for children.

■ ■ Study Guide

1. Distinguish between augmentative and alternative forms of communication (AAC). Provide a broad sketch of children who need augmentative forms versus those who need alternative forms of communication.

2. You are doing your internship in a school that has a special program for children who need AAC. Your clinical supervisor there has assigned two 8-year-old children who may be candidates for AAC. The supervisor has told you that one is more severely limited than the other. She also pointed out that the one who is less severely affected is motorically and intellectually more capable than the other. She wants you to assess the two children, possibly to select a low-technology system for one child and a high-technology system for the other. Design an assessment procedure for these two children. Specify the standardized, criterion-referenced, and client-specific procedures you would use. What kinds of information would you seek from the two families?

3. Some children who currently need an AAC system may be taught functional oral language skills later. In assessing and treating such children, what prognostic signs would you look for that suggest a high or low likelihood for the development of oral speech?

4. Critically evaluate some of the low-technology AAC systems that have received experimental support. Describe how you use each of them.

5. Distinguish between iconic and noniconic systems. Point out the advantages and disadvantages of these systems. State why it is often necessary to experiment with various AAC systems before purchasing one.

6. Compare direct access systems with scanning devices. What child characteristics suggest the appropriateness of each of these two systems?

Glossary

Acceleration-deceleration injuries: Those insults to the brain that are caused by initial violent movement of the head and the subsequent slowing down; these are caused by forces applied to a movable head.

Aided systems of AAC: Systems of AAC that utilize various external aids, such as picture books, alphabet boards, or computerized devices.

Allomorphs: Slight variations of morphemes.

Allophones: Slight variations in production of phonemes.

Alternative form reliability: Consistency of scores on parallel forms of the same test administered to the same individual.

American Sign Language (ASL): A nonverbal language in which the speaker manually gestures to communicate.

Anencephaly: A birth defect caused by the absence of the cranial bones and often the cranial skin.

Antecedent events: Certain aspects of a social situation—isolated or simplified—to serve as specific stimuli that are systematically presented to the child during treatment.

Antonyms: Pairs of words that convey directly opposite meaning.

Aphasia: In adults, a loss or impairment of language skills caused by a recent insult to the brain.

Apraxia of speech: A motor planning disorder in the absence of muscle weakness.

Asperger's syndrome (AS): A pervasive developmental disorder having as its most distinctive feature a severe impairment in social interaction.

Assessment: The overall clinical activities designed to understand the child and the family before a treatment program is established for that child.

Ataxic cerebral palsy: A type of cerebral palsy characterized by ataxia, a balance disorder; characteristics include impaired balance, stumbling and awkward gait, and clumsy and uncoordinated movements.

Athetoid cerebral palsy: A type of cerebral palsy characterized by athetosis, slow, involuntary, and writhing (worm-like) movements

Auditory training program: Teaching children with hearing loss to understand and appreciate the differences in amplified sounds that he or she is perhaps hearing for the first time.

Augmentative and alternative communication (AAC): A set of procedures and processes to either supplement limited oral skills with nonoral methods or provide nonoral methods as the primary means of communication for individuals who are functionally nonverbal. Supplementing limited oral skills with nonoral means is **augmentative;** providing nonoral methods as the primary means of communication is **alternative.** Systems of AAC can be either **aided** or **unaided.**

Autism: A pervasive developmental disorder that varies on a spectrum of mild to profound impairment marked by disinterest in typical social interaction, severely impaired communication skills, and stereotypical movements; also known as autism spectrum disorder (ASD).

Autoclitics: Secondary verbal behaviors that describe or comment upon certain aspects of primary verbal behaviors.

Baseline: A measure of response rates in the absence of treatment.

Behavioral contingency: An abstract relationship between antecedent stimulus events that set the stage for communication, communicative behaviors themselves, and the consequences that follow, usually in the form of listener reactions.

Behavioral treatment: The management of an interdependent relationship between antecedent events, specified language skills, and consequences in the form of listener reactions.

Bidialectal: Proficiency in two variations of a language.

Booster treatment: Treatment offered any time after an initial dismissal.

Bound morphemes: Those suffixes and prefixes which are attached to a root word.

Brain stem injury: An insult to the brain in the area of the brain stem, often resulting in coma.

Briefing: The initial phase of the interpretive process during which the SLP consults with the IT and explains the goals of the upcoming interpretive task.

Case history: A detailed written account of information on the child and the family.

Cerebral palsy: Refers to a complex set of neuromotor and developmental disorders caused by an injury to a still developing nervous system.

Childhood disintegrative disorder (CDD): A pervasive developmental disorder marked by a prolonged (at least 2 years) period of normal development before the child begins to regress, losing social, language, self-help, and motor skills.

Child-specific measurement: Procedures designed to quantify observed behaviors during assessment that a clinician constructs to meet the specific needs of a child; synonymous with **client-specific measurement.**

Client-specific experimental approach: The sequence of language targets specific to the client and experimentally determined; compare to **normative approach.**

Cloze: The classic sentence completion method in which the clinician starts a sentence and pauses waiting for the child to complete it; synonymous with **partial model.**

Cochlear implants: Electronic devices surgically placed in the cochlea and other parts of the ear to directly deliver the sound signal to the auditory nerve endings in the cochlea.

Code-switching: Easily alternating between two languages; a typical process of bilingual acquisition.

Collaborative model: A method of service delivery that emphasizes the interrelatedness of the school SLP with other school personnel.

Coma: A state in which a person is unconscious and unresponsive, following a serious brain injury.

Communication: Exchange of information between two or more persons in verbal, gestural, written, and other forms.

Concurrent validity: A positive correlation between a new test and a well-established old test of the same skill.

Conditioned generalized reinforcement: The method of increasing behaviors with the help of consequences that give access to a variety of reinforcers whose effects are learned.

Conditioned generalized reinforcers: Consequences that have a wide range of effects and do not depend on a state of deprivation.

Conductive hearing loss: Type of hearing loss caused by diminished air conduction of sound to the inner ear due to problems in the ear canal and the middle ear.

Connotative meaning: Emotional meanings words suggest.

Constituent definition: Defines terms with other terms, as does a dictionary.

Construct validity: Expert judgment that given test scores are consistent with a theoretical expectation regarding the skill being measured.

Consultative model: A method of service delivery in which language services are provided indirectly, with the SLP consulting with others in the child's environment, who will then carry out recommendations for intervention.

Content validity: Expert judgment that the contents of a test are relevant, necessary, and sufficient to measure what the test is supposed to measure.

Contingency priming: A technique of drawing out reinforcement (usually attention and positive comments) from ignoring persons; also known as **reinforcement recruitment.**

Continuous schedule of reinforcement: A schedule of reinforcement in which the child receives a reinforcer for every correct response.

Contrecoup injury: Damage to brain tissue that occurs opposite to the point of impact.

Controlled conversation: Verbal interaction between the clinician and the child that is more directed than **spontaneous conversation.**

Controlled research: Scientific research in which treatment is compared against no treatment and may involve either a group experimental design or a single-subject experimental design.

Conversational partner generalization: The production of newly learned skills in relation to people who are not involved in treatment.

Conversational repair strategies: Verbal behaviors both listeners and speakers exhibit when there are breakdowns in communication; a pragmatic language skill.

Conversational turn-taking: Talking and listening in alternative fashion; a pragmatic language skill.

Corrective feedback: A technique to decrease incorrect responses by telling that a given response was wrong, inappropriate, in efficient, and so forth.

Coup injury: Damage to the brain tissue at the point of impact.

Cri du chat syndrome: A genetic syndrome caused by the deletion of a small portion of the short arm of chromosome 5; characterized by a high-pitched cry, low birth weight, slow physical growth and motor development, small head (microcephaly), widely set eyes (hypertelerosim), cleft palate or cleft lip and palate, low-set ears that may also be malformed, partial webbing or fusing of fingers or toes, and low muscle tone.

Criterion-referenced assessment: Assessment instruments that do not offer normative standards; the results are instead described in terms of skills that are present, absent, mastered, not mastered yet, and so forth.

Cross-sectional: A one-time observation of a section of society to observe specified variables, such as prevalence of a disorder.

Dazed: Reduced awareness of the surrounding due to a recent brain injury.

Deaf: Severe to profound hearing loss; those who are cannot effectively use their residual hearing to acquire oral language.

Debriefing: The third and final phase of the interpretive process during which the SLP and the interpreter/translator discuss any problems that were encountered during the interaction along with suggestions for how future interactions can be improved.

Deep structure (D-structure): A hypothetical structure that holds underlying meaning of sentences in the transformational generative grammar.

Delay: A technique used in the milieu approach to teach a child to respond to environmental stimuli other than listener attention as cues for verbalization.

Delayed assistance: Withholding immediate offer of assistance when a child requires assistance in completing a difficult activity; designed to encourage spontaneous action or verbalization.

Delirium: Either reduced level of consciousness or a state of excessive arousal; the result of a severe brain injury.

Derivational bound morphemes: Elements of language that help create entirely new words from root words.

Descriptive classification: A method of classifying language disorders based on observable language behaviors.

Desktop auditory trainer: A desktop instrument that receives the clinician's speech, amplifies it, and feeds it to the children's ears through headphones they wear.

Diagnosis: Determination of the cause of a disorder; in speech-language pathology, the determination that there is (or is not) a disorder based on the results of valid and reliable measurement of relevant skills.

Dialect: A variation in a language due to cultural and regional influences.

Dialogic reading: A method of shared storybook reading that requires the adult to ask open-ended questions, add information to the text, and have the child retell the story.

Differential reinforcement: A procedure in which desirable responses to a specific stimulus are reinforced, and undesirable responses are not reinforced.

Differential reinforcement of alternative behavior (DRA): Replacing an undesirable behavior with a more acceptable, socially more desirable behavior.

Differential reinforcement of incompatible behavior (DRI): A procedure that indirectly reduces undesirable responses by increasing a behavior that is incompatible with it.

Differential reinforcement of low rates (DRL) of responding: A method in which the child is reinforced for reducing the frequency of a troublesome behavior.

Differential reinforcement of other behavior (DRO): A technique in which a particular undesirable behavior will not be reinforced but many alternative, desirable behaviors will be reinforced.

Diffuse axonal injury: A serious neurological consequence of acceleration/deceleration forces of nonpenetrating brain injury, which consists of torn nerve fibers in widespread areas of the brain.

Diffuse vascular injury: Ruptures in the brain's blood vessels, causing bleeding in the brain.

Diplegia: Paralysis or paresis (muscle weakness) that affects like parts on both the sides of the body (e.g., either two legs or the two arms).

Direct access: One of two basic methods of accessing an AAC device in which an individual can directly select symbols from an array either by pointing, touching, with eye gaze, or with the help of an adaptive pointing device; see **scanning** for an explanation of the second basic method.

Direct replication: Treatment research in which the same researcher repeats his or her own earlier study with little or no modification in the treatment procedure to see if the results are reliable.

Direct response-reduction procedures: A method in which a contingency is placed on the behavior that needs to be reduced.

Discourse: The connected and contingent flow of language during social interaction between two or more individuals.

Discrete trials: One structured opportunity to produce a given target response; it is discrete because trials are separated from each other by a short period of time.

Discrimination: The behavioral process of differentiating responses and concepts by differential reinforcement.

Discriminative stimuli: Stimuli in the presence of which a response has been reinforced in the past, and therefore, the response is more likely in its presence.

Down syndrome: A common syndrome of developmental disability due to a chromosomal defect.

Durational measures: Specific time periods for which a skill was sustained.

Dysarthria: A complex set of communication problems due to impaired neural control of muscles involved in speech production.

Dysphagia: A swallowing disorder.

Dysphasia: A dated term that suggested language disorders with a neurological basis.

Echoic: A verbal response that recreates its own causal stimulus; imitative responses.

Echolalia: A speaker's repetition of what has been said, either immediately or in the future, sometimes the far future; a common feature of autism.

Emergent literacy skills: Early skills that precede or are presumed to be prerequisites for later developing reading and writing skills.

Empirical: Pertaining to objective, observable, and measurable events or experiences.

Empirical test: A condition that scientists arrange to experience the truth value of statements.

Empiricism: A branch of philosophy; the belief that sensory experience is the source of knowledge.

Ethnocultural generality: The degree to which a treatment known to be effective with one ethnocultural group also is effective with other ethnocultural groups.

Ethnographic interviewing: A technique that involves seeking out people from a particular culture and asking detailed questions regarding that culture.

Etiological classification: Description of disorders or diseases based on their causes.

Etiology: The study of causes of disorders and diseases.

Evidence-based practice: The use of only those treatment methods that are supported by controlled and replicated research evidence.

Expressive language: Language production.

Extinction: Terminating the reinforcer for a response while no other attempt is made to stop it.

Eye contact: Maintenance of mutual eye gaze during conversation; a pragmatic language skill.

Facilitated communication (FC): A controversial method of AAC in which messages are generated by an individual accessing a keyboard with the help of a "facilitator" who offers physical support to the individual's arm and hand; controlled scientific experimentation has produced evidence that the messages generated are almost always generated by the facilitator.

Fading: A technique in which the special stimulus control of target behaviors is gradually reduced until the child can produce them under typical social stimulus conditions.

Fetal alcohol syndrome (FAS): A congenital syndrome (noticed at birth, but not inherited) caused by maternal alcohol abuse during pregnancy.

Fetal anoxia: Reduced supply of oxygen when the labor is prolonged or the baby fails to cry (and breathe) soon after birth; may cause brain damage.

Fictional narratives: Telling a story, such as a well-known fairy tale or the plot of a popular movie or television show.

Figurative meaning: The meaning phrases or sentences convey that the words used in those productions do not convey.

Final conversational probes: A probe to assess generalized production of a target behavior at the level of conversational speech in the clinic and in natural environments.

Fixed interval schedule: A pattern of reinforcement in which a fixed amount of time should elapse before the child is given an opportunity to earn a reinforcer.

Fixed ratio schedule: A pattern of reinforcement in which a specific number of responses are required to earn reinforcers.

Follow-up assessment: A pure probe of target language skills in conversational speech conducted post-dismissal.

Fossilization: Errors that may remain after acquiring a high level of proficiency in a language although language production is otherwise excellent; a typical process of bilingual acquisition.

Fragile X syndrome (FXS): A genetic syndrome caused by a single-gene mutation on the X chromosome.

Free morpheme: A morpheme that conveys meaning standing alone and cannot be broken down into smaller parts.

Frequency measure: The number of times a behavior is exhibited under specified stimulus conditions.

Frequency modulated (FM) auditory trainer: An amplification system that consists of a transmitting unit and a receiving unit.

Functional response classes: Skills that are independent of each other.

Functional unit: Independent categories of verbal behaviors and their causes.

Function words: A category of words that includes such grammatic morphemes as articles, prepositions, and conjunctions.

Generality: The wider applicability of a treatment procedure or conclusions based on research data.

Generalization: A behavioral process in which learned responses are extended to new stimuli, new situations, and expanded into novel kinds of responses.

Generalized productions: Responses that are given to stimuli not used in training.

Grammatical transformation: An operation that relates the deep and surface structures and yields different forms of sentences.

Grapheme: The smallest part of written language, represented by alphabetic letters.

Guided reading: An instructional method in which the adult requires the child to read aloud while giving the child direct feedback and guidance.

Hard of hearing: Reduced hearing acuity; individuals who are hard of hearing may acquire oral language primarily by hearing the language spoken around them, sometimes with the help of amplication.

Hearing aids: Devices which amplify sound; the main rehabilitation device for most children with hearing loss.

Hearing screening test: A quick measure of hearing done to rule out a hearing loss.

Hemiplegia: Paralysis or paresis of only one side of the body (either the right or the left).

High probability behavior: A method of increasing desirable but infrequently exhibited behavior by making a more frequently exhibited behavior contingent on the former.

Homonyms: words which are identical in pronunciation but have different meanings; synonymous with *homophones*.

Hydrocephaly: An accumulation of cerebrospinal fluid (CSF) in the ventricles (channels or cavities) of the brain, leading to its enlargement and swelling.

Hyperlexia: The presence of precocious reading ability in children with severe language and learning disorders.

Hypothyroidism: An endocrine disorder due to an autoimmune reaction that produces antibodies against the thyroid gland and thus limits the production of thyroxin.

Iconicity: The degree to which a symbol directly resembles the referent that it is meant to represent; the most iconic symbol is the referent itself.

Idioms: Sayings, proverbs, and so forth; a type of figurative language.

Imitation: The child's response that follows a clinician's model.

Incidence: The rate at which a disorder appears in the normal population over a period of time, typically one year.

Incidental teaching: A **milieu teaching** technique that helps teach elaborated language productions to children who independently initiate a communicative interaction with an adult.

Indirect response-reduction techniques: Procedures in which contingencies are placed only on desirable behaviors to increase them while simultaneously decreasing undesirable behaviors as a side effect.

Inferential meaning: That which is not explicitly stated but deduced (presumed) from what is said.

Inflectional bound morphemes: Elements of language that are attached to a root word to add to the meaning of the root word, but not to create a new word.

Informative feedback: Increasing behaviors by providing feedback on the progress a child is making in learning a skill.

Instructions: Verbal directions on how to perform an action.

Interaction: The second phase of the interpretive process which is the actual event at which the IT will be providing services.

Interference: Influence of the first language on phonologic, semantic, syntactic, and pragmatic aspects of second language production; a typical process of bilingual acquisition.

Interjudge reliability: Consistency of scores when two or more observers (clinicians) administer the same test or measurement procedure.

Intermittent schedule of reinforcement: A **schedule of reinforcement** in which reinforcers are given only for some of the correct responses; a certain number of responses go unreinforced.

Intermixed probes: A **probe** in which both trained and untrained stimulus items are alternated in assessing generalized production during the initial stages of treatment.

Interpreter: One who converts an oral message from one language to another.

Interrupted-behavior chain: A child is interrupted from completing a well-established routine or continuing with an activity.

Interval schedule: Describes the relationship between the amounts of time that is allowed to lapse before an opportunity is given for the child to earn a reinforcer.

Interview: A face-to-face conversation with the child, the child's family, and any other relevant individuals in the child's environment, such as teachers.

Intrajudge reliability: Consistency of scores when the same clinician administers the same test to the same person a second time with a reasonable interval between the two administrations.

Intraverbal: Speech caused by speakers' own prior speech.

Irony: A property of statements that mean the opposite of what the words themselves suggest; a type of figurative language.

Joint attention: Two persons paying attention to the same object or event at the same time; often refers to the behavior of a caregiver and child.

Language: From the linguistic viewpoint, an arbitrary system of codes and symbols used to express ideas; from the behavioral viewpoint, language is **verbal behavior.**

Language Acquisition Device (LAD): A hypothetical entity proposed by Chomsky to describe the innate knowledge children have of the universal grammar.

Language differences: Variations mostly in language production (and to some extent in comprehension) that may be associated with a particular linguistic or cultural community.

Language disorders: A lack of acceptable or effective social repertoire to affect the behaviors of other persons in social, educational, and occupational milieu, or to be affected by the verbal behaviors of other persons.

Language production: Speaking or communicating nonverbally.

Language sample: Recording of a child's conversational or naturalistic verbal interaction with the clinician, family member, or both.

Lexical relationships: The different ways in which words are related to each other.

Lexicon: The number of words a child produces and understands; synonymous with **vocabulary.**

Linguistics: An academic discipline concerned with the study of language.

Lipid metabolic disorders: An accumulation of fat in neural tissue, leading to developmental disability and health problems; a well known lipid metabolic disorder is Tay-Sachs disease.

Literacy skills: Reading and writing skills.

Longitudinal method: Repeated observations of children or adults over time to investigate identified variables; a scientific research method.

Macrocephaly: A condition characterized by abnormal largeness of the head and brain in relation to the rest of the body.

Maintenance: The continued production of clinically established skills over time and across situations.

Maintenance strategies: Techniques that help extend treatment to natural settings.

Mand: A group of verbal responses that have motivational states as causes and often specify their own reinforcers.

Mand-model: A **milieu teaching** method to establish joint attention as a cue for verbalization.

Manual guidance: A treatment technique consisting of the clinician providing gentle, but firm, physical assistance to help a child make a movement.

Meaning: In the behavioral view, a relation between a controlling variable (cause) and a verbal production; a relation between antecedents and the responses.

Mean length of utterance: Calculated by counting the total number of morphemes and dividing that number by the total number of utterances in a language sample; a general measure of language development.

Measurement: Procedures that quantify observed objects, events, and their mathematical properties.

Metaphor: A saying that makes a comparison between two or more objects, which are unlike each other (e.g., "The moon was a ghostly galleon . . . ").

Microcephaly: A small head circumference in relation to the rest of the body.

Milieu teaching: A treatment method that embeds behavioral principles into naturalistic settings; the overall goal of milieu teaching is to evoke and reinforce child-initiated communicative interactions in response to environmental stimuli.

Missing-item format: Requires adults to withhold one or more items needed to engage in or complete a desired activity.

Mixed hearing loss: A type of hearing loss caused by dysfunction of both the middle ear and the inner ear.

Mixed type of cerebral palsy: A type of cerebral palsy in which both **spasticity** and **athetosis** may be present in the same child, although typically one or the other will be the dominant symptom.

Model: The production of the target behavior by anyone who wants to teach a child an imitative response.

Molecular genetics: A field of study that isolates specific genes for specific clinical conditions.

Monoplegia: Paralysis or **paresis** in which only one limb is affected.

Morphemes: The smallest units of meaning within a language.

Morphologic component: That component of language which includes the smallest elements of grammar called **morphemes.**

Morphology: The study of word structures.

Multiple contingencies: Combining different techniques of reinforcement to increase their effectiveness.

Multiple meanings: Different meanings that the same word, phrase, or sentence may convey.

Narrative skills: Telling stories or personal experiences with sufficient details, temporal sequence, characterization, and so forth; a pragmatic language skill.

Negative evidence: Research data that fails to support a treatment technique or a research hypothesis.

Neonatal risk factors: Factors that affect an infant's development.

Nonacceleration injuries: Insults to the brain that are caused by forces applied to a fixed (immovable) head.

Nonexclusion time-out: Involves imposing a very brief period of nonreinforcement upon the child—a "frozen moment" of time in which no reinforcing activity takes place.

Nonpenetrating injuries: Those insults to the brain in which no foreign bodies or particles enter the brain; the meninges remain intact; and the brain is damaged with or without skull fracture.

Nonverbal communication: Production of such nonvocal behaviors as signs, gestures, and nonvocal symbols to affect other people.

Nonverbal (physical) prompts: Various signals or gestures the clinician gives to evoke the correct production of a target behavior.

Nonverbal pragmatic language skills: Various physical, emotional, and gestural aspects of communication that supplement, expand, or even contradict what is said in words.

Norm: A standard set by the mean (average) performance from a representative sample of a larger group, giving a range of scores against which a particular child's scores may be compared.

Normative approach: The sequence of language targets according to the known normal sequence of language acquisition.

Obligatory contexts: Situations in which the rules of language dictate the use of a particular language structure.

Occupational therapist (OT): A licensed professional qualified to assess daily living skills, vocational skills, and degrees of sensory/motor impairment in individuals who are limited by physical injury, cognitive deficits, social impairment, or developmental disability.

Onset and rime: In the production of a word, the onset is the initial consonant(s), and a rime is the part of the syllable that contains the vowel and all that follows it.

Operational definition: A definition that describes that which is being defined in observable and measurable terms.

Orofacial examination: Procedures conducted to check the speech structures of the face and mouth to rule out any gross anatomic and physiologic deviations that may be associated with the speech or language disorder.

Overextension: An inappropriately generalized production of a word.

Paralysis: Characteristic of abnormal muscles; muscles cannot be moved.

Paraplegia: Paralysis of only the lower extremities (lower trunk, including legs).

Paresis: Muscle weakness; paretic muscles can move, although inefficiently and with reduced strength.

Partial echoics: Repetitions of only a portion of what is heard.

Partial model: A modeled stimulus that provides only a portion of the correct response; just enough for the child to imitate the response.

Penetrating injuries: Those insults to the brain in which the skull is fractured, the meninges (the brain coverings) are torn, and the brain tissue is damaged.

Perinatal conditions: Factors that may affect the infant during birth.

Personal narratives: Relating personal experiences, such as telling about what happened at their last birthday party or where their family went on vacation.

Pervasive developmental disorders (PDDs): Serious and multiple impairments in child development typically diagnosed in young children, usually before the age of 3.

Pervasive Developmental Disorder—Not Otherwise Specified (PDD-NOS): A diagnostic category used when children have some symptoms of PDD, but not enough to warrant any of the specific diagnoses.

Phenylketonuria: A metabolic disorder caused by a deficiency in metabolizing an amino acid called phenylalanine.

Phone: Any sound a vocal tract is capable of making.

Phoneme: Traditionally defined as the smallest unit of sound that conveys meaning within a language; smallest part of spoken language that affects word meaning.

Phonemic awareness: Skill in discriminatively hearing, identifying, and manipulating individual phonemes, or sounds, in spoken words.

Phonics: A method of reading instruction that emphasizes sound-letter correspondences and skills in "sounding out" (decoding) words.

Phonological awareness: A term that includes phonemic awareness but also involves awareness and manipulation of rhyme, words, syllables, and onsets and rimes.

Phonological component: That component of language that includes the production of speech sounds and the organization of sounds according to the rules of the sound system of a language.

Phonological processes: Speech sound error patterns children typically display when acquiring the sound system of their language.

Phonology: The study of speech sounds, speech production, and the rules for combining sounds to form meaningful words and sentences.

Physical therapist (PT): A licensed professional qualified to assess physical limitations and provide treatment to maximize the independence of people who are physically impaired.

Picture Exchange Communication System (PECS): A system of AAC in which children learn to exchange picture cards for desired items.

Population genetic study: A type of research study that infers the influence of genetic factors in causing clinical conditions based on differential prevalence of disorders in blood relatives contrasted with their prevalence in unrelated individuals.

Postnatal factors: Factors that negatively affect the growth of the child, especially those that affect the child's development.

Post-reinforcement pause: A resting period that occurs after the ratio or interval requirements of the reinforcement schedule have been met and the reinforcer has been delivered.

Prader-Willi syndrome (PWS): A genetic syndrome caused by a deletion of paternal chromosome 15 in the q11-q13 region or when the child receives two copies of chromosome 15 from the mother, and none from the father.

Pragmatics: The study of language production in social contexts.

Predictive validity: Relatively accurate predictions of future performance on a related task from the scores of a test.

Prenatal conditions: Factors that may affect the developing fetus prior to birth, including conditions that may result in premature birth.

Prevalence: The number of individuals who are diagnosed to have a particular disorder at a given time.

Primary language: The language learned by a person first; designated L1.

Primary reinforcement: A method of increasing target skills by arranging consequences that promote the biological survival of a species; **primary reinforcers** such as food and drink are useful in treating childhood language disorders; synonymous with **unconditioned reinforcement.**

Print-referencing: A method of shared storybook reading in which adults use various prompts to draw children's attention to elements on a printed page.

Probe: An assessment of **generalized productions,** based on treatment.

Prognostic statement: A considered professional judgment regarding the course of the disorder under given conditions.

Prompt: A gentle hint; it is another special stimulus that is added or layered over other evoking or modeling stimuli.

Psychologist: A licensed professional who specializes in the study of human behavior, and is the specialist most qualified to determine if a child has any cognitive deficits.

Pull-out model: A method of service delivery in which the children receive either individual or small-group therapy in a clinic room.

Pure probes: A **probe** in which only untrained items are presented.

Quadriplegia: Paralysis or **paresis** in which all four limbs are affected.

Rationalism: A branch of philosophy; the belief that reason is the source of knowledge.

Ratio schedule: Describes a relationship between the number of correct responses the child makes and the delivery of the reinforcer.

Ratio strain: Abrupt and large shifts in reinforcement schedules, a condition in which the correct response rates decrease drastically.

Receptive language: A modality of language having to do with comprehension.

Referential meaning: A simple, concrete meaning of a word that points to (refers to) an object, person, or event.

Reinforcement recruitment: See **contingency priming.**

Reinforcement withdrawal: Weakening behaviors by removing consequences that sustain them.

Reinforcer: Consequences provided contingent upon a correct response that consists of events or objects; the consequence should be delivered immediately after a response is made and should increase the correct response rate.

Relational meaning: Words that express relation between objects and events.

Reliability: The degree to which repeated measures of the same event are consistent.

Replicated: Treatment research that is repeated by either the same researcher or other researchers.

Response cost: Each incorrect response results in the loss of a reinforcer.

Response generalization: Production of novel responses that are similar to those that were trained.

Rett's syndrome (RS): A genetically based neurological disorder that is included under the category of pervasive developmental disorders; affects only females.

Risk factors: Relevant factors that are present in persons from before the time of a clinical diagnosis.

Savant syndrome: The co-occurrence of high-level skills and generally low intelligence.

Scanning: A method to access an AAC device; it is an indirect method of symbol selection in which the individual listens, watches, and, when the desired symbol presents itself, activates a switch to "freeze" the device on that symbol.

Schedule of reinforcement: Describes the relationship between a criterion level for correct response or responses and the delivery of a reinforcer.

Screening procedures: Procedures that are designed to identify children who may face the risk of a language disorder.

Script narratives: Describing a routine series of events.

Scripts: Plans or descriptions of routine events, episodes, and personal experiences that are played out by participants; the basis for *script therapy.*

Secondary language: Language learned after learning a **primary language**; designated L2.

Secondary reinforcement: The use of social consequences to increase skills.

Seizures: A condition that results from abnormal electrical activity in the brain, and manifests itself in symptoms such as loss of consciousness, convulsions, or staring spells.

Self-monitoring: A teachable skill that includes self-evaluation and self-correction.

Semantic component: That component of language which is the element of meaning.

Semantic relations: Contrasting units of meaning that are expressed in different forms of words, phrases, and sentences.

Semantics: The study of the meaning of words and word combinations of a language.

Sensorineural hearing loss: A type of hearing loss due to damage to the cochlea.

Sequential bilingualism: Learning the second language (L2) after having learned a **primary language** (L1).

Setting generalization: Production of responses learned in one setting in new settings that are not involved in training.

Shaping: A treatment procedure designed to teach more complex skills by building upon a series of simple skills; synonymous with *successive approximation.*

Silent period: A period of observational learning in which children listen much but produce little of the second language; a typical process of bilingual acquisition.

Similes: Makes a comparison between two or more objects which are unlike each other and include either the word *as* or *like* (e.g., "My love is like a red, red rose").

Simultaneous bilingualism: Learning two languages at the same time.

Simultaneous speech: A treatment technique in which the clinician and the client produce the target response at the same time.

Spastic cerebral palsy: The most common type of **cerebral palsy** characterized by spasticity, rigidity or stiffness, of the muscles.

Specific language impairment: A language problem in a child who does not have any other clinical condition that would explain it or would be associated with it.

Speech: The production of sounds of a language.

Split-half reliability: Consistency of scores calculated separately for the two halves of a test.

Spontaneous conversation: Discourse evoked by social and natural contexts and stimuli.

Standardized test: A structured assessment tool that has been finalized on the basis of performance of a sample of children drawn from a defined population.

Stimulability: The child's imitation of models provided.

Stimulus generalization: The production of already learned responses in relation to novel but similar stimuli.

Stupor: A state in which a person is unresponsive except for pain and strong stimuli following a serious injury to the brain.

Surface structure (S-structure): Refers to the actual order of words in a sentence; part of Chomsky's theory of syntax.

Syllable: Part of a word containing a vowel; the vowel can stand alone or be surrounded by one or more consonants.

Symbolic play: Play activities in which a child uses one object to represent another.

Symptomatic treatment: Treatment of the symptoms with no clear understanding of the cause.

Syndrome: A constellation of signs and symptoms that are due to morbid genetic and anatomic–physiologic processes.

Synonyms: Different words that convey the same meaning.

Syntactic component: The part of language that refers to syntactic rules.

Syntax: A collection of rules about word combinations and sentence structures within a language.

Systematic replication: Treatment research in which previous studies are repeated in different settings, by different researchers, using different clients to show that the technique will yield similar results under varied conditions and with different clinicians.

Tact: Verbal responses whose cause is a state of affairs in the environment and which are reinforced socially.

Tactile prompts: A special variety of nonverbal prompts involving touch known to be effective with some children, especially those with autism or developmental disability.

Target behavior: Any verbal or nonverbal skill a clinician wishes to teach a child.

Telegraphic speech: A type of condensed speech in which only essential words are used.

Test–retest reliability: Consistency of scores obtained from repeated administration of the same test.

Textual prompts: Printed cues that help evoke a target response.

Textuals: A class of verbal behaviors that are controlled by printed stimuli or writing.

Time-out: A period of nonreinforcement, imposed response contingently, resulting in the reduction of that response.

Topic initiation: The pragmatic language skill of introducing new topics for conversation.

Topic maintenance: Continuous conversation on the same topic without abrupt interruptions or introduction of new topics; a pragmatic language skill.

Transformational generative theory of grammar: A Chomskian theory that states that, through innate knowledge of the rules of grammar and grammatical transformations, language users can generate countless varieties of sentences.

Translator: One who converts a written message from one language to another.

Traumatic brain injury (TBI): Injury to the brain sustained by physical trauma or external force.

Tuberous sclerosis: A genetic disorder, the effects of which include the growth of benign tumors in the brain and other vital organs, epilepsy, mental deterioration, and various skin lesions.

Type-token ratio: A measure of word variety in a child's speech.

Unaided systems of AAC: Systems of augmentative and alternative communication that do not rely upon instruments or other external aids.

Unconditioned reinforcement: A method of increasing target skills by arranging consequences that have biological value to the recipients, synonymous with **primary reinforcement.**

Underextension: Production of words in overly restricted contexts—showing lack of appropriate generalization.

Universal grammar: A set of rules that applies to all human languages and can help generate new sentences with varied word combinations.

Unreplicated: An unreplicated study is the first or the original study on a given procedure or concept.

Validity: The degree to which an instrument measures what it purports to measure.

Variable interval schedule: The time duration allowed to elapse between opportunities to earn a reinforcer is varied around an average.

Variable ratio schedule: The number of correct responses required to earn reinforcers is varied around an average.

Verbal behavior: Behavior reinforced through the mediation of other persons; preferred to the term *language* from the behavioral viewpoint.

Verbal communication: Vocal language production and involves orally produced speech to affect listeners.

Verbal interaction sampling: Behaviors of one or more individuals are measured during social communication.

Verbal pragmatic skills: Various communication skills needed to initiate and sustain conversation, also known as **discourse.**

Verbal prompt: a special verbal stimulus designed to evoke a correct response.

Visual schedules: A pictorial or symbol system to promote receptive language which can be used for several purposes, most frequently to keep children with PDD on task and engaged during classroom activities.

Vocabulary: The number of words a child produces and understands; synonymous with **lexicon.**

Voice output communication aids (VOCAs): An AAC device that, when activated, provides a digitized or synthetic voice to relay a message.

Williams syndrome: A genetic syndrome caused by deleted genetic material on chromosome 7; characterized by developmental disability, low birth weight, slow physical and behavioral development, learning disabilities, attention deficit, visuospatial deficits, irritability during infancy, various kinds of phobias, hypersociability, and speech-language disorders.

Wrong-item format: Handing the child a wrong item that helps teach rejecting or protesting behaviors.

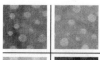

References

Abbeduto, L. (1991). Development of verbal communication in persons with moderate to mild mental retardation. *International Review of Research on Mental Retardation, 17,* 91–115.

Abbeduto, L. (1995). Effects of sampling context on the expressive language of children and adolescents with mental retardation. *Mental Retardation, 33*(5), 279–288.

Abbeduto, L., & Hagerman, R. J. (1998). Language and communication in fragile X syndrome. *Mental Retardation and Developmental Disabilities Research Reviews, 3*(4), 313–322.

Academic Communication Associates. (2004). *Pragmatic communication skills protocol.* Oceanside, CA: Academic Communication Associates.

Adamovich, B. L. (1997). Traumatic brain injury. In L. L. LaPointe (Ed.), *Aphasia and related neurogenic language disorders* (2nd ed.), (pp. 226–237). New York: Thieme Medical Publishers.

Adams, L., & Conn, S. (1997). Nutrition and its relationship to autism. *Focus on Autism and Other Developmental Disabilities, 12,* 53–58.

Adams, M. J. (1990). *Beginning to read: Thinking and learning about print.* Cambridge, MA: MIT Press.

Administration on Developmental Disabilities, U.S. Department of Health and Human Services. (2005). *ADD program overall.* Retrieved January 9, 2005, from www.acf.hhs. gov/programs/add/1385.htm.

Agency for Toxic Substances and Disease Registry. (2004). Alert 970626. Retrieved on August 21, 2004, from www.atsdr. cdc.bov/alerts970626.html.

Ahlander, E. M. (1999). *Effect of pause-and-talk and response cost on stuttering: Social and professional validity.* Unpublished master's thesis, California State University, Fresno, CA.

Algozzine, B., Eaves, R. C., Mann, L., & Vance, H. R. (1993). *Slosson full-range intelligence test.* East Aurora, NY: Slosson Educational Publications.

Alpert, C., & Rogers-Warren, A. K. (1985). Communication in autistic persons. In S. F. Warren & A. K. Rogers-Warren (Eds.), *Teaching functional language* (pp. 123–156). Austin, TX: Pro-Ed.

Alpiner, J. G., & McCarthy, P. A. (2000). *Rehabilitative audiology: Children and adults* (3rd ed.). Philadelphia, PA: Lippincott, Williams, & Wilkins.

American Academy of Pediatrics Committee on Drugs (1998). Neonatal drug withdrawal. *Pediatrics, v101*(6), 1079–1089.

American Association on Mental Retardation. (2005). *Definition of mental retardation.* Retrieved on January 5, 2005, from www.aamr.org/Policies/faq_mental_retardation.shtml.

American Educational Research Association, American Psychological Association, & National Council of Measurement in Education. (1985). *Standards for educational and psychological testing.* Washington, DC: American Psychological Association.

American heritage college dictionary (3rd ed.). (1997). Boston: Houghton Mifflin.

American Psychiatric Association. (2000). *Diagnostic and statistical manual of mental disorders (DSM IV): Fourth edition, text revision.* Washington, DC: American Psychiatric Association.

American Psychological Association. (2001). *Publication manual of the American Psychological Association* (5th ed.). Washington, DC: American Psychological Association.

American Speech-Language-Hearing Association. (1983). Social dialects. *Asha, 25,* 23–27.

American Speech-Language-Hearing Association. (1991). Committee on prevention of speech, language, and hearing problems. *The prevention of communication disorders tutorial.* Washington, DC: Author.

American Speech-Language-Hearing Association. (1996a, Spring). Guidelines for the training, credentialing, use, and supervision of speech-language pathology assistants. *Asha, 38,* 21–34.

American Speech-Language-Hearing Association. (1996b, Spring). Inclusive practices for children and youths with communication disorders: Position statements and technical report. *Asha, 38* (Suppl. 16), 35–44.

American Speech-Language-Hearing Association. (1997–2003). Evidence-based practice. Retrieved on September 20, 2004, from www.asha.org/members/slp/topics/ebp/htm.

American Speech-Language-Hearing Association. (2001). *Roles and responsibilities of speech-language pathologists with respect to reading and writing for children and adolescents: Practice guidelines.* Rockville, MD: Author.

American Speech-Language-Hearing Association. (2003a). Code of ethics (revised). *ASHA supplement, 23,* 13–15.

American Speech-Language-Hearing Association. (2003b). *Highlights and trends: ASHA counts for 2003.* Retrieved

June 6, 2004, from www.asha.org/about/membership-certification/member-counts.htm.

American Speech-Language-Hearing Association. (2004a). *Communication facts: Special populations: Augmentative and alternative communication — 2004 edition.* Retrieved on August 20, 2004, from www.asha.org/members/research/reports/aac.htm

American Speech-Language-Hearing Association. (2004b). *Introduction to augmentative and alternative communication.* Retrieved on August 20, 2004, from www.asha.org/public/speech/disorders/Augmenative-and-Alternative.htm.

American Speech-Language-Hearing Association (n.d.). Child language disorders. Retrieved January 1, 2004, from www.asha.org/members/research/NOMS2/child_language.htm.

American Speech-Language-Hearing Association Ad Hoc Committee on Service Delivery in the Schools. (1993). Definitions of communication disorders and variations. *Asha, 35* (Suppl. 10), 40–41.

Amir, R. E., Van den Veyver, I. B.; Wan, M.; Tran, C. Q., Francke, U., & Zoghbi, H. Y. (1999). Rett syndrome is caused by mutations in X-linked MECP2, encoding methyl-CpG-binding protein 2. *Nature Genetics, 23,* 185–188.

Anastasi, A. (1982). *Psychological testing* (6th ed.). New York: Macmillan.

Anderson, D. M., Keith, J., Novak, P. D., & Elliot, M. A. (Eds.). (2002). *Mosby's medical dictionary* (6th ed.). St. Louis, MO: Mosby.

Anderson, V., & Thompson, S. (1988). *Test of written English (TWE).* Novato, CA: Academic Therapy Publications.

Arndorfer, R., Miltenberger, R., Woster, S., Rortvedt, A., & Gaffaney, T. (1994). Home-based descriptive and experimental analysis of problem behaviors in children. *Topics in Early Childhood Special Education, 14,* 64–87.

Arnold, D. H., Lonigan, C. J., Whitehurst, G. J., & Epstein, J. N. (1994). Accelerating language development through picture book reading: Replication and extension to a video-tape training format. *Journal of Educational Psychology, 86,* 235–243.

Arntzen, E. & Almas, I. K. (2002). Effects of mand-tact versus tact-only training on the acquisition of tacts. *Journal of Applied Behavior Analysis, 35,* 419–422.

Asperger, H. (1944). Die "autistischen psychopathen" im kindesalter. Archiv fur Psychiatrie und Nervenkrankheiten, *117,* 76–136.

Asperger, H. (1979). Problems of infantile autism. *Communication, 13,* 45–52.

Asperger, H. (1991). "Autistic psychopathy" in childhood [Translated and annotated by U. Frith]. In U. Frith (Ed.), *Autism and Asperger syndrome* (pp. 37–92). [Original paper published in 1944.] Cambridge, UK: Cambridge University Press.

Association for Retarded Citizens. (2005). *Mental retardation v. developmental disabilities: Should the ARC change its focus from serving people with mental retardation to serving people with all developmental disabilities?* Retrieved January 9, 2005, from www.rcomo.org/whatismr.htm.

Atherton, S., & Hegde, M. N. (1996). *Experimental enrichment of language in young children.* Paper presented at the Third National Conference on Treatment Research, Rehabilitation Institute of Northwestern University School of Medicine, Chicago, IL (April).

Aylward, E. H., Minshew, N. J., Field, K., Sparks, B. F., Singh, N. (2002). Effects of age on brain volume and head circumference in autism. *Neurology, 59,* 175–183.

Ayres, A. J. (1979). *Sensory integration and the child.* Los Angeles, CA: Western Psychological Services.

Baer, R. A., Williams, J. A., Osnes, P. G., & Stokes, T. F. (1984). Delayed reinforcement as an indiscriminable contingency in verbal/nonverbal correspondence training. *Journal of Applied Behavior Analysis, 17,* 429–440.

Bailey, A., LeCouteur, A. Gottesman, I., Bolton, P. Simonoff, E., Yuzda, E., et al. (1995). Autism as a strongly genetic disorder: Evidence from a British twin study. *Pshycological Medicine, 25,* 63–77.

Bailey, J. S., Shook, G. L., Iwata, B. A., Reid, D. H., & Repp, A. C. (n.d.). *Behavior analysis in developmental disabilities 1968–1985 from the Journal of Applied Behavior Analysis* (Reprint series vol. 1). Lawrence: University of Kansas Department of Human Development: Society for the Experimental Analysis of Behavior.

Bailey, S. L. (1981). Stimulus overselectivity in learning disabled children. *Journal of Applied Behavior Analysis, 14,* 239–248.

Balbani, A. P. S., & Montovani, J. C. (2003). Impact of otitis media on language acquisition in children. *Journal de Pediatria, 79*(5), 391–396. [Available on MEDLINE.]

Baldwin, J. D., & Baldwin, J. I. (1998). *Behavior principles in everyday life* (3rd ed.). Upper Saddle River, NJ: Prentice-Hall.

Ballard, K. D., & Crooks, T. J. (1984). Videotape modeling for preschool children with low levels of social interaction and low peer involvement in play. *Journal of Abnormal Child Psychology, 12,* 95–109.

Barlow, D. H., Hayes, S. C., & Nelson, R. O. (1984). *The scientist practitioner: Research and accountability in clinical and educational settings.* New York: Pergamon.

Barlow, D. H., & Hersen, M. (1984). *Single-case experimental designs* (2nd ed.). New York: Pergamon.

Baroff, G. S. (1999). *Mental retardation: Nature, causes, and management.* Philadelphia, PA: Brunner/Mazel.

Barrera, R. D., & Sulzar-Azaroff, B. (1983). An alternating treatment comparison of oral and total communication training programs with echolalic autistic children. *Journal of Applied Behavior Analysis, 16,* 379–394.

Bartlett, C. W., Flax, J. F., Logue, M. W., Vieland, V. J., Bassett, A. S., Pallal, P., et al. (2002). A major susceptibility locus for specific language impairment is located on 13q21. *American Journal of Human Genetics, 71,* 45–55.

Bates, E. (1976). *Language in context: Studies in the acquisition of pragmatics.* New York: Academic Press.

Bates, E., Bretherton, I., & Snyder, Lynn (1988). *From first words to grammar.* New York: Cambridge University Press.

Battle, D. E. (2002). *Communication disorders in multicultural populations* (3rd ed.). Woburn, MA: Butterworth-Heinemann.

Behavior analysis in developmental disabilities 1968–1985 from the Journal of Applied Behavior Analysis. Reprint Series, Volume 1. Lawrence, KS: Office the Journal of Applied Behavior Analysis.

Beitchman, J., Brownlie, E. B., Inglis, A. L., Wild, J., Mathews, R., Schachter, D., et al. (1994). Seven-year follow-up of speech/language impaired and control children: Speech/language stability and outcome. *Journal of the American Academy of Child and Adolescent Psychiatry, 33,* 1322–1330.

Beitchman, J. H., Nair, R., Clegg, M., & Patel, P. G. (1986). Prevalence of speech and language disorders in 5-year-old kindergarten children in the Ottawa-Carleton region. *Journal of Speech and Hearing Disorders, 51,* 98–110.

Beitchman, J. H., Wilson, B., Brownlie, E. B., Walters, H. & Lancee, W. (1996). Long-term consistency in speech/language profiles: I. Developmental and academic outcomes. *Journal of the American academy of Child and Adolescent Psychiatry, 35*(6), 804–814.

Beitchman, J. H. Wilson, B., Brownlie, E. B., Walters, H., Inglis, A., & Lancee, W. (1996). Long-term consistency in speech/language profiles: II. Behavioral, emotional, and social outcomes. *Journal of the American Academy of Child and Adolescent Psychiatry, 35*(6), 815–825.

Benson, D. F., & Ardila, A. (1992). *Aphasia: A clinical perspective.* New York: Oxford University Press.

Benton, A. (1964). Developmental aphasia and brain damage. *Cortex, 1,* 40–52.

Berard, G. (1993). *Hearing equals behavior.* New Canaan, CT: Keats.

Berenstain, S. & Berenstain, J. (1974). *He bear; She bear.* New York: Random House.

Berenstain, S. & Berenstain, J. (1998). *Old hat, New hat.* New York: Random House.

Berg, W. K., & Wacker, D. P. (1989). Evaluation of tactile prompts with a student who is deaf, blind, and mentally retarded. *Journal of Applied Behavior Analysis, 22,* 93–99.

Berglund, E., Eriksson, M., & Johansson, I. (2001). Parental reports of spoken language skills in children with Down syndrome. *Journal of Speech, Language, and Hearing Research, 44*(1), 179–191.

Bernard, S., Enayati, A., Redwood, L., Roger, H., & Binstock, T. (2001a). Autism: A novel form of mercury poisoning. *Medical Hypotheses, 56,* 462–471.

Bernard, S., Enayati, A., Redwood, L., Roger, H., & Binstock, T. (2001b). The role of mercury in the pathogenesis of autism. *Molecular Psychiatry, 7,* S42–S43.

Bertrand, J., Mars, A., Boyle, C., Bove, F., Yeargin-Allsopp, M., & Decouffle, P. (2001). Prevalence of autism in a United States Population. *Pediatrics, 108,* 1155–1161.

Bettelheim, B. (1967). *The empty fortress.* New York: Free Press

Bettison, S. (1996). The long-term effects of auditory training on children with autism. *Journal of Autism & Developmental Disorders, 26,* 361–374.

Beukelman, D. R., & Mirenda, P. (1998). *Augmentative and alternative communication: management of severe communication disorders in children and adults* (2nd ed.). Baltimore, MD: Paul H. Brookes Publishing Co.

Beukelman, D. R., Yorkston, K., & Dowden, P. (1985). *Communication augmentation: A casebook of clinical management.* Austin, TX: PRO-ED.

Bigler, E. D. (1990). *Traumatic brain injury: Mechanisms of damage, assessment, intervention, and outcome.* Austin, TX: PRO-ED.

Bigler, E. D., Clark, E., & Farmer, J. E. (1997). *Childhood traumatic brain injury: Diagnosis, assessment, and intervention.* Austin, TX: PRO-ED.

Biklen, D. (1990). Communication unbound: Autism and praxis. *Harvard Education Review, 60,* 291–314.

Bishop, D. V. (1989). Autism, Asperger's syndrome, and semantic-pragmatic disorder: Where are the boundaries? *British Journal of Disorders of Communication, 24,* 107–121.

Bishop, D. V., & Edmondson, A. (1987). Language-impaired 4-year-old: Distinguishing transient from persistent impairment. *Journal of Speech and Hearing Disorders, 52,* 156–173.

Bishop, D. V., North, T., & Donlan, C. (1995). Genetic basis of specific language impairment: Evidence from a twin study. *Developmental Medicine and Child Neurology, 37,* 56–71.

Bishop, D. V., North, T., & Donlan, C. (1996). Nonword repetition as a behavioural marker for inherited language impairment: Evidence from a twin study. *Psychology and Psychiatry, 36,* 1–13.

Blackburn, S. (1998). Environmental impact of the NICU on developmental outcomes. *Journal of Pediatric Nursing, 13*(5), 279–289.

Blackstone, S. W., Williams, M. B., & Joyce, M. (2002). Future AAC technology needs: Consumer perspectives. *Assistive Technology, 14,* 3–16.

Bleile, K., & Schwarz, I. (1984). Three perspectives on the speech of children with Down syndrome. *Journal of Communication Disorders, 17,* 87–94.

Bloom, L. (1970). *Language development: Form and function of emerging grammars.* Cambridge, MA: MIT Press.

Bloom, L., & Lahey, M. (1978). *Language development and language disorders.* New York: John Wiley.

Bloomfield, L. (1933). *Language.* New York: Holt, Rinehart & Winston.

Blosser, J. L., & DePompei, R. (1994). *Pediatric traumatic brain injury.* San Diego, CA: Singular Publishing Group.

Bolton, P. F., & Griffiths, P. D. (1997). Association of tuberous sclerosis of temporal lobes with autism and atypical autism. *The Lancet, 349,* 392–395.

Bolton, P. F., Roobol, M., Allsopp, L., & Pickles, A. (2001). Association between idiopathic infantile macrocephaly and autism spectrum disorders. *The Lancet, 358,* 726–727.

Bondurant, J., Romeo, D., & Kretschmer, R. (1983). Language behaviors of mothers of children with normal and delayed language. *Language, Speech, and Hearing Services in Schools, 14*, 233–242.

Bondy, A. S., & Frost, L. A. (1994). *PECS: The Picture Exchange Communication System training manual.* Cherry Hill, NJ: Pyramid Educational Consultants, Inc.

Bondy, A. S., & Frost, L. A. (2001). The Picture Exchange Communication System. *Behavior Modification, 25*, 725–44.

Bonsall, C. (1980). *Who's afraid of the dark?* New York: HarperCollins.

Bosch, S., & Fuqua, R. W. (2001). Behavioral cusps: A model for selecting target behaviors. *Journal of Applied Behavior Analysis, 34*, 123–125.

Bowers, L., Huisingh, R., LaGiudice, & C., Orman, J. (2002). *Test of Semantic Skills—Primary (TOSS-P).* East Moline, IL: LinguiSystems, Inc.

Bowers, P. G. & Wolf, M. (1993). Theoretical links among naming speed, precise timing mechanisms, and orthographic skill in dyslexia. *Reading and Writing, 5*, 69–85.

Brady, N. C., Marquis, J., Fleming, K., & McLean, L. (2004). Prelinguistic predictors of language growth in children with developmental disabilities. *Journal of Speech, Language, and Hearing Research, 47*, 663–677.

Brady, N. C., McLean, J. E., Mclean, L. K., & Johnston, S. (1995). Initiation and repair of intentional communication acts by adults with severe to profound cognitive disabilities. *Journal of Speech and Hearing Research, 38*, 1334–1348.

Brantner, J. P., & Doherty, M. A. (1983). A review of time-out: A conceptual and methodological analysis. In S. Axelrod & J. Apsche (Eds.), The effects of punishment on human behavior (pp. 87–132). New York: Academic Press.

Bremmer, P., Byers, J. F., & Kiehl, E. (2003). Noise and the premature infant: Physiological effects and practice implications. *Journal of obstetric, gynecologic,and neonatal nursing, 32*(4), 447–454.

Brice, A. E. (2002). *The Hispanic child: Speech, language, culture, and education.* Boston: Allyn & Bacon.

Bricker, D. (1993). The, now and the path between. In A. P. Kaiser & D. B. Gray (Eds.), *Enhancing children's communication: Research foundations for intervention* (pp. 11–31). Baltimore, MD: Paul H. Brookes.

Brinton, B., & Fujuki, M. (1991). Response to requests for conversational repair by adults with mental retardation. *Journal of Speech and Hearing Research, 34*, 1087–1095.

Brinton, B., Fujiki, M., Spencer, J. C., & Robinson, L. A. (1997). The ability of children with specific language impairment to access and participate in an ongoing interaction. *Journal of Speech, Language, and Hearing Research, 40*(5), 1011–1025.

British Medical Journal. (1999). Hearing without ears: do cochlear implants work in children? Editorial. *British Medical Journal, 318*, 72–73.

Brown, K. A., Wacker, D. P., Derby, K. M., Peck, S. M., Richman, D. M., Sasso, G. M., et al. (2000). Evaluating the effects of functional communication training in the presence and absence of establishing operations. *Journal of Applied Behavior Analysis, 33*, 53–71.

Brown, L., Sherbenou, R. J., & Johnsen, S. K. (1997). *Test of nonverbal intelligence—Third edition.* Austin, TX: PRO-ED.

Brown, R. (1973). *A first language: The early stages.* Cambridge, MA: Harvard University Press.

Brown, V., Hammill, D., & Wiederholt, J. L. (1995). *Test of reading comprehension (TORC-3).* Austin, TX: PRO-ED.

Brownell, R. (Ed.). (2000a). *Expressive one-word picture vocabulary test (EOWPVT).* Novato, CA: Academic Therapy Publications.

Brownell, R. (Ed.) (2000b). *Receptive one-word picture vocabulary test (ROWPVT).* Novato: CA: Academic Therapy Publications.

Bruck, M., & Tucker, G. (1974). Social class differences in the acquisition of school language. *Merrill Palmer Quarterly, 20*, 205–220.

Bryan, L. C., & Gast, D. L. (2000). Teaching on-task and on-schedule behavior to high-functioning children with autism via picture activity schedules. *Journal of Autism and Developmental Disabilities, 30*, 553–567.

Bryant, B. R., Wiederholt, J. L., & Bryant, d. P. (2004). *Gray diagnostic reading tests (GDRT-2) Second Edition,* Austin, TX: PRO-ED.

Buffington, D. M., Krantz, P. J., McClannahan, L. E., & Poulson, C. L. (1998). Procedures for teaching appropriate gestural communication skills to children with autism. *Journal of Autism and Developmental Disabilities, 28*, 535–545.

Burke, D. (1998). *Street Spanish 2: The best of Spanish idioms.* New York: John Wiley.

California Department of Developmental Services. (2003). *Autism spectrum disorders: Changes in the California caseload. An update: 1999 through 2002.* Retrieved August 11, 2004, from www.autismtreeproject.org/AutismReport2003.pdf.

California State Department of Education. (2004). *Number of English learners in California public schools, by language and grade ranked by total, 2002–2003: Los Angeles Unified.* Retrieved July 15, 2004, from http://data1.cde.ca.gov/dataquest/LEPbyLang3.asp.

Camarata, S. (1993). The application of naturalistic conversation training to speech production in children with speech disabilities. *Journal of Applied Behavior Analysis, 26*, 173–182.

Camarata, S., & Gibson, T. (1999). Pragmatic language deficits in attention-deficit hyperactivity disorder (ADHD). *Mental Retardation and Developmental Disabilities Research Reviews, 5*, 207–214.

Camarata, S., Newhoff, M., & Rugg, B. (1981). Perspective taking in normal and language disordered children. *Proceedings of the Symposium on Research in Child Language Disorders, 2*, 81–88. Madison, WI: University of Wisconsin.

Campbell, C. R., & Stremel-Campbell, K. (1982). Programming loose training as a strategy to facilitate language generalization. *Journal of Applied Behavior Analysis, 15*, 295–301.

Campbell, L. (1993). Maintaining the integrity of home linguistic varieties: Black English vernacular. *American Journal of Speech-Language Pathology, 2,* 11–12.

Campbell, T., Dollaghan, C., Needleman, H., & Janosky, J. (1997). Reducing bias in language assessment: Processing dependent measures. *Journal of Speech, Language, and Hearing Research, 40,* 519–525.

Cans, C., McManus, V., Crowley, M., Gullem, P., Platt, M. J., Johnson, A, & Arnaud, G. (2004). Cerebral palsy of postneonatal origin: Characteristics and risk factors. *Pediatric Perinatal Epidemiology, 18*(3), 214–220.

Caparulo, B., & Cohen, D. (1983). Developmental language studies in the neuropsychiatric disorders of children. In K. E. Nelson (Ed.), *Children's language* (pp. 423–463). Hillsdale, NJ: Erlbaum.

Capelli, R. (1985). *Experimental analysis of morphologic acquisition.* Unpublished master's thesis, California State University, Fresno, CA.

Cardinal, D., & Biklen, D. (1997). Suggested procedures for confirming authorship through research: An initial investigation. In D. Biklen & D. Cardinal (Eds.), *Contested words, contested science: Unraveling the facilitated communication controversy* (pp. 173–186). New York: Teachers College Columbia University

Cardoza, K., & Hegde, M. N. (1996). Discriminative stimulus control in promoting generalized language production. Paper presented at the Third National Conference on Treatment Research, Rehabilitation Institute of Northwestern University School of Medicine, Chicago (April).

Carr, A. M., Bailes, J. E., Helmkamp, J. C., Rosen, C. L., & Miele, V. J. (2004). Neurological injury and death in all-terrain crashes in West Virginia: A 10-year retrospective review. *Neurosurgery, 54*(4), 861–866.

Carr, E. G. (1988). Functional equivalence as a mechanism of response generalization. In R. Horner, G. Dunlap, & R. L. Koegel (Eds.), *Generalization and maintenance: Life-style changes in applied settings* (pp. 221–224). Baltimore, MD: Paul H. Brookes.

Carr, E. G., Binkoff, J., Kologinsky, E., & Eddy, M. (1978). Acquisition of sign language by autistic children: I. Expressive labeling. *Journal of Applied Behavior Analysis, 11,* 489–501.

Carr, E. G., & Dores, P. A. (1984). Patterns of language acquisition following simultaneous communication with autistic children. *Analysis and Intervention in Developmental Disabilities, 1,* 347–361.

Carr, E. G. & Durand, V. M. (1985). Reducing behavior problems through functional communication training. *Journal of Applied Behavior Analysis, 18,* 111–126.

Carr, E. G., & Kologinsky, E. (1983). Acquisition of sign language by autistic children II: Spontaneity and generalization effects. *Journal of Applied Behavior Analysis, 16,* 297–314.

Carr, E. G., Levin, L., McConnachie, G., Carlson, J. I., Kemp, D. C., & Smith, C. E. (1994). *Communication-based intervention for problem behavior.* Baltimore, MD: Paul H. Brookes.

Carroll, R. J., & Hesse, B. E. (1987). The effect of alternating mand and tact raining on the acquisition of tacts. *The Analysis of Verbal Behavior, 5,* 55–65.

Carrow, E. (1973). *Test for Auditory Comprehension of Language.* Austin, TX: Learning Concepts.

Carrow-Woolfolk, E. (1999). *Test for auditory comprehension of language-3 (TACL-3).* Austin, TX: PRO-ED.

Carter-Wagner, J. (1997). *Jenny's TO Thesis. The effectiveness of parent-initiated time-out on the dysfluencies of four stutterers.* Unpublished master's thesis. California State University, Fresno, CA.

Casby, M. W. (1997). Symbolic play of children with language impairment: A critical review. *Journal of Speech, Language, and Hearing Research, 40,* 468–479.

Casby, M. W. (2001). Otitis media and language development: A meta analysis. *American Journal of Speech-Language Pathology, 10,* 65–80.

Cassidy, S. B. (1997). Prader-Willi syndrome. *Journal of Medical Genetics, 34,* 917–923.

Catania, A. C. (1972). Chomsky's formal analysis of natural language: A behavioral translation. *Behaviorism, 1,* 1–15.

Catania, A. C. (1998). *Learning* (4th ed.). Upper Saddle River, NJ: Prentice-Hall.

Catts, H. W., Fey, M. E., Tomblin, J. B., & Zhang, X. (2002). A longitudinal investigation of reading outcomes in children with language impairments. *Journal of Speech, Language, and Hearing Research, 45*(6), 1142–1157.

Catts, H. W., Gillispie, M., Leonard, L. B., Kail, R. V., & Miller, C. A. (2002). The role of the speed of processing, rapid naming, and phonological processing in reading achievement. *Journal of Learning Disabilities, 35*(6), 509–525.

Catts, H. W. & Kamhi, A. (1999). *Language and Reading Disabilities.* Needham Heights, MA: Allyn & Bacon.

Centers for Disease Control and Prevention. (2000). Prevalence of autism in Brick Township, New Jersey, 1998: Community report. Retrieved September 9, 2004, from www.cdc.gov/ncbddd/dd/report/htm.

Centers for Disease Control and Prevention (2004a). Fetal alcohol syndrome (FAS). Retrieved August 20, 2004, from www.cdc.gov/ncbddd.fas.

Centers for Disease Control and Prevention (2004b). About childhood lead poisoning. Retrieved August 21, 2004, from www.cdc.gov/nceh/lead/about/about/htm.

Centers for Disease Control & Prevention (2004c). Economic costs associated with mental retardation, cerebral palsy, hearing loss, and vision impairment—United States. *Morbidity and Mortality Weekly Report, 30,* 53(3), 57–59. [Accessible through www.cdc.gov.]

Chakrabarti, S., & Fombonne, E. (2001). Pervasive developmental disorders in preschool children. *Journal of the American Medical Association, 285,* 3093–3099.

Chambers, M., & Rehfeldt, R. A. (2003). Assessing the acquisition and generalization of two mand forms with adults with severe developmental disability. *Research in Developmental Disability, 24,* 265–280.

Chandler, L. K., Lubeck, R. C., & Fowler, S. A. (1992). Generalization and maintenance of preschool children's social skills: A critical review and analysis. *Journal of Applied Behavior Analysis, 25,* 415–428.

Chapman, R. S., Schwartz, S. E., & Kay-Raining Bird, E. (1991). Language skills of children and adolescents with Down syndrome: I. Comprehension. *Journal of Speech and Hearing Research, 34,* 1106–1120.

Chapman, R. S., Seung, H. K., Schwartz, S. E., & Kay-Raining Bird, E. (1998). Language skills of children and adolescents with Down syndrome: II. Production deficits. *Journal of Speech, Language, and Hearing Research, 41,* 861–873.

Charlop-Christy, M. H., Carpenter, M., Le, L., LeBlanc, L. A., & Kellet, K. (2002). Using the picture exchange communication system (PECS) with children with autism: Assessment of pecs acquisition, speech, social-communicative behavior, and problem behavior. *Journal of Applied Behavior Analysis, 35,* 213–231.

Charlop, M. H., & Milstein, J. P. (1989). Teaching autistic children conversational speech using video modeling. *Journal of Applied Behavior Analysis, 22,* 275–285.

Charlop, M. H., Schreibman, L., & Thibodeau, M. G. (1985a). Increasing spontaneous verbal responding in autistic children using a time delay procedure. *Journal of Applied Behavior Analysis, 18,* 155–166.

Charlop, M. H., Schreibman, L., & Thibodeau, M. G. (1985b). Teaching autistic children conversational speech using video modeling. *Journal of Applied Behavior Analysis, 22,* 275–285.

Charlop, M. H., & Trasowech, J. E. (1991). Increasing autistic children's daily spontaneous speech. *Journal of Applied Behavior Analysis, 24,* 747–761.

Charlop, M. H., & Walsh, M. E. (1986). Increasing autistic children's spontaneous verbalizations of affection: An assessment of time delay and peer modeling procedures. *Journal of Applied Behavior Analysis, 19,* 307–314.

Cheng, L. (1987). Cross-cultural and linguistic considerations in working with Asian populations. *American Speech-Language-Hearing Association, 29*(6), 33–41.

Chin, S. B., Tsai, P. L., & Gao, S. (2003). Connected speech intelligibility of children with cochlear implants and children with normal hearing. *American Journal of Speech-Language Pathology, 12*(4), 440–451.

Chomsky, N. (1957). *Syntactic structures.* The Hague: Mouton.

Chomsky, N. (1965). *Aspects of the theory of syntax.* Cambridge, MA: MIT Press.

Chomsky, N. (1968). *Aspects of the theory of syntax.* Cambridge, MA: MIT Press

Chomsky, N. (1980). *Rules and representations.* New York: Columbia University Press.

Chomsky, N. (1982). *Lectures on government and binding.* New York: Foris.

Chomsky, N. (1999). On the nature, use and acquisition of language. In W. Ritchie & T. Bhatia (Eds.), *Handbook of child language acquisition.* New York: Academic Press.

Choudhury, N., & Benasich, A. A. (2003). A family aggregation study: The influence of family history and other risk factors on language development. *Journal of Speech, Language, and Hearing Research, 46,* 261–272.

Chudley, A. E., Guteirrez, E., Jocelyn, L. J., & Chodirker, B. N. (1998). Outcomes of genetic evaluation in children with pervasive developmental disorder. *Journal of Developmental and Behavioral Pediatrics, 19,* 321–325.

Cipani, E. (1988). The missing item format. *Teaching Exceptional Children, 21,* 25–27.

Clahsen, H., & Almazan, M. (1998). Syntax and morphology in Williams syndrome. *Cognition, 68*(3), 167–198.

Clarke, S., Remington, B., & Light, P. (1988). The role of referential speech in sign learning by mentally retarded children: A comparison of total communication and sign-alone training. *Journal of Applied Behavior Analysis, 21,* 419–426.

Clibbens, J. (2001). Signing and lexical development in children with Down Syndrome. *Down Syndrome Research and Practice, 7,* 101–105.

Cohen, N. J., Barwick, M. A., Horodezky, N. B., Vallance, D. D., & Im, N. (1998). Language, achievement, and cognitive processing in psychiatrically disturbed children with previously identified and unsuspected language impairments. *Journal of Child Psychology and Psychiatry, 39,* 865–877.

Coleman, T. J. (2000). *Clinical management of communication disorders in culturally diverse children.* Boston: Allyn & Bacon.

Constantino, J. N., & Todd, R. D. (2003). Autistic traits in the general population: A twin study. *Archives of General Psychiatry, 60*(5), 524–530.

Conti-Ramsden, G. (1990). Maternal recasts and other contingent replies to language-impaired children. *Journal of Speech and Hearing Disorders, 55,* 252–274.

Conti-Ramsden, G., & Jones, M. (1997). Verb use in specific language impairment. *Journal of Speech and Hearing Disorders, 40,* 1298–1313.

Coplan, J. (2000). Counseling parents regarding prognosis in autistic spectrum disorders. *Pediatrics, 105,* E65.

Cornish, K. M., & Munir, F. (1998). Receptive and expressive language skills in children with cri-du-chat syndrome. *Journal of Communication Disorders, 31*(1), 73–80.

Cornish, K. M., & Pigram, J. (1996). Developmental and behavioral characteristics of cri-du-chat syndrome. *Archives of Disabilities of Children, 75*(5), 448–450.

Costello, J. M. (1975). The establishment of fluency with time-out procedures. Three case studies. Journal of Speech and Hearing Disorders, *40,* 216–231.

Council for Exceptional Children. (2004). The new IDEA: CEC's summary of significant issues. Retrieved January 8, 2005, from www.cec.sped.org/pp/IDEA_120204.pdf.

Courchesne, E. (1997). Brainstem, cerebellar, and limbic neuroanatomical abnormalities in autism. *Current Opinion in Neurology, 7,* 269–278.

Courchesne, E., Carper, R., & Akshoomoff, N. (2003). Evidence of brain overgrowth in the first year of life in autism. *Journal of the American Medical Association, 290,* 337–344.

Courchesne, E., Karns, C. M., Davis, H. R., Ziccardi, R., Carper, R. A., Tigue, Z. D., et al. (2001). Unusual brain growth pattern in early life in patients with autistic disorder: An MRI study. *Neurology, 57,* 245–254.

Coury, D. L., & Nash, P. L. (2003). Epidemiology and etiology of autistic spectrum disorders difficult to determine. *Pediatric Annals, 32*(10), 696–700.

Craft, M. A., Alber, S. R., & Heward, W. L. (1998). Teaching elementary students with developmental disabilities to recruit teacher attention in a general education classroom: Effects on teacher praise and academic productivity. *Journal of Applied Behavior Analysis, 31,* 399–415.

Crago, M., & Gopnik, M. (1994). From families to phenotypes: Theoretical and clinical implications of research into the genetic basis of specific language impairment. In R. Watkins & M. Rice (Eds.), *Specific language impairment in children* (pp. 35–51). Baltimore: Paul H. Brookes.

Craig, H. (1993). Social skills of children with specific language impairment. *Language, Speech, and Hearing Services in Schools, 24,* 206–215.

Craig, H., & Evans, J. (1989). Turn exchange characteristics of SLI children's simultaneous and non-simultaneous speech. *Journal of Speech and Hearing Disorders, 54,* 334–347.

Craig, H. K., Thompson, C., A., Washington, J. A., & Potter, S. L. (2003). Phonological features of child African American English. *Journal of Speech, Language, and Hearing Research, 46,* 623–635.

Craig, H., & Washington, J. (1993). The access behaviors of children with specific language impairment. *Journal of Speech and Hearing Research, 36,* 322–337.

Craig, H. K., & Washington, J. A. (2000). An assessment battery for identifying language impairment in African American children. *Journal of Speech, Language, and Hearing Research, 43,* 366–379.

Crain-Thoreson, C., & Dale, P. S. (1992). Do early talkers become early readers? Linguistic precocity, preschool language, and emergent literacy. *Developmental Psychology, 28,* 421–429.

Cross, T. (1981). The linguistic experience of slow learners. In A. Nesdale, C. Pratt, R. Grieve, J. Field, D. Illingworth, & J. Hogben (Eds.), *Advances in child development: Theory and research* (pp. 110–121). Nedlands: University of Western Australia.

Crossley, R., & McDonald, A. (1980). *Annie's coming out.* New York: Penguin.

Crutcher, D. M. (1993). Parent perspectives: Best practice and recommendations for research. In A. P. Kaiser & D. P. Gray (Eds.) (1993). *Enhancing children's communication: Research foundations for intervention* (pp. 365–374). Baltimore, MD: Paul H. Brookes.

Cunningham, C. E., Siegel, L. S., van der Spuy, H. I., Clark, M. L., & Bow, S. J. (1985). The behavioral and linguistic interactions of specifically language-delayed and normal boys with their mothers. *Child Development, 56,* 1389–1403.

Cunningham, M., & Cox, E. O. (2003). Hearing assessment in infants and children: Recommendations beyond neonatal screening. *Pediatrics, 111*(2), 436–440.

Dabney, K. W., Lyston, G. E., & Miller, E. (1997). Cerebral palsy. *Current Opinion in Pediatrics, 9,* 81–88.

Dale, P. S., & Cole, K. N. (1991). What's normal? Specific language impairment in an individual difference perspective. *Language, Speech, and Hearing Services in Schools, 22*(2), 80–83.

Davis, H., Stroud, A., & Green, L. (1988). Maternal language environment of children with mental retardation. *American Journal of Mental Retardation, 93,* 144–153.

Dawson, J., & Stout, C. (2003). *Structured Photographic Expressive Language Test (SPELT-3).* DeKalb, IL: Janelle Publications.

DeCesari, R. (1985). *Experimental training of grammatical morphemes: Effects on the order of acquisition.* Unpublished master's thesis, California State University, Fresno, CA.

DeFelice, M. L., Ruchelli, E. D., Markowitz, J. E., Strogatz, M., Reddy, K. P., & Mulberg, A. E. (2003). Intestinal cytokines in children with pervasive developmental disorders. *American Journal of Gastroenterology, 98,* 1777–1782.

Delprato, D. J. (2001). Comparisons of discrete-trial and normalized behavioral language intervention for young children with autism. *Journal of Autism and Developmental Disabilities, 31,* 315–325.

Derby, K. M., Wacker, D. P., Berg, W., DeRaad, A., Ulrich, S., Asmus, J., et al. (1997). The long-term effects of functional communication training in home settings. *Journal of Applied Behavior Analysis, 30,* 507–531.

Deutsch, C. K., & Joseph, R. M. (2003). Brief report: Cognitive correlates of enlarged head circumference in children with autism. *Journal of Autism and Developmental Disabilities, 33,* 209–215.

Deutsch, R. M., & Morrill, J. S. (1993). *Realities of nutrition.* Palo alto, CA: Bull Publishing.

Dillard, J. I. (1972). *Black English.* New York: Random House.

DiSimoni, F. (1978). *The Token Test for Children.* Austin, TX: PRO-ED.

Dollaghan, C., & Campbell, T. (1998). Nonword repetition and child language impairment. *Journal of Speech, Language, and Hearing Research, 41,* 1136–1146.

Dougherty, E. H., & Schinka, J. A. (1992). *Mental Status Checklist—Children.* Lutz, FL: Psychological Assessment Resources, Inc.

Douniadakis, D. E., Kalli, K. I., Psarommatis, I. M., Tsakanikos, M. D., & Apostolopoulous, N. K. (2001). Incidence of hearing loss among children with speech-language delay. *Scandinavian Audiology Supplement, 2001*(52), 204–205.

Doyle, T. F., Bellugi, U., Korenberg, J. R., & Graham, J. (2004). "Everybody in the world is my friend" hypersociability in young children with Williams syndrome. *American Journal of Medical Genetics, 124A*(3), 263–273.

Drager, K. D. R., Light, J. C., Carlson, R., D'Silva, K., Larsson, B., Pitkin, L., & Stopper, G. (2004). Learning of dynamic display AAC technologies by typically developing 3-year-olds: Effect of different layouts and menu approaches. *Journal of Speech, Language, and Hearing Research, 47*, 1133–1148.

Drager, K. D. R., Light, J. C., Speltz, J. C., Fallon, K. A., & Jeffries, L. Z. (2003). The performance of typically developing 2½-year-olds on dynamic display AAC technologies with different system layouts on language organizations. *Journal of Speech, Language, and Hearing Research, 46*, 298–312.

Drasgow, E., Halle, J. W., & Ostrosky, M. M. (1998). Effects of differential reinforcement on the generalization of a replacement mand in three children with severe language delays. *Journal of Applied Behavior Analysis, 31*, 357–374.

Dube, W. V., & McIlvane, W. J. (1999). Reduction of stimulus selectivity with noverbal differential observing responses. *Journal of Applied Behavior Analysis, 32*, 25–34.

Duchan, J. F., Calculator, S., Sonnenmeier, R., Diehl, S., & Cumley, G. D. (2001). A framework for managing controversial practices. *Language, Speech, and Hearing Services in Schools, 32*, 133–141.

Ducharme, D. E., & Holborn, S. W. (1997). Programming generalization of social skills in preschool children with hearing impairments. *Journal of Applied Behavior Analysis, 30*, 639–651.

Duker, P. C., Kraaykamp, M., & Visser, E. (1994). A stimulus control procedure to increase requesting with individuals who are severely/profoundly intellectually disabled. *Journal of Intellectual Disability Research, 38*, 177–186.

Dunlap, G., Koegel, R. L., Johnson, J., & O'Neill, R. E. (1987). Maintaining performance of autistic clients in community settings with delayed contingencies. *Journal of Applied Behavior Analysis, 20*, 185–191.

Dunn, L. M., & Dunn, L. M. (1997). *Peabody picture vocabulary test* (3rd ed.). Circle Pines, MN: American Guidance Service.

Durand, M. V., Berotti, D., & Weiner, J. S. (1993). Functional communication training: Factors affecting effectiveness, generalization, and maintenance. In J. Reichle & D. P. Wacker (Eds.), *Communicative alternatives to challenging behavior* (pp. 299–316). Baltimore, MD: Paul H. Brookes.

Durand, V. M., & Carr, E. G. (1991). Functional communication training to reduce challenging behavior: Maintenance and application in new settings. *Journal of Applied Behavior Analysis, 24*, 251–264.

Durand, V. M., & Carr, E. G. (1992). An analysis of maintenance following functional communication training. *Journal of Applied Behavior Analysis, 25*, 777–794.

Dyer, K., Christian, W. P., & Luce, S. C. (1982). The role of response delay in improving the discrimination performance of autistic children. *Journal of Applied Behavior Analysis, 15*, 231–240.

Eadie, P. A., Fey, M. E., Douglas, J. M., & Parsons, C. L. (2002). Profiles of grammatical morphology and sentence imitation in children with specific language impairment an Down syndrome. *Journal of Speech, Language, and Hearing Research, 45*, 720–732.

Eastman, P. D. (1960). *Are You My Mother?* New York: Random House.

Edelson, S. M. (2004). *The candida yeast-autism connection.* Retrieved August 12, 2004, from www.autism.org/candida.html.

Edwards, J., & Lahey, M. (1998). Nonword repetitions of children with specific language impairment: Exploration of some explanations for their inaccuracies. *Applied Psycholinguistics, 19*, 279–309.

Egel, A. L., Richman, G. S., & Koegel, R. L. (1981). Normal peer models and autistic children's learning. *Journal of Applied Behavior Analysis, 14*, 3–12.

Ehlers, S., & Gillberg, C. (1993). The epidemiology of Asperger syndrome: A total population study. *Journal of Child Psychology and Psychiatry, 34*(8), 1327–1350.

Eisenberg, S. L., Fresko, T. M., & Lundgren, C. (2001). The use of MLU for identifying language impairment in preschool children. *American Journal of Speech-Language Pathology, 10*, 323–342.

Eisenson, J. (1972). *Aphasia in children.* New York: Harper & Row.

Eiserman, W. D., Weber, C., & McCoun, M. (1992). Two alternative program models for serving speech-disordered preschoolers: A second year follow-up. *Journal of Communication Disorders, 25*(2–3), 77–106.

Elliott, C. D. (1990). *Differential Ability Scales.* San Antonio, TX: PsychCorp.

Ellis Weismer, S., Tomblin, J. B., Zhang, X., Buckwalter, P., Chynoweth, J. G., & Jones, M. (2000). Nonword repetition performance in school-age children with and without language impairment. *Journal of Speech, Language, and Hearing Research, 43*(4), 865–878.

Enard, W., Przeworski, M., Fisher, S., Lal, C., Wiebe, V., Kitano, T., et al. (2002). Molecular evolution of *FOXP2*, a gene involved in speech and language. *Nature, 418*, 869–872.

Encyclopedia: Black English Vernacular (2004). [On-line]. Retrieved June 5, 2004, from www.nationmaster.com/encyclopedia/Black-English-Vernacular.

Enderby, P. M. (1983). *Frenchay Dysarthria Assessment.* Austin, TX: PRO-ED.

Erickson, J. G., Devlieger, P., & Moon Sung, J. (1999). Korean-American female perspectives on disability. *Journal of Speech-language Pathology, 8*, 99–108.

Erickson, K. A. (2000). All children are ready to learn: An emergent versus readiness perspective in early literacy assessment. *Seminars in Speech and Language, 21*(2), 193–203.

Ervin, M. (2001). SLI: What we know and why it matters. *ASHA LEADER, 6*, 4.

Ezell, H. K., & Goldstein, H. (1991). Comparison of idiom comprehension of normal children and children with mental retardation. *Journal of Speech and Hearing Research, 34,* 812–819.

Ezell, H. K., & Goldstein, H. (1992). Teaching idiom comprehension to children with mental retardation. *Journal of Applied Behavior Analysis, 25,* 181–191.

Fagundes, D. D., Haynes, W. O., Haak, N. J., & Moran, M. J. (1998). Task variability effects on the language test performance of southern lower socioeconomic class African American and Caucasian five-year-olds. *Language, Speech, and Hearing Services in Schools, 26*(1), 82–90.

Farmer-Dougan, V. (1994). Increasing requests by adults with developmental disabilities using incidental teaching by peers. *Journal of Applied Behavior Analysis, 27,* 533–544.

Fazio, B. (1996). Mathematical abilities of children with specific language impairment. *Journal of Language, Speech, and Hearing Research, 37,* 358–368.

Feldman, M. A., Towns, F., Betel, J., Case, L., Rincover, A., & Rubino, C. A. (1986). Parent education project II. Increasing stimulating interactions of developmentally handicapped mothers. *Journal of Applied Behavior Analysis, 19,* 23–37.

Fey, M. (1986). *Language intervention with young children.* San Diego, CA: College-Hill Press.

Fey, M., & Leonard, L. (1984). Partner age as a variable in the conversational performance of specifically language-impaired children and normal-language children. *Journal of Speech and Hearing Research, 27,* 413–423.

Fey, M., Leonard, L., & Wilcox, K. (1981). Speech-style modifications of language-impaired children. *Journal of Speech and Hearing Disorders, 46,* 91–97.

Filipek, P. A., Accardo, P. J., Baranek G. T., Cook, E. H., Dawson, G., Gordon, B., et al. (1999). The screening and diagnosis of autistic spectrum disorders. *Journal of Autism and Developmental Disabilities, 29,* 439–484.

Fisher, S. E., Vargha-Kadem, F., Watkins, K. E., et al. (1998). Localization of a gene implicated in a severe speech and language disorder. *Nature Genetics, 18,* 168–170.

Fisher, W. Piazza, C. C., Bowman, L. G., Hagopian, L. P., Owens, J. C., & Slevin, I. (1992). A comparison of two approaches for identifying reinforcers for persons with severe and profound disabilities. *Journal of Applied Behavior Analysis, 25,* 491–498.

Flax, J. F., Realpe-Bonilla, T., Hirsch, L. S., Brzustowicz, L. M., Bartlett, C. W., Tallal, P. (2003). Specific language impairment in families: Evidence for co-occurrence with reading impairments. *Journal of Speech, Language, and Hearing Research, 46*(3), 530–543.

Fluharty, N. B. (2000). *Fluharty 2: Fluharty Preschool Speech and Language Screening Test.* Austin, TX: PRO-ED.

Forbes, B. J., Christian, C. W., Judkins, A. R., & Kryston, K. (2004). Inflicted childhood neurotrauma (shaken baby syndrome): Ophthalmic findings. *Journal of Pediatric Ophthalmology and Strabismus, 41*(2), 80–88.

Fowler, A. E. (1990). Language abilities in children with Down syndrome: Evidence for a specific syntactic delay. In D. Cichetti & M. Beeghly (Eds.), *Children with Down syndrome: A developmental perspective* (pp. 303–328). New York: Cambridge University Press.

Foxx, R., Faw, G., McMorrow, M., Kyle, M., & Bittle, R. (1988). Replacing maladaptive speech with verbal labeling responses: An analysis of generalized responding. *Journal of Applied Behavior Analysis, 21,* 411–417.

Frattali, C. M. (1998). *Measuring outcomes in speech-language pathology.* New York: Thieme.

Frea, W. D., Arnold, C. L., & Vittimberga, G. L. (2001). A demonstration of the effects of augmentative communication on the extreme aggressive behavior of a child with autism within an integrated preschool setting. *Journal of Positive Behavior Intervention, 3,* 194–198.

Friel-Patti, S., DesBarres, K., & Thibodeau, L. (2001). Case studies of children using Fast ForWord. *American Journal of Speech-Language Pathology, 10,* 203–215.

Fristoe, M., & Lloyd, L. (1979). Nonspeech communication. In N. R. Ellis (Ed.), *Handbook of mental deficiency, psychological theory and research* (2nd ed.) (pp. 401–430). Hillsdale, NJ: Erlbaum.

Frome Loeb, D., & Leonard, L. B. (1991). Subject case marking and verb morphology in normally developing and specifically language-impaired children. *Journal of Speech and Hearing Research, 34,* 340–346.

Fujiki, M., & Brinton, B. (1991). The verbal noncommunicator: A case study. *Language, Speech, and Hearing Services in Schools, 27,* 195–202.

Fuller, D. R. (1997). Initial study in the effects of translucency and complexity on the learning of Blissymbols by children and adults with normal cognitive abilities. *Augmentative and Alternative Communication, 13,* 30–39.

Gaines, R., Leaper, C., Monahan, C., & Weickgenant, A. (1988). Language learning and retention in young language-disordered children. *Journal of Autism and Developmental Disabilities, 18*(2), 281–296.

Gallagher, T., & Darnton, B. (1978). Conversational aspects of the speech of language disordered children: Revision behaviors. *Journal of Speech and Hearing Research, 21,* 118–135.

Garcia, E., Guess, D., & Byrnes, J. (1973). Development of syntax in a retarded girl using procedures of imitation, reinforcement, and modeling. *Journal of Applied Behavior Analysis, 6,* 299–310.

Gathercole, S., & Baddeley, A. (1990). Phonological memory deficits in language impaired children: Is there a causal connection? *Journal of Memory and Language, 29,* 336–360.

Gathercole, S. E., Willis, C., Baddeley, A. D., & Emslie, H. (1994). The children's test of nonword repetition: A test of phonological working memory. *Memory, 2,* 103–127.

Gauger, L. M., Lombardino, L. J., & Leonard, C. M. (1997). Brain morphology in children with specific language impairment. *Journal of Speech, Language, and Hearing Research, 40,* 1272–1284.

Gauthier, J., Joober, R., Mottron, L., Laurent, S., Fuchs, M., De Kimpe,V., et al. (2003). Mutation screening of FOXP2 in individuals diagnosed with autistic disorder. *American Journal of Medical Genetics, 118,* 172–175.

Gauthier, S. V., & Madison, C. I. (1998). *Kindergarten language screening test—Second edition (KLST-2).* Austin, TX: PRO-ED.

Genesee, F. (1988). Bilingual language development in preschool children. In D. Bishop & K. Mogford (Eds.), *Language development in exceptional circumstances* (pp. 62–79). London: Churchill Livingstone.

German, D. (1990). *Test of Adolescent/Adult Word Finding.* Austin, TX: PRO-ED.

German, D. (2000). *Test of Word Finding—2.* Austin, TX: PRO-ED.

Geschwind, N., & Levitsky, W. (1968). Left-right asymmetries in temporal speech region. *Science, 161,* 186–187.

Gibbard, D. (1994). Parental-based intervention with preschool language-delayed children. *Europe Journal of Disordered Communication, 29(2),* 131–150.

Gillam, R. B. (1999). Computer assisted language intervention using Fast ForWord: Theoretical and empirical considerations for clinical decision-making. *Language, Speech, and Hearing Services in Schools, 30,* 363–370.

Gillam, R. B., Cowan, N., & Marler, J. A. (1998). Information processing by school-age children with specific language impairment: Evidence from a modality effect paradigm. *Journal of Speech, Language, and Hearing Research, 41,* 913–926.

Gillam, R. B., Crofford, J. A., Gale, M. A., & Hoffman, L. V. M. (2001). Language change following computer-assisted language instruction with Fast ForWord or Laureate Learning Systems software. *American Journal of Speech-Language Pathology, 10,* 231–247.

Gillam, R. B., & Johnston, J. (1985). Development of print awareness in language-disordered preschoolers. *Journal of Speech and Hearing Disorders, 43,* 521–526.

Gillam, R. B., Loeb, D., & Friel-Patti, S. (2001). Looking back: A summary of five exploratory studies of Fast ForWord. *American Journal of Speech-Language Pathology, 10,* 269–273.

Gillberg, C. (1991). Outcome in autism and autistic-like conditions. *Journal of the American Academy of Child and Adolescent Psychiatry, 30,* 375–382.

Gillberg, C., & de Souza, L. (2002). Head circumference in autism, Asperger syndrome, and ADHD: A comparative study. *Developmental Medicine and Child Neurology, 44,* 296–300.

Gillberg, C., Johansson, M., Steffenburg, S., & Berlin, O. (1997). Auditory integration training in children with autism: Brief report of an open pilot study. *Autism, 1,* 97–100.

Gillette, Y. (2003). *Achieving communication independence.* Eau Claire, WI: Thinking Publications.

Gilliam, J. E. (1995). *Gilliam Autism Rating Scale (GARS).* Circle Pines, MN: AGS Publishing.

Gilliam, J. E. (2000). *Gilliam Asperger's Disorder Scale (GADS).* Circle Pines, MN: AGS Publishing.

Gillis, R. (1996). *Traumatic brain injury: Rehabilitation for speech-language pathologists.* Boston, MA: Butterworth-Heinemann.

Gilpin, W. (1993). *Laughing & Loving with Autism.* Arlington, TX: Future Education, Inc.

Gobbi, L., Cipani, E., Hudson, C., & Lapenta-Neudeck, R. (1986). Developing spontaneous requesting among children with severe mental retardation. *Mental Retardation, 24(6),* 357–363.

Goetz, L., Gee, K., & Sailor, W. (1985). Using a behavior chain interruption strategy to teach communication skills to students with severe disabilities. *Journal of the Association for Persons with Severe Handicaps, 10,* 21–30.

Goldman, R., Fristoe, M., & Woodcock, R. W. (1978). *Goldman-Fristoe-Woodcock Test of Auditory Discrimination.* Circle Pines, MN: American Guidance Service.

Goldstein, B. (2000). *Cultural & linguistic diversity resource guide for speech-language pathologists.* Albany, NY: Thomson Learning.

Goldstein, B. (2001). Transcription of Spanish and Spanish-influenced English. *Communication Disorders Quarterly, 23,* 54–61.

Goldstein, H. (1993). Structuring environmental input to facilitate generalized language learning by children with mental retardation. In A. P. Kaiser & D. B. Gray (Eds.), *Enhancing children's communication* (pp. 317–334). Baltimore, MD: Paul H. Brookes.

Goldstein, H. (2002). Communicative intervention for children with autism: A review of treatment efficacy. *Journal of Autism and Developmental Disabilities, 32(5),* 373–396.

Goldstein, H., & Cisar, C. L. (1992). Promoting interaction during sociodramatic play: Teaching scripts to typical preschoolers and classmates with disabilities. *Journal of Applied Behavior Analysis, 25,* 265–280.

Goldstein, H., & Ferrell, D. R. (1987). Augmenting communication interaction between nonhandicapped and nonhandicapped preschool children. *Journal of Speech and Hearing Disorders, 52,* 200–201.

Goldstein, H., & Hockenberger, E. H. (1991). Significant progress in child language intervention: An 11-year retrospective. *Research in Developmental Disabilities, 12,* 401–424.

Goldstein, H., Kaczmarek, L., Pennington, R., & Shafer, K. (1992). Peer-mediated intervention: Attending to, commenting on, and acknowledging the behavior of preschoolers with autism. *Journal of Applied Behavior Analysis, 25,* 289–305.

Goldstein, H., & Mousetis, L. (1989). Generalized language learning by children with severe mental retardation: Effects of peers' expressive modeling. *Journal of Applied Behavior Analysis, 22,* 245–259.

Goldstein, H., & Wickstrom, S. (1986). Peer intervention effects on communicative interaction among handicapped and nonhandicapped preschoolers. *Journal of Applied Behavior Analysis, 19,* 209–214.

Goldsworthy, C. (1996). *Developmental reading disabilities: A language-based reading approach.* San Diego, CA: Singular Publishing Group.

Gopnik, M., & Crago, M. B. (1991). Familial aggregation of developmental language disorder. *Cognition, 39,* 1–50.

Gough, P., & Tunmer, W. (1986). Decoding, reading, and reading disability. *Remedial & Special Education, 7,* 6–10.

Green, G. (1994). The quality of the evidence. In H. C. Shane (Ed.), *Facilitated communication: The clinical and social phenomenon* (pp. 157–225). San Diego, CA: Singular Publishing Group.

Green, G. (1996). Evaluating claims about treatments for autism. In C. Maurice, G. Green, & S. C. Luce (Eds.), *Behavioral Intervention for Young Children with Autism: A Manual for Parents and Professionals.* Austin, TX: PRO-ED.

Green, G. (2005). Autism and ABA: Applied behavior analysis for autism. Retrieved May 3, 2005, from www.behavior.org/autism/autism_green.cfm.

Green, L. (2004). Research on African American English since 1998: Origins, descriptions, and practice. *Journal of English Linguistics, 32,* 210–229.

Griffin, S. (1979). Requests for clarification made by normal and language impaired children. Unpublished master's thesis, Emerson College.

Grigorenko, E. L., Klin, A., & Volkmar, F. (2003). Annotation: Hyperlexia: disability or superability? *Journal of Child Psychology and Psychiatry, 44,* 1079–1091.

Gronna, S. S., Serna, L. A., Kennedy, C. H., & Prater, M. A. (1999). Promoting generalized social interactions using puppets and script training in an integrated preschool: A single-case study using multiple baseline design. *Behavior Modification, 22,* 419–440.

Guess, D. (1969). A functional analysis of receptive language and productive speech: Acquisition of the plural morpheme. *Journal of Applied Behavior Analysis, 2,* 55–64.

Guess, D., & Baer, D. M. (1973). Some experimental analyses of linguistic development in institutionalized retarded children. In B. B. Lahey (Ed.), *The modification of language behavior* (pp. 3–60). Springfield, IL: Charles C. Thomas.

Guess, D., Sailor, W., Rutherford, G., & Baer, D. M. (1968). An experimental analysis of linguistic development: The productive use of the plural morpheme. *Journal of Applied Behavior Analysis, 1,* 225–235.

Hagberg, B. A. (1989) Rett syndrome: Clinical peculiarities, diagnostic approach, and possible cause. *Pediatric Neurology, 5,* 75–83.

Halle, J. W., Marshall, A. M., & Spradlin, J. E. (1981). Teacher's generalized use of delay as a stimulus control procedure to increase language use in handicapped children. *Journal of Applied Behavioral Analysis, 14,* 389–409.

Halliday, M. A. K. (1973). *Explorations in the functions of language.* New York: Elsevier.

Halliday, M. A. K. (1975). *Learning how to mean: Explorations in the development of language.* New York: Elsevier.

Hamaguchi, P. M. (2001). *Childhood speech, language, and listening problems: What every parent should know* (2nd ed.). New York: John Wiley & Sons.

Hamill, D. D., Pearson, N. A., & Wiederholt, J. L. (1997). *Comprehensive test of nonverbal intelligence.* Austin, TX: PRO-ED.

Hammer, C. S., Detwiler, J. S., Detwiler, J., Blood, G. W., & Qualls, C. D. (2004). Speech-language pathologists' training and confidence in serving Spanish-English bilingual children. *Journal of Communication disorders, 37,* 91–108.

Hammill, D. D. (1998). *Detroit Test of Learning Aptitude—4.* Austin, TX: PRO-ED.

Hancock, T. B., & Kaiser, A. P. (2002). The effects of trainer-implemented enhanced milieu teaching on the social communication of children with autism. *Topics in Early Childhood Special Education, 22,* 39–55.

Haring, T. G., Roger, B., Lee, M., Breen, C., & Gaylord-Ross, R. (1986). Teaching social language to moderately handicapped students. *Journal of Applied Behavior Analysis, 19,* 159–171.

Hart, B. (1985). Naturalistic language training techniques. In S. F. Warren & A. K. Rogers-Warren (Eds.), *Teaching functional language: Generalization and maintenance of language skills* (pp. 63–88). Austin, TX: PRO-ED.

Hart, B., & Risley, T. R. (1974). Using preschool materials to modify the language of disadvantaged children. *Journal of Applied Behavior Analysis, 7,* 243–256.

Hart, B., & Risley, T. R. (1975). Incidental teaching of language in the preschool. *Journal of Applied Behavior Analysis, 8,* 411–420.

Hart, B., & Risley, T. R. (1995). *Meaningful differences in the everyday experience of young American children.* Baltimore, MD: Paul H. Brookes Publishing.

Hart, B., & Risley, T. R. (1999). *The social world of children learning to talk.* Baltimore, MD: Paul H. Brookes.

Hartley, L. L. (1995). *Cognitive-communicative abilities following brain injury.* San Diego, CA: Singular Publishing Group.

Haynes, W. O., & Pindzola, R. H. (2004). *Diagnosis and evaluation in speech pathology* (6th ed.). Boston: Allyn & Bacon.

Heaton, P., & Wallace, G. L. (2004). Annotation: The savant syndrome. *The Journal of Child Psychology and Psychiatry, 45,* 899–911.

Hedrick, D., Prather, E., & Tobin, A. (1995). *Sequenced Inventory of Communication Development—Revised.* Austin, TX: PRO-ED.

Hegde, M. N. (1980). An experimental-clinical analysis of grammatical and behavioral distinctions between verbal auxiliary and copula. *Journal of Speech and Hearing Research, 23,* 864–877.

Hegde, M. N. (1982). Antecedents of fluent and dysfluent oral reading: A descriptive analysis. *Journal of Fluency Disorders, 7,* 323–341.

Hegde, M. N. (1996a). *Pocket guide to assessment in speech-language pathology.* San Diego, CA: Singular Publishing Group.

Hegde, M. N. (1996b). *A coursebook on language disorders in children.* San Diego, CA: Singular Publishing Group.

Hegde, M. N. (1998a). *Treatment protocols in communicative disorders: Targets and Strategies.* Austin, TX: PRO-ED.

Hegde, M. N. (1998b). *Treatment procedures in communicative disorders* (3rd ed.). Austin, TX: PRO-ED.

Hegde, M. N. (2001a). *Hegde's pocketguide to assessment in speech-language pathology* (2nd ed.). Albany, NY: Singular Thomson.

Hegde, M. N. (2001b). *Hegde's pocketguide to treatment in speech-language pathology* (2nd ed.). Albany, NY: Singular Thomson.

Hegde, M. N. (2003a). *Clinical research in communicative disorders: Principles and strategies* (3rd ed.). Austin, TX: PRO-ED.

Hegde, M. N. (2003b). *A coursebook on scientific and professional writing for speech-language pathology* (3rd ed.). Albany, NY: Singular/Thomson Learning.

Hegde, M. N., & Davis, D. (1999). *Clinical methods and practicum in speech-language pathology* (3rd ed.). San Diego, CA: Singular/Thomson Learning.

Hegde, M. N., & Gierut, J. (1979). The operant training and generalization of pronouns and a verb form in language delayed children. *Journal of Communication Disorders, 12,* 23–34.

Hegde, M. N., & McConn, J. (1981). Language training: Some data on response classes and generalization to an occupational setting. *Journal of Speech and Hearing Disorders, 46,* 353–358.

Hegde, M. N., Noll, M. J., & Pecora, R. (1979). A study of some factors affecting generalization of language training. *Journal of Speech and Hearing Disorders, 44,* 301–320.

Hegde, M. N., & Parson, D. (1990). The relative effects of Type I and Type II punishment on stuttering. In L. B. Olswang, C. K. Thompson, S. F. Warren, & N. J. Minghetti (Eds.), *Treatment efficacy research in communication disorders* (p. 251). Washington, D.C.: American Speech-Language-Hearing Foundation.

Hemmeter, M. L., & Kaiser, A. P. (1994). Enhanced milieu teaching: Effects of parent-implemented language intervention. *Journal of Early Intervention, 28,* 269–289.

Hendry, C. N. (2000). Childhood disintegrative disorder: Should it be considered a distinct diagnosis? *Clinical Psychology review, 20,* 77–90.

Herbert, J. D., Sharp, I. R., & Gaudiano, B. A. (2002). *Separating fact from fiction in the etiology and treatment of autism: A scientific review of the evidence.* Retrieved on July 14, 2002, from www.scientificmentalhealth.org/SRMHP/vol1/no1/articles/herbertetal.html.

Heward, W. L., & Eachus, H. T. (1979). Acquisition of adjectives and adverbs in sentences written by hearing impaired and aphasic children. *Journal of Applied Behavior Analysis, 12,* 391–400.

Hoehn, T. P., & Baumeister, A. A. (1994). A critique of the application of sensory integration therapy to children with learning disabilities. *Journal of Learning Disabilities, 27,* 338–351.

Hoffman, L. V. M., & Gillam, R. B. (2004). Verbal and spatial information processing constraints in children with specific language impairment. *Journal of Speech, Language, and Hearing Research, 47,* 114–125.

Hollander, E., King, A., Delaney, K., Smith, C. J., & Silverman, J. M. (2003). Obsessive-compulsive behaviors in parents of multiplex autism families. *Psychiatry Research, 117,* 11–16.

Hollander, E., Phillips, A. T., & Yeh, C. (2003). Targeted treatments for symptom domains in child and adolescent autism. *The Lancet, 362,* 732–734.

Holmes, A. (2002). Heavy metal toxicity in autistic spectrum disorders. Mercury toxicity. In Rimland, B. (Ed.), *DAN! (Defeat Autism Now!) Fall 2001 Conference Practitioner Training,* San Diego, CA: Autism Research Institute.

Hook, P. E., Macaruso, P., & Jones, S. (2003). Efficacy of Fast ForWord training on facilitating acquisition of reading skills by children with reading difficulties—a longitudinal study. *Annals of Dyslexia, 51,* 75–96.

Hook, S. (Ed.). (1969). *Language and philosophy.* New York: New York University Press.

Howlin, P. (2003). Outcome in high-functioning adults with autism with and without early language delays: Implications for the differentiation between autism and Asperger Syndrome. *Journal of Autism and Developmental Disabilities, 33,* 3–13.

Howlin, P., & Rutter, M. (1989). Mothers' speech to autistic children: A preliminary causal analysis. *Journal of Child Psychology and Psychiatry, 30,* 819–843.

Hresko, W. (1996). *Test of early written language-2.* Austin, TX: PRO-ED.

Hutchinson, T. A. (1996). What to look for in the technical manual: Twenty questions for users. *Language, Speech, and Hearing Services in the Schools, 27,* 109–121.

Huer, M. (1988). *The nonspeech test.* Wauconda, WI: Don Johnston, Inc.

Hugdahl, K., Gundersen, H., Brekke, C., Thomsen, T., Rimol, L. M., Ersland, L., et al. (2004). fMRI brain activation in a Finnish family with specific language impairment compared with a normal control group. *Journal of Speech, Language, and Hearing Research, 47,* 162–172.

Hughes, C., Harmer, M. L., Killian, D. J., & Niarhos, F. (1995). The effects of multiple-exemplar self-instructional training on high school students' generalized conversational interactions. *Journal of Applied Behavior Analysis, 28,* 201–218.

Hughes, D., McGillivray, L., & Schmidek, M. (1997). *Guide to narrative language: Procedures for assessment.* Eau Claire, WI: Thinking Publications.

Huisingh, R., Bowers, L., LaGiudice, C., & Orman, J. (1998). *The expressive language test (ELT).* East Moline, IL: LinguiSystems, Inc.

Huisingh, R., Bowers, L., LaGiudice, C., & Orman, J. (2003). *Test of semantic skills—intermediate (TOSS-I)*. East Moline, IL: LinguiSystems, Inc.

Hulit, L. M., & Howard, M. R. (2002). *Born to talk: An introduction to speech and language development*. Boston, MA: Allyn & Bacon.

Hull, R. H. (2001). *Aural rehabilitation: Serving children and adults* (4th ed.). San Diego, CA: Singular.

Hunt, P., Goetz, L., Alwell, M., & Sailor, W. (1986). Using an interrupted behavior chain strategy to teach generalized communication responses. *Journal of the Association for Persons with Severe Handicaps, 11*, 196–204.

Hurlbut, B. I., Iwata, B. A., & Green, J. D. (1982). Nonvocal language acquisition in adolescents with severe physical disabilities: Bliss symbol versus iconic stimulus formats. *Journal of Applied Behavior Analysis, 15*, 241–258.

Hwang, B., & Hughes, C. (2000). Increasing early social-communicative skills of preverbal preschool children with autism through social interactive training. *Journal of the Association for Persons with Severe Handicaps, 25*, 18–28.

Ingenmey, R., & Van Houten, R. (1991). Using time delay to promote spontaneous speech in an autistic child. *Journal of Applied Behavior Analysis, 24*, 591–596.

Inlow, J. K., & Restifo, L. L. (2004). Molecular and comparative genetics of mental retardation. *Genetics, 166*, 835–881.

Isaacs, W., Thomas, J., & Goldiamond, I. (1960). Application of operant conditioning to reinstate verbal behavior in psychotics. *Journal of Speech and Hearing Disorders, 25*, 8–15.

Iwasaki, K., & Holm, M. B. (1989). Sensory treatment for the reduction of stereotypic behaviors in persons with severe multiple disabilities. *Occupational Therapy Journal of Research, 9*, 170–183.

Jamain, S., Betancur, C., Giros, B., Leboyer, M., & Bourgeron, T. (2003). Genetics of autism: From genome scans to candidate genes [article in French; PubMed summary]. *Medical Science, 19*(11), 1081–1090.

James, J. E. (1981). Behavioral self-control of stuttering using time-out from speaking. *Journal of Applied Behavior Analysis, 14*, 25–37.

Janzen-Wilde, M., Duchan, J. F., & Higginbotham, D. J. (1995). Successful use of facilitated communication with an oral child. *Journal of Speech and Hearing Research, 38*, 658–676.

Johnson, C. J., Beitchman, J. H., Young, A., Escobar, M., Atkinson, L., Wilson, B., et al. (1999). Fourteen-year follow-up of children with and without speech/language impairments: Speech-language stability and outcomes. *Journal of Speech and Hearing Research, 42*(3), 744–760.

Johnson, D. L., & Krishnamurthy, S. (1998). Severe pediatric head injury: Myth, magic, and actual fact. *Pediatric Neurosurgery, 28*, 167–172.

Johnston, J., & Ellis Weismer, S. (1983). Mental rotation abilities in language-disordered children. *Journal of Speech and Hearing Research, 26*, 397–403.

Johnston, J. M., & Pennypacker, H. S. (1993). *Strategies and tactics of human behavioral research* (2nd ed.). Hillsdale, NJ: Erlbaum.

Johnston, J. R., & Wong, M. Y. (2002). Cultural differences in beliefs and practices concerning talk to children. *Journal of Speech, Language, and Hearing Research, 45*, 916–926.

Jonas, A. (1997). *Watch William walk*. New York: Greenwillow Books.

Julia, P. (1983). *Explanatory models in linguistics: A behavioral perspective*. Princeton, NJ: Princeton University Press.

Justice, L. M., Chow, S., Capellini, C., Flanigan, K., & Colton, S. (2003). Emergent literacy intervention for vulnerable preschoolers: Relative effects of two approaches. *American Journal of Speech-Language Pathology, 12*, 320–332.

Justice, L. M., & Ezell, H. K. (2000). Enhancing children's print and word awareness through home-based parent intervention. *American Journal of Speech-Language Pathology, 9*, 257–269.

Justice, L. M., & Ezell, H. K. (2002a). Use of storybook reading to increase print awareness in at-risk children. *American Journal of Speech-Language Pathology, 11*, 17–29.

Justice, L. M., & Ezell, H. K. (2002b). *The syntax handbook: Everything you learned about syntax . . . but forgot*. Eau Claire, WI: Thinking Publications.

Justice, L. M., Weber, S. E., Ezell, H. K., & Bakeman, R. (2002). A sequential analysis of children's responsiveness to parental print references during shared book-reading interactions. *American Journal of Speech-Language Pathology, 11*, 30–40.

Kail, R. (1994). A method of studying the generalized slowing hypothesis in children with specific language impairment. *Journal of Speech, Language, and Hearing Research, 37*, 418–421.

Kaiser, A. P. (1993). Parent-implemented language intervention: An environmental system approach. In A. P. Kaiser & D. P. Gray (Eds.), *Enhancing children's communication: Research foundations for intervention* (pp. 63–84). Baltimore, MD: Paul H. Brookes.

Kaiser, A. P., Cai, X., Hancock, B. T., & Foster, E. M. (2002). Teacher-reported behavior problems and language delays in boys and girls enrolled in Head Start classrooms. *Behavioral Disorders, 28*, 23–39.

Kaiser, A. P., & Delaney, E. M. (1996). The effects of poverty on parenting young children. *Peabody Journal of Education, 71*, 66–85.

Kaiser, A. P., & Gray, D. P. (Eds.) (1993). *Enhancing children's communication: Research foundations for intervention*. Baltimore, MD: Paul H. Brookes.

Kaiser, A. P., Hancock, B. T., Cai, X., Foster E. M., & Hester, P. P. (2000). Parent-reported behavior problems and language delays in boys and girls enrolled in Head Start classrooms. *Behavioral Disorders, 26*, 26–41.

Kaiser, A. P., Hancock, T. B., & Nietfeld, J. P. (2000). The effects of parent-implemented enhanced milieu teaching on the social communication of children who have autism. *Early Education and Development, 11*, 423–446.

Kaiser, A. P., & Hester, M. L. (1994). Generalized effects of enhanced milieu teaching. *Journal of Speech, Language, and Hearing Research, 37,* 1320–1340.

Kamhi, A. (1981). Nonlinguistic symbolic and conceptual abilities of language-impaired and normally-developing children. *Journal of Speech and Hearing Research, 24,* 446–453.

Kamhi, A., Catts, H., Koenig, L., & Lewis, B. (1984). Hypothesis-testing and nonlinguistic symbolic abilities in language-impaired children. *Journal of Speech and Hearing Disorders, 59,* 169–176.

Kamhi, A. G., & Johnston, J. R. (1982). Toward an understanding of retarded children's linguistic deficiencies. *Journal of Speech and Hearing Research, 25,* 435–445.

Kamhi, A. G., Pollock, K. E., & Harris, J. L. (1996). Communication development and disorders in African American children. Baltimore, MD: Brookes.

Kaminski, R. A., & Good, R. H. (1996). Toward a technology for assessing basic literacy skills. *School Psychology Review, 25,* 215–227.

Kamps, D. M., Leonard, B. R., Vernon, S., Dugan, E. P., Delquadri, J. C., Gershon, B., et al. (1992). Teaching social skills to students with autism to increase peer interactions in an integrated first-grade classroom. *Journal of Applied Behavior Analysis, 25,* 281–288.

Kanner, L. (1943). Autistic disturbances of affective contact. *Nervous Child, 2,* 217–50.

Karmiloff-Smith, A., Brown, J. H., Grice, S., & Paterson, S. (2003). Dethroning the myth: Cognitive dissociations and innate modularity in Williams syndrome. *Developmental Neuropsychology, 23*(1–2), 227–234.

Kaufman, A. S., & Kaufman, N. L. (2004a). *Kaufman Assessment Battery for Children.* Circle Pines, MN: American Guidance Service.

Kaufman, A. S., & Kaufman, N. L. (2004b). *Kaufman Test of Educational Achievement—II.* Circle Pines, MN: American Guidance Service.

Kavale, K. A., & Mostert, M. P. (2003). River of ideology, islands of evidence. *Exceptionality, 11*(4), 191–208.

Kay-Raining Bird, E., & Chapman, R. S. (1994). Sequential recall in individuals with Down syndrome. *Journal of Speech and Hearing Research, 37,* 1369–1380.

Kay-Raining Bird, E., & Vetter, R. S. (1994). Storytelling in Chippewa-Cree children. *Journal of Speech and Hearing Research, 37*(6), 1354–1368.

Kayser, H. (1995). *Bilingual speech-language pathology: An Hispanic focus.* San Diego, CA: Singular.

Kayser, H. (2002). Bilingual language development and language disorders. In D. E. Battle (Ed.), *Communication disorders in multicultural populations* (3rd ed.) (pp. 202–232). Woburn, MA: Butterworth-Heinemann.

Kazdin, A. E. (1982). Single-case research designs: Methods of clinical and applied settings. New York: Oxford University Press.

Kazdin, A. E. (2001). *Behavior Modification in Applied Settings* (6th ed.). Belmont, CA: Wadsworth Publishing Company.

Kemper, A. R., & Downs, S. M. (2000). A cost-effective analysis of newborn hearing screening strategies. *Archives of Pediatric and Adolescent Medicine, 154*(5), 484–488.

Kennedy Krieger Institute. (2004). *Behavioral disorders/Self-injurious behavior.* Retrieved on August 18, 2004, from www.kennedykrieger.org/kki_diag.jsp?pid+1074.

Kessler, C. (1984). Language acquisition in bilingual children. In N. Miller (Ed.), *Bilingualism and language disability: Assessment and remediation* (pp. 26–54). San Diego, CA: College Hill Press.

Kidd, P. (2002). Autism, an extreme challenge to integrative medicine. Part II: Medical management. *Alternative Medicine Review, 7,* 472–499.

Kinzler, M. (1993). *Joliet 3-minute preschool speech and language screen.* Austin, TX: PRO-ED.

Kinzler, M., & Johnson, C. (1992). *Joliet 3-Minute Speech and Language Screening Test* (Revised). Austin, TX: PRO-ED.

Kirby, K. C., Holborn, S. W., & Bushby, H. T. (1981). Word game bingo: A behavioral treatment package for improving textual responding to sight words. *Journal of Applied Behavior Analysis, 14,* 317–326.

Klin, A. (2003). Asperger syndrome: an update. *Revao Brasil Psiquiatry, 25,* 103–109.

Klin, A., & Volkmar, F. R. (1995). *Asperger's syndrome: Guidelines for assessment and diagnosis.* Retrieved July 14, 2004, from http://info.med.yale.edu/chldstdy/autism/asdiagnosis.html.

Klin, A., Volkmar, F. R., & Sparrow, S. S. (2000). *Asperger Syndrome.* New York: Guilford Press.

Klink, M., Gerstman, L., Raphael, L., Schlanger, B., & Newsome, L. (1986). Phonological process usage by young EMR children and nonretarded preschool children. *American Journal of Mental Deficiency, 91,* 190–195.

Koegel, L. K. (2000) Interventions to facilitate communication in autism. *Journal of Autism and Developmental Disabilities, 30,* 383–391.

Koegel, L. K., Camarata, S. M., Valdez-Menchaca, M., & Koegel, R. L. (1998). Setting generalization of question-asking by children with autism. *American Journal of Mental Retardation, 102*(4), 346–357.

Koegel, R. L., Bimbela, A., & Schreibman, L. (1996). Collateral effects of parent training on family interactions. *Journal of Autism and Developmental Disabilities, 26,* 347–359.

Koegel, R. L., & Frea, W. D. (1993). Treatment of social behavior in autism through the modification of pivotal social skills. *Journal of Applied Behavior Analysis, 26,* 369–377.

Koegel, L. K., Koegel, R. L., & Dunlap, G. (Eds.). (1996). *Positive behavior support: Including people with difficult behavior in the community.* Baltimore, MD: Paul H. Brookes.

Koegel, R. L., O'Dell, M. C., & Koegel, L. K. (1987). A natural language teaching paradigm for nonverbal autistic children. *Journal of Autism and Developmental Disabilities, 18,* 525–538.

Koeppen-Schomerus, G., Spinath, F. M., & Plomin, R. (2003). Twins and non-twin siblings: Different estimates of shared environmental influences in early childhood. *Twin Research, 6*(2), 97–105.

Koman, L. A., Smith, B. P., & Shilt, J. S. (2004). Cerebral palsy. *The Lancet, 363,* 1619–1631.

Koppenhaver, D., Evans, D., & Yoder, D. (1991). Childhood reading and writing experiences of literate adults with severe speech and motor impairments. *Augmentative and Alternative Communication, 7,* 20–33.

Koren, E. (2003). *Very hairy Harry.* New York: Joanna Cotler Books.

Krantz, P. J., MacDuff, M. T., & McClannahan, L. E. (1993). Programming participation in family activities for children with autism: Parents' use of photographic activity schedules. *Journal of Applied Behavior Analysis, 26,* 137–138.

Krantz, P. J., & McClannahan, L. E. (1998). Social interaction skills for children with autism: A script-fading procedure for beginning readers. *Journal of Applied Behavior Analysis, 31,* 191–202.

Kraus, J. K., & McArthur, D. L. (2000). Epidemiology of brain injury. In P. R. Cooper & J. G. Golfinos (Eds.), *Head injury* (4th ed.) (pp. 1–26). New York: McGraw-Hill.

Kravits, T. R., Kamps, D. M., Kemmerer, K., & Potucek, J. (2002). Brief report: Increasing communication skills for an elementary-aged student with autism using the picture exchange communication system. *Journal of Autism and Developmental Disabilities, 32,* 225–230.

Kreimeyer, K. H., & Anita, S. D. (1988). The development and generalization of social interaction skills in preschool hearing-impaired children. *The Volta Review, 90,* 219–231.

Kuhn, S. A. C., Lerman, D. C., & Vorndran, C. M. (2003). Pyramidal training for families of children with problem behavior. *Journal of Applied Behavior Analysis, 36,* 77–88.

Kupperman, P., Bligh, S., & Barouski, K. (2004). *Hyperlexia.* Retrieved July 14, 2004, from www.hyperlexia.org /hyperlexia.html.

Lahey, M. (1990). Who shall be called language disordered? Some reflections and one perspective. *Journal of Speech and Hearing Disorders, 55,* 612–620.

Lahey, M., & Edwards, J. (1999). Naming errors of children with specific language impairment. *Journal of Speech, Language, and Hearing Research, 42,* 195–205.

Lai, C. S. I., Fisher, S. E., Hurst, J. A., Vargha-Kadem, F., & Monaco, A. P. (2001). A forkhead-domain gene is mutated in a severe speech and language disorder. *Nature, 413,* 519–523.

Laing, S. P., & Kamhi, A. (2003). Alternative assessment of language and literacy in culturally and linguistically diverse children. *Language, Speech, and Hearing Services in Schools, 34,* 44–55.

Lainhart, J. E. (2003). Increased rate of head growth during infancy in autism. *Journal of the American Medical Association, 290,* 393–394.

Lancioni, G. E. (1982). Normal children as tutors to teach social responses to withdrawn mentally retarded schoolmates: Training, maintenance, and generalization. *Journal of Applied Behavior Analysis, 15,* 17–40.

Langdon, H. W. (2000). Diversity. In E. P. Dodge (Ed.), *The survival guide for school-based speech-language pathologists* (pp. 367–398). San Diego: Singular Publishing Group/ Thomson Learning.

Langdon, H. W., & Cheng, L. L. (Eds.) (1992). *Hispanic children and adults with communication disorders: Assessment and intervention.* Gaithersberg, MD: Aspen Publishers.

Langdon, H. W., & Cheng, L. L. (2002). *Collaborating with interpreters and translators: A guide for communication disorders professionals.* Eau Claire, WI: Thinking Publications.

Langdon, H. W., & Quintanar-Sarellana, R. (2003). Roles and responsibilities of the interpreter in interactions with speech-language pathologists, parents, and students. *Seminars in Speech and Language, 24* (3), 235–244.

Larson, S. A., Lakin, K. C., Anderson, L., Kwak, L. N., & Anderson, D. (2001). Prevalence of mental retardation and developmental disabilities: Estimates from the 1994/1995 national health interview survey disability supplements. *American Journal of Mental Retardation, 106*(3), 231–252.

Laski, K. E., Charlop, M. H., & Schreibman, L. (1988). Training parents to use the natural language paradigm to increase their autistic children's speech. *Journal of Applied Behavior Analysis, 21,* 391–400.

Laws, G., & Bishop, D. V. M. (2003). A comparison of language abilities in adolescents with Down syndrome and children with specific language impairment. *Journal of Speech, Language, and Hearing Research, 46,* 1324–1339.

Laws, G., & Bishop, D. V. M. (2004). Pragmatic language impairment and social deficits in Williams syndrome: A comparison with Down syndrome and specific language impairment. *International Journal of Communication Disorders, 39*(1), 45–46.

Layton, T. (1988). Language training with autistic children using four different modes of presentation. *Journal of Communication Disorders, 21,* 333–350.

Lazzari, A. M. (1996). *The HELP Test-Elementary.* East Moline, IL: LinguiSystems, Inc.

LeBlanc, L. A., Coates, A. M., Daneshvar, S., Charlop-Christy, M. H., Morris, C., & Lancaster, B. M. (2003). Using video modeling and reinforcement to teach perspective-taking skills to children with autism. *Journal of Applied Behavioral Analysis, 36,* 253–257.

Lenneberg, E. H. (1967). *Biological foundations of language.* New York: Wiley.

Lenski, L. (1937). *The little sailboat.* New York: Random House.

Leonard, H., & Wen, X. (2002). The epidemiology of mental retardation: Challenges and opportunities in the new millennium. *Mental Retardation and Developmental Disabilities Research Review, 8,* 117–134.

Leonard, L. B. (1991). Specific language impairment as a clinical category. *Language, Speech, and Hearing Services in Schools, 22,* 66–68.

Leonard, L. B. (1998). *Children with specific language impairment.* Cambridge, MA: MIT Press.

Leonard, L. B., & Leonard, J. (1985). The contribution of phonetic context to an unusual phonologic pattern: a case study. *Language, Speech, and Hearing Services in Schools, 16,* 110–118.

Leonard, L. B., McGregor, K., & Allen, G. (1992). Grammatical morphology and speech perception in children with specific language impairment. *Journal of Speech and Hearing Research, 35,* 1076–1085.

Leonard, L. B., Miller, C., & Gerber, E. (1999). Grammatical morphology and the lexicon in children with specific language impairment. *Journal of Speech, Language, and Hearing Research, 42,* 678–689.

Leonard, L. H., Silberstein, J., Falk, R., Houwink-Manville, I., Ellaway, C. Raffael, L. S., et al. (2001). Occurrence of Rett syndrome in boys. *Child Neurology, 16,* 333–338.

Lerman, D. C., & Iwata, B. A. (1996). A methodology for distinguishing between extinction and punishment effects associated with response blocking. *Journal of Applied Behavior Analysis, 29,* 231–234.

Lerman, D. C., Iwata, B. A., Shore, B. A., & DeLeon, I. G. (1997). Effects of intermittent punishment on self-injurious behavior: An evaluation of schedule thinning. *Journal of Applied Behavior Analysis, 30,* 187–201.

Lerman, D. C., & Vorndran, C. M. (2002). On the status of knowledge for using punishment: Implications for treating behavior disorders. *Journal of Applied Behavior Analysis, 35,* 431–464.

Lerman, D. C., Vorndran, C. M., Addison, L., & Kuhn, S. A. C. (2004). A rapid assessment of skills in young children with autism. *Journal of Applied Behavior Analysis, 37,* 11–26.

Levy, Y., Tennenbaum, A., & Ornoy, A. (2003). Repair behavior in children with intellectual impairment: Evidence for metalinguistic competence. *Journal of Speech, Language, and Hearing Research, 46,* 368–381.

Lewis, B. A., Freebairn, L., Heeger, S., & Cassidy, S. B. (2002). Speech and language skills of individuals with Prader-Willi syndrome. *American Journal of Speech-Language Pathology, 11,* 285–294.

Lewis, B. A., O'Donnell, B., Freebairn, L. A., & Taylor, H. G. (1998). Spoken language and written expression—Interplay of delays. *American Journal of Speech-Language Pathology, 7*(3), 77–84.

Lieu, J. E. (2004). Speech-language and educational consequences of unilateral hearing loss in children. *Archives of Otolaryngology, Head and Neck Surgery, 130*(5), 524–530.

Light, J. C., Binger, C., & Kelford Smith, A. (1994). The story reading interactions of preschoolers who use augmentative and alternative communication and their mothers. *Augmentative and Alternative Communication, 10,* 255–268.

Light, J. C., & Drager, K. D. R. (2002). Improving the design of augmentative and alternative technologies for young children. *Assistive Technology, 14,* 17–32.

Light, J. C., & Pitkin, L. (2003). *Children's designs for AAC systems for young children.* Unpublished manuscript.

Light, J., Roberts, B., Dimarco, R., & Greiner, N. (1998). Augmentative and alternative communication to support

receptive and expressive communication for people with autism. *Journal of Communication Disorders, 31,* 153–180.

Lindsay, J. (2004). *The Hmong people in the U.S.* Retrieved October 15, 2004, from www.jefflindsay.com/Hmong_tragedy.html.

Linguistic Society of America. (1997). *LSA resolution on the Oakland "Ebonics" issue.* Retrieved January 24, 2004, from www.lsadc.org/resolutions/ebonics.htm.

Loeb, D. F., Stoke, C., & Fey, M. E. (2001). Language changes associated with Fast For Word-Language: Evidence from case studies. *American Journal of Speech-Language Pathology, 10,* 216–230.

Lohr, K. N., Eleazer, K., & Mauskopf, J. (1998). Health policy issues and applications for evidence-based medicine and clinical practical guidelines. *Health Policy, 46,* 1–19.

Long, S. (1994). Language and bilingual-bicultural children. In V. A. Reed (Ed.), *Introduction to children with language disorders* (pp. 290–317). New York: Merrill.

Lonigan, C. J., & Whitehurst, G. J. (1998). Relative efficacy of parent and teacher involvement in a shared-reading intervention for preschool children from low- income backgrounds. *Early Childhood Research Quarterly, 13*(2), 263–290.

Lovaas, I. O. (1966). A program for the establishment of speech in psychotic children. In J. K. Wing (Ed.), *Early childhood autism* (pp. 25–32). London: Pergamon.

Lovaas, I. O. (1987) Behavioral treatment and normal educational and intellectual functioning in young autistic children. *Journal of Consulting and Clinical Psychology, 55,* 3–9.

Love, A. J., & Thompson, M. G. G. (1988). Language disorders and attention deficit disorders in young children referred for psychiatric services: Analysis of prevalence and a conceptual synthesis. *American Journal of Orthopsychiatry, 58,* 57–64.

Lucas, E. (1980). *Semantic and pragmatic language disorders: Assessment and remediation.* Rockville, MD: Aspen.

Luftig, R., & Bersani, H. (1985). An investigation of two variables influencing Blissymbol learnabililty with nonhandicapped adults. *Augmentative and Alternative Commjunication, 1,* 32–37.

Lyovin, A. (1997). *An introduction to the languages of the world.* New York: Oxford University Press.

Madsen, K. M., Hviid, A., Vestergaard, M., Schendel, D., Wohlfahrt, J., Thorsen, P., et al. (2002). A population-based study of measles, mumps, and rubella vaccination and autism. *The New England Journal of Medicine, 347,* 1477–1482.

Magiati, I., & Howlin, P. (2003). A pilot evaluation of the Picture Exchange Communication System (PECS) for children with autism spectrum disorder. *Autism, 7,* 297–320.

Mahoney, G. J., Glover, A., & Finger, I. (1981). Relationship between language and sensorimotor development of Down syndrome and nonretarded children. *American Journal of Mental Deficiency, 86,* 21–27.

Malott, R. W., Malott, M. E., & Trojan, E. A. (2000). *Elementary principles of behavior* (4th ed.). Upper Saddle River, NJ: Prentice-Hall.

Mank, D. M. & Horner, R. H. (1987). Self-recruited feedback: A cost-effective procedure for maintaining behavior. *Research in Developmental Disabilities, 8,* 91–112.

March of Dimes (2004). Infant deaths up in U.S. for first time since 1958: Premature birth is a leading cause. Retrieved April 9, 2004, from www.marchofdimes.com/aboutus/10651_10932.asp.

Markwardt, F. C., Jr. (1998). *Peabody Individual Achievement Test—Revised—Normative Update.* Circle Pines, MN: American Guidance Service.

Martin, F. N., & Clark, J. G. (2003). *Introduction to audiology* (8th ed.). Boston: Allyn & Bacon.

Martin, G., & Pear, J. (1999). *Behavior modification; What it is and how to do it* (6th ed.). Upper Saddle River, NJ: Prentice-Hall.

Martin, R. R., Kuhl, P., & Haroldson, S. K. (1972). An experimental treatment with two preschool children. *Journal of Speech and Hearing Research, 15,* 743–752.

Marvin, C., & Mirenda, P. (1993). Home literacy experiences of preschoolers enrolled in Head Start and special education programs. *Journal of Early Intervention, 17,* 351–367.

Mason, S. M., & Iwata, B. A. (1991). Artifactual effects of sensory-integrative therapy on self-injurious behavior. *Journal of Applied Behavior Analysis, 23,* 361–370.

Matson, J. L., Sevin, J. A., Box, M. L., Francis, K. L., & Sevin, B. M. (1993). An evaluation of two methods for increasing self-initiated verbalizations in autistic children. *Journal of Applied Behavior Analysis, 26,* 389–398.

Matson, J. L., Sevin, J. A., Fridley, D., & Love, S. R. (1990). Increasing spontaneous language in three autistic children. *Journal of Applied Behavior Analysis, 23,* 227–233.

Matsuda, M. (1989). Working with Asian parents: Some communication strategies. *Topics in Language Disorders, 9,* 45–53.

Maurice, C. (1996). *Behavioral intervention for young children with autism.* Austin, TX: PRO-ED.

Maurice, C., Green, G., & Luce, S. (1996). *Behavioral intervention for young children with autism.* Austin, TX: PRO-ED.

McCabe, A., & Bliss, L. S. (2003). *Patterns of Narrative Discourse: A Multicultural, Life Span.* Boston: Allyn & Bacon.

McCabe, A., & Rollins, P. R. (1994). Assessment of preschool narrative skills: Prerequisite for literacy. *American Journal of Speech-Language Pathology: A Journal of Clinical Practice, 3,* 45–56.

McCauley, R. J. (1996). Familiar strangers: Criterion-referenced measures in communication disorders. *Language, Speech, and Hearing Services in Schools, 27,* 122–131.

McCauley, R. J. (2001). *Assessment of language disorders in children.* Mahwah, NJ: Lawrence Erlbaum Associates.

McEachin, J. J., Smith, T., & Lovaas, O. I. (1993). Long-term outcome for children with autism who received early intensive behavioral treatment. *American Journal on Mental Retardation, 4,* 67–73.

McFadden, T. U. (1996). Creating language impairment in typically achieving children: The pitfalls of "normal" normative sampling. *Language, Speech, and Hearing Services in Schools, 27,* 3–9.

McGee, G. G., Almeida, M. C., Sulzer-Azaroff, B., & Feldman, R. S. (1992). Promoting reciprocal interactions via peer incidental teaching. *Journal of Applied Behavior Analysis, 25,* 117–126.

McGee, G. G., Krantz, P. J., Mason, D., & McClannahan, L. E. (1983). A modified incidental-teaching procedure for autistic youth: Acquisition and generalization of receptive object labels. *Journal of Applied Behavior Analysis, 16,* 329–338.

McGee, G. G., Krantz, P. J., & McClannahan, L. E. (1985). The facilitative effects of incidental teaching on preposition use by autistic children. *Journal of Applied Behavior Analysis, 18,* 17–31.

McGee, G. G., Krantz, P. J., & McClannahan, L. E. (1986). An extension of incidental teaching procedures to reading instruction for autistic children. *Journal of Applied Behavior Analysis, 19,* 147–157.

McGhee, R., Bryant, B., Larson, S., & Rivera, D. (1995). *Test of Written Expression (TOWE).* Circle Pines, MN: AGS Publishing.

McLaren, J., & Bryson, S. E. (1987). Review of recent epidemiological studies of mental retardation. *American Journal of Mental Retardation, 92,* 243–254.

McLaughlin, S. (1998). *Introduction to language development.* Albany, NY: Thomson Delmar Learning.

McLean, L. K., Brady, N. C., McLean, J. E., & Behrens, G. A. (1999). Communication forms and functions of children and adults with severe mental retardation in community and institutional settings. *Journal of Speech, Language, and Hearing Research, 42,* pp. 231–240.

McMorrow, M. J., & Foxx, R. M. (1986). Some direct and generalized effects of replacing an autistic man's echolalia with correct responses to questions. *Journal of Applied Behavior Analysis, 19,* 289–297.

McMorrow, M. J., Foxx, R. M., Faw, G. D., & Bittle, R. G. (1987). Cues-pause-point language training: Teaching echolalics functional use of their verbal labeling repertoires. *Journal of Applied Behavior Analysis, 20,* 11–22.

McNeill, D. (1970). *The acquisition of language: The study of developmental psycholinguistics.* New York: Harper & Row.

McNeilly, L., & Coleman, T. J. (2000). Language disorders in culturally diverse populations: Intervention issues and strategies. In T. J. Coleman (Ed.), *Clinical management of communication disorders in culturally diverse populations* (pp. 157–172). Boston: Allyn & Bacon.

McReynolds, L. V., & Engmann, D. L. (1974). An experimental analysis of the relationship between subject and object noun phrases. (ASHA Monograph No. 18). In L. V. McReynolds (Ed.), *Developing systematic procedures for training children's language* (pp. 30–46). Rockville, MD: American Speech-Language-Hearing Association.

Meaburn, E., Dale, P. S., Craig, I. W., & Plomin, R. (2002). Language impaired children: No sign of the FOXP2 mutation. *Neuroreport, 13*(18), 1075–1077.

Mecham, M. J. (1996). *Cerebral palsy* (2nd ed.). Austin, TX: PRO-ED.

Merrick, J., Kandel, I., & Morad, M. (2004). Trends in autism. *International Journal of Adolescent Medicine and Health, 16*(1), 75–8.

Mervis, C. B. (2003). Williams syndrome: 15 years of research. *Developmental Neuropsychology, 23*(1–2), 1–12.

Merzenich, M. M., Jenkins, W. M., Johnston, P., Schreiner, C., Miller, S. L., & Tallal, P. (1996). Temporal processing deficits of language-learning impaired children ameliorated by training. *Science, 271,* 77–80.

Miles, S., & Chapman, R. S. (2002). Narrative content as described by individuals with Down syndrome and typically developing children. *Journal of Speech, Language, and Hearing Research, 45,* 175–189.

Miller, C. A., Kail, R., Leonard, L., & Tomblin, J. B. (2001). Speed of processing in children with specific language impairment. *Journal of Speech, Language, and Hearing Research, 44*(2), 416–433.

Miller, J. F. (1988). The developmental synchrony of language development in children with Down syndrome. In L. Nadel (Ed.), *The psychobiology of Down syndrome* (pp. 168–198). Cambridge, MA: MIT Press.

Miller, J. F. (1992). Lexical development in young children with Down syndrome. In R. S. Chapman (Ed.), *Processes in language acquisition and disorder* (pp. 45–55). St. Louis, MO: Mosby Year Book.

Miller, J. F. (1999). Profiles of language development in children with Down syndrome. In J. F. Miller, M. Lehay, & L. A. Leavitt (Eds.), *Improving the communication of people with Down syndrome* (pp. 11–39). Baltimore, MD: Paul H. Brookes.

Miller, S. J., & Sloane, H. N., Jr. (1976). The generalization effects of parent training across stimulus settings. *Journal of Applied Behavior Analysis, 9*(3), 355–370.

Mira, M. P., Tucker, B. F., & Tyler, J. S. (1992). *Traumatic brain injury in children and adolescents.* Austin, TX: PRO-ED.

Mirenda, P. (1997). Supporting individuals with challenging behavior through functional communication training and AAC: A review. *Augmentative and Alternative Communication, 13,* 207–225.

Mirenda, P. (2003). Toward functional augmentative and alternative communication for students with autism: Manual signs, graphic symbols, and voice output communication aids. *Language, Speech, and Hearing Services in Schools, 34,* 203–216.

Mirenda, P., Wilk, D., & Carson, P. (2000). A retrospective analysis of technology use patterns in students with autism over a five-year period. *Journal of Special Education Technology, 15,* 5–16.

Mobayed, K. L., Collins, B. C., Strangis, D. E., Schuster, J. W., & Hemmeter, M. L. (2000). Teaching parents to employ mand-model procedures to teach their children requesting. *Journal of Early Intervention, 23,* 165–179.

Mockford, C. (2002). *Cleo on the move.* Cambridge, MA: Barefoot Books.

Moerk, E. (1983). *The mother of Eve—As a first language teacher.* Norwood, NJ: Ablex.

Moerk, E. (1992). *A first language taught and learned.* Baltimore, MD: Paul H. Brookes.

Moerk, E. (2000). *The guided acquisition of first language skills.* Stamford, CT: Ablex Publishing Corporation.

Montgomery, J. (1995). Examination of phonological working memory in specifically language impaired children. *Applied Psycholinguistics, 6,* 355–378.

Montgomery, J. (2002). Understanding the language difficulties of children with specific language impairments: Does verbal working memory matter? *American Journal of Speech-Language Pathology, 11,* 77–91.

Montgomery, J. W., & Leonard, L. B. (1998). Real-time inflectional processing by children with specific language impairment: Effects of phonetic substance. *Journal of Speech, Language, and Hearing Research, 41,* 1432–1443.

Moran, M., Money, S., & Leonard, L. (1984). Phonological process analysis of the speech of mentally retarded adults. *American Journal of Mental Deficiency, 89,* 304–306.

Morgan, D., Young, K. R., & Goldstein, S. (1983). Teaching behaviorally disordered students to increase teacher attention and praise in mainstreamed classrooms. *Behavioral Disorders, 8,* 265–273.

Most, T. (2002). The use of repair strategies by children with and without hearing impairment. *Language, Speech, and Hearing Services in Schools, 33*(2), 112–123.

Mouridsen, S. E. (2003). Childhood disintegrative disorder. *Brain & Development, 25,* 225–228.

Moxley, A. (2003). What's your multicultural IQ? *ASHA Leader, 8*(3), 12.

Mudford, O. C., Cross, B. A., Breen, S., Cullen, C., Reeves, D., Gould, J., et al. (2000). Auditory integration training for children with autism: No behavioral benefits detected. *American Journal on Mental Retardation, 97,* 381–384.

Muhle, R., Trentacoste, S. V., & Rapin, I. (2004). The genetics of autism. *Pediatrics, 113,* 472–486.

Murch, S. H., Anthony, A., Casson, D. H., Malik, M., Berelowitz, & M. Dhillon, A. P. (2004). Retraction of an interpretation. *The Lancet, 363,* 750.

Myles, B. S., Jones-Bock, S., & Simpson, R. L. (2000). *Asperger Syndrome Diagnostic Scale.* Circle Pines, MN: AGS Publishing.

National Aeronautics and Space Administration. (NASA; 2004). *A system that 'speaks' the mind.* Retrieved on August 30, 2004, from http://ic.arc.nasa.gov/story.php?sid=139&sec=earth.

National Institute on Deafness and Other Communication Disorders. (2002). *Otitis media (ear infection)* (NIH Pub. No. 974216). Bethesda, MD: Author.

National Institute of Mental Health. (2004). *Autism spectrum disorders (pervasive developmental disorders.* Retrieved July 14, 2004, from www.nimh.nih.gov/publicat/autism.cfm.

National Joint Committee for the Communication Needs of Persons with Severe Disabilities. (2003). Position statement on access to communication services and supports: Concerns regarding the application of restrictive "eligibility" policies. *ASHA supplement, 23,* 19–20.

National Pediatric Trauma Registry of Tufts-New England Medical Center. (2004). *Tramatic brain injury in children.* Retrieved on October 20, 2004, from www.nemc.org/rehab/factshee.htm.

National Reading Panel (2000). *Teaching children to read: An evidence-based assessment of the scientific research literature on reading and its implications for reading instruction* (NIH Pub. No. 00–4769). Washington, D.C.: National Institutes of Child Health and Human Development.

National Reading Panel (2001). *Put reading first: The research building blocks for teaching children to read.* Washington, D.C.: U.S. Department of Education.

Neef, N. A. (1995). Pyramidal parent training by peers. *Journal of Applied Behavior Analysis, 28,* 333–337.

Nelson, K. E. (1977). Facilitating children's syntax acquisition. *Developmental Psychology, 13,* 101–107.

Nelson, K. E., Welsh, J., Camarata, S., Butkovsky, L., & Camarata, M. (1995). Available input for language-impaired children and younger children of matched language levels. *First Language, 43,* 1–18.

Nelson, N. W. (1993). *Childhood language disorders in context: Infancy through adolescence.* New York: Macmillan.

Newbury, D. F., et al., and the International Molecular Genetic Study of Autism Consortium (2002). FOXP2 is not a major susceptibility gene for autism or specific language impairment. *American Journal of Human Genetics, 70,* 1318–1327.

Newbury, D. F., & Monaco, A. P. (2002). Talking genes: The molecular basis of language impairment. *Biologist, 49(6),* 255–260.

Newcomer, P., & Hammill, D. (1997a). *Test of language development—Primary (TOLD-P:3).* Austin, TX: PRO-ED.

Newcomer, P., & Hammill, D. (1997b). *Test of language development—I (TOLD I:3).* Austin, TX: PRO-ED.

Newman, L. (2002). *Dogs, dogs, dogs.* New York: Simon & Schuster.

Nikopoulos, C. K., & Keenan, M. (2004). Effects of video modeling on social initiations by children with autism. *Journal of Applied Behavior Analysis, 37,* 93–96.

Nippold, M. A. (1996). Proverb comprehension in youth: The role of concreteness and familiarity. *Journal of Speech and Hearing Research, 39,* 166–176.

Nippold, M. A. (1998). *Later language development: The school age and adolescent years.* Austin, TX: PRO-ED.

Nippold, M. A., & Taylor, C. L. (1995). Idiom understanding in youth: Further examination of familiarity and transparency. *Journal of Speech and Hearing Research, 38,* 426–433.

Nippold, M. A., Uhden, L. D., & Schwarz, I. E. (1997). Proverb explanation through the life span: A developmental study of adolescents and adults. *Journal of Speech, Language, and Hearing Research, 40,* 245–253.

Oborne, M. (2002). *One beautiful baby.* Boston: Little, Brown.

O'Brien, E. K., Zhang, X., Nishmura, C., Tomblin, J. B., & Murray, J. C. (2003). Association of specific language impairment (SLI) to the region of 7p31. *American Journal of Human Genetics, 72(6),* 1536–1543.

O'Connor N., & Hermelin, B. (1994). Two autistic savant readers. *Journal of Autism and Developmental Disabilities, 24(4),* 501–514.

Odom, S. L., Chandler, L. K., Ostrosky, M., McConnell, S. R., & Reaney, S. (1992). Fading teacher prompts from peer-initiation interventions for young children with disabilities. *Journal of Applied Behavior Analysis, 25,* 307–317.

Odom, S. L., Hoyson, M., Jamieson, B., & Strain, P. S. (1985). Increasing handicapped preschoolers' peer social interactions: Cross-setting and component analysis. *Journal of Applied Behavior Analysis, 18,* 3–16.

Oetting, J. B., & Morohov, J. E. (1997). Past-tense marking by children with and without specific language impairment. *Journal of Speech and Hearing Research, 40,* 62–74.

Oetting, J. B., & Rice, M. L. (1993). Plural acquisition in children with specific language impairment. *Journal of Speech and Hearing Research, 36,* 1236–1248.

Oller, D. K., Eilers, R. E., Neal, A. R., & Schwartz, H. K. (1999). Precursors to speech in infancy: The prediction of speech and language disorders. *Journal of Communication Disorders, 32,* 223–245.

Onslow, M., Packman, A., Stocker, S., van Doorn, J., & Siegel, G. M. (1997). Control of children's stuttering with response-contingent time-out; Behavioral, perceptual, and acoustic data. *Journal of Speech, Language, and Hearing Research, 40,* 121–133.

Oram, J., Fine, J., Okamoto, C., & Tannock, R. (1999). Assessing the language of children with attention deficit hyperactivity disorder. *American Journal of Speech-Language Pathology, 8,* 72–80.

Owens, R. E., Jr. (2004). *Language disorders: A functional approach to assessment and intervention* (4th ed.). Boston: Allyn & Bacon.

Ozonoff, S., Rogers, S. J., & Pennington, B. F. (1991). Asperger's syndrome: Evidence of an empirical distinction from high-functioning autism. *Journal of Child Psychology and Psychiatry, 32,* 1107–1122.

Parrish, J. M., & Roberts, M. L. (1993). Interventions based on covariations of desired and inappropriate behavior. In J. Reichle & D. P. Wacker (Eds.), *Communicative alternatives to challenging behavior: Integrating functional assessment and intervention strategies.* Baltimore, MD: Paul H. Brookes Publishing Co.

Paul, R. (2001). *Language disorders from infancy through adolescence: Assessment and intervention* (2nd ed.). St Louis, MO: Mosby.

Paul, P. (2001). *Language and deafness* (3rd ed.). Albany, NY: Thomson Delmar.

Paul, R. (1966). Clinical implications of the natural history of slow expressive language development. *American Journal of Speech-Language-Pathology, 5,* 5–21.

Paul, R. (1991). Profiles of toddlers with slow expressive language development. *Topics in Language Disorders, 11,* 1–13.

Paul, R., & Alforde, S. (1993). Grammatical morpheme acquisition in 4-year olds with normal, impaired, and late developing language. *Journal of Speech and Hearing Research, 36,* 1271–1275.

Paul, R., & Shriberg, L. (1982). Associations between phonology and syntax in speech-delayed children. *Journal of Speech and Hearing Research, 25,* 536–547.

Payne, J. C. (1997). *Adult neurogenic language disorders: Assessment and treatment.* San Diego, CA: Singular Publishing Group.

Pearson, B. (1990). The comprehension of metaphor by preschool children. *Journal of Child Language 17*(1), 185–203.

Peltola, H., Patja, A., Leinikki, P., Valle, M., Davidkin, I., & Paunio, M. (1998). No evidence for measles, mumps, and rubella vaccine-associated inflammatory bowel disease or autism in a 14-year retrospective study. *The Lancet, 351,* 1327–1328.

Peterson, C., & McCabe, A. (1983). *Developmental psycholinguistics: Three ways of looking at a child's narrative.* New York: Plenum.

Phillips, C. E., Jarrold, C., Baddeley, A. D., Grant, J., & Karmiloff-Smith, A. (2004). Comprehension of spatial language terms in Williams syndrome: Evidence for an interaction between domains of strength and weakness. *Cortex, 40*(1), 85–101.

Piaget, J. (1962). *Play, dreams, and imitation in childhood.* London: Routledge & Kegan Paul.

Pierce, K. L., & Schreibman, L. (1994). Teaching daily living skills to children with autism in unsupervised settings through pictoral self-management. *Journal of Applied Behavior Analysis, 27,* 471–481.

Pierce, K. L., & Schreibman, L. (1995). Increasing complex play in children with autism via peer-implemented pivotal response training. *Journal of Applied Behavior Analysis, 28,* 285–295.

Pierce, K. L., & Schreibman, L. (1997). Multiple peer use of pivotal response training to increase social behaviors of classmates with autism: Results from trained and untrained peers. *Journal of Applied Behavior Analysis, 30,* 157–160.

Pinker, S. (1994). *The language instinct: How the mind creates language.* New York: William Morrow and Company.

Plante, E. (1991). MRI findings in the parents and siblings of specifically language-impaired boys. *Brain and Language, 41,* 67–80.

Plante, E. (1996). Observing and interpreting behaviors: An introduction to the Clinical Forum. Language, Speech, and Hearing Services in Schools, 27, 99–101.

Plante, E., Shenkman, K., & Clark, M. (1996). Classification of adults for family studies of developmental language disorders. *Journal of Speech and Hearing Research, 39,* 661–667.

Plante, E., Swisher, L., Vance, R., & Rapcsak, S. (1991). MRI findings in boys with specific language impairment. *Brain and Language, 41,* 52–56.

Pollock, K. (2001). *Phonological Features of African American Vernacular English (AAVE).* Retrieved January 10, 2005, from www.ausp.memphis.edu/phonology/features.htm.

Polloway, E. A., & Smith, T. (1992). *Language instruction for students with disabilities.* Denver, CO: Love Publishing Co.

Portney, L. G., & Watkins, M. P. (2000). *Foundations of clinical research: Application to practice* (2nd ed.). Upper Saddle River, NJ: Prentice-Hall.

Powell, G. G., & Clibbens, J. (1994). Actions speak louder than words: Signing and speech intelligibility in adults with Down syndrome. *Down Syndrome Research and Practice, 2,* 127–129.

Prizant, B. (1983). Language acquisition and communicative behavior in autism: Toward an understanding of the "whole" of it. *Journal of Speech and Hearing Disorders, 48,* 296–307.

Prizant, B., & Duchan, J. (1981). The functions of immediate echolalia in autistic children. *Journal of Speech and Hearing Disorders, 46,* 241–249.

Prizant, B., & Wetherby, A. M. (1987). Communicative intent: A framework for understanding social-communicative behavior in autism. *Journal of the American Academy of Child Psychiatry, 26,* 472–479.

Qi, K. H., Kaiser, A. P., Milan, S. E., Yzquierdo, Z., & Hancock, T. B. (2003). The performance of low-income African American children on the Preschool Language Scale—3. *Journal of Speech, Language, and Hearing Research, 45,* 576–590.

Rapin, I. (1997). Classification and causal issues in autism. In D. J. Cohen & F. R. Volkmar (Eds.), *Handbook of autism and pervasive developmental disorders* (2nd ed.), (pp. 847–867). New York: John Wiley & Sons.

Redmond, S., & Rice, M. (2001). Detection of irregular verb violations by children with and without SLI. *Journal of Speech, Language, and Hearing Research, 44,* 655–669.

Reichle, J., Anderson, H., & Schermer, G. (1986). *Establishing discrimination between requesting objects, requesting assistance, and helping yourself.* Unpublished manuscript, University of Minnesota, Minneapolis.

Reichle, J., & Wacker, D. P. (Eds.) (1993). *Communicative alternatives to challenging behavior: Integrating functional assessment and intervention strategies.* Baltimore, MD: Paul H. Brookes.

Reichle, J., York, J., & Sigafoos, J. (1991). *Implementing augmentative and alternative communication: Strategies for learners with severe disabilities.* Baltimore, MD: Paul H. Brookes.

Reilly, J., Losh, M., Bellugi, U., & Wulfeck, B. (2004). "Frog, where are your?" Narrative in children with specific language impairment, early focal brain injury, and Williams syndrome. *Brain and Language, 88,* 229–247.

Rescorla, L. (1989). The language development survey: A screening tool for delayed language in toddlers. *Journal of Speech and Hearing Disorders, 54,* 587–599.

Rescorla, L. (2002). Language and reading outcomes to age 9 in late-talking toddlers. *Journal of Speech, Language, and Hearing Research, 45,* 360–372.

Rescorla, L., & Lee, E. (2001). Language impairment in young children. In T. Layton, E. Crais, & L. Watson (Eds.). *Handbook of early language impairment in children: Nature* (pp. 1–55), Albany, NY: Delmar Publishers.

Rescorla, L., Roberts, J., & Dahlsgaard, K. (1997). Late talkers at 2: Outcome at age 3. *Journal of Speech, Language, and Hearing Research, 40,* 556–566.

Restrepo, M. A., & Silverman, S. W. (2001). Validity of the Spanish Preschool Language Scale-3 for use with bilingual children. *American Journal of Speech-Language Pathology, 10,* 382–393.

Rheingold, H. L., Gewirtz, J. L., & Ross, H. Q. (1959). Social conditioning of vocalization in infants. *Journal of Comparative and Physiological Psychology, 52,* 65–72.

Rhode, G., Morgan, D. P., & Young, K. R. (1983). Generalization and maintenance of treatment gains of behaviorally handicapped students from resource rooms to regular classrooms using self-evaluation procedures. *Journal of Applied Behavior Analysis, 16,* 171–188.

Rice, M., & Oetting, J. B. (1993). Morphological deficits of children with SLI: Evaluation of number marking and agreement. *Journal of Speech and Hearing Research, 36,* 1249–1257.

Rice, M., Sell, M., & Hadley, P. (1991). Social interactions of speech- and language-impaired children. *Journal of Speech and Hearing Research, 34,* 1299–1307.

Rice, M., Wexler, K., Marquis, J., & Hershberger, S. (2000). Acquisition of irregular past tense by children with specific language impairment. *Journal of Speech, Language, and Hearing Research, 43,* 1126–1145.

Richard, G. J., & Calvert, L. K. (2003). *Differential assessment of autism and other developmental disorders (DAADD).* East Moline, IL: LinguiSystems.

Rimland, B. (2003). Autism is treatable. Retrieved on January 9, 2005, from www.autismwebsite.com/ari/specialinterest/congressionaltestimony.pdf.

Rincover, A., & Koegel, R. L. (1975). Setting generality and stimulus control in autistic children. *Journal of Applied Behavior Analysis, 8,* 235–246.

Ringdahl, J. E., Kitsukawa, K., Andelman, M. S., Call, N., Winborn, L., Barretto, A., et al. (2002). Differential reinforcement with and without instructional fading. *Journal of Applied Behavior Analysis, 35,* 291–294.

Ripich, D. N., & Craighead, N. A. (1994). *School discourse problems* (2nd ed.). San Diego: Singular Publishing Group.

Risley, T. R., & Reynolds, N. J. (1970). Emphasis as a prompt for verbal imitation. *Journal of Applied Behavior Analysis, 3,* 185–190.

Risley, T. R., & Wolf, M. (1967). Establishing functional speech in echolalic children. *Behavior Research and Therapy, 5,* 73–88.

Roberts, J. E., Mirrett, P., Anderson, K., Burchinal, M., & Neebe, E. (2002). Early communication, symbolic behavior, and social profiles of young males with fragile X syndrome. *American Journal of Speech-Language Pathology, 11,* 295–304.

Roberts, J. E., Wallace, I. F., & Henderson, F. W. (Eds.) (1997). *Otitis media in young children: Medical, developmental, and educational considerations.* Baltimore, MD: Paul H. Brookes.

Robertson, C., & Salter, W. (1997). *Phonological Awareness Test (PAT).* East Moline, IL: LinguiSystems.

Robertson, S. B., & Weismer, S. E. (1997). The influence of peer models on the play scripts of children with specific language impairment. *Journal of Speech, Language, and Hearing Research, 40,* 49–61.

Robison, L. D. (2003). An organizational guide for an effective developmental program in the NICU. *Journal of Obstetric, Gynecologic, and Neonatal Nursing, 32*(3), 379–386.

Rodriguez, B. L., & Olswang, L. B. (2003). Mexican-American and Anglo-American mothers' beliefs about child rearing, education, and language impairment. *American Journal of Speech-Language Pathology, 12,* 452–462.

Rogers-Warren, A., & Warren, S. F. (1980). Mands for verbalization: Facilitating the display of newly trained language in children. *Behavior Modification, 4,* 361–382.

Roid, G. H. (2004). *Stanford-Binet Intelligence Scale—5th Edition.* Itasca, IL: Riverside Publishing Company.

Roid, G. H., & Miller, L. (2004). *Lieter International Performance Scale.* Wood Dale, IL: Stoelting Company.

Roid, G. H., & Sampers, J. L. (2004). *Merrill-Palmer Revised Scales of Development.* Wood Dale, IL: Stoelting Company.

Rolider, A., & Van Houten, R. (1990). The role of reinforcement in reducing inappropriate behavior: Some myths and misconceptions. In A. C. Repp & N. N. Singh (Eds.), *Perspectives on the use of aversive and non-aversive interventions for persons with developmental disabilities* (pp. 119–127). Sycamore, IL: Sycamore.

Rondal, J. A. (1998). Cases of exceptional language in mental retardation and Down syndrome: Explanatory perspectives. *Down Syndrome Research and Practice, 5*(1), 1–15.

Roseberry-McKibbin, C. (2002). *Multicultural students with special language needs: Practical strategies for assessment and intervention* (2nd ed.). Oceanside, CA: Academic Communication Associates.

Roseberry-McKibbin, C., & Eicholtz, G. (1994). Serving children with limited English proficiency in the schools: A national survey. *Language, Speech, and Hearing Services in Schools, 25,* 156–164.

Roseberry-McKibbin, C., & Hegde, M. N. (2005). *An advanced review of speech-language pathology: Preparation for NESPA and comprehensive examination.* (2nd ed.). Austin, TX: PRO-ED.

Rosenberg, S. (1982). The language of the mentally retarded: Development, processes, and intervention. In S. Rosenberg (Ed.), *Handbook of applied psycholinguistics: Major thrusts of research and theory* (pp. 329–392). Hillsdale, NJ: Erlbaum.

Rosner, K. (1996). A review of psychoanalytic theory and treatment of childhood autism. *Psychoanalytic Review, 83,* 325–341.

Ross, S. H., Oetting, J. B., & Stapleton, B. (2004). Preterite HAD + V-ED: A developmental narrative structure of African American English. *American Speech, 79,* 167–193.

Rossetti, L. M. (2001). *Communication intervention: Birth to three* (2nd ed.). Albany, NY: Delmar/Singular/Thomson Learning.

Rossetti, L. M. (2002). Workshop on infants and toddlers. June 27–28, 2002, Fresno, California.

Roth, F. P., & Baden, B. (2001). Investing in emergent literacy intervention: A key role for speech-language pathologists. *Seminars in Speech and Language, 22*(3), 163–173.

Rothman, K. J., & Greenland, S. (1998). *Modern epidemiology* (2nd ed.). Philadelphia, PA: Lippincott Williams & Wilkins.

Rouse, C. E., & Krueger, A. B. (2004). Putting computerized instruction to the test: A randomized evaluation of a "scientifically based" reading program. *Economics of Education Review, 23*(4), 323–338.

Roy, P., & Chiat, S. (2004). A prosodically controlled word and nonword repetition task for 2- to 4-year-olds: Evidence from typically developing children. *Journal of Speech, Language, and Hearing Research, 47,* 223–234.

Ruben, R. J. (2000). Redefining the survival of the fittest: Communication disorders in the 21st century. *Laryngoscope, 110*(2), 241–245.

Ruscello, D., St. Louis, K., & Mason, N. (1991). School-aged children with phonologic disorders: Co-existence with other speech/language disorders. *Journal of Speech and Hearing Research, 34,* 236–242.

Rutter, T., & Buckley, S. (1994). The acquisition of grammatical morphemes in children with Down syndrome. *Down Syndrome: Research and Practice, 2,* 76–82.

Rvachew, S., Ohberg, A., Grawburg, M., & Heyding, J. (2003). Phonological awareness and phonemic perception in 4-year-old children with delayed expressive phonology skills. *American Journal of Speech-Language Pathology, 12*(4), 463–471.

Sacket, D. L., Rosenberg, W. M. C., Gray, J. A. M., Hayes, R. B., & Richardson, R. B. (1996). Evidence-based medicine: What it is and what it isn't. *British Medical Journal, 312,* 71–72.

Sackett, D. L., Straus, S. E., Richardson, W. S., Rosenberg, W., & Hayes, R. B. (2000). *Evidence-based medicine: How to practice and teach EBM.* London: Churchill Livingstone.

Sailor, W., Guess, D., Rutherford, G., & Baer, D. M. (1968). Control of tantrum behavior by operant techniques during experimental verbal training. *Journal of Applied Behavior Analysis, 1,* 237–243.

Sainato, D. M., Goldstein, H., & Strain, P. S. (1992). Effects of self-evaluation on preschool children's use of social interaction strategies with their classmates with autism. *Journal of Applied Behavior Analysis, 25,* 127–141.

Salas-Provance, M. B., Erickson, J. G., & Reed, J. (2002). Disabilities as viewed by four generations of one Hispanic family. *American Journal of Speech-Language Pathology, 11,* 151–162.

Salzberg, C. L., & Villani, T. V. (1983). Speech training by parents of Down syndrome toddlers: Generalization across settings and instructional contexts. *American Journal of Mental Deficiency, 87*(4), 403–413.

Salzinger, K., & Salzinger, S. (Eds.) (1967). *Research in verbal behavior and some neurophysiological implications.* New York: Academic Press.

Sarokoff, R. A., Taylor, B. A., & Poulson, C. L. (2001). Teaching children with autism to engage in conversational exchanges: Script fading with embedded textual stimuli. *Journal of Applied Behavior Analysis, 34,* 81–84.

Scarborough, H. (1998a). Early identification of children at risk for reading disabilities: phonological awareness and some other promising predictors. In B. Shapiro, P. Accoardo, & A. Capute (Eds.), *Specific reading disability: A view of the spectrum.* Timonium, MD: York Press.

Scarborough, H. (1998b). Predicting future achievement of second graders with reading disabilities: Contributions of phonemic awareness, verbal memory, rapid naming, and IQ. *Annals of Dyslexia, 48,* 115–136.

Schalomon, J., Bismark, S. V., Schober, P. H., et al. (2004). Multiple trauma in pediatric patients. *Journal of Pediatric Surgery, 39*(7), 417–423.

Schanen, N. C., Kurczynski, T. W., Brunelle, D., Woodcock, M. M., Dure, L. S., & Percy, A. K. (1998) Neonatal encephalopathy in two boys in families with recurrent Rett syndrome. *Journal of Child Neurology, 13*(5), 229–231.

Schank, R. C., & Abelson, R. P. (1977). *Scripts, plans, goals, and understanding.* Hillsdale, NJ: Lawrence Erlbaum.

Schatschneider, C., Carlson, C. D., Francis, D. J., Floorman, R., & Fletcher, J. M. (2002). Relationship of rapid automatized naming and phonological awareness in early reading development: Implications for the double-deficit hypothesis. *Journal of Learning Disabilities, 35*(3), 245–257.

Schepis, M. M., Reid, D. H., Behrmann, M., & Sutton, K. (1998). Increasing communicative interactions of young children with autism using a voice output communication aid in naturalistic teaching. *Journal of Applied Behavior Analysis, 31,* 561–578.

Schepis, M. M., Reid, D. H., Fitzgerald, J. R., Faw, G. D., van den Pol, R. A., & Welty, P. A. (1982). A program for increasing manual signing by autistic and profoundly retarded youth with the daily environment. *Journal of Applied Behavior Analysis, 15,* 363–379.

Schiefelbusch, R. L. (Ed.) (1973). *Language intervention with the retarded.* Baltimore, MD: University Park Press.

Schiefelbusch, R. L. (Ed.) (1978). *Language intervention strategies.* Baltimore, MD: University Park Press.

Schiefelbusch, R. L., & Lloyd, L. L. (1974). *Language perspectives: Acquisition, retardation, and intervention*. Baltimore: University Park Press.

Schiff-Myers, N. B. (1992). Considering arrested language development and language loss in the assessment of second language learners. *Language, Speech, and Hearing Services in Schools, 23*, 28–33.

Schlesinger, I. M. (1971). Production of utterances and language acquisition. In Dan I. Slobin (Ed.), *The Ontogenesis of Grammar* (pp. 63–101). New York: Academic Press.

Schopler, E., Reichler, R. L., & Renner, B. R. (1998). *Childhood Autism Rating Scale*. Circle Pines, MN: AGS Publishing.

Schreibman, L., & Carr, E. G. (1978). Elimination of echolalic responding to questions through the training of a generalized verbal response. *Journal of Applied Behavior Analysis, 11*, 453–563.

Schreibman, L., Kaneko, W. M., & Keogel, R. L. (1991). Positive effects of parents of autistic children: A comparison across two teaching techniques. *Behavior Therapy, 22*, 479–490.

Schreibman, L., O'Neill, R. E., & Koegel, R. L. (1983). Behavioral training for siblings of autistic children. *Journal of Applied Behavior Analysis, 16*, 129–138.

Schumaker, J., & Sherman, J. A. (1970). Training generative verb usage by imitation and reinforcement procedures. *Journal of Applied Behavior Analysis, 3*, 273–287.

Schumaker, J., & Sherman, J. A. (1978). Parents as intervention agents. In R. L. Schiefelbusch (Ed.), *Language intervention strategies* (pp. 237–326). Baltimore, MD: University Park Press.

Schussler, N. G., & Spradlin, J. E. (1991). Assessment of stimuli controlling the requests of students with severe mental retardation during a snack routine. *Journal of Applied Behavior Analysis, 24*, 791–797.

Scientific Learning Corporation. (1998). *Fast ForWord* [computer software]. Berkeley, CA: Author.

Scudder, R. R., & Tremain, D. H. (1992). Repair behaviors of children with and without mental retardation. *Mental Retardation, 30*(5), 277–282.

Secan, K. E., Egel, A. L., & Tilley, C. S. (1989). Acquisition, generalization, and maintenance of question-answering skills in autistic children. *Journal of Applied Behavior Analysis, 22*, 181–196.

Segalowitz, S. J. (2000). Predicting child language impairment from too many variables: Overinterpreting stepwise discriminant functional analysis. *Brain and Language, 71*, 337–343.

Semel, E., Secord, W., & Wiig, E. H. (2004). *CELF preschool, second edition (CELF Preschool—2)*. New York: Psychological Corporation.

Semel, E., Wiig, E. H., & Secord, W. (2003). *Clinical evaluation of language fundamentals—Fourth edition (CELF-4)*. New York: Psychological Corporation.

Semel, E., Wiig, E. H., & Secord, W. (2004). *CELF-4 screening test*. New York: Psychological Corporation.

Senechal, M., & Cornell, E. H. (1993). Vocabulary acquisition through shared reading experiences. *Reading Research Quarterly, 28*, 360–375.

Shabani, D. B., Katz, R. C., Wilder, D. A., Beauchamp, K., Taylor, C. R., & Fischer, K. J. (2002). Increasing social initiations in children with autism: Effects of a tactile prompt. *Journal of Applied Behavior Analysis, 35*, 79–83.

Shane, H. C. (Ed.). (1994). *Facilitated communication: The clinical and social phenomenon*. San Diego, CA: Singular Publishing Group.

Shapiro, E. S., McGonigle, J. J., & Ollendick, J. H. (1980). An analysis of self-assessment and self-reinforcement in a self-managed token economy with mentally retarded children. *Applied Research in Mental Retardation, 1*, 227–240.

Sheslow, D., & Adams, W. (2002). *Wide Range Assessment of Memory and Learning, Second Edition*. Wood Dale, IL: Stoelting Co.

Shipley, K. G., & McAffee, J. G. (2004). *Assessment in speech-language pathology: A Resource manual* (3rd ed.). Clifton Park, NY: Thomson/Delmar Learning.

Shirley, M. J., Iwata, B. A., Kahng, S., Mazaleski, J. L., & Lerman, D. C. (1997). Does functional communication training compete with ongoing contingencies of reinforcement? An analysis during response acquisition and maintenance. *Journal of Applied Behavior Analysis, 30*, 93–104.

Shprintzen, R. J. (2000). *Syndrome identification for speech-language pathology: An illustrated pocketguide*. San Diego, CA: Singular Publishing Group.

Shriberg, L. D., Friel-Patti, S., Flipsen, Jr., P., & Brown, R. L. (2000). Otitis media, fluctuating hearing loss, and speech-language outcomes: A preliminary structural equation model. *Journal of Speech, Language, and Hearing Research, 43*, 100–120.

Shriberg, L. D., & Kwiatkowski, J. (1994). Developmental phonological disorders I: A clinical profile. *Journal of Speech and Hearing Research, 37*, 1100–1126.

Shriberg, L. D., & Widder, C. J. (1990). Speech and prosody characteristics of adults with mental retardation. *Journal of Speech and Hearing Research, 33*, 627–653.

Siegel, B. (1996). *The world of the autistic child: Understanding and treating autistic spectrum disorders*. New York: Oxford University Press.

Siegel, B. (2004). *Pervasive developmental disorders screening tests-II: Early childhood screener for autistic spectrum disorders*. New York: Psychological Corporation.

Siegel, L., Cunningham, C., & van der Spuy, H. (1979). Interactions of language delayed and normal preschool children with their mothers. Paper presented at the Meeting of the Society for Research in Child Development, San Francisco.

Sigafoos, J. (1999). Creating opportunities for augmentative and alternative communication: Strategies for involving people with developmental disabilities. *Augmentative & Alternative Communication, 15*, 183–190.

Sigafoos, J., Couzens, D., Pennell, D., Shaw, D., & Dudfield, G. (1995). Discrimination of picture requests for missing items among young children with developmental disabilities. *Journal of Behavioral Education, 5,* 295–317.

Sigafoos, J., & Roberts-Pennell, D. (1999). The wrong-item format: A promising intervention for teaching socially appropriate forms of rejecting to children with developmental disabilities? *Augmentative and Alternative Communication, 15,* 135–140.

Silva, P. (1987). Epidemiology: Longitudinal course, and some associated factors: An update. In W. Yule & M. Rutter (Eds.), *Language development and disorders* (pp. 1–15). London: McKeith Press.

Silva, P., Williams, S., & McGee, R. (1987). A longitudinal study of children with developmental language delay at age three: Later intelligence, reading and behavior problems. *Developmental Medicine and Child Neurology, 29,* 630–640.

Sisson, L. A., & Barrett, R. P. (1984). An alternating treatments comparison of oral and total communication training with minimally verbal retarded children. *Journal of Applied Behavior Analysis, 17,* 559–566.

Skinner, B. F. (1953). *Science and human behavior.* New York: Macmillan.

Skinner, B. F. (1957). *Verbal behavior.* New York: Appleton-Century-Crofts.

Skinner, B. F. (1986). The evolution of verbal behavior. *Journal of the Experimental Analysis of Behavior, 45,* 115–122.

Slevin, M., Farrington, N., Duffy, G., Daly, L., & Murphy, J. (2000). Altering the NICU and measuring infants' responses. *Acta Paediatrica, 89*(5), 577–581.

Smalley, S. L, McCracken, J., & Tanguay, P. (1995). Autism, affective disorders, and social phobia. *American Journal of Medical Genetics, 60,* 19–26.

Smith, G. A., Scherzer, D. J., Buckley, J. W., Haley, K. J., & Shields, B. J. (2004). Pediatric farm-related injuries: A series of 96 hospitalized patients. *Clinical Pediatrics, 43*(4), 335–342.

Smith, T., Eikeseth, S., Klevstrand, M., & Lovaas, O. I. (1997). Intensive behavioral treatment for preschoolers with severe mental retardation and pervasive developmental disorders. *American Journal of Mental Retardation, 102*(3), 238–249.

Snow, C. E., Burns, S., Griffin, P. (Eds.). (1998). *Preventing reading difficulties in young children.* Washington, D. C.: National Academy Press.

Snow, C. E., Scarborough, H. S., & Burns, M. S. (1999). What speech-language pathologists need to know about early reading. *Topics in Language Disorders, 20*(1), 48–58.

Sokol, D. K., & Edwards-Brown, M. (2004). Neuroimaging in autistic spectrum disorders (ASD). *Journal of Neuroimaging, 14,* 8–15.

Speech-Ease. (1985). *Speech-Ease screening inventory.* Austin, TX: PRO-ED.

Spitz, R. V., Tallal, P., Flax, J., & Benasich, A. A. (1997). Look who's talking: A prospective study of familial transmission of language impairments. *Journal of Speech, Language, and Hearing Research, 40*(5), 990–1001.

Stackhouse, J., Wells, B., Pascoe, M., & Rees, R. (2002). From phonological therapy to phonological awareness. *Seminars in Speech and Language, 23*(1), 27–42.

Stanovich, K. E., & Siegel, L. S. (1994). Phenotypic performance profile of children with disabilities: A regression-based test of the phonological-core variable-difference model. *Journal of Educational Psychology, 86,* 24–53.

Stark, R. E., & Tallal, P. (1988). *Language, speech, and reading disorders in children.* Boston: Little, Brown.

Steffenburg, S. Gillberg, C., Hellgren, L., Andersson, L., Gillberg, I. C., Jakobsson, G., et al. (1989). A twin study of autism in Denmark, Finland, Iceland, Norway and Sweden. *Child Psychology and Psychiatry, 30,* 405–416.

Stehli, A. (1991). *The sound of a miracle: A child's triumph over autism.* New York: Doubleday.

Stevenson, H. W., & Newman, R. S. (1986). Long-term prediction of achievement and attitudes in mathematics and reading. *Child Development, 57,* 646–659.

Stoel-Gammon, C. (1990). Down syndrome: Effects on language development. *Asha, 32*(9), 42–44.

Stojanovik, V., Perkins, M., & Howard, S. (2001). Language and conversational abilities in Williams syndrome: How good is good? *International Journal of Language and Communication Disorders, 36* (Suppl.), 234–239.

Stokes, T. F., Fowler, S. A., & Baer, D. M. (1978). Training preschool children to recruit natural communities of reinforcement. *Journal of Applied Behavior Analysis, 11,* 285–303.

Stokes, T. M., & Baer, D. M. (1977). An implicit technology of generalization. *Journal of Applied Behavior Analysis, 10,* 349–367.

Stothard, S. E., Snowling, M. J., Bishop, D. V. M., Chipchase, B. B., & Kaplan, C. A. (1998). Language-impaired preschoolers: a follow-up into adolescence. *Journal of Speech, Language, and Hearing Research, 42*(3), 407–418.

Stremel-Campbell, K., & Campbell, C. R. (1985). Training techniques that may facilitate generalization. In S. F. Warren & A. K. Rogers-Warren (Eds.), *Teaching functional language* (pp. 251–288). Austin, TX: PRO-ED.

Stromer, R., McComas, J. J., & Rehfeldt, R. A. (2000). Designing interventions that include delayed reinforcement: Implications of recent laboratory research. *Journal of Applied Behavior Analysis, 33,* 359–371.

Sudhalter, V., & Belser, R. C. (2001). Conversational characteristics of children with fragile X syndrome. *American Journal on Mental Retardation, 106*(5), 389–400.

Sulzby, E. (1985). Children's emergent reading of favorite storybooks: A developmental study. *Reading Research Quarterly, 20,* 458–481.

Sulzer-Azaroff, B., & Mayer, G. R. (1991). *Behavior analysis for lasting change.* San Francisco: Holt, Rinehart & Winston.

Svirsky, M. A., Robbins, A. M., Kirk, K. I., Pisoni, D. B., & Miyamoto, R. T. (2000). Language development in profoundly deaf children with cochlear implants. *Psychological Science, 11*(2), 153–158.

Szatmari, P., Bryson, S. E., Streiner, D. L., Wilson, F, Archer, L., & Ryerse, C. (2000). Two-year outcome of preschool children with autism or Asperger's Syndrome. *American Journal of Psychiatry, 157,* 1980–1987.

Tallal, P. (1999). Children with language impairment can be accurately identified using temporal processing measures: A response to Zhang and Tomblin. *Brain and Language, 69,* 222–229.

Tallal, P., Hirsch, L. S., Realpe-Bonilla, T., Miller, S., Brzusto-wicz, M., Bartlett, C., et al. (2001). Familial aggregation in specific language impairment. *Journal of Speech, Language, and Hearing Research, 44,* 1172–1182.

Tallal, P., Miller, S., Bedi, G., Byma, G., Wang, X., Nagarajan, et al. (1996). Language comprehension in language-learning impaired children improved with acoustically modified speech. *Science, 271,* 81–84.

Tallal, P., Ross, R., & Curtiss, S. (1989). Familial aggregation in specific language impairment. *Journal of Speech and Hearing Disorders, 54,* 167–173.

Tallal, P., Stark, R. E., & Mellits, E. D. (1985). Identification of language-impaired children on the basis of rapid perception and production skills. *Brain and Language, 25,* 314–322.

Talley, J. L. (1995). *Children's Auditory Verbal Learning Test—2.* Lutz, FL: Psychological Assessment Resources, Inc.

Tannock, R. (1988). Mothers' directiveness in their interactions with their children with and without Down syndrome. *American Journal on Mental Retardation, 93,* 154–165.

Taylor, B. A., & Harris, S. L. (1995). Teaching children with autism to seek information: Acquisition of novel information and generalization of responding. *Journal of Applied Behavior Analysis, 28,* 3–14.

Taylor, B. A., & Levin, L. (1998). Teaching a student with autism to make verbal initiations: Effects of a tactile prompt. *Journal of Applied Behavior Analysis, 31,* 651–654.

Taylor, B., Miller, E., Farrington, C. P., Petropoulos, M., Favot-Mayaud, I., Li, J., et al. (1999). Autism and measles, mumps, and rubella vaccine: no epidemiological evidence for a causal association. *The Lancet, 353,* 2026–2029.

Taylor, B., Miller, E., Lingham, R., Andrew, N., Simmons, A., & Stowe, J. (2002). Measles, mumps and rubella vaccination and bowel problems or developmental regression in children with autism: population study. *British Medical Journal, 324,* 393–396.

Teale, W. H., & Sulzby, E. (Eds.). (1986). *Emergent literacy: Writing and reading.* Norwood, NJ: Ablex.

Thal, D., Bates, E., & Bellugi, U. (1989). Language and cognition in two children with Williams syndrome. *Journal of Speech and Hearing Research, 32,* 489–500.

The SLI Consortium (2002). A genomewide scan identifies two novel loci involved in specific language impairment. *American Journal of Human Genetics, 70,* 384–398.

Thiemann, K. S., & Goldstein, H. (2001). Social stories, written text cues, and video feedback: Effects on social communication of children with autism. *Journal of Applied Behavior Analysis, 34,* 425–446.

Thiemann, K. S., & Goldstein, H. (2004). Effects of peer training and written text cueing on social communication of school-age children with pervasive developmental disorder. *Journal of Speech, Language, and Hearing Research, 47,* 126–144.

Tirosh, E., & Canby, J. (1993). Autism with hyperlexia: A distinct syndrome? *American Journal on Mental Retardation, 98*(1), 84–92.

Tirosh, E., & Cohen, A. (1998). Language deficit with attention-deficit disorder: A prevalent comorbidity. *Journal of Child Neurology, 13,* 493–497.

Todd, G. A., & Palmer, B. (1968). Social reinforcement of infant babbling. *Child Development, 39,* 591–596.

Tomblin, B. (1989). Familial concentration of developmental language impairment. *Journal of Speech and Hearing Disorders, 54,* 287–295.

Tomblin, B., & Buckwalter, P. (1994). Studies of genetics of specific language impairment. In R. Watkins & M. Rice (Eds.), *Specific language impairments in children* (pp. 17–35). Baltimore: Paul H. Brookes.

Tomblin, B., Freese, P., & Records, N. (1992). Diagnosing a specific language impairment in adults for the purpose of pedigree analysis. *Journal of Speech, Language, and Hearing Research, 40,* 1245–1260.

Tomblin, J. B., & Buckwalter, P. R. (1998). Heritability of poor language achievement among twins. *Journal of Speech, Language, and Hearing Research, 41,* 188–199.

Tomblin, J. B., Records, N. L., & Zhang, X. (1996). A system for the diagnosis of specific language impairment in kindergarten children. *Journal of Speech, Language, and Hearing Research, 39,* 1284–1294.

Tomblin, J. B., Spencer, L. J., & Gantz, B. J.(2000). Language and reading acquisition in children with and without cochlear implants. *Advances in Otorhinolaryngology, 57,* 300–304.

Tomblin, J. B., Zhang, X., Buckwalter, P., & O'Brien, M. (2003). The stability of primary language disorder: Four years after kindergarten diagnosis. *Journal of Speech, Language, and Hearing Research, 46,* 1283–1296.

Torgesen, J. K., & Wagner, R. K. (1998). Alternative diagnostic approaches for specific developmental reading disabilities. *Learning Disabilities Research and Practice, 13,* 220–232.

Torgesen, J. K., Wagner, R. K., Rashotte, C. A., Burgess, S., & Hecht, S. (1997). Contributions of phonological awareness and rapid automatic naming ability to the growth of word-reading skills in second-to-fifth-grade children. *Scientific Studies of Reading, 1,* 161–185.

Tough, J. (1982). Language, poverty, and disadvantage in school. In L. Feagans & D. Farran (Eds.), *The language of children reared in poverty* (pp. 2–18). New York: Academic Press.

Trapani, I. (1993). *Itsy-bitsy spider.* Watertown, MA: Charlesbridge.

Troia, G. A., & Whitney, S. D. (2003). A close look at the efficacy of Fast ForWord Language for children with academic weaknesses. *Contemporary Educational Psychology, 28,* 465–494.

Tsai, L. Y. (1992). Is Rett syndrome a subtype of pervasive developmental disorders? *Journal of Autism and Developmental Disabilities, 22,* 551–561.

Uchino, J., Suzuki, M., Hoshino, K., Nomura, Y., & Segawa, M. (2001). Development of language in Rett syndrome. *Brain Development, 23*(Suppl.), S233–235.

U.S. Census Bureau. (2000). *U.S. interim projections by age, sex, race, and Hispanic origin. Table 1a. Projected population of the United States, by race and Hispanic origin: 2000–2050.* Retrieved June 4, 2004, from www.census.gov/ipc/www/usinterimproj/.

U. S. Department of Education. (2002). *To assure the free appropriate public education of all Americans: Twenty fourth annual report to Congress on the implementation of the Individuals with Disabilities Education Act.* Retrieved January 29, 2005, from www.ed.gov/about/reports/annual/osep/2002/index.html.

Valdez-Menchaca, M. C., & Whitehurst, G. J. (1992). Accelerating language development through picture book reading: a systematic extension to Mexican day care. *Developmental Psychology, 28,* 1106–1114.

Vallance, D. D., Im, N., & Cohen, N. J. (1999). Discourse deficits associated with psychiatric disorders and with language impairments in children. *Journal of Child Psychology and Psychiatry, 40,* 693–704.

Van der Lely, K. H. J., & Howard, D. (1993). Children with specific language impairment: Linguistic impairment or short-term memory. *Journal of Speech and Hearing Research, 36,* 1193–1207.

van Keulen, J. E., Weddington, G. T., & De Bose, C. E. (1998). *Speech, language, learning, and the African American child.* Boston: Allyn & Bacon.

Van Kleeck, A. (1990). Emergent literacy: Learning about print before learning to read. *Topics in Language Disorders, 10*(2), 25–45.

Van Kleeck, A. (1998). Preliteracy domains and stages: Laying the foundations for beginning reading. *Journal of Children's Communication Development, 20,* 33–51.

Van Kleek, A., & Frankel, T. (1981). Discourse devices used by language disordered children: A preliminary investigation. *Journal of Speech and Hearing Disorders, 46,* 250–257.

Vargha-Khadem, F., Watkins, K., Alcock, K., Fletcher, P., & Passingham, R. (1995). Praxic and nonverbal cognitive deficits in a large family with a genetically transmitted speech and language disorder. *Procedures of the National Academy of Science, United States of America, 92,* 930–933.

Vicari, S., Caselli, M. C., Gagliardi, C., Tonucci, F., & Voltera, V. (2002). Language acquisition in special populations: A comparison between Down and Williams syndromes. *Neuropsychologia, 40*(13), 2461–2470.

Viding, E., Spinath, F. M., Price, T. S., Bishop, D. V. M., Dale, P. S., & Plomin, R. (2004). Genetic and environmental influence on language impairment in 4-year-old same-sex and opposite-sex twins. *Journal of Child Psychology and Psychiatry, 45,* 315–325.

Volkmar, F. R. (1992). Childhood disintegrative disorder: Issues for DSM-IV. *Journal of Autism and Developmental Disabilities, 22,* 627–642.

Volkmar, F. R., & Cohen, D. J. (1991). Debate and argument: The utility of the term Pervasive Developmental Disorder. *Journal of Child Psychology and Psychiatry, 32,* 1171–1172.

Volkmar, F. R., Klin, A., Schultz, R. T., Rubin, E., & Bronen, R. (2000). Clinical case conference: Asperger's disorder. *American Journal of Psychiatry, 157,* 262–267.

Volkmar, F. R., Klin, A., Siegel, B., Szatmari, P., Lord, C., Freeman, B. J. et al. (1994). Field trial for autistic disorder in DSM-IV. *American Journal of Psychiatry, 151,* 1361–1367.

Vollmer, T. R., Iwata, B. A., Cuvo, A. J., Heward, W. L., Miltenberger, R. G., & Neef, N. A. (2000). *Behavior analysis: Applications and extensions 1968–1999 from the Journal of Applied Behavior Analysis* (Reprint Series vol. 5). Lawrence: University of Kansas Department of Human Development: Society for the Experimental Analysis of Behavior.

Vygotsky, L. S. (1967). Play and its role in the mental development of the child. *Soviet Psychology, 5,* 6–18.

Wagner, R. K., Torgesen, J. K., Laughon, P., Simmons, K., & Rashotte, C. A. (1993). Development of young readers' phonological processing abilities. *Journal of Educational Psychology, 85,* 83–103.

Wagner, R. K., Torgesen, J. K., & Rashotte, C. (1999). *Comprehensive Test of Phonological Processing (CTOPP).* Austin, TX: PRO-ED.

Wakefield, A. J., Murch, S. H., Anthony, A., Linnel, J., Casson, D. M., Malik, M. et al. (1998). Ileal-lymphoid-nodular hyperplasia, non-specific colitis, and pervasive developmental disorder in children. *The Lancet, 351,* 637–641.

Walker, D. R., Thompson, A., Zwaigenbaum, L., Goldberg, J., Bryson, S. E., Mahoney, W. J., et al. (2004). Specifying PDD-NOS: A comparison of PDD-NOS, Asperger syndrome, and autism. *Journal of the American Academy of Child and Adolescent Psychiatry, 43,* 172–180.

Wallace, G., & Hammill, D. (2002). *Comprehensive receptive and expressive vocabulary-2 (CREVT-2).* Austin, TX: PRO-ED.

Wallace, G. L., & Treffert, D. A. (2004). Head size and autism. *The Lancet, 363,* 1003–1004.

Waltzman, S. B., Cohen, N. L., Green, J., & Roland, J. T., Jr. (2002). Long-term effects of cochlear implants in children. *Otolaryngology, Head and Neck Surgery, 126*(5), 505–511.

Warren, S. F. (1985). Clinical strategies for the measurement of language generalization. In S. F. Warren & A. K. Rogers-Warren (Eds.), *Teaching functional language* (pp. 197–224). Austin, TX: PRO-ED.

Warren, S. F. (1992). Facilitating basic vocabulary acquisition with milieu teaching procedures. *Journal of Early Intervention, 16,* 235–251.

Warren, S. F., & Gazdag, G. (1990). Facilitating early language development with milieu intervention procedures. *Journal of Early Intervention, 14*(1), 62–86.

Warren, S. F., Gazdag, G. E., Bambara, L. M., & Jones, H. A. (1994). Changes in the generativity and use of semantic relationships concurrent with milieu language intervention. *Journal of Speech and Hearing Research, 37,* 924–935.

Warren, S. F., & Kaiser, A. P. (1986). Incidental language teaching: A critical review. *Journal of Speech and Hearing Disorders, 51,* 291–299.

Warren, S. F., & Rogers-Warren, A. K. (1985). Teaching functional language. In S. F. Warren & A. K. Rogers-Warren (Eds.), *Teaching functional language* (pp. 3–23). Austin, TX: PRO-ED.

Warren, S. F., Yoder, P. J., Gazdag, G. E., Kim, K., & Jones, H. A. (1993). Facilitating prelinguistic communication skills in young children with developmental delay. *Journal of Speech and Hearing Research, 36,* 83–98.

Washington, J. A. (1996). Issues in assessing the language abilities of African American children. In A. G. Kamhi, K. E. Pollock, & J. L. Harris (Eds.), *Communication development and disorders in African American children: Research and intervention* (pp. 35–54). Baltimore, MD: Paul H. Brookes.

Washington, J. A., & Craig, H. K. (2004). A language screening protocol for use with young African American children in urban settings. *American Journal of Speech-Language Pathology, 13,* 329–340.

Wasik, B. A., & Bond, M. A. (2001). Beyond the pages of a book: Interactive book and language development in preschool classrooms. *Journal of Educational Psychology, 93*(2), 243–250.

Wassink, T. H., Piven, J., Vieland, V. J., Pietila, J., Goedken, R. J., Folstein, S. E., et al. (2002). Evaluation of FOXP2 as an autism susceptibility gene. *American Journal of Medical Genetics, 114,* 566–569.

Watkins, K. E., Dronkers, N. F., & Vargha-Khadem, F. (2002). Behavioural analysis of an inherited speech and language disorder: Comparison with acquired aphasia. *Brain, 125,* 452–464.

Watkins, R., & Rice, M. (1991). Verb particle and preposition acquisition in language-impaired preschoolers. *Journal of Speech and Hearing Research, 34,* 1130–1141.

Wechsler, D. (2002). *Wechsler Preschool and Primary Scale of Intelligence—Third Edition.* San Antonio, TX: Harcourt Assessment.

Wechsler, D. (2003). *Wechsler Intelligence Scale for Children—Fourth Edition.* San Antonio, TX: Harcourt Assessment.

Weiner, H. L., & Weinberg, J. S. (2000). Head injury in the pediatric age group. In P. R. Cooper & J. G. Golfinos (Eds.), *Head injury* (4th ed.) (pp. 419–456). New York: McGraw-Hill.

Weisberg, P. (1961). Social and nonsocial conditioning of infant localizations. *Child Development, 34,* 377–388.

Weismer, S. E., Evans, J., & Hesketh, L. J. (1999). An examination of verbal working memory in children with specific language impairment. *Journal of Speech, Language, and Hearing Research, 42,* 1249–1260.

Welch, S. J., & Pear, J. J. (1980). Generalization of naming responses in the natural environment as a function of training stimulus modality with retarded children. *Journal of Applied Behavior Analysis, 13,* 629–643.

Wetherby, A. M., & Prizant, B. M. (2003a). *Communication and symbolic behavior scales developmental profile—First normed edition.* Baltimore, MD: Brookes Publishing.

Wetherby, A. M., & Prizant, B. (2003b). *CSBS DP Infant-Toddler Checklist and Easy-Score.* Chicago: Riverside.

Whitehurst, G. J., Falco, F., Lonigan, C. J., Fischel, J. E., De Barsyhe, B. D., Valdez-Menchaca, M. C., & Caulfield, M. (1988). Accelerating language development through picture-book reading. *Developmental Psychology, 24,* 552–558.

Whitehurst, G. J., & Fischel, J. E. (2000). Reading and language impairments in conditions of poverty. In D. V. M. Bishop & L. B. Leonard (Eds.), *Speech and Language Impairments in Children: Causes, Characteristics, Intervention and Outcome* (pp. 53–71). Philadelphia, PA: Psychology Press.

Whitehurst, G. J., & Lonigan, C. J. (1998). Child development and emergent literacy. *Child Development, 69*(3), 848–872.

Wiig, E. H., Zureich, P. Z., & Chan, H. H. (2000). A clinical rationale for assessing of rapid automatized naming with language disorders. *Journal of Learning Disabilities, 33,* 359–374.

Wild, M. (1994). *Our granny.* Boston: Houghton Mifflin Co.

Williams, G., Donley, C. R., & Keller, J. W. (2000). Teaching children with autism to ask questions about hidden objects. *Journal of Applied Behavior Analysis, 33,* 627–630.

Williams, G., Perez-Gonzalez, L. A., & Vogt, K. (2003). The role of specific consequences in the maintenance of three types of questions. *Journal of Applied Behavior Analysis, 36,* 285–296.

Williams, K. T. (1997). *Expressive vocabulary test (EVT).* Circle Pines, MN: American Guidance Services.

Willis, W. (1998). Families with African American roots. In E. W. Lynch & M. J. Hanson (Eds.), *Developing cross-cultural competence: A guide for working with young children and their families* (2nd ed.) (pp. 165–208). Baltimore: Paul H. Brookes.

Wilson, S. (2003). *A nap in a lap.* New York: Henry Holt.

Wilson, W. F., & Wilson, J. R. (2000). Language learning and behavioral differences in culturally diverse populations. In T. J. Coleman (Ed.), *Clinical management of communication disorders in culturally diverse populations* (pp. 33–50). Boston: Allyn & Bacon.

Windborn, L., Wacker, D. P., Richman, D. M., Asmus, J., & Geier, D. (2002). Assessment of mand selection for functional communication training packages. *Journal of Applied Behavior Analysis, 35,* 295–298.

Windsor, J., & Hwang, M. (1999). Testing the generalized slowing hypothesis in specific language impairment. *Journal of Speech, Language, and Hearing Research, 42,* 1205–1218.

Windsor, J., Milbrath, R., Carney, E., & Rakowski, S. (2001). General slowing in language impairment: Methodological considerations in testing the hypothesis. *Journal of Speech, Language, and Hearing Research, 44,* 446–461.

Wing, L. (1981). Asperger's syndrome: A clinical account. *Psychol Med, 11,* 115–29.

Wing, L. (1988). The continuum of autistic characteristics. In E. Schopler & G. Mesibov (Eds.), *Diagnosis and assessment in autism* (pp. 1–10). New York: Plenum Press.

Wing, L. (1991). The relationship between Asperger's syndrome and Kanner's autism. In U. Frith (Ed.). *Autism and*

Asperger syndrome (pp. 93–121). Cambridge, U.K.: Oxford University Press.

Wing, L. (1993). The definition and prevalence of autism: A review. *European Child and Adolescent Psychiatry, 2*(2), 61–74.

Wing, L., & Gould, J. (1979). Severe impairments of social interaction and associated abnormalities in children: Epidemiology and classification. *Journal of Autism and Developmental Disabilities, 9,* 11–29.

Wing, L., & Potter, D. (2004). Notes on the prevalence of autism spectrum disorders. National Autistic Society. Retrieved on September 9, 2004, from www.nas.org.uk.

Winokur, S. (1976). *A primer of verbal behavior: An operant view.* Englewood Cliffs, NJ: Prentice-Hall.

Wolf, K. E., & Calderon, J. L. (1999). Cultural competence: The underpinning of quality health care and education services. *CSHA Magazine, 28*(2), 4–6.

Wolfensberger, W. (1994). The "facilitated communication" craze as an instance of pathological science: The cold fusion of human services. In H. C. Shane (Ed.), *Facilitated communication: The clinical and social phenomenon* (pp. 57–122). San Diego, CA: Singular Publishing Group.

Wood, A., & Wood, D. (2003). *The napping house.* Orlando, FL: Harcourt Brace Jovanovich.

Woodcock, R. W. (1991). *Woodcock Language Proficiency Battery—Revised.* Chicago: Riverside Publishing.

Woods, J. J., & Wetherby, A. M. (2003). Early identification of and intervention for infants and toddlers who are at risk for autism spectrum disorders. *Language, Speech, and Hearing Services in Schools, 34,* 180–193.

Wulbert, M., Inglis, S., Kriegsmann, E., & Mills, B. (1975). Language delay and associated mother-child interactions. *Developmental Psychology, 11,* 61–70.

Wulz, S. V., Hall, M. K., & Klein, M. D. (1983). A home-centered instructional communication strategy for severely handicapped children. *Journal of Speech and Hearing Disorders, 48*(1), 2–10.

Wyatt, T. (1998). Assessment issues with multicultural populations. In D. E. Battle (Ed.), *Communication disorders in multicultural populations* (2nd ed.), (pp. 379–426). Newton, MA: Butterworth-Heinemann.

Xiang, H., Stallones, L., & Smith, G. A. (2004). Downhill skiing injury among children. *Injury Prevention, 10*(2), 99–102.

Yale Child Study Center. (2004). *Pervasive developmental disorder—not otherwise specified.* Retrieved August 10, 2004, from info.med.yale.edu/chldstdy/autism/pddnos.html.

Yeargin-Allsop, M., Murphy, C. C., Oakley, G. P., & Sikes, R. K. (1992). A multiple-source method of studying the prevalence of developmental disabilities in children: The Metropolitan Atlanta Development Disabilities Study. *Pediatrics, 89*(4), 642–650.

Yeargin-Allsopp, M., Rice, C., Karapurkar, T., Doernberg, N., Boyle, C., & Murphy, C. (2003). Prevalence of autism in a U.S. metropolitan area. *Journal of the American Medical Association (JAMA), 289,* 49–55.

Yoder, P. J., & Layton, T. L. (1988). Speech following sign language training in autistic children with minimal verbal language. *Journal of Autism and Developmental Disabilities, 18,* 217–229.

Yoder, P. J., & Warren, S. F. (2002). Effects of prelinguistic milieu teaching and parent responsivity education on dyads involving children with intellectual disabilities. *Journal of Speech, Language, and Hearing Research, 45,* 1158–1174.

Yoder, P. J., Warren, S. F., Kim, K., & Gazdag, G. E. (1994). Systematic replication and extension (Facilitating prelinguistic communication skills in young children, part 2). *Journal of Speech, Language, and Hearing Research, 37,* 841–852.

Yorkston, K. M., Beukelman, D. R., Strand, E. A., & Bell, K. R. (1999). *Management of motor speech disorders in children and adults* (2nd ed.). Austin, TX: PRO-ED.

Yoshinaga-Itano, C. (2003). Early intervention after universal neonatal hearing screening: Impact on outcome. *Mental Retardation and Developmental Disabilities Research Review, 9*(4), 252–256.

Yoshinaga-Itano, C., Sedey, A. L., Coulter, D. K., & Mehl, A. L. (1998). Language of early- and later-identified children with hearing loss. *Pediatrics, 102*(5), 161–171.

Zafeiriou, D. I. (2004). Primitive reflexes and postural reactions in the neurodevelopmental examination. *Pediatric Neurology, 31*(1), 1–8.

Zanolli, K., & Daggett, J. (1998). The effects of reinforcement rate on the spontaneous social initiations of socially withdrawn preschoolers. *Journal of Applied Behavior Analysis, 31,* 117–125.

Zapella, M., Gillberg, C., & Ehlers, S. (1998). The preserved speech variant: A subgroup of the Rett complex: A clinical report of 30 cases. *Journal of Autism and Developmental Disabilities, 28*(6), 519–526.

Zarcone, J. R., Fisher, W. W., & Piazza, C. C. (1996). Analysis of free-time contingencies as positive versus negative reinforcement. *Journal of Applied Behavior Analysis, 29,* 247–250.

Zeev, B. B., Yaron, Y., Schanen, N. C., Wolf, H., Brandt, N., Ginot, N., et al. (2002). Rett syndrome: Clinical manifestations in males with MECP2 mutations. *Child Neurology, 17,* 20–24.

Zhang, X., & Tomblin, J. B. (1998). Can children with language impairment be accurately identified using temporal processing measures? A simulation study. *Brain and Language, 65,* 395–403.

Zigler, E., & Hodapp, R. M. (1986). *Understanding mental retardation.* New York: Cambridge University Press.

Zimmerman, I., Steiner, V., & Evatt-Pond, R. (2002a). *The preschool language scale—4 (PLS-4).* San Antonio, TX: The Psychological Corporation.

Zimmerman, I. L., Steiner, V. G., & Evatt Pond, R. (2002b). *Preschool Language Scale, Fourth Edition Spanish (PLS-4).* San Antonio, TX: Harcourt Assessment.

Zollweg, W., Palm, D., & Vance, V. (1997). The efficacy of auditory integration training: A double blind study. *American Journal of Audiology, 6,* 39–47.

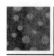

Index

534   Index